Sourcebook of Psychological Treatment Manuals for Adult Disorders

Sourcebook of Psychological Treatment Manuals for Adult Disorders

Edited by

Vincent B. Van Hasselt and
Michel Hersen

Nova Southeastern University
Fort Lauderdale, Florida

PLENUM PRESS • NEW YORK AND LONDON

Library of Congress Cataloging-in-Publication Data

Sourcebook of psychological treatment manuals for adult disorders /
  edited by Vincent B. Van Hasselt and Michel Hersen.
      p.   cm.
  Includes bibliographical references and index.
  ISBN 0-306-45144-1
    1. Psychotherapy--Handbooks, manuals, etc.   I. Van Hasselt,
  Vincent B. II. Hersen, Michel.
  RC480.S633 1996
  616.89'14--dc20   95-48885
                                                          CIP

ISBN 0-306-45144-1

© 1996 Plenum Press, New York
A Division of Plenum Publishing Corporation
233 Spring Street, New York, N. Y. 10013

10 9 8 7 6 5 4 3 2 1

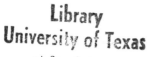

Contributors

Ron Acierno • Center for Psychological Studies, Nova Southeastern University, Fort Lauderdale, Florida 33314

Alan S. Bellack • Department of Psychiatry, Medical College of Pennsylvania, Philadelphia, Pennsylvania 19129; *present address*: Department of Psychiatry, University of Maryland School of Medicine, Baltimore, Maryland 21201–1549

Theo K. Bouman • Department of Clinical Psychology, University of Groningen, Oostersingel 59, 9713 EZ Groningen, The Netherlands

Kelly D. Brownell • Yale Center for Eating and Weight Disorders, Department of Psychology, Yale University, New Haven, Connecticut 06520–7447

Thomas F. Cash • Department of Psychology, Old Dominion University, Norfolk, Virginia 23529

Catherine M. Champagne • Department of Psychology, Louisiana State University, Pennington Biomedical Research Center, Baton Rouge, Louisiana 70803

Thomas P. Dominguez • Department of Psychology, University of New Mexico, Albuquerque, New Mexico 87131

Anthony Eccles • Forensic Behavioural Sciences, Eccles, Hodkinson, and Associates, Kingston, Ontario, Canada K7L 1A8

Paul M.G. Emmelkamp • Department of Clinical Psychology, University of Groningen, Oostersingel 59, 9713 EZ Groningen, The Netherlands

Robert J. Ferguson • Department of Psychiatry, Dartmouth Medical School, Dartmouth–Hitchcock Medical Center, Lebanon, New Hampshire 03756

Edna B. Foa • Department of Psychiatry, Medical College of Pennsylvania, Eastern Pennsylvania Psychiatric Institute, Philadelphia, Pennsylvania 19129

Michael A. Friedman • Yale Center for Eating and Weight Disorders, Department of Psychology, Yale University, New Haven, Connecticut 06520–7447

Jill R. Grant • Virginia Consortium for Professional Psychology, Norfolk, Virginia 23529

W. Kim Halford • Department of Psychology, Griffith University, Queensland, Australia

Michel Hersen • Center for Psychological Studies, Nova Southeastern University, Fort Lauderdale, Florida 33314

Jonathan M. Himmelhoch • Department of Psychiatry, Western Psychiatric Institute and Clinic, University of Pittsburgh School of Medicine, Pittsburgh, Pennsylvania 15213

Lori P. Jackman • Department of Psychology, Louisiana State University, Pennington Biomedical Research Center, Baton Rouge, Louisiana 70803

Michael J. Kozak • Department of Psychiatry, Medical College of Pennsylvania, Eastern Pennsylvania Psychiatric Institute, Philadelphia, Pennsylvania 19129

Kevin T. Larkin • Department of Psychology, West Virginia University, Morgantown, West Virginia 26506

Robert P. Liberman • Clinical Research Center for Schizophrenia, Department of Psychiatry, University of California at Los Angeles School of Medicine, Rehabilitation Services, Veterans Affairs Medical Center, Brentwood Division, Los Angeles, California 90073

Kenneth L. Lichstein • Department of Psychology, University of Memphis, Memphis, Tennessee 38152

William L. Marshall • Department of Psychology, Queen's University, Kingston Sexual Behaviour Clinic, Kingston, Ontario, Canada K7L 3N6

Nathaniel McConaghy • School of Psychiatry, Psychiatric Unit, The Prince of Wales Hospital, Randwick, New South Wales, Australia 2031

Robert J. Meyers • University of New Mexico, Center on Alcoholism, Substance Abuse, and Addictions, Albuquerque, New Mexico 87106

Wiley Mittenberg • Center for Psychological Studies, Nova Southeastern University, Fort Lauderdale, Florida 33314

Suzanne G. Mouton • Department of Educational Psychology, University of Houston, Houston, Texas 77004; and Department of Psychiatry and Behavioral Sciences, University of Texas Mental Sciences Institute, Health Science Center at Houston, Houston, Texas 77030

Brant W. Riedel • Department of Psychology, University of Memphis, Memphis, Tennessee 38152

Agnes Scholing • Department of Clinical Psychology, University of Groningen, Oostersingel 59, 9713 EZ Groningen, The Netherlands

Jane Ellen Smith • Department of Psychology, University of New Mexico, Albuquerque, New Mexico 87131

Melinda A. Stanley • Department of Psychiatry and Behavioral Sciences, University of Texas Mental Sciences Institute, Health Science Center at Houston, Houston, Texas 77030

Michael E. Thase • Department of Psychiatry, Western Psychiatric Institute and Clinic, University of Pittsburgh School of Medicine, Pittsburgh, Pennsylvania 15213

David L. Van Brunt • Department of Psychology, University of Memphis, Memphis, Tennessee 38152

Vincent B. Van Hasselt • Center for Psychological Studies, Nova Southeastern University, Fort Lauderdale, Florida 33314

Patricia Van Oppen • Department of Psychiatry, Free University of Amsterdam, Valeriusplein 9, 1075 BG Amsterdam, The Netherlands

Paula J. Varnado • Department of Psychology, Louisiana State University, Pennington Biomedical Research Center, Baton Rouge, Louisiana 70803

Robert L. Weiss • Oregon Marital Studies Program, Department of Psychology, University of Oregon, Eugene, Oregon 97403

Donald A. Williamson • Department of Psychology, Louisiana State University, Pennington Biomedical Research Center, Baton Rouge, Louisiana 70803

Stephen E. Wong • School of Social Service Administration, University of Chicago, Chicago, Illinois 60637

Claudia Zayfert • Dartmouth–Hitchcock Medical Center, National Center for Post-Traumatic Stress Disorder, Lebanon, New Hampshire 03756

Preface

It is most unlikely that this sourcebook could have been conceptualized or published 20 years ago. Indeed, it is even doubtful that we could have secured and organized the material for a compendium of treatment manuals a decade ago. However, in the last 10 years or so, clinical researchers, consistent with the zeitgeist of empiricism, accountability in treatment, and prescriptive intervention, have developed very comprehensive treatment manuals specifically designed to foster precision and replicability in the therapeutic process. Such precision, of course, is most critical when contrasting approaches in treatment-outcome research. However, accountability and precision now are also called for in the day-to-day clinical enterprise, especially with the increasing mandates and influence of managed care and third-party reimbursers.

The *Sourcebook of Psychological Treatment Manuals for Adult Disorders* is divided into two parts. Part I, Introduction, includes one chapter by Ron Acierno and the editors on basic contemporary issues of accountability in treatment. The bulk of the book appears in Part II, Adult Disorders and Problems, in which there are 17 detailed treatment manuals for use with a large variety of problems presented by adults both as outpatients and inpatients.

Our goal for each chapter is to provide the reader with sufficient information so that the respective approaches can be replicated. A major concern (and complaint) articulated by researchers and clinicians alike is that protocols for interventions developed and implemented in the context of major research programs or funded centers are rarely disseminated. Although some remediation strategies eventually are presented in journal articles, most of these descriptions are usually quite brief. Moreover, they fail to provide readers with the depth of content and detail requisite to employing the technique(s) in their own work.

We also see this volume as one of the first efforts of its kind specifically geared toward bridging the gap between applied clinical research and practice. Each chapter contains current, state-of-the-art treatment methods with numerous specifics as to how they are to be carried out, and with ample clinical illustrations. We expect that there will be considerable interest in this volume from a wide range of mental health professionals, including psychologists, psychiatrists, counselors, social workers, rehabilitation specialists, and graduate students from each of these disciplines.

Many individuals have given of their time and effort to bring this sourcebook to fruition. First, we thank our eminent contributors for refining their treatment manuals for publication herein. Second, we thank Burt G. Bolton, Elissa Miller, and Christine Ryan for their technical assistance. Finally, we again thank our friend and editor at Plenum Press, Eliot Werner, for his perspicacity.

VINCENT B. VAN HASSELT
MICHEL HERSEN

Contents

I
INTRODUCTION

1

Accountability in Psychological Treatment

Ron Acierno, Michel Hersen, and Vincent B. Van Hasselt

INTRODUCTION

Maturation of any science is invariably accompanied by increased demands that its theoreticians and practitioners justify their hypotheses and actions. Indeed, accountability is a defining characteristic of the study of medicine, physics, chemistry, biology, and all other areas of investigation in which funding or compensation is sought in exchange for research or services that endeavor to advance knowledge or reduce suffering. Over the past four decades, psychologists have also been called on to account for their clinical behaviors. Early commentaries on this topic were provided by Eysenck (1952) and Raimy (1950), who both noted that the practical value of psychotherapy was far less than had been assumed. Raimy went so far as to completely refute the conceptualization of psychology as a science when he stated, "Psychotherapy is an undefined technique, applied to unspecified problems, with unpredictable outcomes" (p. 93). Lack of scientific credibility, which described the field 40 years ago and continues to describe it to a limited extent today, is largely attributable to a general schism between basic research and applied psychological procedures. The gap between the laboratory and consulting room was bridged for the first time relatively recently by Wolpe in 1958, with his presentation of the first empirically derived treatment technique: psychotherapy by reciprocal inhibition. Wolpe's introduction of empiricism to the realm of applied clinical psychology, combined with subsequent controlled

Ron Acierno, Michel Hersen, and Vincent B. Van Hasselt • Center for Psychological Studies, Nova Southeastern University, Fort Lauderdale, Florida 33314.

Sourcebook of Psychological Treatment Manuals for Adult Disorders, edited by Vincent B. Van Hasselt and Michel Hersen. Plenum Press, New York, 1996.

3

evaluations of his treatment procedure, was unique in that, for the first time, psychologists were in a position to justify their actions on the basis of data, rather than abstraction and deductively generated theory.

Accountability in psychology has increased tremendously in recent years, following adoption of empiricism as the driving force in *clinical* research. Importantly, whereas problems were once unspecified, we now have highly reliable (albeit not completely validated) diagnostic classification systems, such as the *Diagnostic and Statistical Manual of Mental Disorders*, Fourth Edition (DSM-IV; American Psychiatric Association, 1994). Whereas treatments were largely variable and intuitive, graduate programs are increasingly familiarizing their doctoral students with thoroughly operationalized "teachable" interventions (of which this handbook is wholly comprised). And whereas predictions of change were once uninformed, or worse, random, we now possess scores of treatment-outcome studies, the results of which provide justification for selection of one treatment over another for one type of patient versus another (e.g., Barlow, Craske, Cearny, & Klosko, 1989; Mavissa-kallian, 1987; McKnight, Nelson, Hayes, & Jarrett, 1992; Öst, 1985; Öst, Johansson, & Jerremalm, 1982; Rush, 1983). Interestingly, availability of data from which to base justification for our professional behavior has served to dramatically increase demands that we do just that, leading us into "the current climate of accountability" (Garfield, 1987, p. 99). As Barlow, Hayes, and Nelson (1984) noted, "there is little question that one of the clearest trends in the decade of the 80's is a concerted movement towards greater accountability in the delivery of human services at all levels" (p. 68). In addition to those made by the general public and third-party payers, recent calls for accountability in treatment have originated from within the field by sport psychologists (Smith, 1989), cognitive psychologists (Beck & Haaga, 1992), counseling psychologists (Anderson, 1992; Bishop & Trembley, 1987), child psychologists (Burchard & Schaefer, 1992), family psychologists (Cross, 1985), biofeedback psychologists (Furedy & Shulhan, 1987), and eclectic psychologists (Garfield, 1987). How, then, are applied psychologists to maintain accountability?

FACTORS IN ACCOUNTABILITY

Accountability in clinical psychology and psychiatry demands (1) selection of treatment on the basis of comprehensive assessment, (2) use of interventions with empirically demonstrated efficacy, and (3) repeated evaluation of patient progress during treatment. As for the first point, implementation of psychological treatment must be preceded by thorough assessment of the patient's pathology. Specifically, attention must be directed toward (1) pathological symptoms, (2) etiology, (3) contextual maintaining factors, and (4) subject characteristics and history. Attention to *all* factors permits informed selection of appropriate treatments so that patient gains are maximized. In contrast, measurement of only one area increases the likelihood that patient and treatment will be mismatched, even if empirically validated techniques are chosen. Indeed, assumptions of patient homogeneity are frequently made by clinical researchers, and represent a significant weakness in existing clinical-outcome research (Acierno, Hersen, Van Hasselt, & Ammerman, 1994; Hersen, 1981; Wolpe, 1977). Unfortunately, the DSM-IV, in an effort to avoid theory-specific bias while increasing diagnostic reliability, has been constructed so that patients with decidedly varied phenomenological and etiological presentations receive similar diagnoses. Assessment of the four areas specified above circumvents this diagnostic pitfall.

Assessment

Comprehensive assessment routinely begins with measurement and description of patients' symptomatology. This is effectively accomplished through observation, patient- and significant-other reports, and physiological monitoring. Such tripartite assessment, advocated by Lang (1968) and Hersen (1973), allows clinicians to modify and adapt psychological interventions to the particular pathological presentation of individual patients. Along these lines, Öst et al. (1982) described subjects in their sample of 34 claustrophobics as either physiological or behavioral fear responders on the basis of thorough symptom assessment. Half of each group of responders received a treatment designed to modify physiology, while the other half of each group received a treatment to alter inappropriate behavior. Predictably, physiological responders treated with a physiologically oriented intervention improved to a relatively greater extent than physiological responders treated with a behavioral-oriented intervention. Similarly, behavioral responders receiving behavior-focused treatment evinced greater gains than behavioral responders receiving physiologically based treatment. Comparable benefits of prescriptively matching treatment and pathology on the basis of symptom presentation have been demonstrated with other types of specific phobias as well. For example, although most phobic individuals evince increased heart rate when confronted by phobic stimuli (evolutionary preparation for escape), psychophysiological assessment of symptoms reveals that a small group of phobics, specifically blood phobics, exhibit heart-rate *decreases* when presented with phobic objects (perhaps evolutionary preparation to avoid bleeding to death; Öst, Sterner, & Lindahl, 1984). This diagnostic difference has obvious relevance to treatment of blood phobics, in that typical interventions for phobias that foster eventual heart-rate reductions will be ineffective. In fact, the intervention of choice for blood phobics is applied tension.

Analogous-symptom subtypes of depression (corresponding to etiological subtypes) also exist, and their differential treatment response is well documented (Wolpe, 1990). In addition to clearly distinguishable mood disorder classes (i.e., unipolar and bipolar depression), Wolpe (1979, 1986) posits that depressive subtypes also exist. Specifically, a significant percentage of major depressive patients presents with behavioral, subjective, and physiological symptoms of anxiety. Importantly, the phenomenological experience of these patients differs considerably from those of major depressives who do not experience concomitant symptoms of anxiety. Indeed, patients suffering from "anxious depression" can be physiologically and behaviorally differentiated from nonanxious depressives on the basis of *sedation thresholds* (defined as the level of sodium amobarbital at which known electroencephalogram (EEG) and behavioral nonresponding effects are noted; Wolpe, 1986); that is, individuals experiencing major depression are characterized by higher than average sedation thresholds (as are anxiety-disordered individuals), whereas nonanxious depressives show lower than average sedation thresholds. In this case, tripartite symptom assessment reveals qualitative rather than quantitative differences between these two forms of depression. Note that this finding is in contrast to earlier conceptualizations of depression and current diagnostic practices that place both anxious and nonanxious depressions on a simple quantitative continuum of severity. This is problematic because qualitatively different subtypes of depression appear to require qualitatively different types of specific treatment. For example, Conti, Placidi, Dell'Osso, Lenzi, and Cossano (1987) demonstrated that although nonanxious depressives evinced significant improvement in response to antidepressant medication, anxious depressives respond no better to antidepressant medication than to placebo. For these patients, interventions to reduce anxiety, in addition to treatments for depression, are indicated (Wolpe, 1986).

Clearly, clinicians attempting to remain accountable must thoroughly evaluate patients on the basis of tripartite symptomatology and select treatments with demonstrated efficacy in reducing all aspects of symptomatic presentation; however, symptom assessment is not sufficient to fulfill all requirements for reliable treatment selection. Rather, the contextual and maintaining factors of psychopathology within which symptoms present must also be addressed.

Contextual assessment of maintaining factors, sometimes described as *functional analysis*, involves the delineation of reinforcement contingencies and learned discriminative stimuli in a patient's environment that serve to maintain and evoke, respectively, problem behaviors. Whereas definition and description of target behaviors are achieved through symptom assessment, contextual assessment provides insight into the reasons a group of symptoms may persist. Procedural aspects of contextual assessment of maintaining factors are dictated in large part by each patient's symptomatic presentation. Importantly, however, every assessment must include (1) specification of the antecedents and consequences of problem behaviors, (2) description of the effects of problem behaviors on patient's significant others (and their behavior in response to these effects), and (3) identification of environmental stimuli that vary with the presence or absence of pathological behaviors. As previously mentioned, complexity of contextual assessment of maintaining factors is primarily determined by the class of presenting disorders (e.g., identification of the factors that serve to elicit and maintain a specific phobic response will likely entail less effort than functional assessment of panic disorder without agoraphobia). Kallman, Hersen, and O'Toole (1975) provided an informative case example in which the necessity of complementing symptom assessment with contextual analysis of maintaining factors is clearly illustrated.

The patient, a 42-year-old male, had experienced several 2-week periods of transient paralysis over the 5 years prior to his presentation for treatment. Interestingly, symptom onset coincided with the patient's involuntary early retirement, at which time he was required to assume his wife's household responsibilities so that she could seek employment. Further assessment revealed that periods of paralysis appeared to follow exacerbations of family discord. Finally, investigators determined that the patient received positive reinforcement for his paralytic behavior through social attention, and negative reinforcement through relief from household chores. Initial empirically based treatments were provided on an inpatient basis and included differential reinforcement in the form of social attention provided by attractive research assistants. Consistent with previously reported effects of differential reinforcement strategies, frequency of desired behaviors (standing and walking) increased and was directly related to the level of social praise and attention delivered by research assistants. Unfortunately, treatment gains were short-lived, and the patient was readmitted to the hospital 4 weeks after his initial discharge, again experiencing paralysis. Because contextual assessment of maintaining factors had revealed stimuli that served to trigger pathological behavior (i.e., familial discord) as well as reinforcement contingencies that functioned to maintain this behavior (i.e., interpersonal attention and escape from aversive household chores), a relatively more comprehensive intervention package was implemented and included training family members to provide differential reinforcement for standing and walking, while withholding this reinforcement during periods of paralysis. Appropriate contingency management from family members and hospital staff resulted in lasting treatment gains. Although not performed, even more comprehensive treatment would have involved strategies to reduce familial discord, thereby eliminating occurrence of a major discriminative stimulus for paralysis. This case illustrates the need to address both contingencies that sustain operant as well as conditioned stimuli that serve reliably to elicit problem behaviors; that is, delineation of both instrumental and associative components of the environment within which psychopathology has developed and persists enhances application of comprehensive, multifaceted, empirically based treatment. As noted, however, full accountability also demands etiological assessment, for, as Wolpe (1986) notes, "The most effective treatments of diseases are usually based on knowledge of their etiology" (p. 499). The critical importance of etiological factors in comprehensive behavioral assessment recently has also been underscored by Acierno, Tremont, Last, and Montgomery (1994).

Etiological assessment data enhance the degree to which specific treatments are prescriptively selected and appropriately implemented. However, the DSM's flight from etiological controversy has resulted in formation of diagnostic classes of psychopathology composed of heterogeneous groups of patients. This is particularly problematic when interpreting results of treatment-outcome studies, given that intervention effects may be confounded by possible interactions between etiological differences among subjects (Wolpe, 1977, 1979). However,

> on an a priori basis, it would seem that in cases where faulty habits have been conditioned, a therapeutic strategy directed toward their deconditioning would be most appropriate. On the other hand, where cognitive misperceptions predominate, a therapeutic strategy directed to correcting such misperceptions would seem warranted. (Hersen, 1981, p. 21)

The potential importance of etiological assessment to clinical accountability is demonstrated by existing treatment literature on depression. In a study by Taylor and McLean (1993), patients treated with behavior therapy, amitriptyline, psychodynamic therapy, or relaxation were classified as treatment responders, nonresponders, or responders who relapsed. Results indicated that although behavior therapy produced the largest average gains, each intervention resulted in approximately equal numbers of responders, nonresponders, and responders who relapsed. These findings are similar to those of the major collaborative study on depression (Elkin et al., 1989) and led practitioners to the potentially erroneous conclusion that all treatments for depression are equally efficacious. However, subjects in both these studies were diagnosed almost exclusively on the basis of symptomatic presentation, and thorough differentiation among subjects with differing etiologies (or maintaining factors) was not attempted. Consequently, outcome results are confounded by the probable interaction between etiology and treatment received. Indeed, if etiological subgroups of depression respond to one treatment better than another, then large gains of subjects for whom treatment and etiology were "matched" will be offset by the much smaller gains of those subjects who were "mismatched" within the same experimental condition. As such, lack of between-group differences were, of course, predictable.

Etiological classification schemes for affective disorders most frequently focus on the separation of "biological" or endogenous depression from nonendogenous depression on the basis of several assessment indices (Feinberg, 1992; Kupfer & Thase, 1983; Thase, Hersen, Bellack, Himmelhoch, & Kupfer, 1983; Wolpe, 1986). For example, endogenous depressives are relatively more likely to display symptoms of early morning awakening, lethargy, increased guilt, low levels of anxiety, and diminished coordination than are nonendogenous depressives (Gunther, Gunther, Streck, & Romig, 1988; Wolpe, 1979). In addition, most nonsuppressors on dexamethasone suppression tests are endogenous depressives. Furthermore, endogenous depressives display abnormal EEGs, rapid eye movement (REM) latency, and REM density patterns during sleep (Feinberg, 1992; Jones, Kelwala, Bell, & Dube, 1985; Kupfer & Thase, 1983), and, as mentioned, possess subaverage sedation thresholds (Wolpe, 1986). In contrast to the biological origin of endogenous depression, Wolpe (1986) posits four psychological causes of nonendogenous depression, including depression resulting from (1) severe conditioned anxiety, (2) devaluative or maladaptive cognitions, (3) interpersonal skill deficits, and (4) prolonged bereavement. Of course, differentiation among these depressive subtypes depends on a comprehensive behavioral analysis (see Wolpe, 1990).

Several investigators have demonstrated differential effects of treatment with affective disorder subtypes, particularly those of endogenous and nonendogenous depressives. For example, Raskin and Crook (1976) reported that antidepressant medication and placebo resulted in equivalent levels of improvement for nonendogenous depressives, whereas endogenous depressives improved only following treatment by antidepressant medication. Similarly, Kiloh, Ball, and Garside (1977) found that treatment gains produced by antidepressant medication were maintained to a significantly greater extent in endogenous than nonendogenous depressives. By contrast, Rush (1983) reported that endogenous depressives were unchanged following treatment with cognitive therapy, whereas 89% of nonendogenous depressives in a second sample improved in response to the same treatment. Initial investigations of the differential treatment responses of nonendogenous subtypes of depression have also been conducted. In a study by McKnight et al. (1992), treatment responses of socially unskilled depressed patients who did not present with depressogenic cognitions were compared to socially skilled depressed patients with depressogenic cognitions. Approximately equal numbers of subjects in both groups received social skills training or cognitive therapy. Predictably, patients with social skills deficits improved to a relatively greater extent on measures of both depression and social skills following skills training, whereas patients with depressogenic cognitions showed relatively greater reduction in depressive symptoms and negative thoughts following cognitive therapy. These examples illustrate the potential of comprehensive etiological assessment to facilitate clinicians' informed and appropriate selection of pharmacological and psychological treatments for depression. Importantly, similar theories of etiological heterogeneity have been supported with anxiety disorders (see Acierno et al., 1994).

Rachman (1977) and Wolpe (1981) identify two general etiological classes of phobias: those resulting from irrational thinking or misinformation, and those resulting from conditioning. In addition, social skills deficits leading to social anxiety may constitute a third phobic etiological category. Easily utilized methods to distinguish cognitive from conditioned phobias have been offered by Wolpe, Lande, McNally, and Schotte (1985) and Öst and Hugdahl (1983). According to Wolpe and associates, a specific phobia should be considered cognitive in nature when a patient truly *believes* that the feared object or situation is dangerous, or is very likely to result in physical or mental harm. In contrast, conditioned phobias are those in which patients report feeling "as if" they are in danger, but do not actually believe that feared stimuli carry the potential for significant harm; or patients report fearing panic attacks associated with phobic stimuli, rather than the stimuli themselves (Wolpe et al., 1985; McNally & Steketee, 1985). Using a slightly different etiological classification approach, Öst et al. (1983) differentiated conditioned from cognitive phobias on the basis of subject responses to their Phobic Origins Questionnaire, a test designed to detect the presence or absence of either historical conditioning events or negative information and instruction.

Consistent with the depression literature, an interaction appears to exist between phobic etiology and treatment. Indeed, Öst (1985) found that patients classified as conditioned phobics responded relatively better to interventions directed to counterconditioning or extinguishing learned anxiety responses than similarly assessed subjects treated with cognitive restructuring. Additionally, Trower, Yardley, Bryant, and Shaw (1978) noted that skills training was more effective than systematic desensitization with social phobics displaying skills deficits. In contrast, socially anxious patients demonstrating little or no skills deficits improved to a relatively greater extent after being treated with systematic desensitization. Each of these examples illustrates the potential maximization of treatment effectiveness through etiological assessment of patients who present with very similar overt symptomatology. Failure to perform such assessment diminishes the probability that the most effective treatment for a patient will be selected. As a result, professional accountability is jeopardized.

The final area of assessment necessary for informed and appropriate selection of psychological interventions is that of subject characteristics and history. The inherent relevance of this category to effective prescriptive treatment is reflected by inclusion of subject description in every published clinical-outcome study. Subject characteristics, such as age, sex, socioeconomic status (SES), ethnicity, language, past treatment response, and marital status, provide diagnostic information that facilitates treatment selection and frequently affects treatment outcome. For example, prolonged temporal disorientation and impairment in recent memory in an 80-year-old, nonmedicated male with no history of substance abuse are likely to be indicative of an organically based dementia. In contrast, identical symptoms in a 16-year-old male may indicate an organic disorder, substance abuse or withdrawal, temporal lobe seizures, and so on. Moreover, prevalence rates of many disorders vary as a function of patients' social, economic, and cultural backgrounds, and assessment of these factors may accelerate the diagnostic process. Along these lines, Lonigan, Shannon, Finch, and Daugherty (1991) noted that post-traumatic stress disorder (PTSD) may be more prevalent in African-Americans and Hispanics than in European-Americans. The suicide risk for young Native Americans is significantly greater than for all other ethnic groups (May, 1987). Organic disorders occur with greater frequency in older, rather than younger adults. And patients of low SES status are significantly more likely to suffer any psychological disorder than patients from upper SES levels (B. P. Dohrenwend & B. S. Dohrenwend, 1974).

In addition to predicting the probable presence of one form of psychopathology over another, measurement of subject characteristics and history may also provide insight into a patient's probable treatment response. For example, older depressed adults with weak social-support networks appear to be at significantly greater risk of relapse to depression than similarly diagnosed and treated older adults with extensive social support (George, Blazer, Hughes, & Fowler, 1989). This relationship is particularly strong for males; therefore, appropriate and accountable comprehensive treatments for socially isolated, depressed, elderly males will include strategies to enhance the quality and extent of their social-support structure, in addition to techniques aimed at ameliorating depressive symptomatology.

Subject characteristics and history are also useful in determining the relative appropriateness of one therapy over another. Clearly, interventions that are effective but require some degree of advanced intellectual development may not be completely suitable for use with very young children. Indeed, systematic desensitization, a treatment with strong empirical support for its efficacy, is contraindicated with individuals unable to generate affective imagery. Furthermore, extremely aversive interventions, such as flooding for PTSD, may be inappropriate in patients who are at increased physiological and psychological risk for suffering unacceptably detrimental side effects (e.g., older adults and children). Similarly, delivery of some empirically demonstrated treatments often requires modification for use with particular classes of subjects (e.g., toilet training for retarded vs. nonretarded children). Most important, treatments that have historically proven effective for a particular patient should be selected over interventions lacking such evidence.

Treatment Selection

The second criterion for accountability, selection of an empirically validated treatment over interventions lacking such validation, is indisputable and requires little elaboration. The American Psychological Association's (APA; 1987) Practice Guideline 1.5 states:

> All providers of psychological services attempt to maintain and *apply* current knowledge of *scientific* and professional developments that are clinically related to the services they render. (p. 715, italics added)

Moreover, in their recommendation to the Division 12 Board of the APA, the Task Force on the Practice and Dissemination of Psychological Procedures (September, 1993) suggested that "APA site visit teams make training in empirically validated treatments a criterion for APA accreditation" (p. 8). In addition, several leading scientist–practitioners have advocated selection of empirically validated treatments to assure appropriate and accountable treatment of patients (Garfield, 1987; Wilson, 1984; Wolpe, 1990). Disappointingly, a large percentage of practitioners in the field no longer appear to be active scientists, or even interested in the science of psychology. Indeed, Cohen (1979) pointed out that most practitioners do not even read, much less contribute to empirical clinical research. Unfortunately, failure to select an intervention with empirical support renders practitioners culpable for potentially extending patient suffering and costs. Commenting on this practice in his summary of the Federal Agency Health-Care Policy and Research report, Rush (1993) stated that "there is a wide variation in actual practice [that] is generally believed to reflect unnecessary diversity of practice procedures that raise the cost of care and result in suboptimal outcomes" (p. 484).

Evaluation

Following selection of an empirically validated treatment on the basis of thorough assessment of patient and pathology, the third criterion of accountability, that of repeated measurement of treatment progress, must be addressed. In reference to this point, APA (1987) Practice Guideline 3.3 under "Accountability" stated simply: "There are periodic, systematic, and effective evaluations of psychological services" (p. 719). Consistent with this position, Barlow et al. (1984) noted that "the focus has been on measuring client progress and specifying treatment. These elements are central to any attempt to be accountable" (p. 177). Similarly, Smith (1989) held that "accountability requires that applied psychologists provide data concerning their effectiveness" (p. 169). Furthermore, as Barlow et al. (1984) have illustrated, regular assessment or evaluation of treatment efficacy by practicing psychologists in single-case design formats will significantly complement the existing clinical database with information about idiotypic patient responses. Of course, multiple replication of results is even more imperative in single-case research, and some degree of control above that of the simple case report is desirable. Fortunately, Barlow and Hersen (1984) and Barlow et al. (1984) have outlined methods by which practicing clinicians can conduct and contribute controlled single-case research in professional and clinical settings. Additionally, a special issue of the *Journal of Consulting and Clinical Psychology* (Vol. 61, No. 3, 1993) was devoted to the application of single-case designs to clinical process research. As mentioned, single-case designs have several advantages over group experimental designs. Specifically, single-case research typically involves an exceptionally detailed description of subject and pathology along the parameters of prescriptive, comprehensive assessment outlined earlier. This is in contrast to group designs, in which individual subject and pathology characteristics are intentionally obliterated; that is, single-case research permits emphasis through specificity, rather than nullification through aggregation, of those symptomatic, etiological, contextual, and subject factors that affect treatment outcome. Such specificity, in turn, directs future refinement of interventions. Nevertheless, one single-case report (or group study), however highly controlled, cannot serve as the basis for future treatment selection. Instead, as is the case with group research, replication is essential in establishing the reliability of an effect, and in determining the extent to which the noted effect generalizes to dissimilar situations. Barlow and Hersen (1984), building on the work of Sidman (1960), specified three stages of replication that, when achieved, enable single-case research to greatly contribute to existing clinical knowledge: direct replication, systematic replication, and clinical replication.

Direct replication refers to "administration of a given procedure by the same investigator or group of investigators in a specific setting , on a series of clients homogeneous for a particular behavior disorder" (Barlow & Hersen, 1984, p. 326). Note that in direct replication, the primary aim is to establish the reliability of an effect; thus, an overt effort is made to maintain consistency of all controllable variables (e.g., therapist, setting, patient type, pathology type). Although reliability of a particular treatment effect with a particular type of patient and pathology is established through this form of clinical research, very little is learned about how well (if at all) the treatment works with other patients or pathologies. For this next level of experimental refinement, systematic replication is required. *Systematic replication*, defined as "any attempt to replicate findings from a direct replication series varying setting, behavior, change agents, behavior disorders, or any combination thereof" (Barlow & Hersen, 1984, p. 347), produces data describing treatment potency, or the effectiveness of an intervention *despite* differences in subject, therapist, setting, and so on. It is through systematic replication that, perhaps, the most valuable contribution to clinical research by practitioners is made. Importantly, systematic replication requires that a minimum number of variables be altered from one replication series to the next, thereby strengthening attributions of isolated causality. Simultaneous alteration of multiple variables confounds effects of one modified variable with those of another, thereby preventing matching of prescriptive treatments with particular types of patients and pathologies. Although this concern is relatively great in research settings, it is less important in clinical realms by virtue of the massive number of single-case experiments that are potentially performable; that is, adequate systematic replication, in which only one or two patient, treatment, or pathology variables are changed at a time, will naturally occur if a great number of practicing clinicians conduct and report their single-case research. Note that reports of both failures and successes are necessary for such data to be informative. Although relatively less concise and ordered than multiple-series research emanating from a single laboratory, compilation of results across large numbers of professional clinicians is not impossible, and external validity of treatment-outcome findings is exponentially enhanced. Of course, individual practitioners and researchers should engage in systematic replication only after reliability of a treatment effect is established through direct replication.

Clinical replication is very similar to systematic replication, but involves evaluation of *two* or more combined treatments that have been shown to produce reliable (through direct replication) and generalizable (through systematic replication) improvements when applied individually (Barlow & Hersen, 1984). Whereas systematic replication most resembles work carried out in research settings, clinical replication most reflects efforts of the consulting office. As mentioned, there are no simple cases, and most patients require more than one treatment strategy to completely ameliorate their suffering; however, synergistic (or competing) effects of most treatments are unknown. Clinical replication across classes of patients and pathology types permits evaluation of these "real-world" componental treatment packages. As with systematic replication, practitioners are in a far better position, by nature of their sheer numbers, to perform clinical replication trials with componental treatments than are empirical researchers.

Replication of any type implies that a procedure exists that is reproducible. Moreover, if results are to be meaningful (i.e., if causality is to be established), then some degree of control must characterize the replication process. This text speaks to the first stipulation. In response to the second requirement, a variety of experimental designs exists for use with single subjects that permit inferences of causality (and hence, accountability), which are naturally strengthened through the forms of replication discussed earlier. Barlow and Hersen (1984) and Barlow et al. (1984) specified several general types of single-case designs, seven of which are easily applied to clinical practice. These are the simple phase change, interaction phase change, changing criterion, alternating treatment, multiple baseline, crossover, and constant series designs. The first three (i.e., simple and interaction phase change and changing criterion) are within-series designs. Thus, each score on a particular dependent measure in response to a specific treatment is analyzed in relation to other scores on *that* dependent measure. All scores on the dependent measure constitute a series, and this is graphically represented by a single line. By contrast, the alternating treatment design makes use of between-series comparisons. In this design, scores on a dependent variable in response to one treatment form one series (or graphically, one line) while scores on the *same* dependent variable in response to another treatment form the second series (graphically, a second line). It is to the difference between these two series that attention is directed. The final three single-case designs (i.e., multiple baseline, crossover, and constant series) utilize a combination of within- and between-series analyses to imply causality. Therefore, scores on a dependent variable in response to one treatment (graphically, one line) are concurrently examined in relation to each other, and in relation to a series of scores on another dependent variable in response to additional treatments (graphically, two or more lines).

Simple phase-change designs, also called A–B designs, involve repeated measurement of a dependent variable under one condition (e.g., baseline), followed by repeated measurement of the same dependent variable under a second condition (e.g., treatment). Of course, additional discrete treatment conditions may be added to form A–B–BC designs, and so on. Importantly, a phase change should not occur until a stable trend of at least three data points is obtained (see Barlow & Hersen, 1984, for an extended discussion of baseline stability). In this design, the trend in the second phase is contrasted with the trend in the first phase. A change in trend supports (weakly) the inference that addition of the second phase was responsible for gains or losses; however, simple phase-change designs do not control for effects of time, and noted improvements may have resulted from initiation of the second phase or from some other, unspecified event such as maturation, effects of repeated assessment, or self-monitoring. These drawbacks can be minimized, somewhat, when working with some forms of psychopathology by a reinstitution of the first (typically baseline or A) phase. This is regularly referred to as a withdrawal design, and is most often accompanied by a second treatment phase, producing a double phase change, or A–B–A–B design. Although still attributable to the effects of time, reported changes in trend that repeatedly coincide with changes in phase (in a single within-subject direct replication) strengthen inferences that treatment was responsible for noted gains. The repeated phase change (A–B–A–B) design is appropriate only in evaluating treatments that produce time-limited effects such as reinforcement-contingency structuring. However, ethical implications of treatment withdrawal must be considered when using A–B–A–B or A–B–A phase changes. Obviously, withdrawal of an apparently effective treatment for problems such as self-injurious behavior is obviously unjustified. For treatments that produce enduring effects (e.g., cognitive restructuring), only the A–B simple-phase change is appropriate, hence control and accountability achieved is minimal. Importantly, the simple phase-change design requires very little effort to implement and is very useful in initial evaluations of new treatment techniques.

The interaction phase change is based on the logic of the simple phase-change design, but specifically incorporates a period during which the simultaneous effects of two or more treatments are measured relative to the effects produced by one or more of the treatments (e.g., A–B–A–B–BC–B). As a result, combined effects of multiple treatments are revealed. The second part of the above example design (B–BC–B) demonstrates additive interaction effects of C over and above those of B, following a reversal design in which the effects of B were demonstrated, that is, the first part of the example design (A–B–A–B). In order to more fully clarify the interaction between B and C, direct replication of the experiment must be conducted in which the independent effects of C are isolated (e.g., A–C–A–C) and the effects of B are examined over and above C (e.g., C–CB–C) as in the design A–C–A–C–CB–C. This is because statements regarding interaction effects of a treatment are somewhat inappropriate if made in the absence of an assessment of the treatment's independent effects. Interaction phase-change designs are limited for use with treatment components that do not produce early, enduring effects. Clearly, if any one component of an intervention package produces enduring effects, then removal of that and other components will proceed without a concomitant deterioration in the patient's condition. Consequently, all treatment components, including the one actually responsible for improvement, may erroneously be considered superfluous. Moreover, phase changes must be initiated before maximum gains are attained in order to prevent incorrect conclusions that additional treatment components are ineffective, when, in fact, ceiling effects are responsible for lack of noted progress. Although the effects of time remain uncontrolled, both simple- and interaction-phase designs are strengthened by the inclusion of several phase changes. Notably, interaction phase-change designs are particularly useful in isolating "active ingredients" in treatment packages. As a result, clinicians are able to reject impotent treatment strategies in favor of those that appear to be of particular benefit to the patient.

The final "N of 1" strategy to employ within-series analyses of data is the changing criterion design. The reasoning that underlies this form of single-case evaluation is somewhat different from that of phase-change designs, in which causal inferences are strengthened when trend changes and phase changes are concomitant. In contrast, causality in changing-criterion designs is usually attributed to the changing criterion itself (i.e., the criterion is the treatment) when changes in behavior track changes in specified goal criteria (Barlow et al., 1984). For example, a clinician treating a patient for cigarette-smoking addiction may set a new lowered criterion number of cigarettes to be smoked each week. If observed behavior consistently varies closely with set criteria, casuality inferred to the criterion is supported. However, this design is not limited to assessing effects of "criterion specification" in isolation. Indeed, several psychological treatments lend themselves particularly well to evaluation through changing criterion designs. Exposure and response prevention for compulsive handwashing is an example of one such intervention. Using the changing-criterion design, a clinician may evaluate the efficacy of exposure and response prevention by measuring the patient's ability to consistently engage in compulsive behavior at specified and decreasing frequencies. Close approximation of handwashing frequency to goal criteria would indicate that the combination of treatment and criteria specification are responsible for noted change. Barlow et al. (1984) outline several relevant points to be considered when employing changing-criterion designs: First, multiple criterion shifts are necessary to establish causality to any degree. As with phase changes, each new criterion represents an opportunity to replicate the results obtained with previous criteria. If only one or two criteria are used, then attributions of causality may logically be directed to unknown effects of time, as well as the changing criteria of interest. Second, criteria must be set in a manner that does not imitate natural patterns of the behavior under study. Therefore, both magnitude of criteria and length of time during which they are in effect should vary. Third, because we are interested in the trend of data at each specified period, criteria should be left in effect for at least three assessment periods or until a reasonably stable trend is noted. Interpretation of changing-criterion designs is somewhat more difficult than that of phase-change designs. This is because the focus of the former design is on degree of correspondence between observed behavior and set goals for behavior, rather than on absolute trend change observed in the latter design. Although any change in trend supports inferences of causality in phase-change designs, only those movements in the direction of, and of similar magnitude to, criterion changes support similar inferences in changing-criterion studies.

As mentioned, alternating treatment designs employ between-series analyses to establish causal relationships. Specifically, one treatment's effects on a dependent variable are repeatedly compared with another treatment's effects on the same dependent variable at consecutive points in time. The rate at which interventions are alternated should equal that of the sampling of dependent measures. Consequently, multiple data series are obtained that directly and independently correspond to each treatment. Obviously, if a treatment produces effects that are expected to last 8 days (e.g., a drug trial), measurement after only 2 hours followed by initiation of the second treatment is inappropriate and premature. Alternating treatment designs are most often used to demonstrate the relative efficacy of one intervention over another. Such a demonstration is achieved when a series produced during assessment of one treatment's effects consistently differ in value from that of a second treatment's effects, at corresponding points in time (graphically, the two lines formed by each series do not intersect). In a pure alternating-treatment design, there are no analyses within each series, because each series occurs in only one phase. Rather, attention is directed to the *relative efficacy* of two or more interventions; however, if a baseline is included as one alternating treatment, mildly controlled statements of absolute efficacy can be made. Unfortunately, this design is very susceptible to confounds produced as a result of treatment interaction, or the enduring effects of one intervention combined with effects of another. Advantages of the alternating-treatment design include its ability to establish relative efficacy of two treatments without withdrawal of treatment. In contrast, phase-change designs require an A–B–A–C format in order to permit statements of relative efficacy (and these are severely confounded by time). Alternating research designs also require fewer data points to produce statements of relative effectiveness. Whereas A–B–A–C phase-change design must contain at least 3 data points in each phase to establish trends, or 12 sampling points overall, alternating treatment designs with two groups require only 6 data points. Fewer data points are necessary with alternating treatment designs because, as Barlow et al. (1984) note, they focus on the *variability* of data over its trend. As a result, extraneous events (e.g., maturation, learning) affect each series of data to an approximately equal extent, and stability is not as imperative. Furthermore, effects of any one treatment are not confounded by extraneous events over time because all treatments are rapidly alternating and occurring in the context of all confounding temporal factors. Consequently, these confounds are "washed out." Inferences of causality resulting from alternating-treatment designs are strengthened by using only two or three treatments, by conducting assessments at intervals that account for possible enduring treatment effects, and by adding a phase-change (i.e., baseline) component before treatment alternating has begun.

The most common design to employ both between- and within-series analyses is the multiple baseline. Multiple-baseline designs are actually combinations of multiple phase-change studies, each comprising a different dependent-variable series and different phase lengths. Of the single-subject designs covered thus far, only the multiple baseline controls directly for time. This is accomplished by a delayed, pseudoreplication of each phase-change design across each series. If changes are noted in each series only after a phase change *in that series* (as opposed to concomitant changes in response to phase changes in other series), then attributions of causality are strengthened. Moreover, the greater the number of replication series, the stronger the causal inferences. Note that both within- and between-series analyses contribute to overall impressions. Differences observed in a series following a phase change form the first half of the inference "change has occurred." *Lack* of concurrent change in the other sets of series (which are still in Phase 1) form the second half of the causal inference "change is not due to extraneous factors." These inferences are combined and further strengthened by initiating phase changes in the second series, followed by the third, and so on. Overall, if improvements are noted only after sequential introduction of the phase change across all series, then treatment is assumed to be responsible for change. Of course, it is necessary that the behaviors comprising each series be functionally related but independent of one another. In addition, dependent measures must be continually assessed, because the first phase of the second series serves as the between-series baseline for the second phase of the first series, and so on. Moreover, treatments (phase changes) must be introduced sequentially across all series, rather than concurrently, in order to produce between-series contrasts.

Importantly, phase changes in multiple-baseline designs are not limited to A–B or B–C formats. Indeed, componential treatments (A–B–BC) are also amenable to evaluation through this method, given that phase changes are staggered across each series (e.g., Acierno et al., 1994; Van Hasselt, Hersen, Bellack, Rosenblum, & Lamparski, 1979). Three types of multiple-baseline studies are frequently employed, and include multiple-baseline designs across behaviors, subjects, and settings (Barlow & Hersen, 1984). In multiple-baseline designs across behaviors, "the same treatment is applied sequentially to separate (independent) target behaviors" (p. 213). In this design, one target behavior serves as the relative baseline for another. For example, when treating a multiphobic patient who fears heights, dogs, and elevators, a 4-week stable baseline might be followed by exposure treatment for the first fear area (i.e., heights), while the other two fear areas remain untreated, but assessed. After a trend is evident for the first treated fear, exposure might also be directed to dog fears, while the third fear area remains in baseline phase. Finally, after a trend is also discerned in response to exposure treatment to dog fears, therapy might be implemented for elevator fears. If improvement in each fear area is noted *only* following sequential introduction of exposure treatment, then the inference that this intervention was responsible for change is supported. All assessments for all fear areas should occur simultaneously and repeatedly throughout the study. Moreover, initiation of the second phase for each series is staggered so that effects of treatment (i.e., the trend) in the previous phase are clear. Finally, each behavior targeted must be functionally similar, but independent. Generalized improvement across all behaviors following introduction of treatment to only the first behavior indicates that the design is inappropriate and precludes inferences of causality beyond that of A–B designs.

In the multiple-baseline design across subjects, "a particular treatment is applied in sequence across *matched* subjects, presumably exposed to 'identical' environmental conditions" (Barlow & Hersen, 1984, p. 213). In this design, each subject serves as the other's baseline, and the single treated behavior constitutes the dependent variable of interest. Of course, subjects are assumed to be independent. For example, four patients of the same age and sex diagnosed with hyperventilatory panic that is maintained by a combination of inappropriate breathing and avoidance of interoceptive cues, may be assigned to baselines of varying lengths followed by sequential introduction (across patients) of breathing retraining treatment. If improvement is noted in each patient only after staggered introduction of treatment, attributions of causality are supported. Because individuals do not serve as their own controls, this design is more susceptible to confounds originating from differences across subjects; however, when many patients are employed in a multiple baseline across subjects, and change is consistently noted *only* following sequential introduction of treatment, the potency of the intervention is strongly supported and treatment effectiveness is demonstrated over and above changes attributable to subject differences. Clinicians using this design should assign subjects to varying baselines on a random basis, and should attempt to collect dependent measures from all subjects concurrently to avoid temporal confounds.

In multiple-baseline designs across settings, "a particular treatment is applied sequentially to a single subject ⸳ across independent situations" (Barlow & Hersen, 1984, p. 213). In this design, behavior in one setting serves as the control for the same behavior in another setting. Moreover, events in each setting are assumed to be independent. For example, rate of tic behavior in a child with Tourette's syndrome may be measured at home, in the classroom, and during play. After collection of approximately concurrent baseline assessments in all settings, habit-reversal treatment (Azrin & Peterson, 1987) might be initiated for home tics over several weeks, followed by additional treatment for school tics, and finally for tics that occur during play. If improvement is noted in each setting only after sequential introduction of habit-reversal procedures, inferences that the treatment was responsible for change are supported. As is the case with multiple-baseline designs across subjects, only one dependent variable is employed for each between-series analysis.

In summary, multiple-baseline designs across behaviors involve sequential application of one treatment to independent behaviors in one subject; multiple-baseline designs across subjects involve sequential application of one treatment to similar behavior in several independent (but closely matched) subjects; and multiple-baseline designs across settings involve sequential application of one treatment to one behavior in independent settings in one subject. Importantly, increasing the number of series assessed (i.e., increasing the number of control/comparison phases) strengthens inferences of causality for all multiple-baseline designs. Therefore, a multiple-baseline design across four behaviors is more potent than one across only two behaviors; a multiple-baseline design across six subjects permits stronger causal inferences than one across three subjects; and a multiple-baseline design across four settings is preferable to one across two. Moreover, each multiple-baseline design is flexible in that groups of subjects can be used in the place of each subject. However, Barlow and Hersen (1984) advise investigators to verify that changes in the large majority of individual subjects are consistent with overall averaged changes when several subjects are experimentally conceptualized as a single unit in multiple-baseline designs.

The second single-case design to combine within- and between-series analyses is the constant-series technique. In this evaluative format, two related but independent behaviors are repeatedly and concurrently assessed; however, one behavior remains in the baseline phase while the other undergoes one or more phase changes. Of course, this is the equivalent of a multiple-baseline design in which sequential occurrences of phase changes (i.e., sequential applications of treatment) are not carried out across at least one behavior. As a result, within-subject replication across behaviors found in multiple-baseline designs is absent in simple constant-series designs; however, effects of time are somewhat controlled. Constant-series controls are most useful when combined with other designs. Indeed, they can both aid in controlling confounds produced by order and temporal effects, as well as enhance between-series comparisons during phase changes (Barlow et al., 1984).

The final investigative method to combine within- and between-series analyses is the crossover design. This strategy is nearly identical to the crossover design used in group research. In single-case crossover designs, two phases of equal length across two dependent variables (measuring two behaviors) are implemented simultaneously, each in reverse order (i.e., A–B for one series and, simultaneously, B–A for the other). As such, each series serves as the other's referenced control, and changes following only one phase, regardless of order of implementation, support the causality of treatment in that phase. In this manner, time effects, simple-order effects, and treatment-interaction effects are controlled (within-series). The two phases may be composed of either baseline and treatment, or two different treatments. Moreover, the two behaviors of interest must be functionally similar, but independent. Using the example of the multiphobic patient, relaxation training may be implemented to treat height fears while exposure treatment is concurrently initiated to reduce dog fears. Following several assessments of the dependent variable of each fear series, relaxation is applied to dog fears and exposure is applied to height fears for a duration equal to that of the first phase (as is the case with alternating treatment designs, it is essential to initiate the phase changes before a ceiling effect is produced by any one treatment). Improvement *in both series*, following the introduction of only one of the treatments, regardless of order, indicates that this treatment was responsible for change. Advantages of crossover designs include their ease of use and ability to determine the relative efficacy of treatments without a baseline or withdrawal phase (Barlow et al., 1984).

Clearly, evaluation of treatment through single-case design research both enhances clinical accountability and contributes to the existing clinical database. Importantly, all single-case designs involve collection of repeated measures of patient progress. This is entirely consistent with requirements of professional accountability. Furthermore, as is the case with all empirical research, conclusions based on single-case experiments require direct, systematic, and clinical replication. Finally, single-case evaluations are particularly amenable for use with highly defined, prescriptive treatments. This is because "N of 1" designs are characterized by a high degree of subject and pathology specification, as well as within-subject control. As such, differential efficacy of one prescriptive intervention over that of another can be demonstrated for this particular type of subject with that particular class of pathology in a relatively short amount of time.

SUMMARY

Advancement of contemporary psychology as both a science and practice requires increased efforts on the part of psychologists to remain accountable. To this end, leaders of various clinical subspecialties within the field have joined the general public, the American Psychological Association, and basic researchers in insisting that psychologists justify what it is they do. Such practical justification necessarily involves three specific processes. The first, comprehensive assessment of etiological factors, contextual factors, and subject characteristics and history in *addition* to overt symptomatology, increases the likelihood that appropriate prescriptive interventions will be matched with patient and pathology. The logic underlying the second process is unassailable and directs treatment selection to those publicly detailed interventions that have empirically demonstrated efficacy over those lacking such clarity and support. Finally, maintenance of accountability is achieved through repeated and controlled evaluation of patient progress during treatment. Procedural aspects of each of these processes have been outlined here and elaborated in greater depth elsewhere.

The manualized treatment protocols presented in this text have been generated and refined through empirical evaluations, and represent the most prescriptive interventions available to date. Moreover, several included therapeutic strategies specifically address circumscribed areas of psychopathology. Hence, it is probable that two or more treatments will be necessary and justified for use with any one patient. Indeed, there are only "complex cases" (Hersen, 1981), and patients very rarely present with only one isolated complaint. Moreover, despite their exceedingly high degree of specificity, these treatment manuals are not intended to be used in identical fashion with all patients; therefore, modification may be required for some individuals. Importantly, such changes should be made only after thorough consideration of subject, etiological, and contextual factors. Furthermore, it is imperative that such modifications be subjected to controlled single-case evaluations in order to defend their continued use or abandonment, and to advance knowledge in the field.

REFERENCES

Acierno, R., Hersen, M., Van Hasselt, V. B., & Ammerman, R. (1994). Remedying the Achilles heel of behavioral research: Prescriptive matching of treatment and pathology. *Journal of Behavior Therapy and Experimental Psychiatry, 25*, 179–188.

Acierno, R., Tremont, G., Last, C. G., & Montgomery, D. (1994). Tripartite assessment of the efficacy of eye-movement desensitization. *Journal of Anxiety Disorders, 8*, 259–276.

Anderson, D. (1992). A case for standards of counseling practice. *Journal of Counseling and Development, 71*, 22–26.

Azrin, N. H., & Peterson, A. L. (1990). Habit reversal for the treatment of Tourette syndrome. *Behaviour Research and Therapy, 26,* 347–351.

American Psychiatric Association Committee on Professional Standards (1987). General guidelines for providers of psychological services. *American Psychologist, 42,* 712–723.

American Psychiatric Association. (1994). *Diagnostic and statistical manual of mental disorders* (4th ed.). Washington, DC: Author.

Barlow, D. H., Craske, M. G., Cearny, J. A., & Klosko, J. S. (1989). Behavioral treatment of panic disorder. *Behavior Therapy, 20,* 261–282.

Barlow, D. H., Hayes, S. C., & Nelson, R. O. (1984). *The scientist practioner: Research and accountability in clinical and educational settings.* New York: Pergamon Press.

Barlow, D. H., & Hersen, M. (1984). *Single case experimental designs: Strategies for studying behavior change. (2nd ed.).* New York: Pergamon Press.

Beck, A. T., & Haaga, D. A. (1992). The future of cognitive therapy. *Psychotherapy: Theory, Research and Practice, 29,* 34–38.

Bishop, J. B., & Trembley, E. L. (1987). Counseling centers and accountability: Immovable, objects, irresistible forces. *Journal of Counseling and Development, 65,* 491–494.

Burchard, J. D., & Schaefer, M. C. (1992). Improving accountability in a service delivery system in children's mental health. *Clinical Psychology Review, 12,* 867–882.

Cohen, L. H. (1979). The research readership and information source reliance of clinical psychologists. *Professional Psychology, 10,* 780–786.

Conti, L., Placidi, G. R., Dell'Osso, L., Lenzi, A., & Cassano, G. B. (1987). Therapeutic response in subtypes of major depression. *New Trends in Experimental and Clinical Psychiatry, 3,* 101–107.

Cross, D. G. (1985). The age of accountability: The next phase for family therapy. *Australian and New Zealand Journal of Family Therapy, 6,* 129–135.

Dohrenwend, B. P., & Dohrenwend, B. S. (1974). Social and cultural influences upon psychopathology. *Annual Review of Psychology, 25,* 417–452.

Elkin, I., Shea, M. T., Watkins, J. T., Imber, S. D., Sotsky, S. M., Collins, J. F., Glass, D. R., Pilkonis, P. A., Leber, W. R., Docherty, J. P., Fiester, S. J., & Parloff, M. B. (1989). National Institutes of Mental Health treatment of depression collaborative research program: General effectiveness of treatments. *Archives of General Psychiatry, 46,* 971–982.

Eysenck, H. J. (1952). The effects of psychotherapy: An evaluation. *Journal of Consulting Psychology, 16,* 319–324.

Feinberg, M. (1992). Comment: Subtypes of depression and response to treatment. *Journal of Consulting and Clinical Psychology, 60,* 670–674.

Furedy, J. J., & Shulhan, D. (1987). Specific versus placebo effects in biofeedback: Some brief back to basics considerations. *Biofeedback and Self-Regulation, 12,* 211–215.

Garfield, S. L. (1987). Towards a scientifically oriented eclecticism. *Scandinavian Journal of Behaviour Therapy, 16,* 95–109.

George, L. K., Blazer, D. G., Hughes, D. C., & Fowler, N. (1989). Social support and the outcome of major depression. *British Journal of Psychiatry, 154,* 478–485.

Gunther, W., Gunther, R., Streck, P., & Ronig, H. (1988). Psychomotor disturbances in psychiatric patients as a possible basis for new attempts at differential diagnosis and therapy: III. Cross validation study on depressed patients: The psychotic motor syndrome as a possible state marker for endogenous depression. *European Archives of Psychiatry and Neurological Sciences, 237,* 65–73.

Hersen, M. (1973). Self-assessment of fear. *Behavior Therapy, 4,* 241–257.

Hersen, M. (1981). Complex problems require complex solutions. *Behavior Therapy, 12,* 15–29.

Jones, D., Kelwala, S., Bell, J., & Dube, S. (1985). Cholinergic REM sleep induction response correlation with endogenous major depressive subtype. *Psychiatry Research, 14,* 99–110.

Kallman, W. M., Hersen, M., & O'Toole, D. H. (1975). The use of social reinforcement in a case of conversion reaction. *Behavior Therapy, 6,* 411–413.

Kiloh, L. G., Ball, J. R., & Garside, R. F. (1977). Depression: A multivariate study of Sir Aubrey Lews's data on melancholia. *Australian and New Zealand Journal of Psychiatry, 11,* 149–156.

Kupfer, D. L., & Thase, M. F. (1983). The use of the sleep laboratory in the diagnosis of affective disorders. *Psychiatric Clinics of North America, 6,* 3–25.

Lang, P. J. (1968). Fear reduction and fear behavior: Problems in treating a construct. In J. M. Shlien (Ed.), *Research in psychotherapy* (Vol. 3, pp. 90–102). Washington, DC: American Psychological Association.

Lonigan, C., Shannon, M., Finch, A., & Daugherty, T., (1991). Children's reactions to a natural disaster: Symptom severity and degree of exposure. *Advances in Behaviour Research and Therapy, 13,* 135–154.

May, P. (1987). Suicide and self-destruction among American Indian youths. *American Indian and Alaska Native Mental Health Research, 1,* 52–69.

Mavissakallian, M. (1987). Trimodal assessment in agoraphobia research: Further observations on heart rate and synchrony/desynchrony. *Journal of Psychopathology and Behavioral Assessment, 9,* 89–98.

McKnight, D., Nelson, R., Hayes, S., & Jarrett, R. (1992). Importance of treating individually assessed response classess of depression. *Behavior Therapy, 15,* 315–335.

McNally, R., & Steketee, G. (1985). The etiology and maintenance of severe animal phobias. *Behaviour Research and Therapy, 23,* 431–435.

Öst, L. G. (1985). Ways of acquiring phobias and outcome of behavioral treatment. *Behaviour Research and Therapy, 23,* 683–689.

Öst, L. G., & Hugdahl, K. (1983). Acquisition of agoraphobia, mode of onset and anxiety response patterns. *Behaviour Research and Therapy, 21,* 623–631.

Öst, L. G., Johansson, J., & Jerremalm, A. (1982). Individual response patterns and the effects of different behavioral methods in the treatment of claustrophobia. *Behaviour Research and Therapy, 20,* 445–560.

Öst, L. G., Sterner, U., & Lindahl, I. L. (1984). Physiological responses in blood phobics. *Behaviour Research and Therapy, 22,* 109–117.

Rachman, S. (1977). The conditioning theory of fear-acquisition: A critical examination. *Behaviour Research and Therapy, 15,* 375.

Raimy, V. C. (Ed.). (1950). *Training in clinical psychology (Boulder Conference).* New York: Prentice-Hall.

Raskin, A., & Crook, T. H. (1976). The endogenous–neurotic distinction as a predictor of response to antidepressant drugs. *Psychological Medicine, 6,* 59–70.

Rush, A. J. (1983). A Phase II study of cognitive therapy in depression. In J. B. Williams & R. L. Spitzer (Eds.), *Psychotherapy research: Where are we and where should we go.* (pp. 216–234). New York: Guilford Press.

Rush, A. J. (1993). Clinical practice guidelines: Good news, no news, or bad news? *Archives of General Psychiatry, 50,* 483–490.

Sidman, M. (1960). *Tactics of scientific research,* New York: Basic Books.

Smith, R. E. (1989). Applied sport psychology in an age of accountability. Second annual conference of the Association for the Advancement of Applied Sport Psychology. *Journal of Applied Sport Psychology, 1,* 166–180.

Taylor, S., & McLean, P. (1993). Outcome profiles in the treatment of unipolar depression. *Behavior Research and Therapy, 31,* 325–330.

Task Force on Promotion and Dissemination of Psychological Procedures. (1993). A report to the American Psychological Association, Division 12 Board, September 15, 1993.

Thase, M. E., Hersen, M., Bellack, A. S., Himmelhoch, J. M., & Kupfer, D. J. (1983). Validation of a Hamilton subscale for endogenomorphic depression. *Journal of Affective Disorders, 5,* 267–278.

Trower, P., Yardley, K., Bryant, B., & Shaw, P. (1978). The treatment of social failure: A comparison of anxiety reduction and skills aquisition procedures for two social problems. *Behavior Modification, 2,* 41–60.

Van Hasselt, V. B., Hersen, M., Bellack, A. S., Rosenblum, N. D., & Lamparski, D. (1979). Tripartite assessment of the effects of systematic desensitization in a multi-phobic child: An experimental analysis. *Journal of Behavior Therapy and Experimental Psychiatry, 10,* 51–55.

Wilson, G. T. (1984). Clinical issues and strategies in the practice of behavior therapy. *Annual Review of Behavior Therapy Theory and Practice, 9,* 309–343.

Wolpe, J. (1958). *Psychotherapy by reciprocal inhibition.* Stanford, CA: Stanford University Press.

Wolpe, J. (1977). Inadequate behavior analysis: The achilles heel of outcome research in behavior therapy. *Journal of Behavior Therapy and Experimental Psychiatry, 8,* 1–3.

Wolpe, J. (1979). The experimental model and treatment of neurotic depression. *Behaviour Research and Therapy, 17,* 555–565.

Wolpe, J. (1981). The dichotomy between classically conditioned and cognitively learned anxiety. *Journal of Behavior Therapy and Experimental Psychiatry, 12,* 35–42.

Wolpe, J. (1986). The positive diagnosis of neurotic depression as an etiological category. *Comprehensive Psychiatry, 27,* 449–460.

Wolpe, J. (1990). *The practice of behavior therapy* (4th ed.). New York: Pergamon Press.

Wolpe, J., Lande, S. D., McNally, R. J., & Schotte, D. (1985). Differentiation between classically conditioned and cognitively based neurotic fears: Two pilot studies. *Journal of Behavior Therapy and Experimental Psychiatry, 16,* 287–293.

II
ADULT DISORDERS AND PROBLEMS

2

Panic Disorder and Agoraphobia

Theo K. Bouman and Paul M. G. Emmelkamp

INTRODUCTION

Panic disorder and agoraphobia are among the most frequent referrals in mental health care. The treatment of agoraphobia has received considerable attention from the early days of behavior therapy onward. As of the early 1980s, diagnostic and theoretical refinements led to an increased emphasis on the occurrence and treatment of panic attacks. The *Diagnostic and Statistical Manuals of Mental Disorders*, edited by the American Psychiatric Association, as well as cognitive models of psychopathology, are responsible for these developments. In the present chapter, effective cognitive–behavioral treatment protocols are described, based on these recent insights. After an overview of diagnostic considerations and assessment methods, the treatment of panic disorder is described in detail. Next, strategies in the reduction of agoraphobic avoidance are outlined. Even within the realm of cognitive–behavioral therapy, many treatment approaches have been suggested. In this chapter we focus on the most frequently used variants. Obstacles in the implementation and the conduct of treatment often occur and for that reason deserve ample discussion. Case illustrations and verbatim therapy interactions demonstrate the practical realization of the original treatment plans.

DESCRIPTION OF THE DISORDERS

Panic Disorder

In the *Diagnostic and Statistical Manual of Mental Disorders*, Fourth Edition (DSM-IV); American Psychiatric Association, 1994) *panic* is described as:

Theo K. Bouman and Paul M. G. Emmelkamp • Department of Clinical Psychology, University of Groningen, Oostersingel 59, 9713 EZ Groningen, The Netherlands.

Sourcebook of Psychological Treatment Manuals for Adult Disorders, edited by Vincent B. Van Hasselt and Michel Hersen. Plenum Press, New York, 1996.

a discrete period in which there is a sudden onset of intense apprehension, fearfulness, or terror, often associated with feelings of impending doom. During these attacks, symptoms such as shortness of breath, palpitations, chest pain or discomfort, choking or smothering sensations, and fear of "going crazy" or losing control are present. (American Psychiatric Association, 1994, p. 393; see Table 2.1).

These panic attacks are central phenomena in the panic disorder (see Table 2.2), but also may occur during other DSM-IV anxiety disorders. According to the DSM-IV definition, the central feature of panic disorder is unexpected panic attacks that alter a person's life, which is to say the attacks do not occur immediately before or after exposure to a situation that nearly always causes anxiety. Neither are the attacks solely the result of situations in which the person is the focus of others' attention. Some speak of a "spontaneous" attack, indicating that the phenomena apparently "come out of the blue." In an early phase of treatment, the actual reason for an attack is quite obscure. In the course of psychological treatment, insight will (and should) be gained into the nature of the direct precursor of an attack.

During the attacks, four or more of the following symptoms occur within 10 minutes of the beginning of the first symptom with which the attack commences. A panic attack may lead to the avoidance of situations in which attacks may occur. The DSM-IV distinguishes between panic disorder without agoraphobia and panic disorder with agoraphobia.

Clinical Picture

Physical symptoms of panic, such as sweating, trembling, chest pain, fear of fainting, and sudden changes in temperature, show great similarities with the bodily symptoms of the hyperventilation syndrome (Ley, 1985). The DSM-IV, however, does not mention such a relation. The phenomenon of hyperventilation refers to a breathing pattern that is in excess of the body's demands. During physical exercise, breathing also increases, because more oxygen is used and more carbon dioxide is produced. In this event, the breathing pattern adapts to the needs of the body. When a person is hyperventilating, his or her breathing is

---

Table 2.1. DSM-IV Criteria for Panic Attack

A discrete period of intense fear or discomfort, in which four (or more) of the following symptoms developed abruptly and reached a peak within 10 minutes:

1. Palpitations, pounding heart, or accelerated heart rate
2. Sweating
3. Trembling or shaking
4. Sensation or shortness of breath or smothering
5. Feeling of choking
6. Chest pain or discomfort
7. Nausea or abdominal distress
8. Feeling dizzy, unsteady, lightheaded, or faint
9. Derealization (feelings of unreality) or depersonalization (being detached from oneself)
10. Fear of losing control or going crazy
11. Fear of dying
12. Paraesthesia (numbness or tingling sensations)
13. Chills or hot flushes

Note: Reprinted by permission from *Diagnostic and Statistical Manual of Mental Disorders*, Fourth Edition. Copyright 1994 American Psychiatric Association.

Table 2.2. DSM-IV Criteria for 300.01 Panic Disorder without Agoraphobia

A. Both (1) and (2):
   1. Recurrent unexpected Panic Attacks
   2. At least one of the attacks has been followed by 1 month (or more) of one (or more) of the following:
      (a) Persistent concern about having additional attacks
      (b) Worry about the implications of the attack or its consequences (e.g., losing control, having a heart attack, "going crazy")
      (c) A significant change in behavior related to the attacks
B. Absence of Agoraphobia
C. The Panic Attacks are not due to the direct physiological effects of a substance (e.g., a drugs of abuse, a medication) or a general medical condition (e.g., hyperthyroidism).
D. The Panic Attacks are not better accounted for by another mental disorder, such as Social Phobia (e.g, occurring on exposure to feared social situations), Specific Phobia (e.g., on exposure to feared social situations), Specific Phobia (e.g., on exposure to a specific phobic situation), Obsessive–Compulsive Disorder (e.g., on exposure to dirt in someone with an obsession about contamination), Posttraumatic Stress Disorder (e.g., in response to stimuli associated with a severe stressor), or Separation Anxiety Disorder (e.g., in response to being away from home or close relatives).

Note: Reprinted by permission for *Diagnostic and Statistical Manual of Mental Disorders*, Fourth Edition. Copyright 1994 American Psychiatric Association.

stronger than necessary to provide for those needs. This results in a stronger exhalation of carbon dioxide than is usually the case. A hyperventilation attack with the concomitant bodily sensations often is accompanied by severe anxiety, which by itself may provoke future or chronic hyperventilation. The consequence is a decrease of the carbon dioxide level in the blood and an increase of the acid level, a phenomenon known as "respiratory alkalosis." These resulting symptoms vary considerably over persons, and can be summarized in a number of categories:

- Respiratory complaints (e.g., tightness around the chest, sensation of being unable to breathe)
- Paresthesias (e.g., tingling or numbness of the limbs, especially hands and feet, sometimes also around the mouth)
- Neuromuscular complaints (e.g., stiffness, tremor, or tetanic sensations in the limbs)
- Cerebrovascular complaints (e.g., dizziness, blurred vision, feeling of fainting)
- Cardiac complaints (e.g., a strong increase in heartbeat frequency, irregular heartbeat, pain in the cardiac area)
- Temperature sensation
- Gastrointestinal complaints (e.g., nausea, aerophagy)
- Psychic complaints (e.g., anxiety, feelings of unrest and tension)

There appears to be a considerable diagnostic overlap between panic disorder and the hyperventilation syndrome, ranging from 42% to 92% (Spinhoven, Onstein, Sterk, & De Haen-Versteijnen, 1992). Munjack, Brown, and McDowell (1993) found that 30% of patients with panic disorder were hyperventilating as measured by venous CO_2 levels, in contrast with only 8% of generalized anxiety patients and 4% of normal controls. Until recently, recognition of symptoms in the hyperventilation provocation test (i.e., voluntary overbreathing) has been used as a diagnostic criterion of the hyperventilation syndrome. However, more recent studies cast some doubt on the central role of hyperventilation in panic disorder. Buikhuisen and Garssen (1990) found no evidence of hyperventilation during panic when transcutaneous pCO_2 was monitored during panic attacks in eight patients. Further results of a study by Spinhoven et al. (1992) question the validity of the hyperventilation provocation test.

According to the dyspnea theory of panic disorder (Ley, 1989), fear and panic are the result of severe dyspnea as reflected in difficulty in breathing and a sense of impending suffocation, in combination with a lack of perceived control over its causes. Some evidence was provided that dyspnea usually occurs prior to the experience of fear. Results of other studies, however, suggest that dyspnea is the consequence of fear resulting from catastrophic cognitions regarding bodily sensations, rather than of primary significance (Carr, Lehrer, & Hochron, 1992; Porzelius, Vest, & Nochomovitz, 1992). Results of a recent study by Asmundson and Stein (1994) suggest that there might be a subgroup of panic patients, characterized by lower pulmonary functions, who are most likely to experience respiratory symptoms during panic attacks; however, additional research is needed to investigate whether the respiratory symptoms and fear of dying and losing control are the result of actual airway obstruction in this subgroup of patients.

A considerable number of normal persons in the community experience panic attacks but do not meet criteria for panic disorder. The prevalence rates of nonclinical panic is on average 34.5% (Norton, Cox, & Malan, 1992). Clinical and nonclinical panic differs with respect to coping strategies used. Clinical panic patients take medication, escape the situation, and take alcohol, whereas such strategies are valued as less effective by nonclinical panickers (Cox, Endler, Swinson, & Norton, 1992)

Panic attacks are usually associated with catastrophical misinterpretations (Clark, 1986), most of which are related to immediately impending physical danger and mental catastrophes, and to a lesser extent, to social embarrassment (Westling & Öst, 1993). Patients with chest pain, breathlessness, numbness and tingling, blurred vision, and choking typically have thoughts about having a brain tumor, stroke, or a heart attack. This fear induces patients to make a strong appeal to medical services, such as medical specialists, cardiologists, and neurologists. The latter are unable to demonstrate any organic disorders, leaving the patient increasingly insecure and anxious. Other patients have thoughts about the psychosocial consequences of their anxiety and have thoughts about losing control, acting foolishly, and going crazy. Such patients may be ashamed of sensations that actually occur, such as nervousness, trembling, or wanting to leave. They have thoughts such as "People will find it strange when I leave the meeting unexpectedly," or "People will think I'm mad." Other patients visualize what would happen if they really lost control, although this has never happened. They think, "Just imagine that I'm lying on the ground and everybody is looking at me. I would die."

The acute and intense experience of anxiety is held responsible for the tendency to escape, which is characteristic of the panic attack ("I got to get out of here as soon as possible"). Passive and active avoidance behaviors aim at stopping the attack. When a situation does not allow for an escape (e.g., when the person is at home), some patients start walking about restlessly or talking incessantly. Very often, cognitions are characterized by anticipation of the feared situation ("anticipatory anxiety"). This causes an increase in arousal even before the patient actually enters such a situation. One of our patients once said, "Last time I felt very dizzy, so I'll be unwell the next time. Maybe I'll really faint this time."

Comorbidity is a substantial feature of this condition, because over half of the panic patients with or without agoraphobia also qualify for another anxiety disorder or depression (De Ruiter, Rijken, Garssen, Van Schaik, & Kraaimaat, 1989). The rate of primary depression is about 30% and the range for secondary depression is 30% to 53% (Lesser, 1988). Alcohol abuse is common among panic patients. In a sample of panic patients with agoraphobia gathered from the Epidemiologic Catchment Area Study, nearly 30% qualified for the diagnosis of alcohol abuse or alcohol dependence (Himle & Hill, 1991). Patients with agoraphobia without panic attacks are less likely to have an additional alcohol problem.

Differential Diagnosis

Although panic disorder consists of a number of discrete episodes of fear, it can easily be confused with other disorders, such as hypochondriasis and generalized anxiety disorder. *Hypochondriasis* is the persistent conviction of having a disease, attendant with fear and a tendency to seek reassurance. In panic disorder, the disease conviction (if any) is predominantly restricted to the period of the attacks themselves; between attacks, the patient is capable of feeling less concerned. Furthermore, in panic disorder, somatic preoccupations relate to phenomena occurring during the attack, such as headache, palpitations, or dizziness.

Generalized anxiety disorder (GAD) is characterized by excessive worry and a substantial increase in arousal encompassing a variety of situations. In some cases, panic disorder resembles GAD, for example, with respect to the intensified fear or tension in between the attacks. The fear is mostly caused by anticipation anxiety or anxious expectations concerning a new attack. In contrast, GAD patients worry excessively about minor and/or future issues, and are not solely concerned about panic symptoms.

Panic is often also associated with Borderline Personality Disorder (Friedman & Chiernen, 1994). Patients with Borderline Personality Disorder are at increased risk for suicidal behavior and are characterized by affective instability, fear of abandonment, impulsivity, chronic substance abuse, and relationship instability. In a study by Renneberg, Chambless, and Gracely (1992), 10% of the panic patients met criteria for Borderline Personality Disorder. Friedman and Chiernen (1994) found the following clinical markers to discriminate patients with Borderline Personality Disorder: anger, duration of panic attacks, cognitive fear during panic, and suicidal ideation and attempts. Furthermore, Borderline Personality Disorder patients were more likely to report physical and sexual abuse and family conflict in early life. Discriminating Borderline Personality Disorder patients from Panic Disorder patients may have important treatment implications. Standardized treatment protocols are less suited for Borderline Personality Disorder patients who also suffer from panic attacks given the risk for suicide and chronic substance abuse, and the often difficult therapeutic relationship.

Organic causes of increase in arousal (e.g., hyperthyroidism) should be excluded. Excessive use or abuse of certain substances (e.g., coffee, caffeine-containing products) may lead to a number of panic-related symptoms, such as restlessness, nervousness, increase in heartbeat, and even withdrawal symptoms or a hangover caused by alcohol (with phenomena such as anxiety and autonomic hyperactivity—palpitations, sweating, and hypertension). Finally, the rebound effect of tranquilizers deserves mention. After stopping with tranquilizers, a patient's fear may become (temporarily) greater than before prescription of the medication.

Theo K. Bouman and
Paul M. G.
Emmelkamp

Agoraphobia

The DSM-IV discerns two kinds of agoraphobia: agoraphobia in connection with panic disorder and agoraphobia without a history of panic attacks. Agoraphobia itself is defined according to DSM-IV as presented in Table 2.3.

Many panic patients tend to avoid situations or activities that are supposed to trigger panic attacks, sometimes starting to do so right after their first panic attack. Extensive avoidance behavior may prevent a person from having a panic attack, but at the same time it will prevent him or her from leaving the house. A diagnosis of panic disorder with agoraphobia is made when the complaints meet the criteria of panic disorder and those of agoraphobia as well. The DSM-IV criteria of agoraphobia with panic attack are nearly identical to the criteria for panic disorder without agoraphobia, as can be seen in Table 2.4.

In the absence of panic attack, agoraphobia is defined by DSM-IV as shown in Table 2.5.

This distinction predominantly relates to the patient's motives to avoid situations. *Agoraphobia*, as connected with panic disorder, is described as a fear to be in places or situations from which it is difficult to escape, or in which there is no help at hand in case of a panic attack. In agoraphobia without panic disorder, there is a fear of suddenly emerging symptoms that may cause embarrassment to the person or make him or her need help. Often the theme of the fear is to lose control over bladder or bowels, the urge to vomit, depersonalization or derealization, and dizziness. This fear causes a restriction in traveling or dictates the need for leaving the house only in the company of others. In some cases, the person endures the feared situation, although the anxiety is substantial.

Clinical Picture

Avoidance behavior is one of the most characteristic features of agoraphobia. The number of situations agoraphobics generally consider anxiety-provoking is quite large. The

---

Table 2.3. DSM-IV Criteria for Agoraphobia[a]

A. Anxiety about being in places or situations from which escape might be difficult (or embarrassing) or in which help may not be available in the event of having an unexpected or situationally predisposed Panic Attack or panic-like symptoms. Agoraphobic fears typically involve characteristic clusters of situations that include being outside the home alone; being in a crowd or standing in a line; being on a bridge; and traveling in a bus, train or automobile.

Note: consider the diagnosis of Specific Phobia if the avoidance is limited to one or only a few specific situations, or Social Phobia if the avoidance is limited to social situations.

B. The situations are avoided (e.g., travel is restricted) or else are endured with marked distress or with anxiety about having a Panic Attack or panic-like symptoms, or require the presence of a companion.

C. The Panic Attacks are not better accounted for by another mental disorder, such as Social Phobia (e.g., avoidance limited to social situations because of fear of embarrassment), Specific Phobia (e.g., on avoidance limited to a single situation like elevators), Obsessive–Compulsive Disorder (e.g., avoidance of dirt in someone with an obsession about contamination), Posttraumatic Stress Disorder (e.g., in avoidance of stimuli associated with a severe stressor), or Separation Anxiety Disorder (e.g., avoidance of leaving home or relatives).

Note: Reprinted by permission from *Diagnostic and Statistical Manual of Mental Disorders*, Fourth Edition. Copyright 1994 American Psychiatric Association.

Table 2.4.   DSM-IV Criteria for 300.21 Panic Disorder with Agoraphobia[a]

A. Both (1) and (2):
    1. Recurrent unexpected Panic Attacks
    2. At least one of the attacks has been followed by 1 month (or more) of one (or more) of the following:
        (a) Persistent concern about having additional attacks
        (b) Worry about the implications of the attack or its consequences (e.g., losing control, having a heart attack, "going crazy"
        (c) A significant change in behavior related to the attacks
B. The presence of Agoraphobia
C. The Panic Attacks are not due to the direct physiological effects of a substance (e.g., a drugs of abuse, a medication) or a general medical condition (e.g., hyperthyroidism).
D. The Panic Attacks are not better accounted for by another mental disorder, such as Social Phobia (e.g., occurring on exposure to feared social situations), Specific Phobia (e.g., on exposure to a specific phobic situation), Obsessive–Compulsive Disorder (e.g., on exposure to dirt in someone with an obsession about contamination), Posttraumatic Stress Disorder (e.g., in response to simuli associated with a severe stressor), or Separation Anxiety Disorder (e.g., in response to being away from home or close relatives).

Note: Reprinted by permission from *Diagnostic and Statistical Manual of Mental Disorders*, Fourth Edition. Copyright 1994 American Psychiatric Association.

popular notion that agoraphobia is equal to fear of streets, marketplaces, or open spaces, in fact, neglects the diversity of situations that are indicated as difficult by the patients themselves. Rather, the central theme is "not being able to leave" or "being stuck," and this theme is more important than the open space itself. Sometimes it is not the open spaces but the restricted situation in which a person feels imprisoned.

The following are examples of such situations:

- Standing in a line
- Being in a large shop or a shopping mall
- Traveling by public transportation (bus, train, or airplane)
- Being in crowds, on busy streets, in large gatherings
- Driving a car on a highway (the impossibility to turn on the road)
- Being in a traffic jam
- Crossing a bridge
- Being on a bridge

Table 2.5.   DSM-IV Criteria for 300.22 Agoraphobia without History of Panic Disorder[a]

A. The presence of agoraphobia related to fear of developing panic-like symptoms (e.g., dizziness or diarrhea).
B. Criteria have never been met for Panic Disorder
C. The disturbance is not due to the direct physiological effect of a substance (e.g., a drug of abuse, a medication) or a general medical condition
D. If an associated general medical condition is present, the fear described in Criterion A is clearly in excess of that usually associated with the condition.

Note: Reprinted by permission from *Diagnostic and Statistical Manual of Mental Disorders*, Fourth Edition. Copyright 1994 American Psychiatric Association.

- Sitting at the barber's
- Having a conversation with someone else

The desire to escape prompts some patients to take their precautions. Some of them never leave home without bike or car, because should something happen, they would be able to get home as soon as possible. These and other forms of avoidance behavior should be assessed by the therapist as accurately as possible, because sometimes they are very subtle in nature.

Agoraphobics often avoid being alone and feel less anxious when accompanied by a trusted person, such as a partner or a person who is notified about their complaints. Consequently, an agoraphobic may be able to cope with several kinds of situations as long as he or she is not alone. The anxiety-reducing role of company appears to be one of the most important maintaining factors of agoraphobia. It does matter who this company is, though—preferably a person who knows or understands what it means to be fearful and not to dare that much; however, not all agoraphobics feel comfortable in company. A number of them report quite the contrary. When they are accompanied by a person while outside, they are more nervous and anxious than when they are alone. If they want to escape, they will be "stuck" with this company and have to excuse themselves. For a number of patients, panicking in the company of other people is more embarrassing than having a panic attack when alone. For some agoraphobics, the presence of young children appears to be an additional source of worry instead of being a comfort, especially when the patient feels responsible for the children. The existing tension only increases, which makes it more difficult to leave the house with, instead of without, the children.

Differential Diagnosis

Situational avoidance is not only found in agoraphobia with or without panic attacks, as mentioned earlier, but can also be related to other psychopathology. In depressed patients, one often observes a lack of interest and initiative leading to avoidance of outdoor activities. Due to the fact that depression also involves a certain amount of fear, avoidance behavior can easily be mistaken for agoraphobia. The motive for this behavior, however, is not fear of a possible catastrophe. In a number of cases, depression should not be viewed as an independent disorder, but as the result of the severe restrictions imposed on one's life when one has agoraphobia. Another source of avoidance is social phobia, because many social phobics fear traveling on their own or being in public, because of the fear they experience in being among other people. At first sight, one would consider the diagnosis "agoraphobia"; however, here is another example in which the motive to avoid is crucial. With social phobia, anxiety is triggered by the fear of criticism and negative evaluation. The fear is not for the symptoms as such, but for possible scrutiny by other people. There is also some difference in the symptoms experienced. With agoraphobics, difficulty in breathing, dizziness, and weakness in limbs are common, whereas blushing, sweating, and trembling are more characteristic symptoms of social phobics. It is not always simple to distinguish agoraphobia from obsessive–compulsive disorder (OCD), especially when the OCD patient avoids situations that are characteristic of avoidance in agoraphobics, such as going out or traveling by public transportation; however, the evoking stimuli of obsessive–compulsives differ from those of agoraphobics. In the case of an OCD patient, avoidance of going outdoors and the use of buses and trains may be related to fear of contamination rather than fear of a panic attack.

Interview

In clinical practice, diagnostic criteria are no more than starting points for implementing treatment. The clinical interview is the most commonly employed assessment method. In clinical practice, the frequently used procedure is the unstructured open interview in which the clinician tries to get a clear picture of the complaints and the reasons the patient seeks help. In cognitive–behavioral therapy, the initial interview is dominated by the therapist's intention to formulate a functional analysis of the problem behaviors. At times, the clinician may feel the need for a more formalized diagnosis of anxiety disorders. This is the case when one wants to compose more homogeneous groups in order to conduct research into the effectiveness of treatment.

Anxiety Disorder Interview Schedule

The Anxiety Disorder Interview Schedule (ADIS), developed by DiNardo, O'Brien, Barlow, Wardell, and Blanchard (1983), is an early example of a specific semistructured interview, primarily aimed at the diagnosis of anxiety disorders based on the revised third edition of the *Diagnostic and Statistical Manual of Mental Disorders* (DSM-III-R; American Psychiatric Association, 1987) criteria. The interview starts with a short introduction and explication of its purpose. Next, the patient is questioned about the nuclear symptoms of the specific anxiety disorders. When these nuclear symptoms appear to be present, more detailed manifestations of the complaint are investigated in terms of specific diagnostic criteria. In addition, a short description of the current complaints and their history is obtained. Apart from questions on the anxiety disorder, other information is obtained on depressive phenomena, somatoform disorders (e.g., somatization disorder and hypochondriasis), and substance abuse. DiNardo et al. (1983) conducted research on the interjudge reliability of the ADIS and found a satisfactory level of agreement.

Functional Analysis

Many regard the functional analysis as the core of behavior therapy. We can distinguish two levels of analysis: (1) the analysis of the functional relations *within* the disorder (microanalysis), and (2) the analysis of these relations *between* the disorder and other problem areas (macroanalysis). Information is gathered in an open interview and completed with data from questionnaires, behavioral measures, and diary data. At the initial interview, attention is likely to be focused on the onset, course, and present state of the complaints.

Onset of Complaints. It is very important to obtain a clear picture of the onset of complaints. Is there a clear beginning with a panic attack that can be visually remembered, or is there a gradual development of complaints? Furthermore, it is important to recognize the circumstances at the time of the onset of the complaints, such as distressing events or the accumulation of a number of small stressors—so-called daily "hassles."

Course of Complaints. Have there been any periods in which the panic or agoraphobia worsened, diminished, or disappeared? If so, what were the factors associated with the fluctuations? Are there any other complaints that in the course of time have developed in addition to the panic and agoraphobia or as a consequence of them? The development of these secondary complaints (and the resulting present comorbidity) may pertain, for example, to depression, alcoholism or medication abuse, or marital problems.

Microanalysis

The present state of the panic and/or agoraphobic complaints is schematized in a microanalysis. The therapist now focuses on the stimulus situations, the cognitive processing, emotional and behavioral outcome, as well as the short- and long-term consequences. The following questions may be helpful:

Stimuli. Under which circumstances does the anxiety become manifest? The therapist wants to gain insight into the discriminative stimuli or triggers. These stimuli can be concrete (e.g., situations such as enclosed spaces, shopping malls, or elevators) or imaginary (e.g., anxiety-provoking thoughts). Furthermore, interoceptive triggers (e.g., palpitations, sweating) are often observed in panic disorder. Apart from the direct triggers, contextual parameters (e.g., unemployment, relationship problems, failing an exam) may influence the degree to which a trigger is potentiated or mitigated. Circumstances that lead to a decrease of the complaints also warrant attention. Under which conditions are discriminative stimuli more or less fear provoking?

Cognitive Processing. What are a patient's thoughts and images before, during, and after a period of anxiety or panic, or on confrontation with the feared situations? The therapist should be particularly aware of the characteristic feature of panic: the general preoccupation with thoughts of imminent threat. The elicitation of verbal reports may be difficult in some patients, because they are used to a visual rather than verbal interpretation. Imagery (i.e., a vivid and detailed description of the circumstances and their consequences) may be helpful in these cases.

The patient is prompted to produce implicit or explicit interpretations of the situations. These can be elicited by asking, "What went through your mind when you panicked in the traffic jam?" or "What is the worst thing that could happen when you would collapse in the lecture hall?" or "What image does the light-headedness produce?" In the latter instance, the patient might say, "I see myself fainting and falling to the ground with all these people staring at me." The therapist then wants to know the patient's evaluation of this image (e.g., by asking, "What is so bad about being stared at when you are lying on the ground?") The aim is to gain access to the automatic thoughts and images that explain the anxiety-provoking nature of the particular situation. The therapist may also consider if he or she would become equally distressed or anxious when sharing the same conviction.

Emotional Responses. Although panic and agoraphobia are characterized by anxiety as the central emotion, other emotions may emerge as well. Depression, shame, and irritability are not uncommon in this respect.

Bodily Sensations. Which bodily sensations form part of the experience of fear and panic (e.g., trembling, sweating, and hyperventilating)? Both spontaneous mention and detailed questioning may be helpful. This is an important aspect of the microanalysis, because many bodily sensations are in themselves new interoceptive stimuli (see discussion on hyperventilation).

Behavioral Responses.   What does the patient do when he or she becomes anxious? In this case, the therapist is looking for conditioned avoidance reaction; in agoraphobia this may be the avoidance of being alone in the street. Furthermore, the patient may use drugs or alcohol, or take certain precautions to reduce or prevent anxiety. Other patients feel more relaxed when they take specific comforting objects (e.g., tranquilizers) along when going out. They may resort to going out at set times of the day, when in particular moods, or in certain company. They may take specific routes, avoiding unfamiliar or unsafe places.

Consequences.   In general, it is important to investigate both the costs and the benefits of the avoidance behaviors in a short-term as well as a long-term perspective. The consequences, in turn, may be either desired or aversive by nature and may increase or decrease. For example, most patients mention reduction of anxiety as a relatively immediate effect of their avoidance behaviors (i.e., negative reinforcement); however, when the patient realizes that he or she has given in to avoidance, he or she may become depressed (i.e., punishment). One of the negative consequences is that the patient has not been able to reach his or her goal, such as shopping, paying a visit, or having a hobby (i.e., frustrative nonreward).

An example of the long-term consequences of avoidance behaviors is the development of a continuously increased arousal as a consequence of anticipation anxiety (i.e., punishment). On the other hand, some patients derive certain privileges from their "sick role," such as extra attention and consideration from other people (i.e., positive reinforcement). Increased (and sometimes extreme) dependence on others is a long-term disadvantage that is characteristic of agoraphobia.

Macroanalysis

Anxiety patients often show a certain degree of comorbidity. In most cases, there are functional relations with other more or less clearly defined problems. The macroanalysis addresses the relationship among the various problem areas to determine the role of maintaining factors outside the presenting complaints and to formulate a starting point for treatment. When a patient is suffering from both agoraphobia and depression, for example, it is very important to determine the functional relationship between the two: Has depression been caused by the lack of reinforcers in the patient's limited lifestyle, or is the agoraphobia the result of the depressed patient's lack of motivation and social withdrawal, or are the two problems unrelated?

We find it useful to consider the following potential sources of functional relationships in panic disorder (Emmelkamp & Bouman, 1991):

Social Relationships.   Several studies have found high levels of interpersonal conflict preceding the onset of panic disorder with agoraphobia (cf. Kleiner & Marshall, 1987; Last, Barlow, & O'Brien, 1984). However, because interpersonal problems are also common in the population at large, it may be that certain characteristics (especially dependent, socially anxious, and unassertive behavior) predispose some people to react to these conflicts or to become involved in them. If this is the case, treatment should also focus on social anxiety and unassertiveness (e.g., Emmelkamp, Van den Hout, & De Vries, 1983).

Partner Relationship.   In a number of patients with panic disorder, the relationship with the partner is disturbed, although the evidence is controversial (Emmelkamp & Gerlsma, 1994). A detailed micro- or macroanalysis might reveal whether the relationship problems (if any) are related to the panic disorder and deserve therapeutic attention on their own.

Emotional Processing of Traumatic Events.   In some cases, panic and agoraphobia are related to an inadequate emotional processing of traumatic experiences, such as physical or sexual abuse. In such cases, the therapist must determine whether treatment of the panic disorder will be impeded by the inadequate emotional processing.

Cognitive Style.   Locus of control may be an important variable in the development of panic disorder (Emmelkamp, 1982). Persons with an external-control orientation experiencing panic in a stressful period are likely to misread the anxiety (and its accompanying physical symptoms) as caused by external situations (e.g., crowded areas) or to internal phenomena such as severe illness (e.g., heart attack). Treatment that focuses on changing this cognitive style may have an additional function in preventing posttreatment relapse.

When the treatment plan is based on a comprehensive macroanalysis of the problem behavior, the likelihood of "symptom substitution" will decrease. Both a micro- and a macroanalysis will probably be supplemented by new information gathered during the course of treatment. These analyses should, therefore, be regarded as hypotheses that must be tested by means of the implementation of treatment interventions. When specific interventions do not produce the desired effect, then either the treatment strategy has been inappropriately chosen, or the functional analysis is inadequate. In the latter case, it is necessary to reconsider and to gather new information on the patient and his or her environment.

Self-Report Questionnaires

In past decades, many standardized self-report questionnaires have been published pertaining to global as well as specific aspects of anxiety. Most of these measures are dimensional by nature indicating the *severity* of the complaints; they do not serve to make a discrete or categorical diagnosis. However, in some tests, authors propose cutoff scores to distinguish between pathological and nonpatient groups. In the following sections, we present an overview of some of the most commonly employed instruments used within the realm of panic disorder and agoraphobia.

Anxiety Scale

This self-report scale has been developed to measure specific agoraphobic avoidance behaviors. The original version of Gelder and Marks (1966), and a later improvement by Watson and Marks (1971), consisted of idiosyncratic items that could vary among patients. Emmelkamp, Kuipers, and Eggeraat (1978) formulated five situations relevant for the majority of agoraphobics:

1. A crowded street (alone)

2. Drinking coffee in a crowded cafe or a restaurant
3. Walking from the hospital to the town center (alone)
4. Shopping in a supermarket or department store (alone)
5. Traveling by bus (alone)

Fear Questionnaire

The Fear Questionnaire (FQ) was published in 1979 by Marks and Mathews as a short questionnaire to measure the extent of avoidance. This measure consists of three parts: one is concerned with the patient's most important phobia; the second part, the FQ proper, consists of 15 questions (subdivided into three subscales—Agoraphobia, Social Phobia, and Blood and Injury Phobia); and the third part contains 5 questions assessing the degree of anxiety and depression. The FQ appears to possess adequate psychometric properties (Arrindell, Emmelkamp, & Van den Ende, 1983). Patients with agoraphobia can be discriminated from patients with social phobia (Oei, Moylan, & Evans, 1991). Scores in excess of the cutoff point of 30 identify severe agoraphobics; scores below 10 suggest good response to therapy (Mavissakalian, 1986).

Mobility Inventory

The Mobility Inventory (MI) is also a self-report measure of avoidance, but much more detailed than the FQ. In this 26-item questionnaire, respondents rate the severity of avoidance when alone and when accompanied, which often do not overlap. In addition, ratings of the frequency of panic attacks during the last week are obtained. This measure has been found to be reliable and to discriminate patients with agoraphobia from those with other anxiety disorders (Craske, Rachman, & Tallman, 1986). Factor analysis revealed three reliable subscales accounting for 60% of the variance: (1) fear of public places, (2) fear of enclosed places and (3) fear of open spaces (Cox, Swinson, Kuch, & Reichman, 1993). There is now a version available that assesses severity of avoidance "without medication" (Swinson, Cox, Shulman, Kuch, & Woszczyna, 1992). The advantage of this additional scale is that it identifies situations in which the patient relies heavily on medication. The MI is particularly suited for planning individually tailored *in vivo* exposure treatment.

Agoraphobia Scale

This inventory assesses anxiety and avoidance in 20 typical agoraphobic situations. The internal consistency was found to be good and the questionnaire was able to discriminate between agoraphobics on the one hand and normal controls and simple phobics on the other. There is also evidence of its concurrent validity (Öst, 1990).

Agoraphobia Cognitions Questionnaire and the Body Sensations Questionnaire

Chambless, Caputo, Bright, and Gallagher (1984) designed these questionnaires to assess the cognitive and somatic aspects of anxiety and panic. Both the Agoraphobia Cognitions Questionnaire (ACQ; 14 items) and the Body Sensations Questionnaire (BSQ; 17 items) possess satisfactory psychometric characteristics. There is, however, a considerable intercorrelation between the measures, suggesting that they may measure more or less the same construct. The ACQ was unable to discriminate panic disorder from other anxiety disorders (Craske et al., 1986).

Theo K. Bouman and Paul M. G. Emmelkamp

The Anxiety Sensitivity Index (ASI; Reiss, Peterson, Gursky, & McNally, 1986) is more or less identical to the BSQ, the main difference being that the ASI focuses on discomfort stemming from the bodily sensations specifically associated with anxiety. The ASI has been found to discriminate patients with panic disorder from patients with other anxiety disorders (Apfeldorf, Shear, Leon, & Portera, 1994; Taylor, Koch, & Crockett, 1991). The ASI has been found to be stable over time and to predict the occurrence of panic attacks 3 years later (Maller & Reiss, 1992). Apfeldorf et al. (1994) found that an abbreviated version of merely four of the ASI items was as effective in discriminating panic-disordered patients from other anxiety-disordered patients as the total ASI. In this scale, the Brief Panic Disorder Screen, the following items have to be rated on a zero (very little) to 4 (very much) scale:

1. It scares me when I feel shaky.
2. It scares me when I feel faint.
3. It scares me when my heart beats rapidly.
4. It scares me when I become short of breath.

Catastrophic Cognition Questionnaire

The Catastrophic Cognition Questionnaire (CCQ) assesses catastrophic cognitions as defined by Beck's theory and aims to measure the extent to which patients misinterpret their bodily and emotional reactions and mental states as dangerous. Factor analysis revealed five factors: (1) Emotional Catastrophes, (2) Physical Catastrophes, (3) Mental Catastrophes, (4) Social Catastrophes, and (5) Bodily Catastrophes. Although this questionnaire might be relevant for panic patients, research to date has only been conducted on college students (Khawaja & Oei, 1992).

Self-Monitoring

In both assessment and treatment phases, patient's self-monitoring can be of great value for gaining insight into the course of anxiety complaints. During the admission interview, information is gathered retrospectively, and therefore is subject to distortion of memory, selective perception, social desirability, and so on. For example, patients tend to overestimate the frequency of panic attacks when they have to rate them retrospectively (De Beurs, Lange, & Van Dyck, 1992).

As soon as the therapist, in consultation with the patient, has determined one or more target behaviors, it is recommended that the patient keep a structured diary to ascertain under what conditions these behaviors occur. Inspection of the diary may reveal significant associations between problem behaviors and particular events. It is further suggested that recording forms be tailored to the individual needs of the patient and that they contain specific questions relevant to the each patient. In the case of panic disorder, monitoring of situations in which anxiety and panic occur is especially important. After inspection of the diary, apparently "uncontrollable" panic attacks often turn out to be related to specific events.

The information gathered should be of direct importance for treatment. It must be noted, however, that self-monitoring has a psychometrically unclear status; measures often have no more than face validity. This means that one should be cautious in making interpretations and generalizations. Self-monitoring can be performed in the event that a certain problem behavior occurs, but also as a form of continuous registration. In the former event, the clinician has the frequency and the intensity of the complaints monitored (e.g., avoidance behaviors, panic attacks, anticipatory anxiety, catastrophic thoughts). This method is particularly useful for behaviors and phenomena with a relatively low frequency. The patient can be asked to monitor a certain high frequency phenomenon at fixed times (behavioral sampling), for example, to investigate the course of anxiety and depressed mood over 24-hour periods. The nature and frequency of complaints and the aim of monitoring determine the choice for specific or global measures. A clinician may consider the following options:

• *Direct counts*, such as a tally of the number of times an action has been performed (e.g., having an anxiety attack), are simple to design and implement.

• *Idiosyncratic scales* with standardized response categories can be of great use. In our own clinic, for example, we use blank versions of the aforementioned Anxiety Scale in which the patient records fear-provoking situations prior to treatment. This idiosyncratic scale is completed after treatment as well, allowing an estimate of the amount of change over treatment for the specific patient.

• A *Visual Analogue Scale* (VAS) reflects the intensity or severity of a phenomenon. For example, the degree of anxiety can be indicated by placing a mark on a horizontal line from zero to 100. This type of scale can have various applications.

• *Thought listing* is a widely used method before and during cognitive therapy. The patient receives the instruction: "Please write down what goes though your mind in situation X." During the initial phase of treatment, this method can be utilized for "thought catching," and later as a starting point for formulating alternative thoughts in addition to spontaneous (often irrational or catastrophical) thoughts. Apart from collecting these thoughts in written form, they can also be gathered with the use of other media. Williams and Rappoport (1983), for example, had agoraphobic car drivers speak into the microphone of a tape recorder while driving their cars.

• A *multidimensional diary* may have value when the therapist is interested in more than one aspect of the patient's complaints. A diary could encompass symptom rating, the extent of the avoidance behavior, the description of discrete life events, a VAS for anxiety, and though listing. After the monitoring period, both the patient and therapist are provided with a more detailed picture of the frequency, intensity, and content of the panic attacks and the agoraphobia. To stimulate the use of the diary and keep the recording time within reasonable limits, a tailor-made prestructured version is recommended. An example is provided in Figure 2.1.

Behavioral Avoidance Test

This assessment method is based on the patient's actual performance in a difficult situation, rather than on self-report data outside of such a situation. The procedure implies that the patient is asked to perform a series of actions structured by the therapist. A typical example of a Behavioral Avoidance Test (BAT) in the context of agoraphobia is the "behavioral walk" (Emmelkamp et al., 1978). According to this procedure, the patient is asked to walk a previously determined route. The standardized instruction is as follows: "You are asked to walk a route, and to return to our clinic immediately once you feel tense." The patient is provided with a map on which the route is drawn. The route is divided into a fixed number of segments. The therapist records both the time spent on this test as

1

| Date: _____ / _____ | Did anything special happen today?
If yes, please write down shortly. |

2

How anxious/tensed did you feel today <u>in general</u>?

0......10......20......30......40......50......60......70......80......90......100
not   extreme

3

How many panic attacks did you have today?   None / ......

<u>Symptoms:</u>   **I**   <u>situation</u>   **II**   <u>situation</u>

1. Palpitations
2. Sweating
3. Trembling or shaking
4. Shortness of breath
5. Choking sensations
6. Chest pain or discomfort
7. Nausea
8. Dizziness
9. Feeling unreal
10. Fear of going crazy or losing control
11. Fear of dying
12. Numbness/tingling
13. Hot flushes or chills

Severity of each attack (0–100)

Which thoughts or images went through your mind during the attacks?

Attack I: _____

Attack II:_____

Figure 2.1. Example of a panic diary page.

well as the distance the patient has covered. Although this behavioral measure is rather time consuming, it is particularly interesting because of the extra clinical information it provides. The therapist obtains an actual impression of the way the patient handles a task situation. When debriefing the patient following this task, the therapist has the opportunity to make specific observations based on task performance, such as cognitive and physiological aspects, and subtle types of avoidance.

TREATMENT PROCEDURES

Introduction

In the research literature, as well as in clinical practice, treatment approaches differ with regard to the emphasis on either the agoraphobic avoidance or on discrete panic attacks. In the next sections, a brief overview is given of research on the effects of treatment for both agoraphobia and panic disorder and of effective treatment procedures.

Exposure Treatment in Agoraphobia

Over the past decades, the effectiveness of treatments based on exposure to feared situations has been extensively studied with regard to agoraphobia. In summary, the findings lead to the conclusions that exposure *in vivo* is more effective than exposure in imagination (Emmelkamp & Wessels, 1975), prolonged exposure is more effective than brief exposure (Stern & Marks, 1973), and fast exposure is more effective than slow-paced exposure (Yuksel, Marks, Ramm, & Gosh, 1984). Also, exposure *in vivo* is more effective than rational–emotive therapy and self-instructional training (Emmelkamp et al., 1978; Emmelkamp & Mersch, 1982; Emmelkamp, Brilman, Kuiper, & Mersch, 1986; Michelson, Mavissakalian, & Marchione, 1988). Furthermore, group exposure and individual exposure are about equally effective (e.g., Emmelkamp & Emmelkamp-Benner, 1975; Hafner & Marks, 1976), and treatment can be conducted as a self-help program (Emmelkamp, 1974, 1982; Mathews, Gelder, & Johnston, 1981). In general, the effects of exposure treatment are long lasting (see review by Emmelkamp, 1990). There is also empirical evidence that individual response patterns (e.g., cognitive or behavioral reactors) do not influence the efficacy of exposure *in vivo* (Mackay & Liddell, 1986; Öst, Lindahl, Sterner, & Jerremalm, 1984). Studies show that treatment effectiveness is not enhanced by the spouse's cooperation (Cobb, Mathews, Childs-Clarke, & Blowers, 1984; Emmelkamp, 1990). Arrindell, Emmelkamp and Sanderman (1986) found marital satisfaction not to be a predictor of treatment success with exposure *in vivo*. In conclusion, exposure *in vivo* is generally considered to be the most effective method for the treatment of agoraphobia. However, it would be incorrect to assume that there is only one type of exposure; quite the contrary, there are many variants of this technique.

Variants of Exposure Treatment

In this treatment approach, the patient should be systematically exposed to anxiety-provoking situations in order to facilitate habituation. (In spite of this apparent simplicity, it is still essential to have a sufficiently trained therapist conduct this kind of treatment.) In consultation with the patient, the therapist draws up a list of increasingly difficult situations (a "fear hierarchy"). Next, all situations are practiced via homework assignments; the patient should remain in the feared situation for a certain period of time, which is agreed on beforehand. The objective is to reduce the patient's initial intense fear in the situation to an acceptable level after a period of exposure. In this way, he or she will gradually "unlearn" the avoidant and fear responses and acquire a coping response. After one situation has been exercised satisfactorily (i.e., the patient's fear no longer increases when confronted with the situation), the next situation is assigned as homework.

Although the principle of exposure *in vivo* may seem straightforward, there are many variants of this technique, the choice of which will be determined by the patient's specific needs, psychosocial situation, and severity of complaints:

- Treatment setting (home-based vs. clinic-based)
- Massed versus spaced practice
- Self-directed versus therapist-guided
- Spouse-assisted versus alone
- Gradual exposure versus flooding
- Maximal fear versus controlled escape
- Group versus individual

In this chapter, we largely focus on an individual, self-directed approach with gradual exposure as the basic ingredient. Irrespective of the aforementioned variants chosen, the therapeutic procedure will probably contain the following elements:

1. Explaining the treatment rationale
2. Setting treatment goals
3. Constructing a fear hierarchy
4. Constructing (homework) assignments
5. Carrying out assignments
6. Evaluating assignments and treatment

Explaining the Treatment Rationale

When exposure treatment for agoraphobic complaints is indicated, optimal compliance is a necessary ingredient. A lack or incomplete understanding of the treatment background precludes maximal results. In this phase, at least three elements can be discerned: (1) an explanation of the mechanisms of action, (2) a general overview of treatment procedures, and (3) a check of the patient's understanding of the therapist's explanation.

First, it is important for the patient to learn and understand the principles of exposure *in vivo*. As the example later in this chapter will show, it may be wise to depart from the patient's own experience. The reinforcing role of avoidance behavior should be addressed, as well as the effect of exposure to feared situations or other stimuli. It should be explained that the general aim of therapy is to decrease anxiety by habituating to the original fear-provoking situations and to practice new coping behaviors.

Second, the treatment procedures are discussed in general terms. It should be emphasized that much will be expected from the patient, and that this self-activity will determine to a great extent the effect of the treatment. Therapist and patient discuss what treatment will entail, what is expected from the patient, what is the role of the therapist, and so on. Formal aspects of treatment should also be explained at this point, such as the number of sessions, intersession interval, and the general session agenda.

In many cases, it is advisable to provide the patient with a rationale in writing, since it is a safe assumption that anxious patients have deficits in the retention and reproduction of complex information, such as a treatment rationale. In order to check patients' active understanding, the therapist may ask patients to describe in their own words how the treatment will work. In this way, misunderstandings, doubts, and disbelief will become apparent, enabling the therapist to clarify these points. A mere "Yes, I understand," does not suffice, because the patient may be just polite and not want to "spoil the therapist's good intentions." In addition, the therapist should stimulate patients to fill in their partners or other significant others on the treatment principles, thus enabling those persons sharing the patients' environment to become informed on what to expect; also the patient has another opportunity to rehearse the procedure.

Setting Treatment Goals

After the initial assessment stage, one or more specific treatment goals must be established. Such a goal can be either simple or more complex. An example of a simple goal is the reduction of anxiety in buses, on the streets, and in other public places. A more complex goal for treatment is "becoming independent." Even when a simple goal is selected, it is necessary to formulate precisely what the desired final result is to be (shopping alone in the neighborhood vs. going abroad alone for a holiday). One strategy is to pursue a sequence of simple goals; when one is achieved, a new goal can be identified. It is important to formulate a final goal that can be attained within a reasonable time. In case of severe agoraphobia, for example, patients may learn to carry out their daily activities, such as a job, housekeeping, shopping, engaging in leisure activities, and raising children.

Furthermore, it should be determined which goals are to be reached at the end of treatment and which are to be reached at a later stage. Complex goals, such as "becoming independent," are likely to be achieved over a much longer period than simple goals. At least the short-term goals should be explicitly formulated and agreed on by both patient and therapist.

Another point in this regard is the way in which the attainment of goals should be established and treatment effects evaluated. Questionnaires and specific rating scales can be of use in this evaluation (see an earlier section of this chapter). For example, the patient can rate a number of specific situations on the anxiety and avoidance scales of Watson and Marks (1971) before, during, and after treatment. General anxiety level, mood, and frequency and severity of panic attacks can be monitored daily during treatment. Psychophysiological assessment, however, is cumbersome, costly, and of little use in clinical practice.

Constructing a Fear Hierarchy

After the therapist has explained the rationale, the next step is the construction of a hierarchy of feared and avoided situations. This hierarchy is the starting point of treatment, and therefore, should be formulated with care and specificity.

First, the principle of the "fear thermometer" is explained by pointing to the fact that the patient is not equally fearful across situations and in all circumstances. To rank these situations, it is helpful to position them on a "fear thermometer" with a (arbitrary) scale from zero to 100 (10 = *No Need for Avoidance or Fear at All*, 100 = *Maximal Fear/ Avoidance*). Patients are asked to summarize the principles of the fear hierarchy in their own words. A basic feature of a fear hierarchy is the ranking of situations on the basis of avoidance or fear. Based on initial interview data, and supplemented by an active search, both therapist and patient identify as many situations as possible. However, situations that are only of minor relevance to daily life, or are of an incidental nature may be excluded. The important thing is to accurately determine exactly which stimuli trigger the patient's fear. Although most agoraphobics are afraid of crowds, each has his or her own specific fears. For some patients, quiet streets may be frightening; for others, places near water or unfamiliar places.

During the session, elements of the hierarchy are discussed, and writing down additional situations can be given as a homework assignment. One strategy is to start by asking what situation would be the most difficult (fear = 100; e.g., visiting the city's biggest shopping mall alone at the busiest hour), and what situation could be handled with only minor distress (fear = 15; walking from front door of home to that of next-door neighbor). Intermediate situations can subsequently be elicited. If the patient rarely leaves home, the first items may be exercised in the company of others and may thus be regarded as intermediate assignments. The same situations return higher in the hierarchy, but are then practiced alone. In general, it should be remembered that hierarchy items are to be practiced as daily exercises. Therefore, one situation should be employed that occurs frequently enough and is preferably relevant for the patient's daily life.

After an initial discussion of potential hierarchy items, the question may arise whether to construct one or more hierarchies. For example, is there a single theme in all situations mentioned (e.g., traveling by car and public transport), or are there diverse situations (e.g., those with a clear social element), and those that pertain to individual activities, such as traveling?

Constructing Specific Assignments

After it has been decided which items are included in the fear hierarchy, specific assignments are made. This effort requires a high level of specificity. When formulating an item, both therapist and patient should consider questions such as where, when, what, how, with whom, with what? Such specificity normally leads to the use of, for example, city maps, and is further enhanced by topographical awareness and "house calls" by the therapist. An incomplete assignment would be

> Visiting a busy shop

An adequate assignment would be something like

> Visiting the nearby shopping mall on my own, starting at 3 o'clock in the afternoon after a stroll through Highstreet from the corner of A street to B street and back (about 1 kilometer each way). Fear rating: 60

When adequate assignment appears to be too difficult, intermediate assignments are considered. In the case of agoraphobia, this normally implies the company of a confidant. Therefore, one hierarchy item is split into two separate assignments: the one lower in the hierarchy is the accompanied version, whereas the higher item is the same assignment alone. Very fearful patients are particularly hesitant to formulate items that imply excursions on their own. An additional intermediate step may be necessary in which the company gradually fades away:

> Visiting the local department store while my partner remains on the first floor and I move to the second floor on my own for 30 minutes. Fear rating: 45

Date	Time from–to	Anxiety 0–10*	Which way?	Company (with whom)	Transport**
*0 = No fear at all 10 = maximal fear **Walking, by bicycle, by car, by bus or train					

Figure 2.2. Behavioral diary for exposure exercises.

A clearly formulated homework assignment is pivotal to successful treatment. An adjunct to the daily training program is a self-monitoring form as depicted in Figure 2.2.

Self-monitoring of homework serves as a reminder for evaluating the course of the assignment; it also shows how fear has decreased. This latter observation, in particular, can be a strong point of feedback, just as marking on the map the physical distances that have been covered over a number of weeks. In this way, both therapist and patient have a clear picture of improvements and obstacles. For some patients, the self-monitoring form is the impetus to make them work, since they should return to the therapist with an empty form.

Carrying Out Exposure Assignments

In the conventional view on exposure treatment, the patient is stimulated to spend 1.5 to 2 hours practicing a specific assignment in order to experience a sufficient decrease in anxiety. At times, the exposure is too brief because of the short distances that are covered in the initial phase of treatment. An insufficient fear decrease in these situations can be prevented by giving several consecutive instructions. It should be emphasized that the patient is to remain in the situation until the fear has subsided. Ample time should be taken to make the patient fully aware of the principle that it is very important to experience prolonged exposure to anxiety-provoking stimuli, without having the chance to avoid or escape.

Exposure as homework assignments has a number of advantages over therapist-guided exposure. First, homework assignments are carried out by the patients themselves and, therefore, are more cost effective. Furthermore, generalization of treatment effects can be expected after practicing in the home situation. In some cases, it may be advisable for the therapist to accompany the patient the first time he or she is confronted with a new assignment, and then gradually withdraw. The frequency and interval of patient–therapist contact may vary, depending on the persistence of avoidance behaviors. For some agoraphobics, only one or a few therapist-guided sessions may be sufficient before assignments can be carried out; other patients need more assistance and encouragement before they can do it on their own. Even patients who are perfectly capable of carrying out the procedures will benefit from some encouragement from the therapist by regular telephone calls. Over the course of therapist-guided exposure *in vivo* sessions, the therapist gradually withdraws from the practice situation in order to make the *in vivo* exercises increasingly difficult for the patient. For most agoraphobics, actual exposure to fear-provoking situations does not take place when they know that the therapist is present.

Evaluation of Assignments and Treatment

At the next session, the first item on the agenda is the debriefing of the specific assignment. Two aspects are discussed: (1) What has been successfully accomplished? and (2) What obstacles did the patient encounter? Thus, both success and failure are discussed in a constructive atmosphere. Successful completion of an assignment may indicate a decrease in agoraphobic avoidance, whereas problems during practicing may point to unexpected or unknown difficulties in the situations.

Rather than adopting a punishing or irritated attitude when a patient indicates that an assignment has not been carried out, the first thing to do is to find out what went wrong. Were the instructions unclear? Were there any complicating factors (e.g., relationship turmoil)? Were there specific aspects of the situation that proved to be more difficult than anticipated? With the patient's "hands-on" experience, a new assignment can be formulated, or the same assignment can be carried out under less ambiguous conditions.

After all items of a hierarchy have been mastered, results up to that point should be evaluated. How much gain has been made? When treatment consisted of more than one hierarchy, evaluation takes place after the last hierarchy has been completed. At the end of a treatment block (i.e., one or more hierarchies), the therapist should return to the original treatment goals to check whether they have been reached. If so, did new problems emerge? In some patients, relational or social problems come to light after agoraphobia has subsided. Other patients may question what to do with their lives now that they are free of severe avoidance behaviors. Agoraphobia may have had such an influence on daily life that the patient needs additional support (or even problem-solving therapy) to cope with the new demands of life. It would be unwise to terminate treatment too early, because there is a danger of relapse.

Panic Management

In recent cognitive models (e.g., Clark, 1986), a *panic attack* is conceptualized as the consequence of a misinterpretation of innocuous bodily sensations. As outlined earlier in this chapter, many panic patients experience symptoms of hyperventilation and interpret these as signs of imminent threat, such as a heart attack, stroke, or collapse. The consequence will be the experience of increased anxiety and panic. A positively accelerating vicious circle emerges, resulting in a panic attack, which in itself provokes more bodily reactions of anxiety (e.g., palpitations, sweating, trembling). The treatment developed for patients with panic attacks is based on the model presented in Figure 2.3. The aim of panic management is to challenge catastrophic attributions and replace them with more realistic ones; in this way, the vicious circle will be broken. Furthermore, coping with bodily processes, such as hyperventilation, is also included in many panic management approaches (e.g., Craske & Barlow, 1993).

Several studies show that this approach leads to a significant decrease in the number of panic attacks (Clark, Salkovskis, & Chalkley, 1985; Salkovskis, Jones, & Clark, 1986).

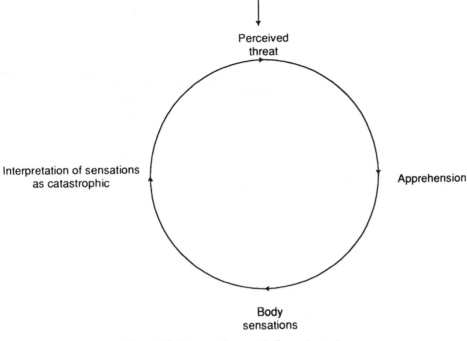

Figure 2.3. The cognitive model of a panic attack.

Bonn, Readhead, and Timmons (1984) compared exposure *in vivo* alone with exposure *in vivo* in combination with breathing exercises. At the end of treatment, both groups made similar gains. After 6 months, however, it appeared that the group with combined treatment had improved more. A more behavioral approach to panic was demonstrated by Griez and Van den Hout (1986), who exposed panic patients to CO_2 inhalation. The result after repeated exposure was a decrease in fear for interoceptive stimuli. It is remarkable that many strategies contain an exposure component; exposure can be applied to external situations as well as to interoceptive stimuli, such as palpitations or feeling faint. There presently are a number of approaches that are variants of the procedure described in this chapter. Treatment is distinguished by the following steps:

1. Inventory of bodily symptoms and cognitions
2. The hyperventilation provocation test
3. Training in abdominal breathing
4. Decatastrophizing
5. Using behavioral experiments
6. Modifying panic triggers

Inventory of Bodily Symptoms and Cognitions

An important first step is a detailed inventory of the nature and severity of bodily and cognitive symptoms associated with a panic attack. It should be mentioned here that during the admission interview, an inventory is to be drawn up of the patient's physical condition (e.g., asthma, bronchitis, cardiac abnormalities, and epilepsy) and of his or her previous experiences with other forms of treatment (e.g., many of our patients have received prior physiotherapy).

The therapist asks the patient for specific symptoms preceding and during a panic attack. Occasionally, patients may need some prompting ("What sensations do you feel in the upper part of your body, ... in your chest, ... in your arms and legs, ... in the rest of your body?"). Assessing interpretations is next; this involves the elicitation of the meaning the patient attaches to each symptom or groups of symptoms. Some characteristic combinations of symptoms and catastrophic misinterpretations are:

Chest pain	Cardiac attack
Pain radiating to the left arm	Cardiac attack
Wobbly knees	Fainting
Dizziness	Fainting
Light-headedness	Fainting
Breathlessness	Choking
Smothering sensations	Choking
Inability to think clearly	Insanity

This assessment elucidates two of the most important elements in the vicious circle, as depicted in Figure 2.3. The therapist can easily appreciate that anxiety will be strong if the credibility of such a specific catastrophic misinterpretation is high.

Hyperventilation Provocation Test

It is safe to assume that verbal information provides a distorted picture of the actual circumstances during a panic attack. Therefore, in many cases the next treatment strategy is a hyperventilation provocation test. The aim of this procedure is to gain insight into the similarities between the attributions of the symptoms resulting from a "spontaneous" panic attack, and the sensations of artificially provoked bodily sensations. For this reason, the therapist introduces the provocation test in neutral terms in order to preclude fear induction or specific expectations concerning effects of the procedure. It is preferable to refer to a "diagnostic test" rather than to a "hyperventilation provocation." It should be mentioned that before conducting the test for the first time, the therapist should practice the breathing test him- or herself. The resulting experience is illustrative for the impact of hyperventilation phenomena. Careful preparation will produce an optimal effect with the patient during the therapy session.

The procedure itself is rather simple: Patients are asked to breathe through their nose and mouth deeply and quickly (about 30 inhalations a minute) for a period of 2 minutes. Patients should be reminded that they are allowed to stop sooner if they want to; the most information will be yielded, however, if they continue for the full 2 minutes. Discussion of possible symptoms should be postponed until after the test; some patients try to avoid the test by engaging the therapist in an elaborate discussion. If patients understand the procedure, overbreathing commences. During the 2 minutes, the therapist utters reinforcing remarks (e.g., "Okay," "You're doing fine," "Carry on").

After the test, the point is to determine similarities between these provoked symptoms and the those of a "spontaneous" panic attack. It is helpful to use a symptom list on which patients can indicate their severity. Subsequently, the therapist marks the similarities between these symptoms and those of a panic attack on a scale from zero (*No Accordance*) to 10 (*Perfect Accordance*). The two checklists form a starting point for discussing the similarities to and differences from a real panic attack. The following questions may be useful: "What symptoms did you have in both situations?" "What symptoms did you have during the test and not during a panic attack?" and "What symptoms did you have during a real panic attack that you did not experience during the test?" Many patients report less fear in the test situation than in a real-life panic attack, although symptoms may be quite similar. They explain this by saying, for example, "You wanted me to do this," or "If it were dangerous, you would not expose me to this test," or "If something should go wrong, help is at hand." Most patients need some time before they arrive at the conclusion that their interpretations, rather than their bodily sensations, are responsible for the panic attacks.

By now, the moment has come to draw the vicious circle of Figure 2.3. Both therapist and patient recapitulate the course of an attack. While talking, the therapist takes notes and constructs the circle step by step. With each step, the therapists checks whether the patient recognizes the description ("Am I right in understanding that you are feeling dizzy then?"). This active questioning is meant to set the patient thinking and to clarify the course of the panic attack.

There is one part of the procedure that should be elucidated through a didactic explanation: the phenomenon of hyperventilation. The patient's knowledge and intellectual sophistication determines how detailed this explanation should be. Of course, therapists must be sufficiently informed themselves on this phenomenon in order to explain this clearly. There are several essential points that certainly should be discussed. One of them is the obvious presence of irregular breathing, the subsequent decrease in CO_2 level, and the consequent bodily sensations (see earlier section for further details).

After this explanation, the therapist checks the patient's understanding of the panic model. This can be done by asking, for example, "Imagine you would want to explain the model to your partner; how would you do that?" In this active (or even role-played) manner, the information will be better assimilated. In addition, the therapist is able to deal with potential misunderstandings or doubts, because an adequate understanding is a *conditio sine qua non* for further treatment.

Training in Abdominal Breathing

One of the conclusions from the previous discussion may be that the patient should adopt a more relaxed and regular breathing pattern. In the case of hyperventilation, the use of the muscles of the thorax is too strong, whereas the abdominal muscles are kept too tense. The aim of breathing exercises is to acquire a relaxed abdominal breathing pattern. Clark (1986) recommends a pace of 8 to 12 breaths per minute, in which the (nasal) inhalation is as long as the exhalation. It is helpful if the patient uses an audiotape on which the words "In" and "Out" are recorded in the required pace. The therapist demonstrates the correct breathing position (i.e., one hand placed on the stomach and the other on the chest, with only the hand on the stomach moving during respiration).

Homework consists of practicing with the audiotape three times a day for about 20 minutes while undisturbed and wearing comfortable clothing. The first practice sessions at home can be held in front of a mirror, enabling the patient to check the breathing position. After several days, the tape may be faded out, while the patient keeps on breathing at the same pace. In the next sessions, the progress of breathing training is discussed. As an adjunct, the patient is asked to overbreathe for a short period (approximately 15 seconds), after which he or she is encouraged to perform the newly trained breathing pattern.

In some patients, the somatic-tension component is unduly high and persistent. The addition of other techniques (e.g., applied relaxation) to modify the somatic responses should then be considered in order to enable the patient to control the ongoing flow of tension (see Öst, 1987, for a detailed discussion of this procedure).

Decatastrophizing

The primary aim of cognitive treatment is teaching the patient to develop adequate (i.e., noncatastrophic) cognitions. The list of cognitions that the therapist has obtained before the provocation test is an important point of departure. Patients' misinterpretations are challenged by asking them to give evidence of the imminent catastrophe. More specifically, the discussion starts with the bodily sensations and the interpretations that patients attach to them. Patients often appear to be very preoccupied with the possible consequences of a panic attack and seem to disregard its triggers. An important first step, therefore, consists of "thought catching" (i.e., the identification of panicogenic attributions). To this end, the patient is provided with a homework sheet on which to note:

1. A specific situation (either external or interoceptive)
2. Panic symptoms
3. Thoughts or images that occur in this situation
4. Credibility of these thoughts or images (0% to 100%).

When retrospective verbal techniques fail to provide a sufficient degree of detail, the therapist asks patients to close their eyes and concentrate on a typical attack. Next, this situation is described as if it were occurring right now. At first, patients may find it difficult to recognize the panic mechanism, because they may experience fear or tension by talking about the panic attack. Often, the therapist will refer to the model of the vicious circle and ask patients to fit in their experiences.

Considerable time must be devoted to challenging catastrophic misinterpretations, and two ways of challenging can be discerned: verbally (to be discussed) (see below) and behaviorally (see previous section). Verbal techniques imply the investigation of the tenability of misinterpretations. The following are typical questions:

- "What is the evidence in favor of your interpretation of these symptoms?"
- "What is the evidence against your interpretation of these symptoms?"
- "Would everybody interpret these symptoms in the same way?"
- "Did you always (or under all circumstances) interpret these symptoms as catastrophic?"

The first two questions lead patients to doubt their strong conviction that something fatal is about to happen, because nothing of that kind has occurred to date. It emerges that there is no conclusive evidence for chest discomfort to equal a heart attack, for breathlessness to mean choking, or for wobbly knees to indicate fainting. It is important not only to garner disconfirming evidence, but also confirmative data. What leads patients to stay with their conviction? Very often a confirmatory bias will become evident, implying that the patients emphasize information in favor of the feared explanation, and at the same time neglect conflicting information.

The third and fourth questions prompt the search for alternative interpretations of panic symptoms. If other interpretations are conceivable, based on the experiences of other people, or of the patients themselves in other circumstances, what does this imply for the strong catastrophic conviction? The ensuing discussion gradually yields more than a single explanation of the panic symptoms; this will normally require a few sessions. Results of the hyperventilation provocation test, for example, may suggest the irregular breathing pattern as a potential alternative mechanism as compared to cardiac problems. In this line of reasoning, it is often helpful to produce several alternatives and to investigate the evidence for and against all of them. This will present patients with something to think about for the period between the sessions.

Behavioral Experiments

In addition to verbal challenging techniques, Beck and Emery (1985), Clark (1986), and many others consider behavioral experiments to be a substantial part of cognitive therapy. Essentially, the patient is challenged to perform certain activities aimed at testing his or her catastrophic interpretations. The patient, for example, has to expose him- or herself to something that may at least be considered exciting or fear provoking and that allows for both a catastrophic and an alternative explanation.

After the experiment, the therapist and patient agree on which of the hypotheses is actually supported by the experiment: the patient's catastrophic hypothesis or the more realistic one advocated by the therapist (or even by the patient him- or herself). It is neither necessary nor likely that patients abandon all of their irrational cognitions as a result of only one behavioral experiment; rather, a gradual shift takes place toward the desired noncatastrophic direction.

In clinical practice, behavioral experiments are often a powerful tool to guide the patient into discovering the untenability of the original (and long-held) catastrophic attributions. It is of great importance that the experiment be designed in such a way that it is a relevant test of precisely the misinterpretation held by the patient in connection with a specific sensation. Behavioral experiments should, therefore, be tailor made and carefully chosen to fit the patient's situation.

Modifying Panic Triggers

Panic triggers often are hardly noticed at first sight, although they are the actual causes of the panic attack. One of our female patients, for example, reported having had a limited symptom attack while wearing high-heeled shoes to which she was not accustomed. When discussing this event, she discovered that she automatically associated this unsteady feeling with one of the first symptoms of her panic attacks (i.e., feeling faint). Another patient thought he experienced the first symptoms of a panic attack when he wore a friend's glasses with strong lenses, although he himself did not wear spectacles. The blurred vision made him nearly panic.

These examples illustrate that panic attacks may be triggered by minor (changes in) bodily sensations. The problem is, however, that patients are so preoccupied with the phenomena of a panic attack and the associated anxiety, that the actual onset of the attack becomes obscured. In the course of treatment, in which the detection of triggers is an important issue, antecedents of panic attacks are gradually revealed. Careful questioning brings the triggers to the foreground and encourages patients to look for these and other triggers themselves. In this way, the assumption that panic attacks just "come out of the blue" or that they are being caused by some serious disease, eventually disappear. Identification of panic triggers is facilitated by the use of a diary (Figure 2.1) in which the patient records the occurrence and intensity of the (limited) attacks on a day-to-day basis. Cognitions during an attack should also be recorded. The therapist and the patient use the diary to discover triggers and catastrophic cognitions in order to modify both. After a number of sessions, the patient becomes increasingly aware of the onset of panic; its "spontaneous" nature will then be viewed in a different light.

Evaluation of Assignments and Treatment

Similar to the guidelines described in earlier, every assignment in the treatment of the panic disorder should be carefully evaluated as to its results and the impact on the patient's beliefs. One of the main treatment goals is the reduction of panic attack by modifying panicogenic interpretations.

MAINTENANCE AND GENERALIZATION STRATEGIES

Maintenance

Maintenance of therapeutic results implies that gains acquired during treatment are consolidated in the next (posttreatment) phase. The basis of such consolidation is laid down during treatment, particularly its final stage.

To promote maintenance, a number of considerations are worth mentioning. At the end of treatment, it is sensible to gradually increase the interval between sessions, allowing the patient to become more self-reliant and less dependent on the therapist. A clear understanding of treatment rationale, both principle and procedure, is important during treatment and after termination.

The therapist should (1) discuss the patient's doubts in connection with continuation of treatment gains, and (2) address irrational future expectations (e.g., when a patient expects no obstacles or minor relapses). This can also be challenged in cognitive–behavioral style by asking how likely the perfect situation (no anxiety at all) would be and how disastrous a temporary setback (an incidental panic attack) is.

Making use of setbacks during therapy as an exercise in prevention and/or coping with relapses can be illustrative and models the attitude toward coping with future setbacks. What has the patient learned thus far about how to handle these adverse situations when complaints (avoidance behaviors, panic attacks) seem to increase?

Furthermore, carrying out self-prescribed exercises after treatment has terminated is another constructive maintenance strategy. In the final few sessions, the patient is encouraged to devise a plan to further increase treatment gains. It may be beneficial to plan at fixed time intervals some assignment to counter the inclination to avoid situations. Self-control strategies posttreatment can be suggested in which continued practicing is reinforced with something pleasant (going out for dinner, buying something desirable), and failing to do so with the engagement in something less pleasant (e.g., cleaning out the attic).

A support system involving significant others (e.g., partner, parent) may stimulate further progress. Some patients need such a catalyst to maintain their training schedule.

Problem-solving interventions appear to enhance the effects of exposure *in vivo*, although they are not effective when used alone (e.g., Cullington, Butler, Hibbert, & Gelder, 1984). Similar to the application of assertiveness training in nonassertive agoraphobics (Emmelkamp et al., 1983), problem-solving therapy appears to prevent posttreatment relapses.

51

**Panic Disorder and
Agoraphobia**

Generalization

Because treatment is time limited, it is unlikely that all phobic situations (external or interoceptive) will be targeted within this period. Treatment should, therefore, include attention to generalization of the results to other situations, persons, times, and moods. During treatment, it is sensible to have the patient practice in various situations (in particular, his or her own living environment), with various persons, at disparate times of the day and week, and in different moods (not only when feeling alright). Having the patient carry out assignments in his or her own living environments is assumed to enhance generalization of treatment effects. After treatment, the patient is encouraged to vary the practice conditions started during treatment.

PROBLEMS IN IMPLEMENTATION

Dealing with Problems

It sometimes occurs, both in the exposure program and in the panic-management programs, that homework assignments have not been carried out satisfactorily. Criticizing patients who have not completed their assignments will usually have no effect and may even be counterproductive. The therapist should instead ascertain *why* the patient has not done his or her homework: perhaps the instructions have been unclear or too difficult, too easy, or viewed as irrelevant. Such a discussion might reveal that the patient does not really understand the treatment rationale. If this is the case, the therapist should explain the rationale more thoroughly. In some cases, therapists might blame themselves for not having clearly explained the purpose of an assignment or the treatment as a whole. As a general strategy, it is recommended that therapists thoroughly analyze the patient's failure to comply with a certain assignment or with treatment in general, and only after that analysis consider a course of action, because partial or noncompliance may be part of the disorder. Details of common problems in the treatment of agoraphobia and panic are discussed elsewhere (Emmelkamp & Bouman, 1991).

Personality Factors

In a number of patients, panic disorder and agoraphobia are complicated by a personality disorder. The avoidant and dependent personality disorders are the most prevalent among panic patients (Van Velzen & Emmelkamp, 1994). As yet, there are no indications that treatment is less effective with patients demonstrating a personality disorder, although treatment usually takes longer. It has yet to be determined whether such personality disorders precede, or are merely epiphenomena, of the panic disorder. Some patients with a dependent personality disorder are inclined to cling to the therapist. For example, with exposure *in vivo*, they are able to perform the exercises when the therapist is nearby, but are unable to carry them out on their own when at home. In such cases, a fading program might be appropriate. In this procedure, the therapist first writes down assignments on cards; later on, he or she gives only oral instructions. Next, the patient him- or herself devises assignments and discusses these with the therapist. As an additional help, the therapist might initially instruct the patient by phone to do his or her homework assignment and then call again to reinforce the patient after successful assignment completion. After having prompted the patient to complete the assignments on his or her own, the therapist shifts the responsibility for homework assignments to the patient after a few successful attempts. In the final phase, treatment progress is left entirely to the patient. The patient has to devise assignments him- or herself and carry them out without consulting the therapist. At the end of treatment, the therapist may offer a few booster sessions that the patient may receive when needed; however, it should be made clear to the patient that no more treatment sessions will be available after the agreed number of sessions have been ended.

In patients with a comorbid avoidant personality disorder, it is often important to include social situations in the treatment program, because most of the avoidance is related to social situations. Furthermore, it might be important to deal with the underlying social fears. For clinical guidelines, the reader is referred to Chapter 4 by Scholing, Emmelkamp, and Van Oppen in this volume.

In cases of a comorbid borderline personality disorder, a standard exposure *in vivo* program, or cognitive program dealing only with panic attacks, will usually not be appropriate, given the often turbulent therapeutic relationship and suicide threats. In case of chronic alcohol abuse, a standard exposure program is also usually less effective. In such cases a comprehensive treatment program is often needed.

Technique-Related Problems: Exposure in Vivo

It is not necessary to maintain the highest possible level of fear. Prolonged exposure can be carried out with the help of a hierarchy of fear-provoking situations. It is essential, however, that all situations during one session should evoke more or less the same amount of anxiety. It is strategically incorrect to assign a difficult task first and then an easy one, because it will prevent habituation to the fear-provoking stimuli. Patients will feel relieved when they receive an easy task that arouses no fear, rather than feeling relief as a result of habituation.

Inexperienced therapists often instruct their patients to go for a short walk, then take the bus for a short period, and so on, until the session is over. Although this can be considered a prolonged session, the actual exposure to each individual situation remains relatively brief. It is not surprising that this kind of exposure often fails, because the patient is still anxious when leaving the situation. It is important for the patient *to remain in the situation until his or her fear has subsided* before proceeding to the next situation. These guidelines imply that exposure *in vivo* should be tailored to individual patient needs.

Subtle avoidance may remain a concealed threat to an effective exposure *in vivo* treatment (Emmelkamp, 1982). Subtle forms of avoidance behavior may include carrying medicine, wearing sunglasses, talking with passersby, carrying a bag, or running in the street. Besides, real exposure can be prevented by cognitive avoidance, for example, by thinking, "There is a hospital," "My sister lives there," "The doctor lives nearby," "At least there will be help when something goes wrong." It is often very difficult to trace these subtle forms of avoidance behavior, because many patients themselves are not aware of them. Careful analyses of unsuccessful homework assignments are often very instructive as to the more subtle mechanisms of the disorders.

One of the major problems encountered with exposure *in vivo* is that the exposure is not to the idiosyncratic stimuli that provoke anxiety in a particular patient. This is especially relevant in patients with a comorbid anxiety disorder that might be related to the agoraphobia. For example, for some of our socially anxious agoraphobics, exposure assignments did not produce the desired level of habituation. When discussing the course of exposure, it appeared that these patients had continually avoided making eye contact and in doing so had escaped exposure to the most threatening aspects of the situation. In the next session, they were asked to walk the same route again and to make eye contact with passersby. Even though the exposure initially caused much more anxiety than the first experience, the fear eventually subsided. In a substantial proportion of agoraphobics, social phobia plays an important maintaining role. We consider it to be a therapeutic mistake if this social phobia is not dealt with separately, because it may eventually trigger another agoraphobic or panic episode.

In a number of cases, agoraphobia and panic is associated with post-traumatic stress disorder, which may complicate treatment. In one of our cases, standard exposure to agoraphobic stimuli was not successful because the patient avoided stimuli that were related to a traumatic war experience. Such stimuli included cemeteries, a gun shop, policemen, and soldiers. In a case of a sexually victimized agoraphobic, female-patient exposure *in vivo* failed because the anxiety experienced in typical agoraphobic situations turned out to be related, in part, to prior sexual abuse. In other patients, the panic and agoraphobia were fed by unresolved grief, which interfered with a standard exposure *in vivo* program. In all such cases, a good functional analysis conducted at the start of treatment (and updated periodically) provides directions for the next step in treatment and suggests potential obstacles.

There are also a number of potential problems with exposure *in vivo* as a homework-based therapy. It may, for example, be disturbing for the patient to pass his or her neighbor's house a number of times each day, especially when he or she lives in a small town. This problem may be solved by having the patient practice from a different starting point (e.g., the place of treatment). Another problem involving this type of exposure is that the patient can spend time avoiding the difficult situation. Explicit instructions, detailing not only the content of the homework assignment, but also day and exact time when the assignment has to be completed, may prevent such problems.

Technique-Related Problems: Cognitive Therapy

It is often difficult to elicit cognitions from patients. The question: "What do you think when you are in situation X and you are feeling anxious?" does not always yield the desired information. Examples of alternative questions are "What went through your mind?"; "What did you think could happen?"; "How did you think it would end?"; "What were you afraid of?" It also helps to have the patient close his or her eyes, imagine a situation, and think aloud. In particular, the latter technique enhances the likelihood of obtaining a detailed picture of the anxiety-inducing situation.

When challenging catastrophic interpretations, many patients report that they do not feel differently, although they think more realistically. This is probably due to the fact that they can produce a noncatastrophic thought, but that its degree of credibility is only low. It is also quite conceivable that only one misinterpretation has been challenged; others may still remain in operation. A careful analysis of additional beliefs is necessary to challenge the entire belief system.

The therapist's expectations as to the rate of cognitive change should also be realistic; it is a slow process allowing patients to learn to change their thinking styles.

Theo K. Bouman and
Paul M. G.
Emmelkamp

CASE ILLUSTRATIONS

Panic Disorder

Richard (aged 33, married, with a 2-year-old daughter) was referred by the family doctor to our office because of severe complaints of anxiety. For several years, he has been employed as an office clerk. He is satisfied with his job and is known to be a hard and conscientious worker. Approximately 8 months ago, after a summer vacation, his complaints began. While he was taking a relaxing stroll in the woods, he was seized by great anxiety and felt such a terrifying pain in his heart that he believed he was going to die. The general practitioner examined him thoroughly but could find nothing out of the ordinary. Richard felt relieved; however, he kept feeling worried about the cause of his symptoms. According to the doctor, his troubles were psychic; he was "working too hard" and was "too meticulous." He still kept worrying that it would happen again and, indeed, he did have recurrent attacks. Due to these attacks, Richard avoids going too far from home. Because he has lost control of his behavior, he has become considerably depressed, cannot concentrate, sleeps badly, and has withdrawn socially.

From the initial interview it was concluded that Richard was suffering from a panic disorder with mild agoraphobia and that he makes high demands on himself. His greatest fear was that he would die from a heart attack. Since Richard was able to rationalize this fear between attacks, the diagnosis "hypochondriasis" was not applicable. In view of the temporal relationship between panic and depression, the therapist hypothesized that his mood would improve as the fear subsides.

Symptom Assessment

In the second session, an inventory was made of the bodily sensations and thoughts Richard experienced just before, during, and after a panic attack. In order to gather complete information, Richard was asked to describe a typical (preferably recent) panic attack. The therapist recorded both Richard's thoughts and his bodily sensations during the attack, with the intention of returning to them later on in the session. The most prominent symptoms were chest discomfort and pain, breathlessness, choking sensations, sweating, and trembling. These symptoms were associated with thoughts and images about heart attacks and fainting.

Hyperventilation Provocation

The therapist (T) started treatment with a hyperventilation provocation test. The test was introduced as follows:

> **T:** I would like to ask you to do a diagnostic test. This test is quite simple and it may provide us much information about the symptoms we have just discussed. I would like you to breathe deep and fast through your mouth for 2 minutes. I will tell you when to stop. All right, is this clear? Let me show you first how to do it.

(The therapist briefly demonstrates the overbreathing procedure.)

> **T:** During these two minutes, you may possibly feel certain sensations. Some people experience them as pleasant, others do not. As soon as you feel different from the way you normally do, raise your hand while continuing with the test. After the 2 minutes we will return to it.

If Richard wants to stop before time is up, he can do so by resuming normal breathing. Since there are no questions regarding the test itself, the therapist presses the chronometer and for a few seconds breathes together with the patient to help him keep the right pace and depth of breathing. Richard continues on his own while the therapist makes some encouraging remarks, such as "Good," "Fine," and "Carry on." After 2 minutes, Richard is asked to rise from his seat, close his eyes, and describe all of the bodily sensations he feels at the moment. Next, he is asked to sit down and try to regain his normal breathing pattern. When the therapist (T) observes that Richard (P) has recuperated, he starts to debrief him on the overbreathing experiment.

T: Can you tell me what symptoms you have had during a panic attack and which ones also occurred during the previous test?
P: Well ... as a matter of fact, I didn't feel so anxious this time.
T: Right, not so anxious." (*Writes it down*) Are there any more symptoms you didn't have this time?
P: Another thing is that I wasn't perspiring that much, and I was feeling less insecure.
T: Hmm ... less perspiration and less feelings of insecurity. (*Writes this down as well*) Are there any more differences?
P: (*Pauses*) No, I don't think so, only that the symptoms were less serious.
T: Let me summarize: You were feeling less anxious and insecure just now, you perspired less, and the symptoms were less severe.
P: I believe that's right.
T: It's quite remarkable, isn't it? Can you explain these differences between a panic attack and the diagnostic test?
P: (*Pause*) I don't think I can.
T: It seems hard to explain. Let's try to find out. When you made the test, what made you feel less anxious?
P: I'm not sure, perhaps I was aware that it was only a test.
T: Only a test. ... Was there anything else that went through your mind?
P: Well. ... I guessed that if something might go wrong, I would be in good hands, since we are on the hospital premises.
T: So that's what you were thinking just now. What are your thoughts when you have a panic attack?
P: I only feel terribly frightened!
T: All right, you feel frightened, and what goes on in your mind when the attack comes?
P: What I think of then ... I always think that I'll faint, that I'll collapse, and that when I come to, people will just stand there staring into my face. It makes me sick just to think of it.
T: And the symptoms you had here strongly resemble the symptoms of a panic attack, don't they? (*looks at his notes, patient nods*) You were also just saying that you gave them 7 points on the scale from zero to 10, concerning their similarities. You also told me that you believed you were in good hands here, whereas in the panic attack situation you were afraid to faint and to be embarrassed. What do you make of that difference?
P: I'm doing this to myself, aren't I? It's the way I think that frightens me!

Discussing the role of hyperventilation in panic attacks is a next step in treatment. Since Richard is not well informed about this phenomenon, the therapist provides specific information.

T: Hyperventilation means that one's respiration is too strong in comparison to the needs of the body. When you're exercising your body in sport, you need to breathe faster. The reason for this is that body needs to get rid of a lot of waste gases, mostly carbon dioxide (CO_2). When

Theo K. Bouman and Paul M. G. Emmelkamp

you hyperventilate, you also exhale a great deal of this gas without any physical exertion. In doing so, the level of carbon dioxide in the blood will drop and consequently change the acidity: The blood becomes less acid. This causes a number of bodily sensations, some of which you have experienced during the test. Many people actually think that a lack of oxygen is the cause of hyperventilation and of the choking sensations, but hyperventilation is a decrease in carbon dioxide level, let's say expired air.

Cognitive Restructuring

At their next meeting, Richard tells the therapist that he has had another panic attack the evening before the session: without warning, and apparently without any cause. He was sitting on the couch, watching television, enjoying a drink, and expecting his wife to come home half an hour later.

T: What happened then?

P: I felt terribly bad, my heart was pounding like mad, and I felt dizzy, nauseous, as if were going to faint any minute. I don't understand how it could happen, I was just watching television.

T: What is it exactly you don't understand?

P: Well, that such a thing can happen without reason. All was well at the office, no stress at all.

T: What was the next thing you were thinking of then?

P: Then I started to wonder whether there was something wrong with my heart after all!

T: It really unsettled you, didn't it? Let's try to use this attack to your advantage and see what we can make of it. Let's start at the beginning. Try to recollect what happened as precisely as possible, what you were doing and what you were thinking of. You may close your eyes if you like.

P: (*Closes his eyes*) I was watching television and wasn't worrying about a thing.

T: What were you watching?

P: All kinds of programs, I think, nothing in particular.

T: And what program was on just before the panic attack?

P: I think it was a detective series on Channel 2 ... yes ... it was exciting this time ...

T: So, it was exciting? ... Indeed ... did you get carried away?

P: Yes, I suppose so.

T: What happens normally when you get excited?

P: (*Hesitates*) Well ... you get involved, is that what you mean?

T: That's exactly what I mean. How do you notice this involvement?

P: What do you mean?

T: Can you describe your bodily reactions when you're watching something exciting?

P: Oh well ... I sit tight and get carried away. If it's really thrilling, my heart starts pounding in my throat ... it's as if I'm actually there.

T: Your heart starts pounding in your throat. ... What was it like yesterday evening?

P: (*Reflecting*) Yes ... now you come to mention it, I believe it was exactly the same way.

T: What did the panic attack begin with?

P: With palpitations?

T: What crossed your mind then?

P: I was thinking ... oh my God ... I'm all alone now. ... What will happen if I have a heart attack?

T: How were you feeling then?

P: Frightened to death!

T: And what happened then?

P: Everything went wrong, I panicked completely.

T: What can we conclude after retracing the course of your "spontaneous" panic attack? It seems that you have misinterpreted a normal fast heartbeat due to an exciting movie, and thought you were going to have a heart attack. This catastrophic view, in turn, triggered a fear reaction and the attendant bodily sensations. (*The therapist illustrates this point by showing the vicious circle that he has drawn.*)

P: I believe I got so worked up that I had this attack. … Was it really because of a movie?

T: That's a very good question indeed: Was it because of the movie or was it your own doing?

P: (*Reflecting*) I think it was my own doing. I've been worrying about ordinary palpitations.

Richard's homework assignment was to write down what he usually thinks as soon as the first symptoms of the panic attack set in. Beside each catastrophic thought, he is to indicate a realistic thought. In the following sessions, he notices an increased ability to challenge the catastrophic thoughts by generating alternative noncatastrophic cognitions. Over the course of treatment, he improves this skill. Every now and then he is bothered by distressing bodily sensations; however, in contrast to earlier periods, he is now capable of handling them, thus preventing undue anxiety and situational avoidance.

Behavioral Experiments

Richard devoted several sessions to breathing exercises and reinterpretation of his bodily symptoms. Yet, he still worried about going into the street alone, for fear of becoming sick or fainting. When he told the therapist of his fears, the therapist used it as an opportunity for a behavioral experiment. The following week Richard was to go to town several times on his own and find out what happens. He had acquired the breathing correction and it is likely that he would have an opportunity to practice it during the experiment. Richard is not very keen on carrying out the experiment, but agrees to proceed. At the next session, it appears that he has been to town twice. The first time he felt dizzy, insecure, and anxious; after a short while, he went home. He considered the trip a failure. On the next occasion, he pulled himself together and went again. After 20 minutes, the first symptoms of panic occurred, after which he applied his breathing correction and encouraged himself to keep it up ("Just continue to breathe normally and everything will be all right. I won't faint and even if I do, so what?").

The experiment demonstrated to Richard that he was able to cut short an attack; furthermore, he discovered that there were no catastrophic consequences. Similar experiments were repeated several times and increased Richard's belief that he has only innocuous symptoms with which he can now cope adequately.

Modifying Panic Triggers

At the admission interview, Richard indicated that he was very meticulous at work and easily annoyed when things went wrong. After some time in treatment, his panic subsided and he learned to cope with it adequately. In this phase, the therapist suggested taking a closer look at his more "structural" sources of stress. In general, Richard appeared to place high demands on himself. This was shown in his work (he did not allow himself any mistake) as well as in social contacts (he wanted to be friends with everybody). This caused considerable stress and tension in his daily life. The next couple of sessions, therefore, were devoted to cognitive therapy of his excessive demands. The therapist explained that his panic attacks evidently did not come "out of the blue," but were directly or indirectly influenced by his own lifestyle and personal rules. During each of the subsequent sessions, a particular theme or situation was analyzed. The particular situations, the automatic thoughts, and the behavioral and emotional consequences were specified.

In the third session, for example, Richard's tendency to try to be friends with everybody was discussed. This implicit rule caused him to rarely oppose anyone, even if he did not like the way things were going. When a colleague at work took a few days off in a busy period, Richard did not dare say anything about it, although it annoyed him significantly. He was very angry and inwardly swore at his colleague, but was outwardly very friendly every time they met. The therapist investigated the advantages of being good friends with everyone. After some thought, Richard remarked that in the case of his colleague, it was only Richard himself who was bothered; his colleague did not seem to be aware of his annoyance. In challenging the irrational thought, "I must be liked by everybody," Richard concluded that this was an impossible demand. The costs of this belief exceeded the benefits, because avoiding confrontations with other people gave him considerable stress and tension. He gradually shifted toward the belief that it is not absolutely necessary to be liked by everybody.

After five sessions both patient and therapist agreed that Richard was quite capable of making his own rational analyses. His mood improved considerably and he felt more cheerful. Six months after termination of therapy, the therapist received a letter from Richard in which he reported having had only a few panic attacks, with which he was able to cope by using cognitive modification and breathing exercises. Furthermore, he related that his attitudes toward his job had changed, making him more productive and even eligible for promotion.

Richard's treatment emphasized the need for an adequate micro- and macrolanalysis of the problem behaviors. The high demands can be regarded as a more structural problem. Therefore, they were dealt with later in therapy, when the acute panic problems had subsided. Furthermore, treatment results supported the therapist's estimation that the depressed mood was only secondary to the incapacitating effects of panic. The patient's original failure to meet his own high demands also were considered depressogenic.

Agoraphobia

Clinical Picture and Background

The course of an exposure *in vivo* treatment for agoraphobia will be illustrated by the case of Paula, 34 years of age, who was married with two children (a 10-year-old boy and a 7-year-old girl). Over the last 5 years, she has become increasingly afraid to go into the street; walking in the street makes her feel nervous, and she is afraid to become sick or faint. She experienced her job as a saleswoman as rather exacting and her complaints started at a time when she was overstressed. At first she found it difficult to go to work by bus because she often felt the urge to get off. She remembers her first moment of great fear when she was sitting in the back of the bus, short of breath and feeling dizzy and anxious. After this incident she called in sick regularly.

At the beginning of treatment, it appeared that she hardly ever left the house unless her husband accompanied her. Her social contacts were limited, because she was afraid to pay a return visit after someone had come to see her. Paula made a rather gloomy impression and she was convinced that there was little point in going on this way. Moreover, she and her husband often quarreled and at home the atmosphere was tense. During the initial interview, her husband seemed to understand little of his wife's complaints. Even though he tried to help her as much as possible, his wife showed no improvement. Because Paula insisted on his presence at home after work, he felt restricted in his movements.

After the admission phase, a functional analysis was conducted from which it appeared that exposure *in vivo* would be the most appropriate treatment for this strong avoidance behavior. On the basis of the macroanalysis, the therapist concluded that the depressed mood, social isolation, and marital problems resulted from the agoraphobia. Her husband's supporting role functioned as a maintaining factor for the phobic complaints.

Explaining the Treatment Rationale

The explanation of the treatment rationale is illustrated by a portion of the second treatment session.

T: Last time we discussed all kinds of situations you are avoiding nowadays. This session I want to talk about the treatment itself. You told me that in the course of the last 5 years you have become more and more afraid to go out. First, you were afraid to go by bus, so you went by bike; later on you stopped going by bike and then you hardly walked anywhere far from home. Your husband accompanied you more often and he did the shopping as well. The striking thing is that your circle has become smaller and smaller. Let's, therefore, try to figure out how your phobia has come so far. Could you tell me why you stopped going by bus in the first place?

P: Well ... I was afraid of what would happen in case I couldn't get off.

T: And then you started to avoid the bus?

P: Yes.

T: Did the avoidance make it easier or more difficult for you to take the bus the next time?

P: More difficult, that's for sure.

T: So, after you have avoided a fearful situation, it becomes more difficult to face the same situation the next time. The avoidance has become a habit because it makes you feel less anxious in the short term. In the long run, this strategy of avoiding has caused even greater problems: By escaping all fearful situations, you hardly ever go out by yourself now. You also told me that it has *gradually* become more difficult to go far away from home, Am I right?

P: Yes, that is how things are.

T: Well now, in treatment, you are *gradually* going to extend your radius again, starting with less difficult situations. In order to do so, we will draw up a list of situations in which you feel anxious, starting from a little anxious to very anxious. After the list has been completed, you are to practice the situations as homework assignments. The object is to stay in each situation for quite some time, about 90 minutes, and not leave. In doing so, you will have the opportunity to experience that situation and you will become less anxious. After a period of practice, when you are no longer afraid in a particular situation, the idea is to move on to the next situation on the list. By proceeding this way you will eventually be able to tackle all situations and to cope with the anxiety, which in turn decreases. Is it clear how the treatment works?

P: Yes, I think so. But ... will the anxiety just disappear?

T: You might say that the strategy of avoidance has increased the agoraphobia. You have never given fear itself the chance to subside, because you have constantly pulled the emergency brake by escaping or by staying indoors. Now we're going to work the other way round.

Defining a Treatment Goal

After the therapist has explained the treatment principles, he and Paula formulated a final goal. In her opinion the primary goals included being able to do the shopping by herself, paying her brother a visit, and going through town without fear. This meant that all of the situations took place in town. Because the therapist was not familiar with the surroundings, Paula brought a map on which all distances and important routes were drawn.

Constructing the Fear Hierarchy

During the third session, she and the therapist agreed on the composition of the hierarchy and its theme: increasing Paula's radius within the town.

> **T:** We are now going to compare several situations regarding the fear they evoke. It is therefore helpful to make use of a "fear thermometer" on a 10-point scale. Zero means that you have no fear at all, and 10 means that you experience the greatest possible fear. Most situations discussed so far can be indicated somewhere on this fear thermometer. So, the higher the mark, the greater the fear you have in the situation. The situations will be written down on a number of cards and subsequently be arranged according to the extent of fear they arouse. It is important for us to check whether the fear decreases during the treatment. Consequently, it is necessary to describe the situations as accurately as possible. Only then we will know which situation we're dealing with. Let me give an example. Let's say we write down the situation: "Going to the shop." Does this seem specific enough for you?
>
> **P:** No, because you don't know which shop.
>
> **T:** Exactly, but will it be entirely clear if you mention the shop?
>
> **P:** (*Pause*) I don't think so, because it also depends whether it's busy or not.
>
> **T:** Fine, this means we'll have to write down several things on the list about each situation, what we're dealing with, what time; it may also matter if someone goes with you (this can occur in the beginning) and the means of transport, walking, by car, on the bike. Furthermore, it is important to note the object of the excursion: Is it because you want to cover a certain distance, or is it because you want to buy something or mail a letter?

At home, Paula engaged her husband in the selection of the specific situations in the hierarchy. In the next session, she produced a dozen situations, some of which needed more specification. Generally speaking, it appeared that she understood the treatment rationale, the role of the fear hierarchy, and the need for specific assignments.

Formulation Homework Assignments

Before the next session, Paula practiced the first assignment, (i.e., walking around the block according to a defined route). The therapist gave her a homework monitoring form (see Figure 2.2) on which she indicated the time, fear, company, and means of transport (walking, car, bicycle). At the next session, Paula reacted somewhat enthusiastically. The walk in the neighborhood was quite exacting. The first few days before going outdoors she felt nervous, but after a few days the period of anticipatory fear had gradually become shorter. In the street she felt very uneasy. She kept up a rapid pace and came home feeling very tense. They also discussed the way Paula had taken the route, feeling chased and walking very fast. The therapist advised her to go more slowly next time. It was explained that in doing so, she would come closer to her goal, that is, walking about and feeling at ease.

Actually, she was not satisfied about her activities. The therapist wanted to know the reason for her discontent. Paula replied that she wanted things to go faster. It seemed, in the therapist's opinion, that she received more attention for her shortcomings than for her relative gains over the week. Paula (similar to many other patients) was inclined to neglect the progress she made. The therapist countered this by labeling her efforts positively, thus serving as a model for an alternative way of interpreting events, a method that proves to be more productive than negative labeling.

In the next session, Paula was much more enthusiastic. She became aware of her pace, stopped to look around, and even deviated from her route. She was more aware of her surroundings and, consequently, felt less tense. During one of her walks, she suddenly felt quite dizzy. According to the exposure paradigm, she suppressed the inclination to go home, stopped to sit on a bench, and proceeded with her walk later on.

Course of Treatment

Paula devoted 15 sessions to working in the hierarchy. First, she went through the town on her bicycle; later on, she went walking. Next, she visited the small shops and the supermarket, and then she and her husband went for a spin in the countryside. Paula's husband did not attend sessions, but she told him how he could be helpful. Currently, Paula is becoming less dependent on her husband. She goes out alone and does most of the shopping. Both of them consider their relationship to have improved since treatment. For the first time in years, they are making plans for the holidays, even though the idea still frightens her. Paula no longer feels depressed; she engages in a variety of activities, visits her brother in town, and has even considered working as a volunteer in a home for the elderly. The gains in the latter areas support the functional analysis the therapist made at the onset of treatment.

REFERENCES

American Psychiatric Association. (1987). *Diagnostic and Statistical Manual of Mental Disorders* (3rd ed. rev.). Washington, DC: Author.

American Psychiatric Association. (1994). *Diagnostic and Statistical Manual of Mental Disorders* (4th ed.). Washington DC: Author.

Apfeldorf, W. J., Shear, M. K., Leon, A. C., & Portera, L. (1994). A brief screen for panic disorder. *Journal of Anxiety Disorder, 8*, 71–78.

Arrindell, W. A., Emmelkamp, P. M. G., & Van der Ende, J. (1984). Phobic dimensions: Reliability and generalizability across samples, gender, and nations. The Fear Survey Schedule (FSQ-III) and the Fear Questionnaire (FQ). *Advances in Behaviour Research and Therapy, 6*, 207–254.

Arrindell, W. A., Emmelkamp, P. M. G., & Sanderman, R. (1986). Marital quality and general life adjustment in relation to treatment outcome in agoraphobia. *Advances in Behaviour Research and Therapy, 7*, 139–185.

Asmundson G. G., & Stein, M. B. (1994). A preliminary analysis of pulmonary function in panic disorder: Implications for the dyspnea–fear theory. *Journal of Anxiety Disorders,, 8*, 63–69.

Beck, A. T., & Emery, G. (1985). *Anxiety disorders and phobias: A cognitive perspective.* New York: Basic Books.

Bonn, J. A., Readhead, C. P. A., & Timmons, B. H. (1984). Enhanced adaptive behavioural response in agoraphobic patients pretreated with breathing retraining. *Lancet, 2*, 665–669.

Buikhuisen, M., & Garssen, B. (1990). Hyperventilation and panic attacks. *Biological Psychology, 31*, 280.

Carr, R. E., Lehrer, P. M., & Hochron, S. M. (1992). Panic symptoms in asthma and panic disorder. *Behaviour Research and Therapy, 30*, 251–261.

Chambless, D. L., Caputo, G. C., Bright, P., & Gallagher, R. (1984). Assessment of fear in agoraphobics: The Body Sensations Questionnaire and the Agoraphobia Cognitions Questionnaire. *Journal of Consulting and Clinical Psychology, 52*, 1090–1097.

Clark, D. M. (1986). A cognitive approach to panic. *Behaviour Research and Therapy, 24*, 461–470.

Clark, D. M., Salkovskis, P. M., & Chalkley, A. J. (1985). Respiratory control as a treatment for panic attacks. *Journal of Behavior Therapy and Experimental Psychiatry, 16*, 23–30.

Cobb, J. P., Mathews, A. A., Childs-Clarke, A., & Blowers, C. M. (1984). The spouse as co-therapist in the treatment of agoraphobia. *British Journal of Psychiatry, 144*, 282–287.

Cox, B. J., Endler, N. S., Swinson, R. P., & Norton, G. R. (1992). Situations and specific coping strategies associated with clinical and nonclinical panic attacks. *Behaviour Research and Therapy, 30*, 67–69.

Cox, B. J., Swinson, R. P., Kuch, K., & Reichman, J. T. (1993). Dimensions of agoraphobia assessed by the mobility inventory. *Behaviour Research and Therapy, 31*, 427–431.

Craske, M. G., & Barlow, D. H. (1993). Panic disorder and agoraphobia. In D. H. Barlow (Ed.), *Clinical handbook of psychological disorders* (pp. 1–47). New York: Guilford.

Craske, M. G., Rachman, S. J., & Tallman, K. (1986). Mobility, cognitions and panic. *Journal of Psychopathology and Behavioral Assessment, 8*, 199–210.

Cullington, A., Butler, G., Hibbert, G., & Gelder, M. (1984). Problem-solving: Not a treatment for agoraphobia. *Behavior Therapy, 15*, 280–286.

De Beurs, E., Lange, A., & Van Dyck, R. (1992). Self-monitoring of panic attacks and retrospective estimates of panic: Discordant findings. *Behaviour Research and Therapy, 30*, 411–414.

De Ruiter, C., Rijken, H., Garssen, B., Van Schaik, A., & Kraaimaat, F. (1989). Comorbidity among the anxiety disorders. *Journal of Anxiety Disorders, 3*, 57–68.

DiNardo, P. A., O'Brien, G. T., Barlow, D. H., Waddell, M. T., & Blanchard, E. B. (1983). Reliability of DSM-III anxiety disorder categories using a new structured interview. *Archives of General Psychiatry, 40*, 1070–1075.

Emmelkamp, P. M. G. (1974). Self-observation versus flooding in the treatment of agoraphobia. *Behaviour Research and Therapy, 12*, 229–237.

Emmelkamp, P. M. G. (1982). *Phobic and obsessive–compulsive disorders: Theory, research and practice.* New York: Plenum Press.

Emmelkamp, P. M. G. (1990). Anxiety and fear. In A. S. Bellack, M. Hersen, & A. E. Kazdin (Eds.), *International handbook of behavior modification and therapy* (pp. 283–305). New York: Plenum Press.

Emmelkamp, P. M. G., & Bouman, T. K. (1991). Psychological approches to the difficult patient. In J. R. Walker, G. R. Norton, & C. A. Ross (Eds.), *Panic disorder and agoraphobia: A compehensive guide for the practitioner* (pp. 398–429). Pacific Grove: Brooks/Cole.

Emmelkamp, P. M. G., Brilman, E., Kuiper, H., & Mersch, P. P. (1986). The treatment of agoraphobia: A comparison of self-instructional training, rational emotive therapy and exposure in vivo. *Behavior Modification, 10*, 37–53.

Emmelkamp, P. M. G., & Emmelkamp-Benner, A. (1975). Effects of historically portrayed modeling and group treatment on self-observation: A comparison with agoraphobics. *Behavior Research and Therapy, 13*, 135–139.

Emmelkamp, P. M. G., & Gerslma, C. (1994). Marital functioning in the anxiety disorders. *Behavior Therapy, 25*, 407–429.

Emmelkamp, P. M. G., Kuipers, A., & Eggeraat, J. (1978). Cognitive modification versus prolonged exposure in vivo: A comparison with agoraphobics. *Behaviour Research and Therapy, 16*, 33–41.

Emmelkamp, P. M. G., & Mersch, P. P. (1982). Cognition and exposure *in vivo* in the treatment of agoraphobia: Short-term and delayed effects. *Cognitive Therapy and Research, 6*, 77–90.

Emmelkamp, P. M. G., Van den Hout, A., & De Vries, K. (1983). Assertive training for agoraphobics. *Behaviour Research and Therapy, 21*, 63–68.

Emmelkamp, P. M. G., & Wessels, H. (1975). Flooding in imagination versus flooding *in vivo*: A comparison with agoraphobics. *Behaviour Research and Therapy, 13*, 7–16.

Friedman, S., & Chiernen, L. (1994). Discriminating the panic disorder patient from patients with borderline personality disorder. *Journal of Anxiety Disorders, 8*, 49–61.

Gelder, M. G., & Marks, I. M. (1966). Severe agoraphobia: A controlled prospective trial of behaviour therapy. *British Journal of Psychiatry, 113*, 53–73.

Griez, E., & Van den Hout, M. A. (1986). CO_2 inhalation in the treatment of panic attacks. *Behaviour Research and Therapy, 24*, 245–250.

Hafner, R. J., & Marks, I. M. (1976). Exposure *in vivo* in agoraphobics: Contributions of diazepam, group exposure, and anxiety evocation. *Psychological Medicine, 6*, 71–88.

Himle, J. A., & Hill, E. M. (1991). Alcohol abuse and the anxiety disorders: Evidence from the Epidemiologic Catchment Area Survey. *Journal of Anxiety Disorders, 5*, 237–245.

Khawaja, N. G., & Oei, T. P. S. (1992). Development of a catastrophic cognition questionnaire. *Journal of Anxiety Disorders, 6*, 305–318.

Kleiner, L., & Marshall, W. L. (1987). Interpersonal problems and agoraphobia. *Journal of Anxiety Disorders, 1*, 313–323.

Last, C. G., Barlow, D. H., & O'Brien, G. T. (1984). Precipitants of agoraphobia: Role of stressful life events. *Psychological Reports, 54*, 567–570.

Lesser, I. M. (1988). The relationship between panic disorder and depression. *Journal of Anxiety Disorders, 2,* 3–15.

Ley, R. (1985). Blood, breath and fears: A hyperventilation theory of panic attacks and agoraphobia. *Clinical Psychology Review, 5,* 271–285.

Ley, R. (1989). Dyspneic-fear and catastrophic cognitions in hyperventilatory panic attacks. *Behaviour Research and Therapy, 27,* 549–554.

Mackay, W., & Liddell, A. (1986). An investigation into the matching of specific agoraphobic anxiety response characteristics with specific types of treatment. *Behaviour Research and Therapy, 24,* 361–364.

Maller, G., & Reiss, S. (1992). Anxiety sensitivity in 1984 and panic attacks in 1987. *Journal of Anxiety Disorders, 6,* 241–247.

Marks, I. M., & Matthews, A. M. (1979). Brief standard self-rating for phobic patients. *Behaviour Research and Therapy, 13,* 135–139.

Matthews, A. M., Gelder, M. G., & Johnston, D. W. (1981). *Agoraphobia: Nature and treatment.* London: Tavistock.

Mavissakalian, M. (1986). Clinically significant improvement in agoraphobia research. *Behaviour Research and Therapy, 24,* 369–370.

Michelson, L., Mavissakalian, M., & Marchione, K. (1988). Cognitive, behavioral and psychophysiological treatments of agoraphobia: A comparative outcome investigation. *Behavior Therapy, 19,* 97–120.

Munjack, D. J., Brown, R. A., & McDowell, D. E. (1993). Existence of hyperventilation in panic disorder with and without agoraphobia, GAD, and normals: Implications for the cognitive theory of panic. *Journal of Anxiety Disorders, 7,* 37–48.

Norton, G. R., Cox, B. J., & Malan, J. (1992). Nonclinical panickers: A critical review. *Clinical Psychology Review, 12,* 121–139.

Oei, T. P. S., Moylan, A., & Evans, L. (1991). Validity and clinical utility of the fear questionnaire for anxiety-disorder patients. *Psychological Assessment, 3,* 391–397.

Öst, L. G. (1987). Applied relaxation: Description of a coping technique and review of controlled studies. *Behaviour Research and Therapy, 25,* 397–409.

Öst, L. G. (1990). The agoraphobia scale: An evaluation of its reliability and validity. *Behaviour Research and Therapy, 28,* 323–329.

Öst, L-G., Lindahl, I.-L. Sterner, U., & Jerremalm, A. (1984). Physiological responses in blood phobics. *Behaviour Research and Therapy, 22,* 109–177.

Porzelius, J., Vest, M., & Nochomovitz, M. (1992). Respiratory functions, cognitions, and panic in chronic obstructive pulmonary patients. *Behaviour Research and Therapy, 30,* 75–77.

Reiss, S., Peterson, R. A., Gursky, D. M., & McNally, R. J. (1986). Anxiety sensitivity, anxiety frequency, and the prediction of fearfulness. *Behaviour Research and Therapy, 24,* 1–8.

Renneberg, B., Chambless, D. L., & Graceley, E. J. (1992). Prevalence of SCID-diagnosed personality disorders in agoraphobic outpatients. *Journal of Anxiety Disorders, 6,* 111–118.

Salkovskis, P. M., Jones, D. R. G., & Clark, D. M. (1986). Respiratory control in the treatment of panic attacks: Replication and extension with concurrent measurement of behaviour and pCO_2. *British Journal of Psychiatry, 148,* 526–532.

Spinhoven, Ph., Onstein, J., Sterk, P. J., & De Haen-Versteijnen, D. (1992). The hyperventilation provocation test in panic disorder. *Behaviour Research and Therapy, 30,* 453–462.

Stern, R. S., & Marks, I. M. (1973). A comparison of brief and prolonged flooding in agoraphobics. *Archives of General Psychiatry, 28,* 210–216.

Swinson, P., Cox, B. J., Shulman, I. D., Kuch, K., & Woszczyna, C. B. (1992). Medication use and the assessment of agoraphobic avoidance. *Behaviour Research and Therapy, 30,* 563–568.

Taylor, S., Koch, W. J., & Crockett, D. J. (1991). Anxiety sensitivity, trait anxiety and the anxiety disorders. *Journal of Anxiety Disorders, 5,* 293–312.

Van Velzen, C. J. M., & Emmelkamp, P. M. G. (submitted). Comorbidity of personality and anxiety disorders.

Watson, J. P., & Marks, I. M. (1971). Relevant and irrelevant fear in flooding—A crossover study of phobic patients. *Behavior Therapy, 2,* 275–293.

Westling, B. E., & Öst, L.-G. (1993). Relationship between panic attack symptoms and cognitions in panic disorder patients. *Journal of Anxiety Disorders, 7,* 181–194.

Williams, S. L., & Rappoport, A. (1983). Cognitive treatment in the natural environment for agoraphobics. *Behavior Therapy, 14,* 299–313.

Yuksel, S., Marks, I., Ramm, E., & Ghosh, A. (1984). Slow versus rapid exposure *in vivo* of phobics. *Behavioural Psychotherapy, 12,* 249–256.

3

Obsessive–Compulsive Disorder

Michael J. Kozak and Edna B. Foa

INTRODUCTION

Definition of Obsessive–Compulsive Disorder

According to the *Diagnostic and Statistical Manual of Mental Disorders*, Fourth Edition (DSM-IV; American Psychiatric Association, 1994), the essential features of obsessive–compulsive disorder are recurrent obsessions or compulsions of significant severity. *Obsessions* are "persistent ideas, thoughts, impulses, or images that are experienced as intrusive and inappropriate and that cause marked anxiety or distress" (APA, 1994, p. 418). *Compulsions* are "repetitive behaviors … or mental acts … the goal of which is to prevent or reduce anxiety or distress" (p. 418). This DSM-IV conceptualization of OCD offers no fundamental reformation of the previous construct, but there have been some noteworthy shifts of emphasis that reflect recent thinking about the disorder.

Foa and Kozak (1991) noted that DSM-III-R (American Psychiatric Association, 1987) criteria for OCD can be understood as reflecting three traditional views:

1. Obsessions are mental events and compulsions are behavioral events,
2. Obsessions and compulsions may be either connected or may occur independently.
3. Those with OCD recognize the senselessness of their obsessions.

The DSM-IV update reflects more recent views about these issues.

The view that obsessions and compulsions are functionally related has empirical support and is increasingly recognized (Rachman & Hodgson, 1980). Foa and Tillmanns (1980), for example, proposed that obsessions and compulsions be *defined* on the basis of their functional relationship on the modality in which they are expressed (mental or

Michael J. Kozak and Edna B. Foa • Department of Psychiatry, Medical College of Pennsylvania, Eastern Pennsylvania Psychiatric Institute, Philadelphia, Pennsylvania 19129.

Sourcebook of Psychological Treatment Manuals for Adult Disorders, edited by Vincent B. Van Hasselt and Michel Hersen. Plenum Press, New York, 1996.

behavioral). Accordingly, *obsessions* are defined as thoughts, images, or impulses that *generate* anxiety or distress, and *compulsions* are defined as overt (behavioral) or covert (mental) actions that are performed in an attempt to *alleviate* the distress brought on by the obsessions. Behavioral rituals are equivalent to mental rituals (such as silently repeating numbers) in their functional relationship to distressing obsessions; both serve to reduce obsessional distress. In summary, both behavioral and mental rituals may be performed to prevent harm, restore safety, or reduce distress.

The "functional" view of the relationship of obsessions and compulsions is more evident in the DSM-IV criteria than in the previous edition, and is supported by results of a recently completed DSM-IV field study indicating that 90% of compulsions are viewed by OCD individuals as functionally related to obsessions, and only 10% are perceived as unrelated to obsessions (Foa & Kozak, 1995). Data from the DSM-IV field study indicate that the vast majority (over 90%) of obsessive–compulsives manifest both obsessions and behavioral rituals. When mental rituals are included, only 2% of the sample reported obsessions only.

We have argued elsewhere (Kozak & Foa, 1994) that a continuum of "insight" or "strength of belief" more accurately represents the clinical picture of OCD than the previously prevailing view that obsessive–compulsives recognize the senselessness of their obsessions. There has been a growing consensus about this issue over several years (Insel, & Akiskal, 1986; Foa & Kozak, 1995; Lelliott, Noshirvani, Basoglu, Marks, & Monterio, 1988), and DSM-IV has accommodated this by allowing a subtype of OCD to include those patients "with poor insight" into the senselessness of their obsessional fears.

Prevalence and Course of OCD

No longer thought to be a rare disorder, OCD is now estimated to occur in about 2.5% of the population (Karno, Golding, Sorensen, & Burnam, 1988). Slightly more than half of those suffering from OCD are female (Rasmussen & Tsuang, 1986). Age of onset of the disorder ranges from early adolescence to young adulthood, and with earlier onset in males (modal onset 13- to 15-years-old) than in females (modal onset 20- to 24-years-old; Rasmussen & Eisen, 1990). Development of the disorder is usually gradual, but acute onset has been reported in some cases. Chronic waxing and waning of symptoms is typical; however, episodic and deteriorating courses have been observed in about 10% of patients (Rasmussen & Eisen, 1989).

Many individuals with OCD suffer for years before seeking treatment. In one study, individuals first presented for psychiatric treatment over 7 years after the onset of significant symptoms (Rasmussen & Tsuang, 1986). The disorder is frequently associated with impairments in general functioning, such as disruption of gainful employment and of marital and other interpersonal relationships (Emmelkamp, de Haan, & Hoogduin, 1990; Riggs, Hiss, & Foa, 1992).

Associated Disorders

Symptoms such as depression, anxiety, phobic avoidance, and excessive worry are often comorbid with OCD (Tynes, White, & Steketee, 1990). Rasmussen and Tsuang (1986) found that in a sample of OCD patients, the lifetime incidence of simple phobia was about 30%, for social phobia 20%, and for panic disorder 15%. Approximately 30% of OCD sufferers also meet criteria for major depression, and sleep disturbances have been found in roughly 40% (Karno et al., 1988). Severe depression may impede the efficacy of behavioral treatment of OCD (Foa, 1979; Foa, Grayson, & Steketee, 1982).

A relationship of OCD with eating disorders has also been reported. About 10% of women with OCD had a history of anorexia nervosa (Kasvikis, Tsakiris, Marks, Basoglu, & Noshirvani, 1986), and over 33% of bulimics had a history of OCD (Hudson, Pope, Yurgelun-Todd, Jonas, & Frankenburg, 1987; Laessle, Kittl, Fichter, Wittchen, & Pirke, 1987).

Tourette's syndrome and tics also appear related to OCD. Twenty to thirty percent of individuals with OCD reported a current or past history of tics (Pauls, 1989). Estimates of the comorbidity of Tourette's syndrome and OCD range from 36% to 52% (Leckman & Chittenden, 1990; Pauls, Towbin, Leckman, Zahner, & Cohen, 1986). Interestingly, whereas incidence of OCD among Tourette's sufferers is quite high, the converse is not true, with 5% to 7% of those with OCD thought to suffer from Tourette's syndrome (Rasmussen & Eisen, 1989).

Differential Diagnosis

The high comorbidity of OCD with other disorders sometimes leaves difficult diagnostic questions. The co-occurrence of depression with OCD can give rise to questions about depressive rumination versus obsessions. Mood-congruent ruminations are common in depressed individuals, and their confounding presence can make it difficult to evaluate the severity of obsessive intrusions. Distinctions can be made according to the content of the thoughts and the patients' resistance. Mood-congruent ruminations are pessimistic ideas about the self or the world and, in contrast to obsessions, are not characterized by patients' attempts to ignore or suppress them.

The high rate of a variety of anxiety symptoms among individuals with OCD can complicate diagnosis. For example, generalized anxiety disorder (GAD) is characterized by excessive worries that bear a strong formal resemblance to obsessions, but which, unlike obsessions, are excessive concerns about real-life circumstances and are experienced as appropriate. In contrast, obsessive thinking is more likely to be unrealistic or magical, and obsessions experienced as inappropriate. This algorithm does not obviate all ambiguity, however, for in some cases an obsession involves a real-life threat, but with a greatly exaggerated likelihood estimate. Fortunately, the problem of distinguishing obsessions from worries assumes diagnostic significance primarily when there are no compulsions, and pure obsessionals have been found to be quite rare (Foa & Kozak, 1995).

An analogous situation arises with the symptom of phobic avoidance, which in the absence of rituals can give the diagnostic impression of specific phobia. For example, obsessive fear of germs can lead to avoidance of public rest rooms. Avoidance can become so severe that daily activity is minimized and the individual becomes housebound and appears agoraphobic. Notably however, OCD differs clearly from specific phobia. Specific phobics can successfully reduce distress by escape or avoidance of the feared situation. In contrast, ideas of threat (i.e., obsessive fears) continue to intrude in OCD, despite the absence of the feared situation. This gives rise to those rituals that are the hallmark of most OCD. Thus, the obsessive–compulsive, but not the specific phobic, will exhibit ritualistic behavior.

Hypochondriasis is formally quite similar to OCD. It has been suggested that patients with obsessive concerns about their health who also exhibit somatic checking or excessive physician visits should be diagnosed with OCD and treated accordingly (Rasmussen &

Tsuang, 1986; Rasmussen & Eisen, 1989). A useful way of differentiating the two disorders is by the presence or absence of compulsions. Thus, obsessions about illness combined with rituals such as excessive handwashing would indicate OCD, whereas preoccupation with health without actions taken in pursuit of this concern would indicate hypochondriasis.

A related diagnostic issue arises with body dysmorphic disorder (BDD), the essential feature of which is concern with an imagined physical defect. This preoccupation is sometimes coupled with compulsive checking behavior. The formal parallel with OCD is obvious.

It can sometimes be difficult to differentiate the stereotyped motor behaviors that characterize Tourette's syndrome and tic disorder from compulsions. These behaviors can usually be distinguished from compulsions, in that they are generally experienced as involuntary and are not aimed at neutralizing distress brought about by an obsession. There is no conventional way of differentiating them from "pure" compulsions, but fortunately, OCD with compulsions only is rare (Foa & Kozak, in press).

Individuals with OCD may present with obsessions that are of a delusional intensity (see Kozak & Foa, 1994, for review). It is important not to discount a diagnosis of OCD simply because of such obsessions. Such recognition is reflected in the DSM-IV in the addition of a subtype of OCD "with poor insight." Differentiation of delusional disorder, characterized by persistent nonbizarre delusions, from OCD can depend on the presence of compulsions in OCD. Because OCD is typically characterized by both obsessions and compulsions, obsessions of delusional intensity may be distinguished from delusions of delusional disorder by presence of compulsions.

It is important to recognize that the content of obsessions in OCD may be quite bizarre, as in the delusions of schizophrenia, but that this does not in itself counterindicate OCD. To indicate a diagnosis of schizophrenia, such bizarre ideas must be accompanied by other symptoms of formal thought disorder, such as loose associations, hallucinations, flat or grossly inappropriate affect, and thought insertion or projection. Of course, symptoms of both OCD and schizophrenia can justify a dual diagnosis.

THEORIES

Conditioning Theories

Mowrer's (1939, 1960) two-stage theory for acquisition and maintenance of fear and avoidance behavior has helped learning theorists to understand OCD. Accordingly, a neutral event comes to elicit fear after by being experienced along with an event that itself causes distress, and discomfort can be conditioned to mental events, such as thoughts and images, as well as physical events, such as snakes and spiders. Once fear is acquired, escape or avoidance patterns emerge in the service of fear reduction and are maintained when successful. This is the second, or operant stage, of the hypothesized process.

Mowrer's theory was adopted by Dollard and Miller (1950) to understand obsessive–compulsive neurosis. Unlike the foci of specific phobias, obsessions cannot readily be avoided, because they often occur spontaneously. Thus, passive avoidance tactics used by phobics are often ineffective with obsessional distress, and active avoidance (i.e., compulsive rituals) is developed to counter the obsessions.

Although it is clear that Mowrer's theory is too simple to account for fear acquisition (Rachman & Wilson, 1980), it maps well onto observations about the maintenance of obsessive–compulsive rituals: Obsessions give rise to anxiety/discomfort and compulsions reduce it. Obsessions, as well as confrontation with situations that prompt obsessions, provoke reports of discomfort and elevated cardiac and electrodermal activity (Boulougouris, Rabavilas, & Stefanis, 1977; Hodgson & Rachman, 1972; Hornsveld, Kraaimaat, & van Dam-Baggen, 1979; Kozak, Foa, & Steketee, 1988; Rabavilas & Boulougouris, 1974). Furthermore, obsessive distress routinely decreases following the performance of a ritual (Hodgson & Rachman, 1972; Hornsveld et al., 1979; Roper & Rachman, 1976).

Cognitive Theories

Cognitive theories of OCD abound. Carr (1974), for example, noting that obsessions typically involve exaggerated concerns about health, death, welfare of others, sex, religion, and so on, argued that OCD is founded in ideas of exaggerated negative consequences. This view of obsessions as mistaken beliefs that are similar to the those of generalized anxiety disorder, agoraphobia, and social phobia resembles Beck's (1976) notion that obsessions are mistaken beliefs about harm. McFall and Wollersheim (1979) also observed that obsessive–compulsives harbor mistaken ideas that lead to erroneous perceptions of threat, associated distress, and ritualized attempts to reduce it.

There are several difficulties with these theories that feature mistaken beliefs in a prominent explanatory role in OCD. Not only has presence of specific ideas common to OCD not been established, but the clinical observations suggest that the sort of pessimistic ideas about outcomes, and about perfectionistic criteria for self-worth, are typical in other anxiety disorders, as well as in depression. Curiously, none of the theories addresses the distinctive intrusive character of obsessions that differentiates them from the fearful beliefs of simple phobia. Finally, because the mistaken ideas invoked to account for OCD are so much a part of the obsessive symptoms themselves, those cognitive theories that explain OCD via mistaken beliefs have a faint ring of circularity.

Salkovskis (1985) has offered an elaborate cognitive analysis of OCD. Accordingly, obsessional intrusions are supposed to stimulate certain self-critical beliefs that then cause mood disturbances. Both covert and overt rituals are attempts to reduce such guilt. Furthermore, frequently occurring thoughts about unacceptable actions may be perceived by the obsessive–compulsive individual as representative of the actions themselves.

Salkovskis proposed that five specific assumptions are specifically characteristic of OCD:

1. Thinking of an action is tantamount to its performance.
2. Failing to prevent (or failing to try to prevent) harm to self or others is morally equivalent to causing the harm.
3. Responsibility for harm is not diminished by extenuating circumstances.
4. Failing to ritualize in response to an idea about harm constitutes an intention to harm.
5. One can and should exercise control over one's thoughts.

An interesting implication of this scheme is that whereas obsessive intrusions may be seen by the patient as unacceptable, the mental and overt rituals that it prompts will not. Another implication is that identification and modification of these mistaken assumptions should be a useful treatment approach. Experimental support for this approach is yet unforthcoming.

Other cognitive theorists have focused not so much on mistaken ideas as on impaired cognitive processes. For example, Reed (1985) hypothesized that OCD is characterized by impairments in the organization and integration of experiences, and that certain symptoms (e.g., excessive structuring of activities, strict categorizations) constitute compensatory efforts. Other investigators have found specific memory deficits for actions in compulsive checkers (Sher, Frost, & Otto, 1983; Sher, Frost, Kushner, Crews, & Alexander, 1989) that might play a causal role in OCD.

Patients' doubts about having performed an action may not reflect a memory deficit, but rather, as suggested by Foa and Kozak (1985), an impairment in the way inferences are made about danger. Specifically, they hypothesized that obsessive–compulsives often conclude that a situation is dangerous based on absence of evidence for safety, and fail to make inductive leaps about safety from information about the absence of danger. Consequently, rituals that are performed to reduce the likelihood of harm can never really provide safety and must be repeated. Regardless of whether cognitive deficits lie in memory processes or in transformational rules, it is an open question whether such impairments are general or specific to the processing of threat related information.

In Foa and Kozak's (1985) cognitive approach to anxiety disorders, specific impairments in emotional memory structures were postulated. Following Lang's (1979) bioinformational theory, Foa and Kozak construed anxiety as founded in informational structures in memory that represent fear stimuli, responses, and their meanings. Accordingly, disordered fear memories are characterized by erroneous estimates of threat, high negative valence for the feared event, and excessive response elements that are preparatory for escape or avoidance.

The puzzling persistence of unrealistic fear may reflect failure to access the fear network, either because of active avoidance or because the content of the fear network precludes spontaneous encounters with situations that evoke anxiety. Anxious memories may also persist because of some impairment in the mechanism of extinction. Cognitive defenses, excessive arousal with failure to habituate, faulty premises, and erroneous rules of inference are all potential impairments that could hinder the processing of corrective information.

Foa and Kozak (1985) noted several types of fear structures that occur in obsessive–compulsives. Associations between the stimuli (e.g., toilet seats) and meaning (e.g., a high probability of contracting a venereal disease) are evident in the patient with unrealistic fears of public bathrooms. For other obsessive–compulsives, certain harmless stimuli are strongly associated with distress, without regard to harm. For example, some patients reduce distress about disarray by rearranging objects but do not anticipate any harmful consequences of the disorganization, except that it "just doesn't feel right."

Biological Models

Neurochemical Factors

The prevailing biological account of OCD hypothesizes that abnormal serotonin metabolism is expressed in OCD symptoms. The efficacy of serotonin reuptake inhibitors (SRIs) with OCD has provided the primary impetus for this hypothesis. SRIs have been found more potent with OCD than placebo and several other antidepressant medications such as imipramine, nortriptyline, and amitriptyline (Zohar, & Insel, 1987). Significant correlations between clomipramine (CMI) plasma levels and improvement in OCD suggest that serotonin function mediates obsessive–compulsive symptoms, thus lending further support to the serotonin hypothesis (Insel et al., 1983; Stern, Marks, Wright, Luscombe, 1980).

Studies that directly investigated serotonin functioning in obsessive–compulsives have not been conclusive (Joffe & Swinson, 1991). High correlations between improvement in OCD symptoms and a decrease in the serotonin metabolite 5-hydroxy indoleacetic acid (5-HIAA) were reported in two studies (Flament et al., 1985; Thoren et al., 1980). These results are consistent with the hypothesis that the antiobsessional effects of CMI are mediated by the serotonergic system. Lucy, Butcher, Clare, & Dinan (1993) found that responses to a serotonin agonist, d-fenfluramine, significantly attenuated in OCD, while pituitary response to hypothalamic stimulation (protirelin challenge) was normal. These results point to central serotonergic dysfunction in OCD, rather than pituitary hyperactivity.

There are, however, troubling inconsistencies in the literature on serotonin involvement in OCD. Serotonin platelet uptake studies have failed to differentiate obsessive–compulsives from controls (Insel, Mueller, Alterman, Linnoila, & Murphy, 1985; Weizman et al., 1985). In two studies, Zohar and his colleagues (Zohar, & Insel, 1987; Zohar, Mueller, Insel, Zohar-Kaduch, & Murphy, 1987) found an increase in obsessive–compulsive symptoms following administration of serotonin agonist metachlorophenylpoprazine (mCPP), which disappeared after treatment with CMI. However, administration of mCPP intravenously did not produce an increase in OCD symptoms (Charney et al., 1988).

Neuroanatomical Factors

Several studies suggest a neuroanatomical abnormalities in OCD. Some neuropsychological results have pointed to frontal lobe abnormalities (e.g., Behar, et al., 1984; Cox, Fedio, & Rappaport, 1989; Head, Bolton, & Hymas, 1989), but there have also been inconsistent neuropsychological findings (Insel, Donnely, Lalakea, Alterman, & Murphy, 1983). The success of capsulotomy and cingulotomy with OCD also hints at frontal lobe involvement (Ballentine, Bouckoms, Thomas, & Giriunas, 1987).

Additional evidence for neurobiological abnormalities comes from several positron-emission tomographic studies of cerebral metabolism that have revealed elevated metabolic rates in the prefrontal cortex in OCD (e.g., Scarone et al., 1993). Also suggestive is the association of OCD symptoms with disorders stemming from basal ganglia problems: encephalitis lethargica (Schilder, 1938), Sydenham's chorea (Swedo et al., 1989), and Tourette's syndrome (Rapoport & Wise, 1988).

TREATMENTS

OCD was formerly considered quite intractable: Neither psychodynamic psychotherapy, nor a wide variety of pharmacotherapies has been successful with it (Black, 1974; Perse, 1988). Now, however, there are two treatments of established efficacy: behavior therapy by prolonged exposure and pharmacotherapy with SRIs.

Behavioral Treatments

Early Behavioral Treatments

Despite initial claims of the efficacy of systematic desensitization with OCD, case reports indicated that it helped only 30% of patients (Beech & Vaughn, 1978; Cooper, Gelder, & Marks, 1965). A number of other exposure-oriented procedures has also yielded generally unimpressive results (e.g., paradoxical intention, imaginal flooding, satiation, and aversion relief).

Other learning-based procedures aimed at blocking or punishing obsessions and compulsions, such as thought stopping, aversion therapy, and covert sensitization have also been relatively unsuccessful with OCD. Thought stopping was found to be largely ineffective in several case studies and one controlled study (Emmelkamp & Kwee, 1977; Stern, 1978; Stern, Lipsedge, & Marks, 1975). Aversion procedures such as electric shocks, rubber-band snaps, and covert sensitization have fared somewhat better (Kenny, Mowbray, & Lalani, 1978; Kenny, L. Solyom, & C. Solyom, 1973), but their long-term efficacy has not been determined.

Exposure and Response Prevention

Meyer (1966) successfully treated two cases of OCD with prolonged exposure to obsessional cues and strict prevention of rituals (response prevention), which were subsequently found highly successful in 10 of 15 cases and partly effective in the remainder; only two patients relapsed after 5 to 6 years (Meyer & Levy, 1973; Meyer, Levy, & Schnurer, 1974). Both uncontrolled and controlled studies of exposure and response prevention have been remarkably consistent: 65% to 75% of patients are responders at posttreatment and follow-up (Foa and Kozak, in press).

This treatment entails repeated, prolonged (45 minutes to 2 hours) confrontation with situations that provoke discomfort, and abstinence from rituals, despite strong urges to ritualize. Exposure is usually gradual, with situations provoking moderate distress encountered before more upsetting ones, and treatment sessions often include both imaginal and actual (*in vivo*) exposures. Many hours of additional exposure between treatment sessions are also prescribed. Detailed descriptions of the procedures of exposure treatment are available (e.g., Steketee, 1994).

Exposure. The differential contributions of exposure and response prevention have been determined in a series of studies with obsessive–compulsive patients. The effects of exposure only, response prevention only, and their combination have been evaluated, and the combination treatment was found to be more potent at both posttreatment and follow-up than were the two individual components. Moreover, the two components affect symptoms differently: Exposure reduced obsessional distress, whereas response prevention reduced rituals (Foa, Steketee, Grayson, Turner, & Latimer, 1984; Foa, Steketee, & Milby, 1980; Steketee, Foa, & Grayson, 1982).

The combination of *in vivo* and imaginal exposure seems to afford no advantage over *in vivo* exposure immediately posttreatment, but does at follow-up, where there is somewhat less relapse after the combined procedure (Foa, Steketee, Turner, and Fischer, 1980). *In vivo* exposure alone is sometimes practically insufficient to address the feared catastrophes that characterize some obsessions (e.g., eternal hellfire) that can be realized imaginally. Also, supplementing *in vivo* exposure with imagery exercises might circumvent the counterproductive defensive tactics of "cognitive avoiders."

In principle, fear reduction does not depend on whether anxiety-provoking stimuli are presented hierarchically, beginning with the least distressing stimulus and proceeding to the most distressing, or if the most distressing stimulus is presented at the outset of treatment (Hodgson, Rachman, & Marks, 1972). In practice, however, it appears that patients prefer a gradual approach. Typically, situations of moderate difficulty are confronted first, followed by several intermediate steps before the most distressing exposure is accomplished. If a patient underestimates the difficulty of certain situations, additional intermediate steps can be interpolated. It is important, however, not to delay the most difficult exposures until the end of the treatment, lest insufficient time be available for habituation to these most distressing situations.

It has been difficult to document the therapist's contribution to successful outcome of exposure therapy. Although patients often seem more willing to confront feared situations in the presence of the therapist, particularly if the therapist confronts the situation first, the therapist's modeling of the exposure exercises has not been demonstrated to help (Rachman, Marks, & Hodgson, 1973). Evaluations of the contribution of a therapist have yielded inconsistent results. In one study, patients who received therapist-aided exposure fared better immediately posttreatment than a group who received clomipramine and self-exposure, but this advantage disappeared at the 1-year follow-up (Marks et al., 1988). In another study, no immediate posttreatment differences were found between the effects of self-exposure and those of 10 sessions of *in vivo* exposure conducted by a therapist (Emmelkamp & van Krannen, 1977). In both conditions, however, the therapist developed a list of exposure items, and the patient determined the exposure schedule.

Failure to demonstrate therapist's contributions in exposure therapy for OCD is surprising, particularly in light of the demonstration by Öst and Salkovskis (1991) that the therapist does indeed facilitate improvement via exposure treatment with specific phobias. Several factors might account for the inconsistent findings about the absence of analogous therapist's effects with OCD. First, there was some therapist's involvement even in the self-exposure conditions, thus decreasing potential effect size. Second, sample size of the studies was relatively small, so that power to detect anything less than large therapist's effect sizes was limited. Third, sessions were less frequent (weekly) and less numerous (10) than is typical in the intensive programs that have achieved the most impressive outcomes, and thus may have afforded less therapist's contact time than might have been optimal for detecting therapist's effects. Given these complications, it would be premature to draw strong conclusions about therapist's contributions in exposure therapy for OCD from the available studies of this phenomenon.

Duration of exposure definitely matters: Prolonged continuous exposure is better than short, interrupted exposure (Rabavilas, Boulougouris, & Stefanis, 1976). However, there is still the question: "How much time is time enough?" The simple answer is not some optimal time parameter, but rather that exposure should be long enough for a noticeable decrease in distress to occur. The required exposure time seems to differ among anxiety disorders as well as among individuals. For OCD, there is no fast rule about required exposure duration, but 90 minutes is a useful rule of thumb (Foa & Chambless, 1978; Rachman, DeSilva, & Roper, 1976).

Ideal frequency of exposure sessions has not been ascertained. The intensive behavior-therapy programs that have achieved the most impressive results typically involve daily sessions, but favorable outcomes have also been achieved with more widely spaced meetings.

Response Prevention. In some inpatient facilities, actions are taken to actually prevent the patient from performing rituals (e.g., turning off water supply in patient's room). But in outpatient treatment, it is primarily the patient's responsibility to *choose* to abstain from rituals. Thus, the term "response prevention" is really a misnomer for the voluntary abstinence that is usually part of outpatient behavior-therapy programs for OCD. Even with the daily 2-hour sessions that often characterize intensive outpatient programs, there are still 22 hours per day remaining in which the patient must practice the self-discipline of abstinence. Thus, it is vitally important to persuade the patient of the necessity of this component of the program, so that there is sufficient motivation for its successful completion.

Although exposure reduces obsessional distress, it does not in itself eliminate compulsions, which can develop some independent habit strength. To reduce the urges to ritualize, patients must practice refraining from ritualistic behavior. Self-monitoring of both urges to ritualize and of violations of the abstinence rules can be used to enhance awareness of the processes surrounding ritualization. In addition, a friend or family member can be designated as a support person who can encourage the patient to resist urges to ritualize by offering reminders of its rationale (but not by coercion).

Abstinence from rituals is of demonstrated importance, but procedures have differed from study to study, ranging from normal washing without supervision to complete abstinence from washing for several days under continuous supervision. The level of supervision does not appear to significantly affect treatment outcome, but the strictness of the rules themselves may matter. We have observed that, perhaps counterintuitively, patients better comply with strict instructions that minimize demands to decide if a particular action is normal or ritualized.

Mental rituals can be harder to overcome than overt motor acts if the patient has difficulty distinguishing between two related mental events: the urge to perform the ritual and the ritual itself. In such cases, the patient will perceive little capacity for self-control. Therapists can help patients distinguish obsessional intrusions from mental rituals aimed at getting rid of obsessions. Once this distinction is clear to the patient, he or she can choose to abstain from the mental rituals. The distinction is also important, because behavior therapy requires deliberate confrontation with obsessive intrusions, but systematic abstinence from rituals.

Repeated requests for assurances about safety are common in OCD but may not be recognized as rituals, because not every inquiry is compulsive; however, when multiple inquiries yield no new information and are motivated by obsessional fear, they are indeed compulsions, and must be proscribed along with all other rituals. Accordingly, the patient should be enjoined by the therapist from assurance *seeking*, and customary assurance providers in the patient's social environment should be enjoined by the patient from assurance *giving*.

A noncompliant social environment, although therapeutic, often initially prompts anxiety, anger, or both in the patient when requests for assurance are denied. It can be helpful if the therapist prepares the patient for this by rehearsal of such refusals. For example, a man who was concerned with perfectionistic actions routinely asked his spouse to wait for him while he performed very subtle rituals. Prior to treatment, they agreed that if he asked her to wait for him, she would first ask if he were having an urge to ritualize. Upon his acknowledgment of a compulsive urge, she would remind him of their mutual understanding that his best interest would be served by her refusal to wait and by his resistance of the urge, and that she would then go on without him, in the hope that he would be able to do what was best for himself.

Cognitive Therapy

The efficacy of cognitive procedures used in conjunction with exposure techniques for OCD has been suggested by case reports of successful outcomes (Salkovskis & Warwick, 1985; Kearney & Silverman, 1990). Emmelkamp and colleagues found that the effects of six sessions of cognitive therapy, based on Ellis's (1962) ABC techniques, did not differ from those of self-controlled exposure and response prevention (Emmelkamp, Visser, & Hoekstra, 1988), and that exposure plus response prevention was not enhanced by the addition of cognitive therapy (Emmelkamp & Beens, 1991). Thus, evidence on the efficacy of formal cognitive therapy with OCD is sketchy, and does not clearly support its use with this disorder.

Serotonergic Medications

Pharmacotherapy with certain SRIs has proven to be effective for OCD. The trycyclic antidepressant clomipramine (Anafranil) was the first FDA-approved compound with an indication for OCD, and its usefulness has been documented in several double-blind controlled trials (DeVeaugh-Geiss, Landau, & Katz, 1989; Marks, Stern, Mawson, Cobb, & McDonald, 1980; Thoren, Asberg, Chronholm, Jornestedt, & Traskman, 1980; Zohar & Insel, 1987). More recently, fluoxetine (Prozac) has also been established as an effective antiobsessive agent (Fontaine & Chouinard, 1985; Jenike, Buttolph, Baer, Ricciardi, & Holland, 1989; Montgomery et al., 1993). Another SRI, fluvoxamine (Luvox), has also been found effective (Goodman et al., 1989b; Montgomery & Manceaux, 1992; Price, Goodman, Charney, & Heninger, 1987; Perse, Griest, & Jefferson, Rosenfeld, & Dor, 1987).

The various studies of SRIs revealed responder rates of up to approximately 60%, but symptom reductions are quite modest, averaging 5–8 points on the Yale–Brown Obsessive–Compulsive Scale (Y–BOCS). Conclusions about the relative efficacy of the different SRIs are difficult in the absence of head-to-head comparisons. However, Greist, Jefferson, Kobak, Katzelnick, and Serlin conducted a meta-analysis of large-scale, double-blind controlled studies that suggests clomipramine is superior to fluoxetine, fluvoxamine, and sertraline, which do not themselves differ from one another in efficacy.

Improvements with SRIs seem to depend heavily on continuation of the pharmacotherapy, and relapse is evident after discontinuation (Thoren et al., 1980). Ninety percent of a group who had improved with clomipramine were found to relapse within a few weeks after a blind drug withdrawal (Pato, Zohar-Kadouch, Zohar, & Murphy, 1988). Notwithstanding the somewhat lower relapse rate that has been found after withdrawal from fluoxetine (Fontaine & Chouinard, 1989; Mallya, White, Waternaux, & Quay, 1992), the problem is substantial for this compound as well.

Combined Behavioral and Pharmacotherapies

The availability of two treatments that are partially effective individually has spawned a handful of investigations of their combined efficacy. Major improvement following behavior therapy, with a small additive effect of clomipramine, was found in 40 obsessive–compulsives immediately posttreatment by Marks and associates (1980). However, the drug-only period was too short (4 weeks) to allow for optimal assessment of the efficacy of clomipramine alone. In a subsequent comparison of clomipramine and exposure treatment in 49 obsessive–compulsives, Marks et al. (1988) found that adjunctive medication had a small transitory (8 week) additive effect: Again, exposure was more potent than clomipramine. Although the design of the study did not allow evaluation of the long-term effects of behavior therapy, a 6-year follow-up of 34 of the patients included in the aforementioned study revealed no drug effect, and long-term improvement was associated with better compliance during exposure treatment (O'Sullivan, Noshirvani, Marks, Monterio, & Lelliott, 1991).

Fluvoxamine and behavior therapy have been found to produce comparable reductions in obsessive–compulsive symptoms immediately after treatment and at 6-month follow-up, and behavior therapy plus fluvoxamine produced slightly greater improvement in depression than did behavior therapy alone (Cottraux et al., 1990). The superiority of the combined treatment for depression, however, was not evident at follow-up.

At the Medical College of Pennsylvania, an uncontrolled study examined the long-term effects (mean 1.5 years posttreatment) of intensive behavior therapy and fluvoxamine or clomipramine in 62 patients with OCD (Hembree, Cohen, Riggs, Kozak, & Foa, 1992). Patients had been treated with serotonergic drugs, intensive behavior therapy, or behavior therapy plus one of the two medications. Patients who were taking medication at follow-up ($N = 25$) did equally well regardless of whether they had received behavior therapy plus medication or medication alone. However, patients who were medication-free at follow-up ($N = 37$) showed a different pattern: Those who had received behavior therapy alone or behavior therapy plus medication were less symptomatic than those who had received medication alone. Thus, patients treated with behavior therapy maintained their gains more than patients treated with serotonergic medication that was subsequently withdrawn.

ASSESSMENT

In addition to conducting a diagnostic interview to ascertain presence of OCD, it is valuable to quantify the severity of OCD symptoms with valid and reliable instruments in order to evaluate how successful treatment was for a given patient. In our clinic, we use the following assessment instruments:

The Yale–Brown Obsessive–Compulsive Scale

The Yale–Brown Obsessive–Compulsive Scale (Y–BOCS; Goodman et al., 1989a,b) is a commonly used instrument for assessing the nature and severity of OCD symptoms. This is a semistructured interview consisting of a symptom checklist and a severity rating scale. The severity scale has five items about obsessions and five about compulsions, each rated on a 5-point scale ranging from 0 (No Symptoms) to 4 (Severe Symptoms). Overall severity is rated according to time spent on obsessions and compulsions, interference with functioning, distress associated with obsessive–compulsive symptoms, resistance to the symptoms, and control over the symptoms. The Y–BOCS has satisfactory interrater reliability, internal consistency, and validity (Goodman et al., 1989a, 1989b) and has been found sensitive to treatment effects in many studies of OCD.

Assessor Ratings

Clinicians rate the patient's three primary target fears, avoidances, and rituals on on 8-point Likert-type rating scales. For example, if the main contaminant is feces, the primary avoidance item selected for rating might be sitting on toilets in public rest rooms. The primary ritual might be handwashing. Severity rating of rituals is based on both the frequency and duration of the ritualistic behavior. For example, the severity rating of a ritual that occurs 75 times a day and lasts only 30 seconds each time would be based on the high frequency, whereas the severity of a ritual that occurs only twice a day and takes 90 minutes to complete would be determined by the time spent on the ritual.

Although researchers have used these and similar ratings in treatment-outcome studies of OCD (e.g., Emmelkamp & Beens, 1991; Foa et al., 1983-b; Foa, Grayson, & Steketee, 1982; Marks et al., 1988; O'Sullivan et al., 1991), information about their psychometric properties is scarce. The scales appear to have adequate interrater agreement when completed by two independent assessors (Foa et al., 1983b), but there is less agreement between the ratings of therapists and patients (Foa, Steketee, Kozak, & Dugger, 1985). Support for the validity of these rating scales is derived mainly from their demonstrated sensitivity to therapeutic change.

Obsessive–Compulsive Checklist

This 38-item questionnaire version of the Compulsive Activity Checklist (CAC) has been found to be reliable, valid, and sensitive to treatment change (Freund, 1986). It was derived from the Obsessive–Compulsive Interview Checklist (Philpott, 1975; Marks, Hallam, Connelly, & Philpott, 1977), an assessor–rated measure of the extent to which OCD interferes with daily functioning.

Several other questionnaire measures of OCD symptoms are available, but have the disadvantage that they assess only certain forms of obsessive–compulsive behavior and/or include items unrelated to OCD symptoms (Leyton Obsessional Inventory (LOI); Kazarian, Evans, & Lefave, 1977; Lynfield Obsessional–Compulsive Questionnaire (LOCQ); Allen & Tune, 1975; Maudsley Obsessive–Compulsive Inventory (MOCI); Hodgson & Rachman, 1977).

TREATMENT PLANNING

Before beginning the exposure exercises, 4 to 6 hours are required for treatment planning with the patient. Several goals must be achieved during these sessions. First, information necessary for treatment planning must be obtained. Specific situations that prompt obsessional distress, avoidance, and rituals must be enumerated for the purpose of developing a list of exposure exercises. Second, feared consequences of not performing rituals must be identified, so that imaginal exposure scripts can be developed. Third, the rationale and therapy procedures must be reiterated so that the patient is thoroughly persuaded of their importance, rather than intimidated into compliance. Finally, it is during the treatment-planning hours that good rapport with the patient should be developed. A caring and honest approach by the therapist may help to encourage the patient to confront feared situations despite the resulting distress.

Obsessional distress may be provoked by either physical events in the patient's external environment, or by mental events (thoughts, images, or impulses that the person experiences). Avoidance and rituals are both aimed at minimizing distress associated with the threatening events. Avoidance and rituals may be covert (i.e., cognitive avoidance or rituals) and thus not directly observable, or overt.

Information about OCD Symptoms

Environmental Cues (Objects, Situations, Places)

Most obsessive–compulsives react to discernible physical events (objects, persons, or situations) that evoke obsessional distress. The specific details of the precipitants, however, differ among patients. For example, two individuals who fear contracting human immuno-deficiency virus (HIV) may have quite different ideas of what constitutes dangerous situations. One patient may fear only contact with individuals suspected to be high risk for HIV, whereas another may fear all surfaces contacted by individuals of uncertain HIV status. Similarly, two patients may be afraid of causing auto accidents, whereas only one of them may be especially concerned with hitting small children.

It is important to identify the perceived threat associated with fear cues. Otherwise, exposure exercises might not adequately address obsessional fear. Confronting situations that actually provoke obsessional fear is essential for successful exposure treatment of OCD, and understanding what the patient perceives as threatening about the feared situations permits development of exposure exercises that correct such perceptions.

If mistaken perceptions or beliefs of harm are not corrected during exposure treatment, the patient is probably at elevated risk for relapse, because such perceptions will engender anxiety and distress that will motivate avoidance and rituals. For example, a patient whose fear of driving during daytime on bright city streets decreased via practice with the therapist may relapse upon returning home where he or she must drive on dark country roads at night. The opposite situation may hold for the patient who successfully practices driving on uncrowded suburban streets and returns fearfully to busy, urban congestion. These examples illustrate why it is important to ascertain what the person perceives as dangerous about driving: Is it crowds of pedestrians or dark deserted roads? The answer has implications for planning the exposure exercises.

An exhaustive inquiry about what evokes obsessional distress is an important part of treatment planning. The patient can be asked to rate how evoking different situations are in subjective units of distress (SUDs) ranging from 0 to 100. The following dialog exemplifies this type of inquiry:

T: When do you get the urge to repeat certain actions?
P: Everywhere. It happens all the time.
T: In what situations does it happen more often than others?
P: Well, when I am moving from place to place, or picking up objects.
T: How upset do you get when you have to pick up an object on the distress scale?
P: That's bad. I guess about a 70.
T: Can you tell me what is upsetting about that?
P: Not really, it just has to feel right when I do it, and it usually doesn't feel right the first time.
T: How do you know when it feels right?
P: Well, there isn't anything in particular. It just feels that way.
T: What is upsetting about moving from place to place?
P: The same thing. It usually doesn't feel right.
T: What would feel right?
P: Well, I have to pause at certain objects, like a chair, or a doorway, before going on, or else it just doesn't feel right.
T: So, if you walked quickly from place to place without pausing, it would be distressing for you, and you would get an urge to go back and retrace your steps and pause, until it feels right?
P: Yes, that's it. It doesn't make any sense, really, but that's how I feel at the time.
T: Have you tried to move quickly from place to place without pausing at objects?
P: Not really.
T: What would you rate your distress when you feel that you haven't paused properly?
P: 85.

It is clear from this interchange that the patient did not fear objects or places. Rather, the object or situation gave rise to a perception than an action had been done "wrong," and this perception is the most important aspect of the fear.

Mental Fear Cues (Thoughts, Images, Impulses)

Certain unacceptable thoughts, images, or impulses can themselves provoke obsessional fear, shame, or disgust. Examples include impulses to harm a loved one, thoughts of accidental injury to a loved one, or images of blasphemous sexual activity with sacred personages. Of course, such mental events may be prompted by the patient's environment, but the unacceptability of a thought is the focus of the distress. Interoceptive events may also prompt obsessive distress. For example, a headache could prompt the patient's fear of going insane, along with urges to seek assurances from others about his sanity.

Sometimes patients hesitate to describe an obsession because they fear that just thinking about it or describing it is in itself harmful. It can be useful to tell the patient that many people with and without OCD have unwanted thoughts (as many as 85% of normal individuals; Rachman & DeSilva, 1978), and to state clearly that merely having an abhorrent thought is not dangerous, and is not tantamount to acting according to the thought. Without accurate descriptions of the obsessions, relevant exposure exercises cannot be designed. The following interchange illustrates an inquiry designed to encourage a patient to disclose unacceptable thoughts.

T: So tell me, when is it that you feel the urge to pray?
P: When I have bad thoughts?
T: What kind of thoughts?
P: I don't want to say them.
T: What would happen if you say them?
P: God wouldn't like it.
T: What would be troublesome about that for you?
P: I'd be punished.
T: How?
P: I'm not sure, but I could go to hell.
T: I understand now how talking about the bad thoughts would be difficult and uncomfortable for you, but if I am to know how to help you, it will be important that you let me know what specific thoughts are bothering you. Many people with OCD have problems with unwanted thoughts that they find unacceptable, and people without OCD also get unacceptable ideas. I am accustomed to this kind of difficulty and have been able to help people with it. The first step, however, is for you to describe the thoughts, even though you feel anxious about this. As long as you keep trying to keep the thoughts out of your mind, they will continue to bother you. On the other hand, if you are willing to tell me what they are, I might be able to help you overcome them.
P: I'd really rather not. Can't we talk about something else.
T: It is important that I know what the thoughts are in order to plan your treatment. I'll try to help you. Do the thoughts involve hurting someone?
P: No, not really.
T: Do you have bad thoughts about God or religious figures?
P: Yes, but I hate to have those kind of thoughts.
T: Are you a religious person?
P: I don't go to church, but I believe in God.
T: Could you give me an example of one of the bad thoughts so that I can start to understand what is bothering you?

P: Well, I get different images; sometimes I get images of doing something I'm not supposed to do and sometimes images of others doing bad things. I really don't want to say anymore.

T: I know this is scary, but if you don't tell me more about what is bothering you, I won't know how to help with it. What do you imagine yourself doing that is bad?

P: It is sexual.

T: Other people have had sexual thoughts that are sacrilegious. Sometimes they imagine religious figures having sex, or themselves having sex with religious figures. What sort of distressing images are you having?

P: One of the bad ones is the virgin Mary having sex with the devil.

T: It is good that you were willing to describe that image to me, even though it was uncomfortable for you. You said that you see yourself in the images? What are you doing with them?

P: That's even worse, because I have sex with Jesus and the devil at the same time.

T: How do you feel when these images occur?

P: Anxious, disgusted, and guilty.

T: It is not surprising that you don't want to have these images, and that you try to avoid them or get rid of them if they make you feel so bad about yourself. We will develop exposure exercises that will reduce how much they bother you.

Anticipated Harm (e.g., Feared Disastrous Consequences)

The idea that harm will ensue from exposure to feared situations or from failure to perform rituals is often an important component of obsessive fear. Ideas of illness, disability, or death are frequently associated with contaminants for individuals with washing compulsions. Ideas of harm consequent to acts of omission or commission can provoke excessive checking of performance and its aftermath. However, not all individuals with OCD articulate clear hypotheses of harmful consequences associated with their obsessions. Some report only vague notions of harm, or they are mainly concerned that their own anxiety will harm them. Others completely deny ideas of harm and are puzzled about why they are so intensely distressed by patently harmless situations.

Identification of anticipated harm is prerequisite to developing a useful exposure agenda. Exposure situations that do not provoke the patient's obsessional ideas about harm, when such ideas are present, will not be very useful. For example, if a patient is concerned that children, but not adults, are vulnerable to incompetent driving, practicing driving near adults will probably not be beneficial. It is also important to match the patient's anticipated disasters with those detailed in imaginal exposure scripts, and such matching can sometimes be subtle. For example, imagery of *contracting* a disease from contaminants would not be very helpful for a patient whose primary concern is *communicating* a disease to others.

Strength of Belief

Some obsessive–compulsives do not regard their symptoms as unreasonable or excessive, and the traditional assumption that all patients have this insight is subject to revision. Recognition that irrational, fixed beliefs can characterize obsessive–compulsive thinking has led to consideration of the presence of overvalued ideas (OVIs) and delusions in patients diagnosed with OCD (for review, see Kozak & Foa, 1994).

A recent attempt to clarify the distinctions can be found in the DSM-IV. *Obsessions* are defined as "persistent ideas, thoughts, impulses, or images that are experienced as intrusive and inappropriate," and there are "attempts to ignore or suppress such thoughts or neutralize them with some other thought or action" (p. 418). An *overvalued idea* is an "unreasonable and sustained belief or idea that is maintained with less than delusional intensity" (p. 769), and about which the person can acknowledge the possibility of its falsehood. By implication however, it differs from an obsessional thought in that the person does not recognize its absurdity and thus does not struggle against it. Thus, the OVI is an *almost* unshakable belief that can be acknowledged as potentially unfounded only after considerable discussion. A *delusion* is defined as a false personal belief based on an incorrect inference about external reality that is firmly sustained in spite of what almost everyone else believes, and despite what constitutes incontrovertible and obvious proof or evidence to the contrary" (p. 765). It follows that OVIs are distinguished from delusions by their *less* than delusional intensity: OVIs are strongly held, unreasonable beliefs that are not as firmly held as delusional ideas.

Janet (1908) and, later, Schneider (1925) specified the following criteria for OCD: 1) subjective feeling of being forced, or compelled to think, feel, or act; 2) content of the obsession is perceived as absurd or nonsensical and ego alien; 3) the obsession is resisted. These criteria notwithstanding, studies of strength of belief in OCD have revealed that many obsessive–compulsives do not "fit" this definition (Foa & Kozak, in press; Insel & Akiskal, 1986).

Following Lewis (1935), Solyom, Sookman, Solyom, and Morton (1985) noted that not all obsessive patients report the subjective feeling of forced thoughts or action, nor do they all recognize the senselessness of their obsessions or rituals. Solyom et al. (1985) noted Schneider's observation that in some patients with OCD, insight was present only "upon quiet reflection." Clinicians experienced with OCD recognize that insight into the senselessness of obsessive–compulsive fears is often situation-bound: An individual is more likely to demonstrate insight under nonthreatening conditions, that is, when there is no impending contact with the feared situation. Thus, when patients are asked during a clinical interview how they assess danger "objectively," they seem more likely to show insight than when they are afraid.

Some studies of "atypical" obsessive–compulsives (i.e., those with very strongly held obsessional beliefs) have suggested poorer prognoses (Foa, 1979; Solyom et al., 1985), whereas others have found no relationship between strength of belief and treatment outcome (Eisen & Rasmussen, in press; Lelliott et al., 1988; Basoglu, Lax, Kasvikis, & Marks, 1988).

It is important to note that insight into the senselessness of obsessions varies across and within patients. Some readily acknowledge that their obsessional beliefs are irrational but nevertheless distressing, whereas others firmly believe that their obsessions and compulsions are rational. In most patients, though, the strength of belief seems to fluctuate across situations, thus complicating the assessment. The following dialogue exemplifies an inquiry about the strength of a patient's obsessional belief.

T: If you don't retrace your route, do you really think that you will miss seeing someone that you've injured on the road?

P: Well, that's how I feel.

T: So, do you really believe that you are killing people on the roads, and that if you don't check, you won't see the trail of bodies that you are leaving behind?

P: Well, I'm not sure, but I guess when you put it that way it doesn't sound very rational, does it?

T: It is very unlikely that you would hit someone with your car and not know it.

P: It is hard to explain. When I'm here I can see that it doesn't make sense, but when I'm driving on the road, I can't tell whether my fear is realistic. It feels like I really could have hit someone and I get very anxious and I have to check.

T: Do you think that you are an especially bad driver?

P: I'm not sure. No, I guess I drive okay.

T: Have you ever hit someone while you were driving?

P: I don't think so, but I'm not really sure.

T: Do you think that other people retrace their routes to check for accidents?

P: I guess not.

T: If you drove home after the session, and did not look in your mirror for accidents, and did not drive back at all to check, would that be negligent on your part?

P: I'm not sure. This is confusing. I can see right now that what I do isn't rational, but it seems rational to me when I'm driving, and I get very anxious then. That's when I get stuck doing the checking.

Avoidance and Rituals

Because the practice of avoidance and rituals sustains obsessive fear, it is important that they be carefully listed and eliminated. Because it is unlikely that the therapist's inquiry can elicit every avoidance or ritual that the patient does, it is important to help the patient understand their function in maintaining fear, and to encourage the patient to notice specific instances and to report them to the therapist spontaneously. If the patient can confront a situation he or she usually avoids without distress, the avoidance is probably irrelevant to the OCD, and need not be addressed further in therapy. The more strongly a patient protests such an experiment, the more likely it is that the avoided situation is related to obsessional fear, and the more important it is to confront it during exposure therapy.

Many forms of fearful avoidance are readily understood by both the patient and the therapist (e.g., squatting over a toilet seat or avoiding public toilets completely, avoiding driving, avoiding sharp objects). However, subtle avoidance is also common and must be addressed as well. For example, a patient may limit his or her excursions from home according to how long it takes to develop a full bladder, because only the toilet at home is used. Tab-top beverage cans may be avoided in favor of capped bottles, and dented cans or marred boxes in supermarkets may be taboo. Socks may be avoided in favor of loose slippers only, because donning socks requires touching the feet. Even astute observation by the therapist will not reveal every subtle avoidance, so training the patient in self-observation to recognize such avoidance is essential for its elimination.

As with avoidance, both blatant and subtle forms of rituals must be identified and eliminated for successful therapy. Detection of mental rituals relies primarily on the patient's self-observation. Therefore, the therapist must teach the patient to recognize and report them so that they can be addressed during treatment. The majority of patients with OCD exhibit some mental rituals (Foa & Kozak, 1995), and their neglect during assessment and treatment can seriously compromise treatment outcome.

Sometimes patients find the act of ritualizing to be distressing, rather than anxiety reducing, as is commonly supposed. This can yield paradoxical situations when the patient avoids certain situations or actions because they involve distressing rituals. For example, someone who is excessively concerned with cleanliness may live in filthy surroundings, because ritualized cleaning is an ordeal to be avoided. Someone who is excessively concerned with neatness and order might leave belongings in a clutter of unpacked boxes because the perfectionistic unpacking, sorting, and arranging of the items would be too distressing.

Because of the aversiveness of some rituals, avoidance may expand to the point that the patient falsely appears to be agoraphobic. When feelings of contamination entail 3-hour showers, sterilization or discarding of clothing, and painstaking cleaning of all surfaces in the home, the patient sometimes just gives up venturing outside, where contaminants abound.

In some cases, new rituals emerge to replace those that have been eliminated, thus calling to mind that *shibboleth* of psychodynamic theorists, "symptom substitution." For example, a patient who stops decontaminating with alcohol might use chlorine bleach instead. Subtler switches are evident in the driving phobic who gives up checking for accidents in the rearview mirror, replacing this with avid monitoring of radio news programs for reports of hit-and-run accidents, or with systematic reliance on a passenger's silence as an indirect assurance that no accident has occurred.

History Taking

Patients often cannot describe the circumstances surrounding onset of their OCD symptoms, either because such onset was so gradual that there was no obvious starting point, or because it began so long ago that the memory has since faded. Obtaining detailed information about onset of OCD symptoms is not prerequisite to successful treatment by behavior therapy; however, such information may lead to hypotheses about the nature of the patient's fear, and thus point to exposure exercises that may be useful.

Inquiry about outcome of previous pharmacotherapy and/or psychotherapy is important. Sometimes patients have received inadequate treatments. For example, some have received medications that have not been found useful with OCD, or nonstandard dosages or durations of SRIs. In such cases, communication with the treating physician is essential if the therapist is to ascertain the rationale and outcome of previous treatments, and to help the patient understand his or her treatment options. Alternatively, patients may have been told by their psychotherapist that their OCD stems from internal conflicts dating from childhood, and that discussing their anger, (e.g., at a parent) is a preferred therapeutic technique. For patients who have found either pharmacotherapy or psychotherapy unsatisfactory, it may be advisable to summarize the evidence on the efficacy of various treatments for OCD, so as to provide encouragement and clear direction for therapeutic efforts.

If the patient has received behavioral therapy, it was inadequate unless it involved prolonged exposure to the patient's most feared situations and abstinence from rituals. Examples of inadequate behavioral therapy include weekly exposure sessions between which the patient returns to avoidance and rituals, exposure regimens that do not address the most feared situations (e.g., discarding junk mail without discarding amassed hoards of other junk), and a regimen of ritual abstinence that neglects to address mental rituals.

A good working hypothesis about failure of any previous behavioral therapy can help minimize duplication of insufficiencies in a behavioral retreatment. Ignorance of the nature of a patient's previous difficulties and an attendant lack of systematic efforts to help the patient circumvent such problems can condemn the retreatment to repetition of an unsuccessful history. Thus, if the patient did not comply with previous instructions for ritual abstinence, a hypothesis about this should be developed and a corrective procedure implemented. If the patient dutifully performed assigned exposure exercises but did not achieve relief, the inadequacy of the exposure tasks should be understood, and more effective exercises developed.

It is not unusual that an adequate prior treatment has yielded a partial response, and the patient is seeking additional relief. This is often the experience of patients treated successfully with SRIs, the best of which generally produce symptom reductions of about 40%. Such patients frequently seek behavioral treatment either to augment the gains achieved with the medication or to allow medication withdrawal to eliminate side effects. Some simply do not want to continue taking the medicine indefinitely.

Daily Functioning

Obsessive–compulsive symptoms may severely disrupt routine activities and thus impair general functioning; and this impact should be assessed. Exposure exercises targeted at symptoms that cause such impairments can be coupled with instructions to resume adaptive functioning in the previously disrupted area. For example, one patient experienced difficulties making sales calls because of retracing his path when driving, and had therefore avoided sales assignments in favor of office work. Treatment included driving practice, and he was instructed to resume making sales calls. Self-maintenance tasks and tasks involved in the care of children (e.g., laundry, cooking, shopping, etc.) can also be practiced in conjunction with exposure exercises. Simulation of occupational performance can be a less satisfactory but useful therapy technique when actual job duties cannot be realized during the treatment period.

Assessment should include an evaluation of how others cooperate in the maintenance of the patient's symptoms. If the patient demands assurances of safety from others, or cooperation in avoidance or rituals (e.g., family members must remove their shoes before entering the house, or check locks or appliances for the patient), this must be addressed. The patient must enter an agreement with the other people involved not to seek to involve them in OCD symptoms, and the interested others must agree not to cooperate in such symptoms. The therapist can role-play appropriate responses to prohibited requests to prepare the patient's friends or family for situations in which the patient seeks collaboration in OCD despite the agreement not to do so.

Mood State

Although some research has suggested that depression may limit the efficacy of behavior therapy for OCD (Foa, et al., 1982; Foa, Grayson, Steketee, & Doppelt, 1983a; Marks, 1977; Rachman & Hodgson, 1980), other findings have indicated that moderately depressed patients respond well to exposure-based therapy (Foa, Kozak, Steketee, & McCarthy, 1992). Highly depressed patients can be expected to have difficulty adhering to a challenging behavioral therapy regimen, and premedication of such patients with an established antidepressant, particularly one of the SRIs with demonstrated antiobsessive effects, is usually advisable.

Choice of Treatment

How should a patient choose among the available treatments? Prolonged exposure and SRIs are the only established treatments, so the choice is between either of these or their combination. No therapy is effective with all patients, and no useful predictors of individual outcome with the different therapies are available. Uncontrolled comparisons of exposure and SRIs suggest stronger and more durable effects for BT (Hembree et al., 1995), but definitive, controlled trials have not been published. Preliminary findings of a controlled double-blind multicenter comparison of clomipramine, behavioral therapy, and their combination indicate that behavioral therapy has stronger effects than clomipramine, and that both procedures instigated simultaneously are equivalent to behavioral therapy alone (Foa et al., 1993). Pretreatment with clomipramine, followed by behavioral therapy, has been found marginally superior to behavioral therapy alone (Marks et al., 1980; 1988), but because premedication periods were short, the additive contribution of initial pharmacotherapy might have been underestimated. Based solely on considerations of efficacy, monotherapy with behavioral therapy is preferable to pharmacotherapy alone. It remains unclear whether a combination of behavioral therapy plus pharmacotherapy yields generally superior outcome to that of behavioral therapy alone. As mentioned earlier, for seriously depressed patients, pretreatment with an established SRI should be considered. The following text provides a model for offering treatment recommendations to patients.

T: The purpose of our interview is for me to give you the results of your evaluation and to help you decide what, if any, treatment you would receive.

It is clear that the difficulties you are having fit into the category of obsessive–compulsive disorder. You may have already been aware of that, but our first task is to discover whether the problems you are having match the treatments in which we specialize, so that we know how to advise you. Your OCD is of (mild, moderate, severe) intensity, compared to others we have evaluated. It is considered (mild, moderate, severe) because (specify details of comparative distress and impairment). Your future experience with OCD, if it is not treated, is difficult to predict, because there is almost no evidence about spontaneous recovery over the long term. We do know that in the short term there is very little spontaneous improvement—probably in about 5% of individuals. Some people who come for treatment have described a gradual worsening of OCD symptoms over years, and many have said that their symptoms are variable—getting worse or better from time to time, particularly depending on stressful events in their lives.

It makes sense to assume that unless you receive treatment, you will continue to have problems with your OCD. Because your OCD symptoms impair your functioning and decrease your quality of life, I recommend that you seriously consider receiving treatment for your OCD.

Many people would like to know how they developed OCD. There are a number of guesses, some better than others, about why some people get OCD, but there is no satisfactory theory of its development. Fortunately, despite our lack of knowledge about development of OCD, there is good information available about treatment.

There are two types of treatment that have been found helpful for OCD: behavior therapy and pharmacotherapy. Both have been studied extensively with hundreds of patients in centers in different parts of the world, and both are established treatments for OCD.

What treatment is right for you?

There are advantages and disadvantages to both types of treatments. I'll describe each treatment to you, along with its advantages and disadvantages, to help you make a choice.

I said that pharmacotherapy has been found helpful. It is important to note that not just any drug is helpful. Particular drugs called serotonin reuptake inhibitors are a class of antidepressant drugs that are of use with OCD. It is not clear why they work, but it is clear that they do indeed often help to reduce OCD symptoms. The idea is that these drugs act on a chemical in the brain called serotonin, and when pharmacotherapy is successful, obsessional distress decreases, urges to ritualize decrease, and along with these, rituals and avoidance also decrease. The frequency and persistence of obsessive intrusions decrease as well, although most patients say that they still have some obsessive intrusions even after successful drug treatment.

There are several drugs that fall into the class of SRIs that have been found helpful for OCD, but I'll focus only on the ones that are approved by the FDA with an indication for OCD. Depending on the particular drug, evidence is more or less strong for its helpfulness. The most well-established drug is clomipramine, whose brand name is Anafranil. It has been studied with hundreds of patients it has been found that about half of those who take it do well with it. The average amount of OCD symptom reduction has been about 40%. Thus, you can see that clomipramine is a good drug: Half of those who take it improve enough that they say it makes an important difference in their lives. The other FDA-approved drug for OCD is fluoxetine (brand name Prozac). It is more recently available than clomipramine, but has also been studied very extensively and has been established as helpful with OCD. It is hard to say with confidence which of the SRIs is best for OCD, but it seems like clomipramine produces somewhat larger improvements.

The drugs have the clear benefit that they are helpful for many people. They also have an advantage in that they do not require much effort to take. After a few psychiatrist visits, and once you have worked up to an effective dosage of the drug, you meet with your psychiatrist only occasionally for monitoring. Of course these are averages, and in choosing a treatment, you are betting on averages. You could do much better than the average or might not improve at all with the drug. We don't know how to predict who will do well with a particular treatment, and who will not.

What are the disadvantages of the drug therapy? Well, even though many people do well with pharmacotherapy, about half of those who take medication do not improve, and of those who do improve, most still experience noticeable OCD symptoms. In addition, drugs do not usually do only what you want them to do: decrease OCD symptoms. They usually also have some unwanted side effects. These are readily tolerated by many people, but can sometimes be unpleasant or intolerable. For example, side effects from clomipramine can include dry mouth, sleep changes, weight gain, and sexual dysfunction. Although you would probably have some side effects, it is difficult to predict how tolerable they will be for you. One other disadvantage of the medications is that although while you keep taking them, you will probably continue to do well, most people who withdraw from them have a return of OCD symptoms. Many people are not concerned about taking a medication for a long period, but some people prefer not to do this. (Women who wish to get pregnant are generally advised to withdraw from their medication because so little is known about how it may affect the pregnancy.)

The other established treatment for OCD is behavior therapy. This has also been studied very extensively with hundreds of patients in different countries and has been found very helpful. The idea behind behavior therapy is different from that behind drug therapy. With drug therapy, you ingest a chemical, it gets into your brain and changes your neurochemistry, and your experience improves. Behavior therapy is based on the idea that obsessive intrusions, distress, and rituals are habitual ways of reacting, and that as habits, they can be weakened. Behavioral therapy is a learning-based therapy that consists of a series of exercises designed to weaken certain thinking habits, feeling habits, and overt habits. The exercises are called prolonged exposure and response prevention, which actually means abstaining from rituals.

Exposure means that you purposely confront situations that prompt obsessions, distress, and urges to ritualize, and that you stay in the situation for a long period of time, until the symptoms decrease spontaneously. Response prevention means abstaining from using rituals as a way to reduce obsessions and discomfort.

We have found excellent results with an intensive behavioral therapy program, with daily, 90-minute sessions for a month, including exposure practice at your home, guided by the therapist. This is important, because OCD habits are often especially strong in the home. In addition, this program involves daily homework practice with the exposure exercises and concentration on abstaining from rituals.

There are some clear advantages to behavior therapy. First, it has been found to be more helpful than drugs for individuals who complete it. About three out of four patients who complete behavior therapy improve substantially and maintain their gains years after therapy has been completed; the average symptom reduction is about 65%. Second, you need not concern yourself with medication side effects from behavior therapy.

There are some drawbacks to behavior therapy that you should know about. First of all, just as with medication, there is no guarantee of improvement. Even though it is a very effective treatment, 20% to 25% of patients do not improve significantly and maintain the gain over time. Furthermore, those who do benefit are not usually completely symptom free. They do, however, say that the therapy made an important difference in their life.

Second, although one doesn't usually think of psychotherapy as having side effects, there is one unpleasant "side effect" of behavior therapy. This is the distress that occurs when you confront situations that provoke your obsessions. Typically, when a person first confronts a feared situation, he or she reacts with distress, but this then decreases gradually over the course of a session. The next time you confront that situation, you experience less distress, and so on, with repeated exposure practice until the situation prompts little discomfort. The distress is a kind of side effect in that the goal of the therapy is really to reduce distress, but during the exposure practice, distress increases temporarily. If you choose to participate in intensive behavioral therapy program, you should expect to experience discomfort during the exposure exercises. It is difficult to predict how uncomfortable you would feel: Some people are intensely distressed and others experience minimal discomfort.

A third thing to consider about the behavior therapy program is that it requires substantial effort on your part. Unlike the drug treatment, in which a chemical does most of the work, in behavioral therapy, you do most of the work, practicing exposure both in sessions with the therapist and on your own for "homework." Thus, for the behavior therapy to work as well as it does, you must dedicate enough time and energy to practice. The payoff from behavior therapy depends heavily on your investment of time and effort in the program. This cost in your own time and effort can be seen as a disadvantage of behavioral therapy, compared to drug therapy.

In summary, there are two good treatments for OCD. Behavior therapy seems to produce more improvement than medication, and this improvement is more lasting after treatment is stopped. Drug therapy takes less time and effort in the short run than behavioral therapy, but would probably have to be continued indefinitely if you are to keep your improvement. Behavior therapy is usually emotionally challenging and requires your determination to continue even when the exposure is distressing. Drug therapy requires your willingness to tolerate various medication side effects.

On the whole, behavior therapy would seem to be the preferred option, both because it produces more improvement, and because the improvement is more lasting. Therefore, I recommend that you seriously consider this treatment as your first choice. A second-choice recommendation would be one of the FDA-approved serotonergic drugs. If you choose pharmacotherapy, the specific drug choice would be decided by you and your psychiatrist.

This model is idealized in that it assumes that the patient has had no prior experience with any of the treatments, and begs the question of combination treatments. Prior response or nonresponse to one of the treatments would complicate the recommendation, as would also a history of relevant drug allergies or other physical conditions that would counterindicate a particular pharmacotherapy. Women of childbearing potential need to consider that medication withdrawal is generally recommended before pregnancy.

The long-term efficacy of combined treatment by behavioral therapy and medication is yet unclear. Therefore, we are hesitant to offer any strong recommendations about such combined treatment. Because antidepressants, including the SRIs have been found not to compromise behavioral therapy, patients need not withdraw from such medication, particularly if it has reduced depressive or obsessive–compulsive symptoms. Furthermore, as mentioned earlier, severely depressed patients would be well advised to consider premedication with an effective antidepressant before starting behavior therapy.

Some patients are motivated to maximize their treatment outcome by simultaneous treatment with both SRIs and behavioral therapy. Because definitive results on specific augmentation tactics are unavailable, the decision about whether to pursue this approach is somewhat arbitrary. In most cases, we do not favor starting or stopping *any* medication immediately before, immediately after, or during behavior therapy, because the salutary or adverse effects of such changes are confounded with those of behavior therapy, thus making decisions about modifying either behavior therapy procedures or medication regimens more difficult. Patients who have had an adequate trial of a medication to which they have not responded should usually be withdrawn from it before behavior therapy begins, so that any physical and emotional consequences of medication withdrawal do not compromise the behavior therapy.

INTENSIVE BEHAVIORAL THERAPY

The treatment program consists of three phases: (1) treatment planning, (2) exposure and response prevention (i.e., abstinence from rituals) and (3) maintenance.

Treatment Planning

The obvious prerequisite for treatment planning is a diagnostic evaluation indicating OCD. The second step is determination of candidacy for behavioral therapy. Drug or alcohol abuse should be resolved before behavioral therapy begins. Formal thought disorder also counterindicates exposure-based therapy. Individuals with severe major depressive disorder should probably receive pharmacotherapy for depression before beginning treatment for OCD.

The patient's motivation to comply with the requirements of treatment must be high. A detailed discussion of these requirements is essential, so that the patient can make a well-informed choice about whether to pursue the treatment. If the patient does not agree to comply with the treatment procedures, the pharmacotherapy alternatives can be recommended. Few highly motivated patients are actually enthusiastic about the prospect of behavioral therapy, either because they anticipate the exposure and ritual prevention fearfully, or because they are not confident they can complete the treatment. However, the patient must agree in advance to make a best attempt to complete the therapy, without insisting on *à priori* exceptions to the requirements. Willingness to participate in what promises to be a challenging therapy often depends on the patient's understanding its rationale and noncoercive nature.

The requirement that the patient refrain from all rituals after confronting distressing situations means that the experience will be aversive. The intensity of discomfort experienced during exposure therapy varies from patient to patient and can be quite severe for some. If a patient does not know to expect some discomfort as a side effect of therapy, or is not optimistic about treatment efficacy, he or she will probably experience more difficulty performing the exercises. The following is a model description and rationale.

T: You can think of obsessive–compulsive symptoms as a set of habits. They are thinking, feeling, and action habits that are distressing, wasteful, and difficult to get rid of. Usually these habits involve thoughts, images, or impulses that come to mind even though you don't want them, and are connected with bad feelings. We call these obsessional intrusions, intrusive thoughts, or just obsessions. Naturally, people try to avoid or eliminate unwanted thoughts and feelings, and in OCD, people find various special thoughts or actions, called rituals, that sometimes help temporarily to get rid of the unwanted thoughts and feelings.

Unfortunately, the rituals don't work very well, and at best, the distress decreases for a short time and then returns. Then you do more ritualizing to try to reduce anxiety, but the pattern is repeated. You can spend so much time and energy ritualizing that other areas of your life are disrupted.

The treatment procedures we will use are confrontation with situations that provoke obsessions and abstinence from rituals. You must practice both of these together; it is not good enough to confront feared situations and then to do your rituals afterward. If you practice diligently, you should notice some important changes in your obsessive–compulsive reactions as early as few days after the beginning of treatment. First, anxiety connected with the feared situations decreases and doesn't return as strongly when you confront the situation the next time. Second, urges to do rituals decrease as well.

It might seem puzzling that this is expected to help you with your OCD. But we know that when people confront situations they fear, first they get anxious, but if they stay in the situation for a long period, anxiety gradually declines. Doing this repeatedly weakens the link between your anxiety reaction and the situation that bothers you. That link is weakened for you because you stay in the situation long enough to get accustomed to it, and this forms a new experience about the situation. This is what it takes to weaken the obsession: repeated, prolonged confrontation with bothersome situations until they lose their power to provoke discomfort for you. Unfortunately, when you first confront the bothersome situations, they are usually distressing. This is a side effect of the therapy that you can expect. It is important that you be so determined to weaken your obsessions that you are willing to stay in the bothersome situations for prolonged periods without ritualizing, even though you want to leave or do a ritual.

For many people, anticipation of feared situations or consequences is as bad or worse than the actual situations. Most often, the actual feared consequences never arise. One way of looking at this is that the person has a very vivid imagination that gets him or her into trouble when anticipatory fear images get too strong. Some obsessions seem to be like vivid fear images. Repeated, prolonged imaginal confrontation with feared situations can weaken the emotional quality of these images, so that they no longer bother you so much. In your therapy, we will develop some imagery for you to practice here and at home. One advantage to imaginal exposure is that one can purposely confront all kinds of disasters that are not practical to confront in real life. For example, if just the thought of getting cancer is excessively upsetting for you, you can weaken this reaction by imagining that you have cancer. This kind of practice will not make you not care if you got cancer. Getting it would still be upsetting, but the imagery practice can help you weaken the anticipatory fear so that the thought of having cancer in the future does not ruin your day-to-day life. For you, we will develop images having to do with (specify consequences), so that just getting the idea that this could happen would not upset you very much any more.

When an obsession arises, it is distressing, and a person naturally wants to reduce this discomfort. Avoidance of certain situations and various rituals is usually an attempt to avoid or escape discomfort. Unfortunately, this does not work very well in OCD. It may put off or reduce discomfort temporarily, but it comes back. Unfortunately, it also seems to strengthen the fear in the long run, so that you feel even more discomfort and urges to ritualize. Therefore, in treatment, it will be essential that you give up doing rituals, even though you have strong urges to do them. By confronting bothersome situations and tolerating the discomfort without doing rituals, you will weaken your obsessive–compulsive habits, including the habitual discomfort that arises with your obsessional intrusions. When the discomfort that accompanies the obsessions decreases, you won't think about them as much.

When the patient understands the nature of the therapy and what is required, a schedule of specific exposure exercises and rituals prevention must be formulated. This phase typically takes of 4–6 hours of interviews directed at detailed inquiry about the obsessive–compulsive symptoms. During these sessions, the rationale for treatment is reviewed until the patient has learned it well. Also during this time, the patient is taught to monitor rituals, and a treatment plan is explicated.

Accurate information about frequency and duration of rituals is necessary for evaluating the progress and useful for illustrating changes to the patient. In cases in which the rituals have become automatic, in that the habit has become so overlearned that the patient has become unaware of their performance, the monitoring can be an active intervention. It increases the awareness of rituals that is prerequisite for systematic prevention of the rituals.

A sample self-monitoring form is included in Appendix A. A model for instructing the patient in self-monitoring is next presented.

> **T:** I am going to ask you to keep a record of any rituals that you do. This self-monitoring can be somewhat burdensome, but it serves two important purposes for your therapy. The first value of self-monitoring is that it provides accurate information, providing that you do it diligently. The second advantage to the self-monitoring is that it helps you to be more aware of your urges to ritualize, and of whether you give in to them. Refraining from rituals can be difficult, and the self-monitoring is a tool that can help you with self-control. Here is an example of a form for recording your thoughts and rituals.

The therapist should specify the rituals to be monitored and have the patient complete the monitoring form based on the previous day's rituals. If the patient has numerous rituals, the two main ones should be selected for monitoring (e.g., washing, checking). The monitoring form should be carried by the patient at all times, and rituals should be recorded at the time they occur. Notations should be quite brief, and perfectionistic patients should be instructed to make each notation incomplete in some small way. All targeted rituals should be recorded, without exception. Monitoring forms should be brought to each session for inspection by the therapist.

It can be useful if, before treatment, the patient identifies someone who can assist him or her during the course of therapy. If the patient experiences difficulty resisting an urge to ritualize, this person can be contacted and should be asked to remind the patient of the importance of adherence to the procedures. Also, this person should be available to collaborate in various activities that help the patient overcome urges to ritualize. In addition, the support person can provide valuable information to the patient and the therapist about obsessive–compulsive patterns that are evident to an observer but overlooked by the patient, and thus are not reported in therapy sessions.

The therapist should help the support person and the patient reconcile difficulties that arise during the course of treatment and offer suggestions to facilitate the support person's role. Any historical patterns of angry interactions between the two should be identified, and alternative patterns should be discussed and role-played in the session. It is important that the support person avoid trying to "make" the patient adhere to the therapy regimen. The interpersonal conflict that is likely to ensue from such attempts will probably disrupt therapy and impede progress toward reduction of OCD symptoms. If such a pattern cannot be circumvented, it may be preferable to relieve the support person of the designated role.

At the onset of the second treatment-planning session, the therapist should inspect and discuss the patient's self-monitoring record. Constructive criticism should be offered, as well as acknowledgment of any efforts the patient has made to comply with the self-monitoring procedure.

The next step in developing a treatment plan is to make a list of events that provoke obsessive distress, and this will constitute the exposure material for the treatment.

Guidelines for selecting exposure situations are as follows:

- Exposure items (i.e., objects, situations or thoughts evoking discomfort and urges to ritualize) are chosen based on the patient's report.
- Exposure items are ordered according to how distressing the patient expects them to be, and will be confronted in ascending order, beginning with items of at least moderate difficulty.
- Confrontation with the most difficult situations should occur well before the projected end of treatment, so that there remains ample time for many sessions of repeated practice with these situations.
- The treatment plan can be modified to accommodate distressing situations that are discovered to have been overlooked during the initial assessment and treatment planning.

Guidelines for imaginal exposure are as follows:

- Image scripts of scenes of gradually increasing anxiety-evoking potential are prepared. Image scripts of scenes should include a description of the feared situation that evokes obsessional distress, as well as a description of the anticipated disastrous consequences.
- Provocation of obsessional distress by image scripts indicates that relevant affective memory has been accessed and is available for modification if it is maintained for a prolonged period, during which habituation can occur.
- Image scripts that do not match fears of the patients are unlikely to provoke obsessional distress. If the patient denies feeling anxious during imaginal exposure, either the script should be modified or the patient's way of forming images might be incorrect. For example, some patients purposely avoid including certain scripted material in images, or distract themselves during the image, to reduce distress. Patients who do not engage emotionally in the image should be questioned about the details of their imagery and reminded that the imagery must be distressing if it is to be useful.
- Therapist should be willing to change a script if necessary; otherwise treatment effectiveness can be compromised.
- Some patients can better produce fear images *without* the distraction of a therapist's narrative. Having the patient simultaneously describe and practice imagery can reveal disparities between the therapist's script and the patient's image. If the therapist's script contains material that is incongruent with essential elements of the patient's fear memory, or if it has important omissions, the script should be modified. If the patient is compromising or the "softening" the image in some way, the patient should be encouraged to allow the image be more distressing. The therapist's

task is to help the patient access his or her fear memory, *not* simply to follow some prearranged script in a rote fashion. A sample image is given in Appendix B.

Homework Instructions

Homework exposure is an essential component of a successful treatment program. During treatment planning, the therapist must emphasize the essential role of homework exposure and describe the homework that will be included in the treatment program. Homework exposure is an extension of the exposure that has been done in sessions and should generally occupy at least as much time/day as is spent in a session. It consists of additional exposure exercises to be carried out between treatment sessions (at the patient's or a relative's home, at shopping malls, etc.).

In practice, time spent on homework varies widely from day to day and from patient to patient. Sometimes, a homework-exposure task may continue throughout the entire period between sessions, when a patient maintains contact with a contaminant at all times. Other homework tasks may be more limited, such as driving a car for an hour each day. Homework self-exposure practice should be prolonged and persist as long as is practical, or until the patient notices significant decrease in discomfort. In cases in which prolonged exposure is practically difficult, the therapist should arrange a plan that will allow sufficient exposure. For example, in lieu of sitting for an hour on the toilet seat of a public facility, a patient could touch the toilet seat with a cloth or a paper and continue the exposure for hours, using this derivative contaminant.

Treatment Phase

An intensive exposure program at our clinic typically consists of 15 two-hour sessions conducted daily for 3 weeks. Clinical observations suggest that massed sessions are superior to spaced practice. The mechanism of any such superiority is unclear, especially in view of the likely efficacy of extensive daily self-exposure in the absence of sessions with the therapist. We believe that frequent sessions help the patient to comply with the program requirements and allow the therapist to discover errors that the patient is making, and offer corrective instruction before the patient becomes demoralized.

Sessions customarily begin with an inspection of self-monitoring records and discussion of experiences (successes and difficulties) with self-exposure and ritual abstinence. The therapist should recommend how to circumvent difficulties if they arise. Such discussion is usually followed by a review of the planned exposures for the session. The remainder of the session consists of exposure, typically 45 minutes imaginal, and 45 minutes *in vivo*. Toward the end of the session, new homework is assigned. Sometimes an *in vivo* exposure exercise requires that the therapist and patient travel outside the office, and an entire session will be devoted to this activity. At other times, an entire session might be devoted to imaginal exposure. Imaginal exposure procedures may be abandoned entirely if a script that evokes OCD-relevant affective images cannot be developed.

Instructions for imaginal exposure are as follows:

> **T:** Today's exposure will include some imagery practice. As we discussed when we were planning treatment, you will imagine (summarize situation). I'll ask you to close your eyes so that you won't be distracted. The imagery practice will be useful to you only if you can imagine the situation vividly and realistically enough that you feel some of the distress you would feel if the situation were actually happening to you. So when you are doing the imagery, it is important that you let yourself feel the way you do when you are having an

obsessive concern. Also, it is important that you do not perform any rituals in your mind during the imagery. After you maintain the image for a while, I will ask you do describe aloud what you are seeing, thinking, feeling, and doing in the image. Also, I'll ask you from time to time to indicate how uncomfortable you feel. You can use the zero–100 scale that I taught you to describe your discomfort, with 100 being the most severe distress.

Imaginal exposure sessions are audiotaped and used by the patient for homework imaginal exposure outside the session.

Instructions for *in vivo* exposure are as follows:

> **T:** (*Instructions for Washers*) Today, we will be working with (specify item(s)). Your task will be to confront this for a prolonged period of time and to stay with it even if you feel uncomfortable. You may start by touching it with a finger or two, but then it will be useful for you to touch it to your face and hair and clothing, all over yourself, so that there are no spots on you that you have kept "protected." It is also important not to do any washing or cleaning to rid yourself of the contamination. For exposure to be helpful, you must touch the item knowing that you won't do anything to "undo" what you are doing. I know that it can be difficult to do this, but it will get easier as you continue with the practice.

The therapist can give the contaminated item to the patient and ask him or her to touch it, or touch the item first and then ask the patient to touch it. The item itself or the "contaminated" hands are then touched to the face, hair, and clothing. The patient should be asked periodically about level of distress using the zero–100 SUDs scale.

> **T:** (*Instructions for Checkers*) Your task is to address and mail some envelopes without checking the mailbox afterwards. You can address them right here, and we will walk to the mailbox and mail them right away without checking even once after you've done it. Then we will do a similar practice with purchasing an item and receiving change from your payment without counting it. While doing these exercises, I would like you to recognize that you are taking a chance that you could make a mistake, mismail the envelopes, or get the incorrect change. There is no guarantee that you will not make a mistake, and your task is to take the risks in these situations, without checking to try and make sure that you've done things correctly.

Instructions for abstinence from rituals should be offered in detail on the first day of exposure practice and reiterated daily during treatment. A printed copy of the rules for abstinence from rituals is sometimes a useful adjunct to oral instruction. Sample rules are offered later, but must be individually adapted to the pattern of rituals of each patient.

A target of total cessation of all rituals on Day 1 of treatment is achievable for many patients, but for some it is unrealistic. For example, patients who have either a large variety of different rituals that pervade all their activities, or whose rituals are brief and have become automatized, will probably not be able to stop them all immediately (e.g., someone who, in a practically unconscious manner, briefly checks hundreds of items daily). For such patients, focus on stopping one or two primary rituals before attending to others can be most practical.

Rules for Ritual Abstinence

Ideally, washers should not use water in any way that is decontaminating (i.e., no handwashing, no rinsing, no wet towels or washcloths). Use of creams and other toiletry articles (bath powder, deodorant, etc.) is permitted *except* when use of these items reduces discomfort about contamination. Shaving may be done using an electric razer to circumvent the need to use water. Water can be drunk or used to brush teeth, with care not to get any on the face or hands. Supervised showers lasting no more than 10 minutes usually may be permitted every 3 days. Ritualistic washing of specific areas of the body (e.g., genitals, hair) and ritualistic washing orders (e.g., "top down" or genital or anal area last) are prohibited, and the patient must recontaminate immediately after the shower.

At home, ritual prevention may be aided by predesignated relatives or friends who are instructed to be available to the patient should he or she have difficulty resisting an urge to wash. The patient is advised to report any such concern to the support person, who should remain with the patient until the urge decreases to a manageable level. The support person should report observed rituals to the patient, with encouragement to discuss them with the therapist. The support person should remind the patient of the importance of adhering to the therapy regimen, but should not argue with the patient or try to force compliance. Water supplies may be shut off by the support person if the patient gives prior consent to such a plan. Although the support person is encouraged to assist the patient in timing of handwashing and showers, it is not necessary to observe him or her directly during the shower.

Exceptions to these rules may be necessary in certain circumstances (e.g., medical conditions necessitating cleansing), but in any case, any needed washing should not serve to "decontaminate" the patient. Recontamination immediately after any washing is a useful technique.

Ideally, for checkers, beginning with the first session of exposure, the patient should abstain from all checking. For example, after turning off a faucet or switch, no checking is permitted. After locking a door, no checking is permitted. At home, ritual abstinence can be aided by a support person who should be available at the patient's request when an urge to check is difficult to resist. That person is to stay with the patient until the urge decreases to a manageable level. Patients are often encouraged by a reminder of the importance of resisting urges to ritualize. The support person should not argue with the patient nor should he or she attempt to force compliance.

Once obsessional fear has been weakened substantially, strict abstinence rules may be modified to promote learning of nonritualistic patterns. Toward the end of treatment, patients may be introduced to routine washing, cleaning, or checking. Guidelines for such "normal" behavior are presented in Appendix C. We typically suggest that washers restrict themselves to one 10-minute shower daily and handwash only when soil can be seen, smelled, or felt, without careful examination. Long-term maintenance that includes some special restrictions is advisable for many patients.

The final treatment session follows the same format as previous sessions. The therapist should instruct the patient in the role of self-exposure to previously avoided situations in preventing relapse. For example, the therapist could suggest to a woman with an obsessive fear of germs that she continue to engage systematically in activities that she had previously avoided, such as touching all doorknobs, using public restrooms and waiting areas, eating at restaurants, and so on. Additionally, she should visit the waiting area of a hospital periodically, even though her scheduled treatment sessions are finished.

Home Visit

Visits made by the therapist to the patient's home are often quite helpful, particularly when obsessive–compulsive habits are especially strong there. It is important that learning that occurs in office sessions be generalized to the patient's local environment. Often, homework assignments are sufficient for this purpose, but a home visit by the therapist affords valuable opportunities for direct observation of patient functioning. A visit to the patient's place of employment is sometimes important for the same reasons.

For those patients whose obsessional fears are especially salient at home, home visits are routinely conducted, if practical. Exposure practice during the home visit is conducted the same as during office sessions. Because the prospect of in-home exposure is often so daunting for patients with OCD we customarily conduct home visits at the end of the intensive treatment period, after the patient has had a substantial amount of guided exposure in the office and related self-exposure at home. However, scheduling of such exposure practice is somewhat arbitrary, and can be conceptualized simply as *in vivo* exposure in the home locale, and thus, is not essentially dissimilar to other out-of-the-office exposure, such as that done in markets, automobiles, on sidewalks, and so on.

A typical home visit takes several hours on each of two consecutive days, usually at the end of a series of outpatient sessions. Exposures to feared situations are performed in and around the patient's home or workplace, and the therapist offers suggestions for further exposure. For example, the therapist might observe the patient contaminating or disordering the house, or the local grocery store. With the patient's explicit permission, the therapist can model the exposure exercises to be done. Many patients will report little or no discomfort when doing these exposures because of their similarity to previous exercises. Others, however, will find such exercises distressing. During a home visit, the therapist may discover some areas in the patient's home or work environment that have not been contaminated or disordered, either inadvertently or by systematic avoidance. The therapist's careful observation of the details of the patient's actions is a most important element of the home visit.

Follow-up Sessions

Follow-up sessions may help patients to maintain gains achieved during intensive therapy. We have found that 1 week of daily sessions devoted to relapse prevention followed by eight brief (10-minute) weekly telephone contacts inhibited relapse (Hiss, Foa, & Kozak, 1994).

Therapeutic Setting

It is preferable that patients remain in their natural environments during intensive treatment. This can be particularly important for patients whose obsessions and compulsions would not arise in other environments, such as an inpatient setting. For example, patients with driving fears would be prohibited from driving while inpatients because of potential institutional liability for driving accidents. Alternatively, the hospital may be an artificially "safe" environment for checkers, who may feel relieved of the responsibilities that concern them. Hospitalization is indicated only for suicidal patients, those with psychosis, and those who need close supervision and cannot receive such supervision at home.

If a patient's symptoms are work related, it is usually desirable that the patient continue working during the treatment period, so that work-related exposure exercises can be implemented readily. Because treatment entails daily 2-hour sessions, part-time work hours during the treatment period are often the most practical arrangement.

Michael J. Kozak and
Edna B. Foa

Therapist Variables

Successful exposure treatment requires that the therapist maintain a delicate balance between encouraging the patient to confront feared situations and preserving the patient's sense of choice in the matter. Patients who feel coerced into exposure exercises are unlikely to comply with treatment procedures, either in-session or after they leave the session. Rabavilas, Boulougouris, and Perissaki (1979) found that a respectful, understanding, encouraging, explicit, and challenging therapist will be more successful than a permissive, tolerant therapist, but clinical observations suggest that such firmness of style must not devolve into rigidity or argumentativeness.

Patient Variables

Because exposure exercises are distressing, patients must be highly motivated for treatment to be completed successfully. Motivation is partly related to symptom severity, in that severe impairment may motivate the patient to comply with treatment in face of the distress it generates.

Some individuals agree to participate in treatment to appease a spouse or parent. These patients are at risk for noncompliance with the therapy, because their motivation depends on interpersonal contingencies that are not in force when the person is alone. Since successful outcome depends substantially on completion of homework exercises, self-motivation is important.

Treatment is unlikely to eliminate all OCD symptoms. As noted earlier, intensive behavior therapy yields 65% reduction in OCD symptoms on average (and pharmacotherapy, about 40% reduction). It is therefore important to inform the patient that although anxiety and the urges to ritualize will diminish and become more manageable, complete elimination of symptoms is unlikely immediately posttreatment. Maintenance of treatment gains achieved with behavioral therapy usually requires that the patient continue to apply techniques learned in sessions, over a period of time following the intensive treatment.

PROBLEMS ARISING DURING TREATMENT

Persistent Ritualizing

Although patients are instructed to cease all ritualizing from Day 1 of intensive treatment, they rarely achieve this goal. Even when a patient is highly motivated to refrain from rituals, the habit of ritualizing is so strong that lapses occur. These should be recorded on the self-monitoring forms and reported to the therapist daily. Such lapses should be carefully addressed by therapist. The patient should be reminded of the crucial role of ritual prevention, but also cautioned against self-devaluation stemming from imperfect attainment of the goals of therapy.

The patient should continue to strive for complete abstinence from rituals, but must not become demoralized because of occasional lapses that can be countered with subsequent self-reexposure. This constitutes a useful way of coping with lapses. If the patient perceives the therapist as a supportive ally in solving problems of lapses, rather than as a punitive authority figure, needless interpersonal conflicts about the patient's failure to comply with instructions may be avoided.

Sometimes a patient's support person will notice violations of ritual-prevention rules. Coaching the support person and the patient in handling such violations can be helpful. One approach is to have the support person report directly to the therapist any observed violations. This entails some risk of provoking conflicts if the patient perceives him- or herself as subordinate to the support person and the therapist. An alternative tactic is to have the support person speak directly to the patient about observed violations. This approach can also provoke conflicts. A third alternative is for the therapist to meet conjointly with the patient and support person for discussion of progress and problems. The therapist can then train both the patient and the support person (S) in how to communicate about violations. The following is a model dialogue.

T: I have asked to meet with both of you so that we could discuss your progress in the program so far, including any problems. I like to speak with both the patient and the support person from time to time, because the support person sometimes notices important things that the patient may not have paid much attention to, and so may not have reported to me. For example, sometimes a patient may have become so accustomed to a certain ritual that it is taken for granted and not even noticed, even though another person would notice. So, I'd like to ask what you've noticed about how (patient's name) is doing with obsessive–compulsive habits since the program began.

S: Well, she's definitely doing a lot of things she didn't do before. She sits in places she wouldn't sit before, and we've gone to some restaurants and museums and stuff. We went to the movies, too, and she wouldn't do that before. Also, we were able to get out of the room in time to make the movie, and there was no way we would have been able to do that before.

T: I am glad to hear this. You know that she was instructed to stop performing all rituals. Have you noticed her doing any rituals since we began the program?

S: Well, I'm not sure if they're rituals, but something was going on when we went to the movie. We had to sit in the back and she made us wait until everyone else left the movie until we could leave. That seemed a little strange.

T: What did you do when you noticed this?

S: Well, I didn't really know what to do. I know she's not supposed to be washing, but this wasn't washing so I wasn't sure whether I should have said anything about it. You know she gets mad sometimes if I say anything.

T: (*To patient*) I'd like to ask you about what happened in the movie. Do you remember that situation?

P: Yes, but I didn't think it was a ritual. I guess I just always do that, you know.

T: Could you tell us what was going on there?

P: Well, first I wanted to make sure that the place we sat wasn't filthy. You know how people dump their filth all over the seats and floors in movies, and the seats in the back were okay. The other thing was that I don't like people rubbing against me because they could be dirty, so if you wait till they all leave, you can get out without getting squashed into that crowd. Now, I really didn't think about it at all when I was there. I just always did it that way when I used to go to a movie. Before this week, its been a long time since I've been in one, but I always looked for a clean seat in the back and waited till people went out before leaving.

T: So did you know this was an obsessive–compulsive habit?

P: I can see it now, but I didn't think of it then. I just did it.

T: I'd call what you did avoidance, rather than ritualizing, because you tried to stay away from contaminants. I think its interesting that (support person) noticed what you were doing but you just did it automatically, out of habit, without noticing that it was an avoidance. Can you think of a way (support person) could have helped you with it at that time?

P: I guess tell me to stop ritualizing, right?

T: (*To patient*) Actually, I'd suggest something a little bit different. For one thing, (support person) figured you were doing something obsessive–compulsive, but wasn't sure whether it was ritualizing, and in fact, it was more like avoidance than ritualizing. Second, you weren't even aware that you were avoiding, so I'm not confident that telling you to stop ritualizing would have been so helpful. Usually, a helpful thing for your support person to do if she notices that you are performing something you shouldn't be doing is first gently to tell you that she noticed you doing it, and to *ask* you whether you think that it was an obsessive–compulsive habit. If you recognize that it is, the support person can ask you if it is one of things she has discussed with me, and whether she's supposed to be working on it. If you say it is part of your homework, she can remind you that it is important for to follow the program to get better, and ask if she can do anything to help her through it. It is also good to suggest that you discuss the event with me, so that we can work on it together. Is that clear?

S: I think so.

T: (*To the support person*) It is generally best not to try to order (patient) around, or to try to make her do what she's supposed to do. People often don't respond well to being told strongly what to do, so if you ask questions and make suggestions, and offer to help, it will probably work better than just telling her to stop.

When a patient acknowledges a violation and agrees to continue efforts at compliance, little further discussion is required. However, if ritualizing occurs repeatedly, especially if the ritualizing is prolonged and intentional rather than brief and automatic, the therapist should reiterate the rationale for these rules and alert the patient to the implication of a pattern of violations: unsatisfactory outcome. Consideration of treatment discontinuation because of the likelihood of poor outcome can communicate seriousness of the problem of a pattern of ritualizing during treatment and sometimes can be a powerful motivator for the patient. However, raising the issue of treatment discontinuation must be done carefully, in a supportive manner, lest the patient react with anger or depression to perceived rejection by the therapist.

Persistent Avoidance

Some patients may engage in unreported fearful avoidance. The preceding example of the precautions taken by the patient in the movie theater is illustrative of this pattern. Such avoidance may simply constitute strong habits that my have become automatized, but could reflect an ambivalence about exposure. Such ambivalence is neither unusual nor surprising, and if it is evident, direct discussion of it with the patient may promote compliance with the treatment regimen. Because it predicts poor outcome, a pattern of continuing avoidance merits the same sort of serious consideration that should be given to a pattern of continuing rituals.

T: I'd like to address an issue that can become a problem for people who are going through this therapy. The reason I'm bringing it up is that I've noticed some things you are doing that might cause trouble for you later, and I'd like to alert you about them. It has to do with the way a person does the homework exposure. If you continue to avoid situations, even in small ways, after we have completed a relevant exposure practice, then you will probably have continuing difficulty with your obsessive fear. So for example, we had already gone to the public market and brushed up against people in the crowded aisles, but when you went to the movies, you avoided brushing up against people. Can you see how this goes against what we are trying to do here?

P: Yes.

T: So what would have been a helpful thing for you to do there?

P: I guess purposely sit somewhere dirty and get up and leave when everybody else did.

T: Exactly. If you just confront the very specific situations that we do in our sessions, but don't apply what you learn here to other situations that come up, you won't be very successful with this therapy. You have to understand the principle of exposure and apply it, rather than just do the specific exposure practices that we discussed at the session. In other words, it is like following the spirit of the thing, rather than just the letter. This means that when you are not here in a session, you should be looking actively for opportunities to do exposure practice with situations that are related to those we are working with. Is that clear?

Arguments

It is important not to argue with patients about their doing the exposure tasks. Most patients have a history of argument with others about the unreasonableness of their obsessions and compulsions, and these arguments have not provided relief from the symptoms. Time spent on argument is time taken from the exposure practice that is of demonstrated efficacy. Invoking the prearranged treatment plan is a useful way to circumvent arguments. Thus, it is important to have agreed previously about how the therapy will proceed. Patients must agree to follow the arranged schedule of exposure without argument. If new, feared situations are discovered, the schedule should be revised by agreement before the therapy proceeds. If a patient refuses to carry out a planned exposure, the therapist should acknowledge the patient's difficulty but encourage him or her to proceed.

The therapist can circumvent a struggle with the patient about an exposure task by describing the challenge as an opportunity for a courageous choice by the patient, and reminding the patient of the relationship between exposure practice and outcome. Thus, it is made clear to the patient that it is not the therapist who needs the patient to do the exposure, but rather the patient who needs to carry out the exposure. If the therapist needs the patient to do the exposure task and becomes frustrated and or angry when the patient hesitates or refuses, the consequent interpersonal conflict will probably detract from progress.

One way to help a patient confront a particularly difficult situation is to introduce a less difficult version of that task as an intermediate step. This can be construed to the patient as a method of preparation for the more difficult step, and can function both to decrease fear by a process of generalization of the exposure effect, but also to increase the patient's confidence, so as to increase the likelihood of a decision to confront the more difficult item. Therapist modeling of the exposure task sometimes will encourage patients to advance, but attempts to document this experimentally have been relatively unsuccessful.

Emotional Obstacles to Functional Exposure

Sometimes emotional reactions, such as anger or sadness, occur in response to exposure exercises that have been supposed to be anxiety provoking. Theoretical considerations suggest caution about the mechanism of such reactions in fear reduction with exposure. Specifically, if we want to change a fear memory, evocation of such fear during a related exposure is taken as evidence that the targeted memory has been accessed and is available for modification. Clinical observations and some experimental evidence (Foa et al., in press) suggest that other emotional reactions, such as anger, may be counterindicated and interfere with efficacy of exposure therapy.

If one construes nontarget emotions as forms of avoidance, it follows that the therapist should alert the patient that such emotional reactions might impede progress and help the patient focus on those aspects of the exposure that provoke fear. Failing this, therapist and patient should reevaluate the treatment plan. Inflexible pursuit of a schedule of exposures that produces anger or sadness in the absence of evidence for fear habituation would be highly undesirable.

Family Involvement

A variety of problems that interferes with the progress of exposure therapy can emerge from family interactions. Because family members often have a history of intense affect surrounding the patient's OCD symptoms, such affect frequently emerges in family interactions during the course of the therapy and can distract the patient from the exposure tasks at hand. It is important that the therapist advise both the patient and interested family members or friends to minimize such distraction. Sometimes family members are so motivated by the therapy prospect of relieving them from hardships incurred from entanglement with the patient's OCD symptoms that their behavior during therapy is governed by fear, frustration, or anger. Alternatively, family members may have an intense commitment to the patient's welfare, which leads to counterproductive attempts to control progress. Alertness by the therapist to these processes and appropriate interventions upon their discovery can probably influence course of treatment.

Sometimes family members will themselves have habits that reinforce the patient's obsessive–compulsive patterns. When the family behavior has been developed in response to the patient's OCD, family members should be advised by the therapist *and* the patient to stop these patterns. For example, a wife who has been trained by her husband to respond to repeated requests for assurances of safety (e.g., that the doors are locked) must learn that such assurances are counterproductive. The husband should solicit her agreement to refuse to cooperate in such rituals.

If a superstitious pattern of family behavior developed somewhat independently of the patient's OCD symptoms, the situation can become somewhat more difficult. For example, if a wife is concerned with contamination, and the husband is as well, but to a much less disruptive extent, the wife could encounter opposition from the husband to some of the exposure exercises. Particularly difficult are situations in which there is strong cultural support for ritualistic behavior relevant to the patient's OCD, as in the ritualistic observance of some religious dietary rules. Unfortunately, there is no convenient solution to the problem of highly motivated family or cultural support for generally innocuous rituals that steer the patient down a slippery slope of obsessive–compulsive superstition.

Posttreatment Adaptation

Some patients are unskilled or disorganized in pursuing satisfying and/or productive activity. For such individuals, the posttreatment transition from ritualizing to fulfilling, functional activity can be particularly difficult. The therapist should assess the patient's capacity for planning new social or occupational goals and offer skills training or help in problem solving if indicated.

Patients usually welcome a therapist's guidance about appropriate washing, checking, repeating, or ordering. Because some obsessive intrusions or urges to ritualize typically recur, patients can be well served by general rules for relevant behavior. For example, a handwasher might adopt the rule "Wash only if you can see, feel, or smell something on your hands without close inspection." Such a rule can bear the burden of many decisions that could arise in response to obsessive intrusions and associated discomfort. A checker might live with the rule "Never more than one check."

CASE DESCRIPTION

In this section we illustrate the process of gathering information relevant to planning the treatment program and conducting exposure sessions, using a composite case constructed from material drawn from cases seen in our clinic. This will allow convenient demonstration of a variety of OCD symptoms that a clinician might encounter.

Jake, a 37-year-old married man with a degree in engineering, sought treatment for OCD with a primary obsession of AIDS-related contamination. He lived far a way from our clinic but was referred to us by his psychiatrist because of our expertise with behavioral treatment of OCD. He was moderately depressed at the time of his referral, and had been taking Prozac 60 mg/day for 8 weeks, and lower doses off and on previously, but had no prior exposure treatment.

This information was collected during a telephone inquiry by the patient, and an in-person evaluation was scheduled. The patient's travel arrangements entailed air travel to Philadelphia and an overnight stay. At his in-person evaluation, a psychiatric history was obtained, as well as a thorough study of the scope and severity of his OCD symptoms. The Y–BOCS checklist and severity scales were administered (Y–BOCS total = 31). The patient showed no evidence of formal thought disorder and denied current and past alcohol and other substance abuse. He did report some depressive symptoms (17-item Hamilton Depression Scale (HAM-D) = 9) but denied suicidal intent and history. His diagnosis and history indicated that he was likely to benefit from intensive exposure treatment, and the rationale and procedures were explained in detail, including examples of high-difficulty exposure items. He was very reluctant to pursue the treatment because of his belief that he would be at serious risk for contracting HIV infection by doing some of the exposure items, especially visiting the local AIDS library. Nevertheless, he decided to participate in the treatment program and was scheduled to begin his sessions one month later.

Information Gathering

Current Symptoms

Obsessional content, fear cues, beliefs about consequences, passive avoidance patterns, and types of rituals were ascertained in a series of interviews, as exemplified in the following interchange.

T: I understand from what you told us at your evaluation that you are having difficulty with washing and cleaning. Can you tell me specifically what you are doing that is troublesome?

P: I wash my hands all the time and I clean everything too much. My wife is fed up with me and I don't know if we'll stay together. She is also fed up with the alcohol.

T: What is the problem with the alcohol?

P: I sterilize everything with rubbing alcohol. I go through a case a week. I always have a spray bottle and I sterilize everything around me.

T: How do you mean everything? I did not notice you sterilizing anything here in the office.

P: No, I didn't do the office, but I sprayed in the waiting room when I went in there and sprayed on the chair when I sat down. There wasn't anyone in there then; I try to spray when no one is around. When I got to the clinic there was someone in the waiting room. I waited outside until they left, then I went in and sprayed the air and the chair where I was going to sit. I wanted to spray in the office here because I don't know who was sitting here before, but I don't want everyone to see me spraying, so sometimes I don't sterilize, even when I want to. Then I keep thinking about what could be on the chair. You know, somebody could have had a cut on their hand or something.

T: I noticed an odor of alcohol when you came in.

P: That's cause I spray myself, too, my clothes. I do my hands after I've touched things.

T: And how often do you use the alcohol?

P: All the time.

T: I'd like to get a more specific guess about your alcohol use. Tell me how many times/day that you use alcohol.

P: I don't know. I never really counted. I use it a lot. I guess I go through a case every week.

T: How many bottles are in a case, and how many ounces does each bottle hold?

P: A dozen bottles, about 16 ounces, I think. They are like the one over there on your sink. You can look and see how much that holds.

T: I understand that you do not count the number of times you use alcohol each day, but it is important that I get a better idea of the frequency than "all the time." One way to do this is for you to think about today. Remember the last hour, and guess how many times you used alcohol, then think about the hour before, and so on, until you get back to when the day started for you. If your alcohol use today is typical, we can then guess how many times you use it each day. If today is not a typical day, then remember what yesterday was like, and we'll make a guess that way.

P: Well, there are two kinds of days. Days when I stay inside, and days when I go out. I use more alcohol if I go out. I guess I use it two or three times in an hour, except when I first get up. Then I just rinse my mouth with it.

T: With rubbing alcohol?

P: Yes. When I get up and whenever I brush my teeth.

T: So two or three times/hour throughout the day comes to about 45 times per day. Is that a good estimate?

P: Its about right for days that I go outside, I think.

T: How long does each alcohol use take?

P: Not long, just a few seconds to spray it, unless I'm washing my hands with it, then it takes longer.

T: How many times/day do you wash your hands, and how long does each wash take?

P: I can't really say. It depends on the day.

T: Think about how often you washed yesterday, and tell me about that.

P: I'd say five times yesterday.

T: How long does one wash take?

P: Well, it varies.

T: How long does an average wash take?

P: Well, not long usually.

T: How long in minutes would you say a wash takes?

P: I guess a minute or two.

This interchange is not untypical of inquiries regarding the details of patient behavior. Patients often do not monitor their behavior carefully, or are reluctant to venture general characterizations of their behavior, and the therapist must be very persistent to obtain estimates of the target behavior. Some patients are especially concerned with being inaccurate, and so will consistently avoid offering clear statements. Sometimes the therapist must reinstruct the patient about the importance of offering best-guess (i.e., less than perfect estimates of the behavior at issue). Once the primary rituals have been assessed, details of other rituals should be ascertained in a similar manner.

T: Do you do anything else to make yourself feel clean?
P: Yes, I use tissues to handle things.
T: What kind of things?
P: Things that feel dirty.
T: Can you tell me how much you do that?
P: Whenever I can.

Here the therapist must chose whether to pursue the details of the use of barriers to contamination, or to inquire about other rituals.

T: I know that it is difficult for you to make guesses about how often you do some of the things we're discussing, but it important for you to make a guess, even it is not quite right. Remember, your guess is bound to be better than mine, because I don't know at all how much you do these things. So, even though guess won't be exactly accurate, it will give me a rough idea of how much you are doing a particular ritual. So, please give me a guess about the number of times you used a tissue yesterday.
P: I used a tissue about 20 times yesterday.
T: Good, that helps. What about other rituals?
P: I don't know if this counts, but I do have trouble throwing things away.
T: Do you save up a lot of useless items?
P: I guess so. I have stuff I should get rid of.
T: What would bothers you about getting rid of it?
P: I'd have to go near trash cans.
T: Are you concerned that you might need the stuff that you throw away?
P: No, not really. I just don't want to get near trash cans.

This inquiry revealed that the problem of discarding items is not hoarding of collectibles, but rather avoidance of contamination. After the details of all the rituals have been assessed, the therapist turn to inquiry of the patient's obsessions.

T: What situations get you anxious about being dirty?
P: Anything unknown.
T: When you don't know where something has been, what could it have touched that would bother you?
P: Well, you know, something dirty.
T: What would be a dirty thing that would be the hardest for you to touch?
P: I don't even want to say it. I don't like to even think about it. I feel anxious just thinking about it, and if I tell you are going to make me touch it, so I'm not sure I should say it.
T: There is something that you said that I'd like you to rethink. You said that I was going to make you touch something. It is important that you know that the therapy does not work that way. I do not make you do anything. I will tell you what I think you must do get better with your OCD symptoms through exposure exercises, and that will involve touching some things you don't want to touch. But I will not try to force you to do the exercises. If you are afraid to describe to me the things that bother you most because you are afraid that I'll make you touch these things, we won't be able to develop a plan of exposure exercises that will work well for

you. Remember, after we develop a treatment plan, it will be your choice whether to do the exposures. Is that clear?

P: Yes.

T: Good. So please go on and tell me what you were hesitating to describe.

P: You mean what I don't want to touch?

T: Yes.

P: Ok. I know I'll regret this later, but here goes. Its anything that comes from inside someone's body.

T: So things like saliva, urine, feces, and blood would bother you.

P: Yes.

T: What is the worst thing?

P: Its hard to say. All those things terrify me.

T: What do you worry might happen if you contacted one of those things?

P: Are you kidding? You could pick something up. A disease. You know. There are germs. You never know what somebody has and you could pick it up. Alcohol kills germs, right?

T: Is there any particular disease that concerns you?

P: Well, AIDS is the worst, isn't it? Aren't you worried about AIDS?

T: Do you think you touching these things will give you AIDS?

P: Well you get it from germs, don't you, and these things are really dirty, full of germs. If they get into you, you could get it.

T: You're right that germs do cause many diseases, and that saliva, urine, feces, and blood can contain germs, but just touching them doesn't usually make you sick. These things are not very dangerous. This is especially true for AIDS. Just touching these things has not been found to give anyone AIDS. To get AIDS, it seems that you have to get blood or semen inside your body, generally through a break in the skin or other opening in the body. Has anyone ever told you that?

P: I've heard that you can't get AIDS from touching stuff, but you never know. Scientists don't know everything. They could be wrong and then later you could get AIDS.

T: So even though researchers agree that you don't get AIDS just from touching things, you think you can?

P: Well, I'm not positive, but I feel that way, and you can never be too careful about AIDS.

The next interchange illustrates assessment of the patient's strength of obsessional belief. One approach is to inquire about the patient's subjective sense of the conditional probability of a disastrous consequence, given contact with the feared situation without subsequent rituals.

T: Let's say that you did actually get a fluid from someone else's body on your hand, and you weren't aware of it, so you didn't wash to remove it. What is the likelihood that you would get AIDS from this?

P: I'm not sure what you mean. I feel it really could happen.

T: The likelihood means how much of a chance there is. For example, there is a chance that you will get hit by lightning during your lifetime, but it is very small. If only one person out of 100,000 ever gets hit by lightning, the chance would be 1 in about 100,000. There is no certainty about this, but it is pretty clear that there is a low risk of getting hit by lightning. I understand that when you feel contaminated you get anxious, and you worry that you will get a disease. What I want you to do now though is to think about it calmly, when you are not in the situation, and give me your best guess about the chances that if you contact something from inside someone else's body, that you will get AIDS? For example, if 100 people touched some saliva, how many of them would get AIDS from it?

P: I don't know. All of them could, especially if they got it in a cut or something.

T: Do you really believe that just from touching saliva all 100 people will get AIDS, even if they don't have cuts on their hands? Do you think that all 100 will have cuts on their hands?

P: I don't know. This is confusing. How can you be sure the AIDS doesn't get into a cut? What if I have a small cut that I don't see? You know how you get little cuts around your fingernails. It could get inside you there. You can't be sure. If I use alcohol and it burns a little I know I have a cut. You can have cuts in your mouth, too. My gums bleed sometimes. You could get it on your hands and then eat something and get it in your mouth. That's why I rinse my mouth with alcohol. My lips get dry and I get cuts there, too. You could get cuts anywhere. You know it could get in through your penis, too, at the opening. Everybody must have some kind of little cut or some way for it to get into them.

It is clear that the patient strongly believes that contact with the feared contaminants is very risky. The patient's initial subjective likelihood estimate is 100% and does not change readily with questioning. A significant minority of patients with OCD have strongly held obsessional beliefs in harm. However, some patients with less strongly held beliefs are unable even to identify a specific feared consequence. Checkers often fear they will forget or discard something, but sometimes do not know what this would be. Repeaters often fear that something bad will happen to a loved one but sometimes cannot specify any particular disaster. Information obtained about feared consequences is used later for construction of imagery scripts.

The following interchange illustrates further inquiry about other situations that prompt obsessional fears.

T: Now I'd like you to tell what situations are difficult for you because of your concern with germs. What things are very difficult for you to do because of the OCD?

P: Everything is difficult. There are lots of things I don't do. Like I don't go very far from home because I might have to go to the bathroom and I only use my bathroom at home.

T: How were you able to travel all the way to Philadelphia if you can only use the bathroom at home?

P: Well I didn't like it and I had to use the alcohol a lot. This trip has been pretty hard and I've been using a lot of alcohol. If I really have to I can use a public toilet, I spray it first with alcohol and spray myself afterward.

T: What other situations cause difficulties?

P: Restaurants are bad. You know a lot of those waiters are gay and they could have AIDS. I don't like them handling things I'm going to eat. That makes me nervous, so I try to stay away from restaurants. Also, buying food that is right out in the open, like at supermarkets, the fruits that everybody touches. And I don't like people on the street getting too close to me. You know how they rub against you when you are walking. Sometimes these dirty looking people come up and ask you for money and I don't want them around me either. So I don't go out much. It makes it hard for me to get things done. Any public place is a problem.

T: So how do you manage on a daily basis?

P: My wife has to do a lot things for me. She's fed up with it, too. She does the shopping and takes care of the kids.

T: What conflicts with your wife occur because of your fears?

P: We fight a lot about it. I get really angry when she doesn't pay enough attention to keeping things clean. And she just let's the kids run around and come in and go all over the place. They don't care where they've been or what they touch. I'm always on them about it but they forget all the time. She thinks its wrong for me to be on them all the time. She really doesn't understand what its like for me. The kids don't understand either. If they would just keep away from the clean areas I could deal with it better.

T: So you have some clean areas at home?

P: Well, not too much, but some places are clean. Like my chair in the living room and the bed. Nobody's allowed to get near my chair. The bed is clean, too.

T: How do you keep the bed clean?

P: I shower before I go to bed.

T: What does your wife do?

P: She has to shower, too. She doesn't want to but she does, so I can deal with the bed okay. Once she forgot and we had a big fight, so she remembers all the time now.

To plan the specific exposure exercises, the therapist develops with the patient a list of objects and situations that provoke obsessive distress and has the patient estimate the relative difficulty of confronting each situation (without subsequent reutilizing). Although in principle there is no limit to the number of such items that can be developed, practical constraints usually limit the length of the list to about 10 to 20 items. The list should include examples of the most troublesome situations related to each obsessional fear content, but need not specify each of the many possible variations of each item. The following interchange illustrates the development of such a list.

T: We need to make a plan about what specific exposure exercises you will do for this therapy. A good way to do this is to make a list of what situations would get your obsessions going. These will be the situations that you confront during the therapy, and we will want to include the most difficult situations as well as some situations of moderate difficulty, because you will start your practice with the less difficult practices. A convenient way for me to know how the situations compare in difficulty for you is if you rate each one on a zero–100 scale of discomfort. Zero indicates no distress at all and 100 means you'd be extremely upset. So I'll make up the first situation based on what you've told me, and then you can add some more until we have a usable list.

P: Okay.

T: How about going down the hall into the waiting room and sitting right down in a chair but without any spraying of alcohol and without any close inspection of the chair to make sure it is okay? What would you rate doing that?

P: Could I at least wash my hands afterwards?

T: No. The idea is that when you do an exposure practice, you will not do anything afterward to reduce your discomfort. If you don't let the discomfort decrease on its own, the exposure exercise doesn't work so well to reduce your fear. So after you sit in the chair, you shouldn't use alcohol, wash, change your clothes, or do anything else to make yourself feel less contaminated.

P: Oh that's bad, 100.

T: I'm a bit puzzled about this. I would have thought that there were more difficult situations for you than sitting in a chair in the waiting room, but you rated this 100, which is the highest rating. Does that mean that sitting in the waiting-room chair would be just as difficult for you as handling books in the AIDS library in downtown Philadelphia?

P: You're not going to make me do that are you? You mean without washing? There's no way I'd go near that place.

T: It sounds like that would be more distressing than sitting in the chair in the waiting room, but since you rated the waiting room chair as 100, there was no room left to rate the AIDS library higher. What would you rate going to the AIDS library?

P: I'm not going in there. That would be 1,000.

T: Do you see how you have to save the highest ratings for the things that would be the worst? Do you still want to rate the waiting room chair as 100 or would you like to change that?

P: Okay, so that's not really 100. Maybe 75. But I'm not going in that AIDS place. No way. You can't make me do that.

This dialogue illustrates how a patient may need a little training beyond just description of the endpoints in the use of the SUDS rating scale. It also shows how strongly motivating are obsessional beliefs about harmful consequences. The following dialogue illustrates a model response to such strong opposition to a particular exposure exercise.

T: When you were talking about the AIDS library you said some things that I wanted to talk more about with you, because they are pretty important. First, you asked if I were going to make you go to the AIDS library, and then you said that I couldn't make you do that. That is not how this therapy works. I do not expect to make you do anything, and I won't try to force you to do anything. It is important to get that clear from the very start of this therapy. If you see me as an opponent who is trying to make you do things you aren't willing to do, we will waste a lot of energy and you won't profit much from the therapy.

The second thing is that you said there was no way you would go near the AIDS library. Well, I'm not going to try to force you to go there, but one thing I will do is to give you accurate information about what you must do if you are to get relief from your OCD through this therapy. If you decide in advance that there is no way you will try to do some of the exposure exercises, then our treatment will not be of much help to you. You must at least be willing to try as hard as you can to do the exposures. If you do this and find something too difficult, at least you have made a strong effort. If you're extremely afraid of something, we can develop some exercises to help you work up to doing most difficult one, but you have to be determined to try. Is that clear?

P: I'm not sure I can do that AIDS thing. I really don't want to do it.

T: It isn't surprising that you don't want to do something that is extremely frightening to you. To go on with this program, you don't have to be sure that you can do it, but you must be willing to try as much as you can. It will take a lot of courage on your part to confront things that you are very scared to do. I'm accustomed to helping people do this, encouraging them to do what they need to do to get relief. Sometimes I can help by explaining more about the exercise, sometimes by doing it first, and sometimes by devising some intermediate exposures. So, are you willing to try to do whatever exposures are needed, even if you really don't want to do them?

P: I guess so. I'm still not sure I can do this.

The inquiry is continued until a satisfactory list has been developed. Care must be taken to develop items that address each of the content areas of the patients obsessions. For example, a list that includes contamination and checking items but neglects items related to hoarding would be inadequate for a patient with all three types of obsessional concerns.

Asking the patient to describe in detail a typical day's activities can yield useful information relevant to developing exposure items. Such interviewing can alert the patient to troublesome situations that were taken for granted. Bathroom routines are often of particular difficulty, and detailed inquiry, as well as direct observation, can be informative. For example, just observing the way a patient brushes teeth, turns on and off faucets, and flushes toilets, can reveal avoidant or ritualistic patterns that require correction. Additional inquiries should be made about other routine activities such as shopping, eating out, housecleaning, preparing meals, working, etc.

Information obtained from interviewing can be supplemented by the patient's self-monitoring of the frequency and duration of compulsions. Not only can this information be useful, it can also enhance the patient's awareness of ritualistic behavior, and this is important for choices about abstinence from rituals.

A routine history is usually taken at the first session. Inquiries should be made about symptoms whose form to some extent parallels that of OCD, as well as about commonly co-occurring symptoms (e.g. depression, anorexia nervosa, body dysmorphia, hypochon-driasis, other anxiety disorders, superstitions, and tics). The relationship of any such symptoms to the OCD should be ascertained, and addressed during therapy.

Treatment Planning

The second session usually begins with a review of the patient's self-monitoring homework, with corrective instruction as needed. Then assessment continues as needed to complete the history taking, or the development of the list of exposure situations. When these are completed, a summary of the treatment plan is articulated, including the specifics of what exposure exercises are to be done in sessions, and at home. The following interchange illustrates such a summary.

T: I want to summarize our plan for the therapy. You will confront in imagination and in reality all of the things we put on our list, as well as any new troublesome situations that we may discover as we go along. In conjunction with the exposure practice, you will stop all rituals. To help you do this, you will follow a schedule of limited washing. Specifically, you will not touch water except for a brief shower every 3 days.

P: You mean I can't even take a shower? I've got to at least take a shower. Nobody doesn't take a shower for 3 days.

T: It is important that you don't take a shower for 3 days, even though many people routinely shower more often than that. You have a very difficult habit to weaken. That is the excessive washing. Going without washing for 3 days is a somewhat exaggerated exercise, and after you finish the program, you will return to a more frequent washing schedule. Nevertheless, we have found this exercise helpful in weakening the connection between contamination and washing, and that is your goal here. When you do wash after 3 days, it will be very brief, and you will recontaminate yourself immediately afterwards, so that the washing doesn't provide relief from obsessive fear.

P: Well, what about brushing my teeth? And I wear contact lenses. I have to clean them.

T: Unless you have been doing rituals during brushing, you can still brush your teeth, but you may not wash or rinse your hands while doing this. You can bring your toothbrush tomorrow to the session, and I can coach you on doing it properly. Do you have a pair of glasses you can use during the therapy instead of the contacts?

P: No, I just have the contacts.

T: Then you should clean them properly. Please bring in your lens-cleaning materials tomorrow, and we will work out a way for you to clean them without any ritualizing.

Complete abstinence from washing relieves the patient of the burden of making judgments about what is an appropriate time and period for washing. Once the intensity of the obsessive fear has been weakened by exposure practice and the washing habit has been weakened via abstinence from washing, the patient can be instructed to begin practicing more frequent washing, but without rituals. Customarily, patients resume more frequent washing during the last week of the intensive program (see Appendix C for "normal" washing rules). In the case example, the practical need to clean contact lenses was accommodated by allowing the patient to touch water briefly during this time, but with immediate recontamination. Alternative methods might have been substituting the use of eyeglasses during the treatment period or using surgical gloves for the lens cleansing, so that no incidental personal decontamination would occur during the lens cleansing. Direct observation of the patient's behavior can reveal whether the toothbrushing or lens cleansing can be done without rituals, and whether measures such as rubber gloves should be introduced.

Illustration of treatment planning is continued below.

T: Now I'd like to discuss the exposure schedule. We will do both imaginal and actual exposure in a gradual manner. You will confront the situations on the list we made, starting with those that you rated as being moderately difficult (i.e., about 50 on the scale). You will work up the list until you get to the most difficult items by the sixth day. According to the list, that means you will start with things like sitting in the waiting room without sterilizing the chair and move up to sitting on the floor; then we'll touch items at supermarkets and surfaces in bathrooms. The highest items are touching books and other surfaces at the AIDS library and touching a residue of blood.

P: I don't know if I can do those last things. Not that AIDS library or the blood. You can't make me do those things.

T: We already discussed these exercises, and we agreed that you did not have to be sure that you would do those exposure exercises, but that you did have to be determined to try, even though they would be very difficult. It seems that you still have the idea that I will make you do things. Do you remember that we talked about it and I assured you that I will not try to force you to do things?

P: Yes.

T: It is clear that you are very hesitant about confronting the most difficult situations, but if they were easy for you, you would not be seeking help with your fear. Are you still willing to give this your best try?

P: I guess so.

T: Good. Very often, the exposure practice with the less difficult items reduces fear of more difficult items, so that you are better prepared to confront them. The imaginal exposure might be helpful with that, too. In this exposure exercise, you will confront the distressing situations in imagination, including harm that you fear will happen, like getting AIDS. You will picture yourself touching something that bothers you, not washing or sterilizing with alcohol, and then becoming ill. The scenes that we use will be based on the list of situations we developed, and we will begin with moderately difficult images and work up to the most difficult ones by the sixth day.

An extremely important part of the program will be what you do in between the times when you meet with me. We call that part of the program your homework. We already discussed your refraining from rituals, including the no-washing part. In addition to this, you will do exposure practice on your own between the sessions. Each day you will practice the exposure that you have done during the session, and sometimes you will have additional exposure homework as well. This homework is as important as the exposure that you do during the sessions.

Intensive Treatment

Jake was seen for 15 outpatient-treatment sessions, many of which involved confrontation with situations *in vivo*, such as public markets, public toilets, and a library. During these visits, Jake, under the therapist's supervision, confronted all the situations on the list. Thereafter, weekly telephone follow-up sessions were conducted to promote maintenance of gains.

Michael J. Kozak and
Edna B. Foa

As planned, exposure began with moderately difficult items on the hierarchy and progressed to the most disturbing ones by the beginning of the second week. The major distressing items are repeated during the remainder of the second and third week. The following interchange exemplifies problems sometimes encountered when the most difficult item is to be confronted.

T: Today you are scheduled to work with blood residue. I have a cloth with some dried blood on it in the other room. May I bring it in here so that we may get started with the exposure?

P: I'm still not ready to touch that blood. Do you know who it came from? Can you guarantee that I won't get AIDS from it? I don't think I should touch that because I can't be sure that its safe.

T: Do you remember that before we began the therapy I told you that none of the exposure tasks would be dangerous?

P: Yes.

T: Well, touching a spot of blood on a cloth isn't dangerous.

P: Can you guarantee 100% me that its safe?

T: No, but it is a mistake to try to get 100% certainty. I am confident that this is a very low-risk thing to do, but I don't have absolute certainty of safety. Whenever you try to get such certainty, you will get into trouble, because it is virtually impossible to achieve. If I refused to drive an auto or travel by plane unless I had 100% certainty of safety, I'd never go anywhere, because there are some risks involved with auto and air travel. The risks are low, but they are real. Accidents do occur, and people are sometimes injured or killed. It is clear that you are willing to do many things that are low risk and are not 100% guaranteed safe. But you make an exception when it comes to the risk of infectious disease. It will be important for you to learn to confront low-risk situations related to your fear of disease. This means touching things that are low risk, but not guaranteed to be completely risk free. This dried blood spot is one of those things that is low risk.

P: You mean I have to touch this even though it might give me AIDS? A normal person wouldn't do that.

T: If you want to reduce this obsessional fear with this therapy, you must touch this spot even though you don't have a guarantee that it is safe. It might help to know that there are no documented cases of someone getting AIDS from touching a spot of blood, but that still doesn't give you a 100% guarantee. To demonstrate it, I will touch the spot. May I touch it to show you?

P: Okay, as long as you don't spread it to me. (*Therapist then touches spot with finger.*)

T: So when I touch the spot like this, I'm taking a risk that in my mind is so low as to not matter much. It is true that I can't guarantee that I won't get AIDS from this, but I don't try to get that kind of a guarantee because it would be too difficult.

P: You are going to wash now, right?

T: No, and I won't wash after you leave either, because it would be a waste of time. There isn't anything important to wash off my finger. The risk is so low that I'm not going to waste time trying to make it even lower, or trying to make absolutely sure I'm safe. Now it is your turn to touch the spot. What is your rating of discomfort now?

P: 100.

T: It is time for you to touch the bloodspot. The more you procrastinate and think about it, the more difficult it gets to do it. Just reach over and touch the spot.

P: I can't do it.

T: Remember, what you do is by your own choice. Clearly, you can reach over and touch the spot. You know how to do it, but you are choosing not to do it because you are anxious. It take courage to touch it even though this scares you. You have done this with other exposure tasks so far, but this one is the most difficult one, so you are hesitating, but you really can do it, if that's what you choose to do. It calls for taking a chance now in order to reduce the obsessive fear in the long run.

P: Are you sure its safe? If you would just tell me its safe, I think I could do it.

T: We already discussed this. It is low risk. If I tell you I'm sure its safe, that might help you think that there is some kind of a guarantee. It is safe, but not absolutely, and you need to touch it anyway if you are to get better with this therapy. That is the worst part of this therapy. You have to confront things like this that give you a lot of distress, and if you don't do it, the therapy doesn't work. So touch the spot now.

P: Its too hard. I can't do it.

T: You saw that I did it. Can you try just touching my finger?

P: Well, maybe I can touch your finger.

T: (*Holds out finger.*) Just touch the tip of my finger. (Patient quickly touches tip of therapist's finger and withdraws hand; patient holds hand away from his body.) Good. You did it. How do you feel?

P: 1,000. I don't believe you made me do this. This is ridiculous. What am I going to do about this blood on my finger? How am I going to clean it off without spreading it to everything?

T: What I want you to do is to just stay here awhile, until you don't feel so bad about it. What usually happens when you confront a really difficult item is that it bothers you a lot for a little while, then later it isn't as bad. But it doesn't work if you decide to use alcohol or wash, so try as hard as you can not to do that. Some people get angry when they do an exposure because they feel caught in the situation. If they touch the item, they feel bad, and if they don't touch the thing, they feel bad. The best thing to do is go ahead with it. I'm going to touch the spot again, and spread it around on myself, including onto my face. Watch what I'm doing. What is your rating of discomfort about what is on your finger?

P: Still 1,000. I don't like this at all.

Exposure should continue until a noticeable decrease in distress occurs. Session length can be adjusted according to the needs of the individual. If anxiety has not decreased by the end of an available session period, the patient can be instructed to remain in the clinic for an extended period for prolonged exposure and intermittent monitoring by the therapist.

During prolonged exposure in the session, the patient's focus should be on the exposure practice. Thus, if the conversation is about topics other than the exposure task at hand, the therapist should frequently redirect the patient's attention to this task.

Periodic inquiries about the patient's level of distress can indicate whether the expected fear reduction is occurring.

T: How do you feel now?

P: 100.

T: So do you notice any difference at all in how you feel now compared to when you first touched the spot?

P: No.

T: I'm a little puzzled about that, because you look a little less anxious. When you first touched the spot, your rating was 1,000 and you were pushing yourself way back in the chair, and you held your finger held out as far away from you as you could reach. Now you aren't pushing back, and your face looks a bit more relaxed. Does my description fit your experience?

P: Well, when you put it that way, I guess it is a little bit better than when before, but it is almost no difference.

T: So, do you still rate your discomfort as 100?

P: Well, maybe 95.

T: So far it has been about 25 minutes since you touched the spot. It can take awhile before you experience much of a decrease in discomfort, so let's keep working with the spot. I'm going to touch it again. (*Therapist touches spot again.*) You already did this once. Try touching it again now. Very good. Is it just as hard to do as it was before?

P: (*Patient touches spot again.*) Yes, it's about the same.

It is notable that although the patient said that retouching the spot was as uncomfortable as it was the first time, the arguing and attempts at delaying the exposure declined. Such observations can be useful indicators of fear reduction and should supplement the patient's introspective reports.

T: How do you feel now about having touched the spot?

P: Maybe I'm down to 85.

T: Good. This is how the therapy is expected to be. When you first confront the spot, it bothers you a lot and if you continue to do the exposure for a long-enough time, you start to feel better.

P: How much longer do I have to do this?

T: I don't know exactly. People differ in how long they have to do an exposure before they get so used to it that it doesn't bother them. It often takes at least an hour or two before you notice much difference, and it can take several hours. Sometimes a person has to keep doing it all day before it gets much better. Your job is to stay with this until you notice a clear decrease in discomfort. So far, you've just noticed a very small difference, so you should keep doing it for a while longer. What is your rating now?

P: Maybe a little less, I'll say 82.

Imaginal Exposure

Forty-five minutes of imaginal exposure preceded *in vivo* exposure on most days of the intensive treatment period. Several strategies can be used to develop image scripts. One approach is to prepare the patient for the day's *in vivo* exposure with imaginal exposure immediately prior to that very situation. The difficulty of imaginal exposure can often be manipulated by regulating the inclusion of disastrous consequences in the narrative. If the patient's discomfort has decreased to a relevant disaster scenario, the subsequent actual exposure can become less difficult by contrast. Imaginal exposure can be particularly useful for situations that are impractical to realize *in vivo*. For example, it may be impractical to confront feared nuclear waste products in reality during each session; the patients can imagine daily exposure to nuclear waste. For Jake, imaginal exposure involved contact with HIV-infected blood, but the blood used for *in vivo* exposure was not infected.

Habituation of Obsessional Distress

After 10–15 exposure sessions, discomfort, frequency, and persistence of obsessive intrusions, as well as urges to ritualize, are expected to decrease considerably. Jake required a longer than usual time to experience substantial decreases in discomfort. Typically, decreases of 50% in self-rated distress occur within a 2-hour session. Jake, however, reported only a 20% decrease for several days, and was persistently troubled by beliefs that several of the low-risk exposure tasks were indeed high risk. By the end of 15 sessions, however, strength of those beliefs had weakened considerably, and self-rated discomfort for the highest items decreased from 100 to 40.

To facilitate transition to routine washing, the therapist instituted a "normal washing" regimen during the last week of intensive treatment. One daily 10-minute shower was permitted; brief (30-second) handwashes (not more than five per day) were also permitted, but only if the hands were actually dirty. A convenient rule of thumb is that a wash is permitted only if one can readily see, smell, or feel that the hands are soiled. The patient should be cautioned, however, that the soil must be obvious without close inspection, and that perfectionistic checking of the hands for soil is prohibited.

Follow-up Sessions

Jake left Philadelphia and returned to his hometown after the intensive treatment period. Brief telephone sessions were scheduled weekly for 1 month and biweekly for another month. His wife had decided to pursue divorce proceedings, and he found the return to his home stressful. Telephone sessions were devoted to assessment of Jake's progress in applying principles of exposure and ritual prevention to situations that arose in his day-to-day life. Over the 2 months following his intensive treatment, he reported many lapses into avoidance and cleaning rituals, but the overall frequency, duration, and subjective intensity of his obsessive–compulsive symptoms decreased by about 75% compared to pretreatment levels.

Rarely do patients eliminate 100% of their obsessive–compulsive symptoms after behavior therapy. Occasional obsessive intrusions typically recur, but the intense discomfort and strong urges to ritualize that were present before treatment do dissipate. Because of the substantially reduced obsessional discomfort, there is usually little avoidance and ritualizing. Nevertheless, it is important to help patients anticipate recurrent obsessive intrusions, so that they know not to strengthen them through avoidance and rituals. Such recurrences seem particularly likely to emerge in stressful circumstances, such as during interpersonal, occupational, or health crises. Some women have reported noticing recurrences premenstrually, and with pregnancy.

CONCLUSIONS

Exposure treatment produces marked improvement in the large majority of obsessive–compulsive patients who complete it, both immediately after treatment and at longer term follow-up. The fundamental principles of such treatment have been established through the studies, but many of the details of their successful implementation depend on creative ingenuity of the skilled therapist.

In this chapter we have described a basic intensive program that we have found to be highly effective: 15 sessions of intensive treatment for a short period of time, followed by 8–10 weekly sessions. The extent to which departure from this protocol would degrade outcome is unclear. For some patients, fewer sessions seem adequate; for others, not. The concentrated efforts required during the intensive treatment phase may not be feasible for every therapist and patient in clinical practice, but our clinical experience suggests that once-weekly sessions are generally inadequate for all but those with very mild symptoms. Perhaps three sessions weekly would suffice for many patients. Definitive studies evaluating the various interesting permutations of the protocol would be expensive affairs and have not been done.

Although most patients show immediate posttreatment improvement, about 15% to 20% relapse to various degrees. Those at greatest risk for relapse are the moderately improved at the end of treatment (Foa et al., 1983b). This suggests that anything but a full course of treatment, with no degradation of outcome, is undesirable.

The high efficacy of exposure treatment notwithstanding, about 25% of patients we evaluate decline to accept this treatment. Thus, an intent-to-treat analysis would reveal considerably less satisfactory outcome than that obtained with treatment completers. Efforts to understand the factors influencing the acceptability of exposure treatment are indicated, so that more patients may profit from this powerful remedy.

APPENDIX A: SELF-MONITORING OF RITUALS

Name _____ Date _____

In the second column of the table below please describe the activity or thought that evokes a ritual. In the third column, specify what the ritual was. In the fourth column, record the anxiety/discomfort level (zero–100). In the fifth column write the number of minutes you spend in performing rituals during the time stated in Column 1. Record SUDS for each homework assignment, when treatment is in progress.

Time of day	Activity or thought that evokes the ritual	Ritual	Discomfort (0–100)	Number of minutes spent on ritual
6:00–6:30 A.M.				
6:30–7:00				
7:00–7:30				
7:30–8:00				
8:00–8:30				
8:30–9:00				
9:00–9:30				
9:30–10:00				
10:00–10:30				
10:30–11:00				
11:00–11:30				
11:30–12:00 P.M.				
12:00–12:30				
12:30–1:00				
1:00–1:30				
1:30–2:00				

2:00–2:30				
2:30–3:00				
3:00–3:30				
3:30–4:00				
4:00–4:30				
4:30–5:00				
5:00–5:30				
5:30–6:00				
6:00–6:30				
6:30–7:00				
7:00–7:30				
7:30–8:00				
8:00–8:30				
8:30–9:00				
9:00–9:30				
9:30–10:00				
10:00–10:30				
10:30–11:00				
11:00–6:00 A.M.				

APPENDIX B: EXAMPLE OF AN IMAGINAL EXPOSURE SCENE

T: "I want you to imagine the following scene as vividly as you can, as if it is actually happening, and to experience the feelings as you imagine. I want you to imagine that you are sitting here in the chair, and I am with you. The door opens and your mother comes in. She enters the room, she sees you, and she says, 'Hello, it has been a long time.' She comes to you and she touches you. She wants to hug you. Your mother is astonished that you let her hug you, and she says, 'I am allowed to hug my daughter again.' Now you feel the contamination spreading all over you. You can feel her hands on your back. You begin to feel that it will never go away. It can never be washed. You would like your mother to leave and you want to take a shower or a bath so you can feel clean again. You can't say anything. You just let her hold your hand and let her hug you. You can't move, you are overwhelmed by the feeling of being contaminated. Your mother is standing beside you, and she is holding your hand and you can feel how she becomes even more contaminating. You would like her to take her hand off. And she is asking you, 'Are you afraid of me?', and you would like to explain to her how much afraid of her you are, but you don't say anything. You just let her hold your hand and let her hug you. You let her sit beside you, real close, and she is contaminating you. You can feel the contamination all over your body. You wish you could run out and scream and never come in contact with her again. But you stay here, you stay beside her as she contaminates you more and more. you feel that you will never be clean again. You realize that your mother is contaminating you. You feel the contamination on your skin. You feel the burning spots on your back and hands. It is the feeling of contamination, creeping up your arms, creeping up your face, it's all over your body. You try to keep your hand close to your body to make sure that the parts which are not contaminated now will remain clean. But it is spreading over your whole body. And your mother is still beside you, still contaminating you. She is contaminating you more and more. She is telling you something but you can't really listen to her. You are so upset, your heart is beating, you can feel your heart beating really fast. You feel as though you are going to faint. But something forces you to stay and listen to her. You would like to run to the next room, but you realize that you have to fact the fact that you can't avoid your mother any longer. You feel trapped. She will never go away, she will go on contaminating you forever, more and more. You will never feel free again. You have the urge to leave the room and to forget everything about your mother. But her touch is everywhere on your body. How are you feeling now?''

APPENDIX C: GUIDELINES FOR "NORMAL BEHAVIOR"

Washing

1. Do not exceed one 10-minute shower daily.
2. Do not exceed 5 handwashings per day, 30 seconds each.
3. Restrict handwashing to when hands are visibly dirty or sticky.
4. Continue to expose yourself deliberately on a weekly basis to objects or situations which used to disturb you.
5. If objects or situations are still somewhat disturbing, expose yourself twice weekly to them.
6. Do not avoid situations that cause discomfort. If you detect a tendency to avoid a situation, confront it deliberately at least twice a week.

Checking

1. Do not check more than *once* any objects or situations that used to trigger an urge to check.
2. Do not check even once in situations that your therapist has advised you do not require checking.
3. Do not avoid situations that trigger an urge to check. If you detect a tendency to avoid, confront these situations deliberately twice a week and exercise control by refraining from checking.
4. Do not assign responsibility for checking to friends or family members in order to avoid checking.

Other Rules: _____

REFERENCES

Allen, J. J., & Tune, G. S. (1975). The Lynfield obsessional/compulsive questionnaire. *Scottish Medical Journal*, *20*, 21–24.

American Psychiatric Association. (1952). *Diagnostic and statistical manual of mental disorders* (1st ed.). Washington, DC: Author.

American Psychiatric Association. (1968). *Diagnostic and statistical manual of mental disorders* (2nd ed.). Washington, DC: Author.

American Psychiatric Association. (1980). *Diagnostic and statistical manual of mental disorders* (3rd ed.). Washington, DC: Author.

American Psychiatric Association. (1987). *Diagnostic and statistical manual of mental disorders* (3rd ed., rev.). Washington, DC: Author.

American Psychiatric Association. (1994). *Diagnostic and statistical manual of mental disorders* (4th ed.). Washington, DC: Author.

Baer, L., Jenike, M. A., Ricciardi, J. N., Holland, A. D., Seymour, R. J., Minichiello, W. E., & Buttolph, M. L. (in press). Standardized assessment of personality disorders in obsessive–compulsive disorder. *Archives of General Psychiatry.*

Ballentine, H. T., Bouckoms, H. A., Thomas, E. K., Giriunas, I. E. (1987). Treatment of psychiatric illness by stereotactic singulotomy. *Biological Psychiatry, 22,* 807–809.

Basoglu, M., Lax, T., Kasvikis, Y., & Marks, I. M. (1988). Predictors of improvement in obsessive–compulsive disorder. *Journal of Anxiety Disorders, 2,* 299–317.

Baxter, L. R., Phelps, M. E., Maziotta, J. C., Guze, B. H., Schwartz, J. M., & Selin, C. E. (1987). Local cerebral glucose metabolic rates in obsessive and compulsive disorder: A comparison with rates of unipolar depression and normal controls. *Archives of General Psychiatry, 44,* 211–218.

Beck, A. T. (1976). *Cognitive therapy and the emotional disorders.* New York: International Universities Press.

Beech, H. R., & Vaughn, M. (1978). *Behavioral treatment of obsessive states.* New York: Wiley.

Behar, D., Rapoport, J. L., Berg, C. J., Denckla, M., Mann, L., Cox, C., Fedio, P., Zahn, T., & Wolfman, H. (1984). Computerized tomography and neuropsychological test measures in adolescents with obsessive–compulsive disorder. *American Journal of Psychiatry, 141,* 363–369.

Black, A. (1974). The natural history of obsessional neurosis. In H. R. Beech (Ed.), *Obsessional states* (pp. 19–54). London: Methuen.

Boulougouris, J. C., Rabavilas, A. D., & Stefanis, C. (1977). Psycho-physiological responses in obsessive–compulsive patients. *Behaviour Research and Therapy, 15,* 221–230.

Carr, A. T. (1974). Compulsive neurosis: A review of the literature. *Psychological Bulletin, 81,* 311–318.

Charney, D. S., Goodman, W. K., Price, L. H., Woods, S. W., Rasmussen, S. A., & Heninger, G. R. (1988). Serotonin function in obsessive–compulsive disorder: A comparison of the effects of tryptophan and m-chlorophenylpiperazine in patients and healthy subjects. *Archives of General Psychiatry, 45,* 177–185.

Cooper, J. E., Gelder, M. G., & Marks, I. M. (1965). Results of behaviour therapy in 77 psychiatric patients. *British Medical Journal, 1,* 1222–1225.

Cottraux, J., Mollard, E., Bouvard, M., Marks, I., Sluys, M., Nury, A. M., Douge, R., & Ciadella, P. (1990). A controlled study of fluvoxamine and exposure in obsessive–compulsive disorder. *International Clinical Psychopharmacology, 5,* 17–30.

Cox, C. S., Fedio, P., & Rapoport, J. L. (1989). Neuropsychological testing of obsessive–compulsive adolescents. In J. L. Rapoport (Ed.) *Obsessive–compulsive disorder in children and adolescents* (pp. 73–85). Washington, DC: American Psychiatric Press.

DeVeaugh-Geiss, J., Landau, P., & Katz, R. (1989). Treatment of OCD with clomipramine. *Psychiatric Annals, 19,* 97–101.

Dollard, J., & Miller, N. E. (1950). *Personality and psychotherapy: An analysis in terms of learning, thinking and culture.* New York: McGraw-Hill.

Eisen, J., & Rasmussen, S. (in press). Obsessive–compulsive disorder with psychotic features. *Journal of Clinical Psychology.*

Ellis, A. (1962). *Reason and emotion in psychotherapy.* New York: Lyle Stuart.

Emmelkamp, P. M. G., & Beens, H. (1991). Cognitive therapy with obsessive–compulsive disorder: A comparative evaluation. *Behaviour Research and Therapy, 29,* 293–300.

Emmelkamp, P. M. G., de Haan, E., & Hoogduin, C. A. L. (1990). Marital adjustment and obsessive–compulsive disorder. *British Journal of Psychiatry, 156,* 55–60.

Emmelkamp, P. M. G., & Kwee, K. G. (1977). Obsessional ruminations: A comparison between thought-stopping and prolonged exposure in imagination. *Behaviour Research and Therapy, 15,* 441–444.

Emmelkamp, P. M. G., & van Kraanen, J. (1977). Therapist-controlled exposure *in vivo*: A comparison with obsessive–compulsive patients. *Behaviour Research and Therapy, 15,* 491–495.

Emmelkamp, P. M. G., Visser, S., & Hoekstra, R. J. (1988). Cognitive therapy vs. exposure *in vivo* in the treatment of obsessive–compulsives. *Cognitive Therapy and Research, 12,* 103–114.

Esquirol, J. E. D. (1838). *Des maladies mentales: Volume 2.* Paris: Bailliere.

Flament, M. F., Rapoport, J. L., Berg, C. J., Sceery, W., Kilts, C., Mellstram, B., & Linnoila, M. (1985). Clomipramine treatment of childhood obsessive–compulsive disorder: A double-blind controlled study. *Archives of General Psychiatry, 42,* 977–983.

Foa, E. B. (1979). Failure in treating obsessive–compulsives. *Behaviour Research and Therapy, 17,* 169–176.

Foa, E. B., & Chambless, D. L. (1978). Habituation of subjective anxiety during flooding in imagery. *Behaviour Research and Therapy, 16,* 391–399.

Foa, E. B., Grayson, J. B., & Steketee, G. (1982). Depression, habituation and treatment outcome in obsessive–compulsives. In J. C. Boulougouris (Ed.), *Practical applications of learning theories in psychiatry* (pp. 129–141). New York: Wiley.

Foa, E. B., Grayson, J. B., Steketee, G. S., & Doppelt, H. G. (1983a). Treatment of obsessive–compulsives: When do we fail? In E. B. Foa & P. M. G. Emmelkamp (Eds.), *Failures in behavior therapy* (pp. 10–34). New York: Wiley.

Foa, E. B., Grayson, J. B., Steketee, G., Doppelt, H. G., Turner, R. M., & Latimer, P. R. (1983b). Success and failure in the behavioral treatment of obsessive–compulsives. *Journal of Consulting and Clinical Psychology, 51,* 287–297.

Foa, E. B., & Kozak, M. J. (1985). Treatment of anxiety disorders: Implications for psychopathology. In A. H. Tuma & J. D. Maser (Eds.), *Anxiety and the anxiety disorders* (pp. 421–451). Hillsdale, NY: Erlbaum.

Foa, E. B., & Kozak, M. J. (1991). Emotional processing: Theory, research and clinical implications for anxiety disorders. In J. Safran & J. Greenberg (Eds.), *Emotion and therapeutic change* (pp. 21-49). New York: Guilford Press.

Foa, E. B., Kozak, M. J., Goodman, W. K., Hollander, E., Jeniko, M. A., & Rasmussen, S. (1995). DSM-IV field trial: Obsessive–compulsive disorder. *American Journal of Psychiatry, 1,* 116–120.

Foa, E. B., Kozak, M. J., Liebowitz, M., Gorfinkle, K., Campeas, R., Stehle, S., Street, L., Riggs, D., Franklin, M., Davies, S., Hearst, D., Del Bene, D., & Nixon, W. (1993). *Treatment of obsessive–compulsive disorder by behavior therapy, clomipramine, and their combination: Preliminary findings of a multicenter double blind-controlled trial.* Poster presented at annual meeting of the Association for the Advancement of Behavior Therapy, Atlanta, GA.

Foa, E. B., Kozak, M. J., Steketee, G., & McCarthy, P. R. (1992). Treatment of depressive and obsessive–compulsive symptoms in OCD by imipramine and behavior therapy. *British Journal of Clinical Psychology, 31,* 279–292.

Foa, E. B., Riggs, D. S., Massie, E. D., & Yarczower, M. (in press). The impact of fear activation and anger on the efficacy of exposure treatment for PTSD. *Behavior Therapy.*

Foa, E. B., Steketee, G. S., & Grayson, J. B. (1985). Imaginal and *in vivo* exposure: A comparison with obsessive–compulsive checkers. *Behavior Therapy, 16,* 292–302.

Foa, E. B., Steketee, G., Grayson, J. B., Turner, R. M., & Latimer, P. (1984). Deliberate exposure and blocking of obsessive–compulsive rituals: Immediate and long-term effects. *Behavior Therapy, 15,* 450–472.

Foa, E. B., Steketee, G. S., Kozak, M. J., & Dugger, D. (1985, September). *Effects of imipramine on depression and on obsessive–compulsive symptoms.* Paper presented at the European Association for Behavior Therapy, Munich, Federal Republic of Germany.

Foa, E. B., Steketee, G. S., & Milby, J. B. (1980). Differential effects of exposure and response prevention in obsessive–compulsive washers. *Journal of Consulting and Clinical Psychology, 48,* 71–79.

Foa, E. B., Steketee, G. S., & Ozarow, B. (1985). Behavior therapy with obsessive–compulsives: From theory to treatment. In M. Mavissakalian (Ed.), *Obsessive–compulsive disorder: Psychological and pharmacological treatment* (pp. 49–129). New York: Plenum Press.

Foa, E. B., Steketee, G., Turner, R. M., & Fischer, S. C. (1980). Effects of imaginal exposure to feared disasters in obsessive–compulsive checkers. *Behaviour Research and Therapy, 18,* 449–455.

Foa, E. B., & Tillmanns, A. (1980). The treatment of obsessive–compulsive neurosis. In A. Goldstein & E. B. Foa (Eds.), *Handbook of behavioral interventions: A clinical guide* (pp. 416–500). New York: Wiley.

Foa, E. B., & Wilson, R. (1991). *Stop obsessing: How to overcome your obsessions and compulsions.* New York: Bantam.

Fontaine, R., & Chouinard, G. (1985). Fluoxetine in the treatment of obsessive–compulsive disorder. *Progress in Neuropsychopharmacology and Biological Psychiatry, 9,* 605–608.

Fontaine, R., & Chouinard, G. (1989). Fluoxatine in the long-term maintenance treatment of OCD. *Psychiatric Annals, 19,* 88–91.

Freund, B. (1986). *Comparison of measures of obsessive–compulsive symptomatology: Rating scales of symptomatology and standardized assessor- and self-rated.* Unpublished dissertation, Southern Illinois University, Carbondale, Ill.

Goodman, W. K., Price, L. H., Rasmussen, S. A., Delgado, P. L., Heninger, G. R., & Charney, D. S. (1989a). Efficacy of fluvoxamine in obsessive–compulsive disorder: A double blind comparison with placebo. *Archives of General Psychiatry, 46*, 36–44.

Goodman, W. K., Price, L. H., Rasmussen, S. A., Mazure, C., Delgado, P., Heninger, G. R., & Charney, D. S. (1989b). The Yale–Brown obsessive–compulsive scale. II. Validity. *Archives of General Psychiatry, 46*, 1012–1016.

Goodman, W. K., Price, L. H., Rasmussen, S. A., Mazure, C., Fleischmann, R. L., Hill, C. L., Heninger, G. R., & Charney, D. S. (1989a). The Yale–Brown obsessive–compulsive scale. I. Development, use, and reliability. *Archives of General Psychiatry, 46*, 1006–1011.

Greist, J. H. (1990). Treatment of obsessive–compulsive disorder: Psychotherapies, drugs, and other somatic treatments. *Journal of Clinical Psychiatry, 51*, 44–50.

Greist, J. H., Jefferson, J. W., Kobak, K. A., Katzelnick, D. J., & Serlin, R. C. (in press). Efficacy and tolerability of serotonin transport inhibitors in obsessive–compulsive disorder: A meta-analysis. *Archives of General Psychiatry*.

Head, D., Bolton, D., & Hymas, N. (1989). Deficit in cognitive shifting in patients with obsessive–compulsive disorder. *Biological Psychiatry, 25*, 929–937.

Hembree, E. A., Cohen, A., Riggs, D. S., Kozak, M. J., & Foa, E. B. (1995). *The long-term efficacy of behavior therapy and serotonergic medications in the treatment of obsessive–compulsive ritualizers.* Unpublished manuscript.

Hiss, H., Foa, E. B., & Kozak, M. J. (1994). Relapse prevention program for treatment of obsessive–compulsive disorder. *Journal of Consulting and Clinical Psychology, 62*, 801–808.

Hodgson, R. J., & Rachman, S. (1972). The effects of contamination and washing in obsessional patients. *Behaviour Research and Therapy, 10*, 111–117.

Hodgson, R. J., & Rachman, S. (1977). Obsessional–compulsive complaints. *Behaviour Research and Therapy, 15*, 389–395.

Hodgson, R. J., Rachman, S., & Marks, I. M. (1972). The treatment of chronic obsessive–compulsive neurosis: Follow-up and further findings. *Behaviour Research and Therapy, 10*, 181–189.

Hornsveld, R. H. J., Kraaimaat, F. W., & van Dam-Baggen, R. M. J. (1979). Anxiety/discomfort and handwashing in obsessive–compulsive and psychiatric control patients. *Behaviour Research and Therapy, 17*, 223–228.

Hudson, J. I., Pope, H. G., Yurgelun-Todd, D., Jonas, J. M., & Frankenburg, F. R. (1987). A controlled study of anorexia nervosa and obsessive nervosa. *British Journal of Psychiatry, 27*, 57–60.

Insel, T. R., & Akiskal, H. (1986). Obsessive–compulsive disorder with psychotic features: A phenomenologic analysis. *American Journal of Psychiatry, 12*, 1527–1533.

Insel, T. R., Donnelly, E. F., Lalakea, M. L., Alterman, I. S., & Murphy, D. L. (1983). Neurological and neuropsychological studies of patients with obsessive–compulsive disorder. *Biological Psychiatry, 18*, 741–751.

Insel, T. R., Mueller, E. A., Alterman, I. S., Linnoila, M., & Murphy, D. L. (1985). Obsessive–compulsive disorder and serotonin: Is there a connection? *Biological Psychiatry, 20*, 1174–1188.

Insel, T. R., Murphy, D. L., Cohen, R. M., Alterman, I. S., Kilts, C., & Linnoila, M. (1983). Obsessive–compulsive disorder: A double-blind trial of clomipramine and clorgyline. *Archives of General Psychiatry, 40*, 605–612.

Janet, P. (1908). *Les obsessions et la psychasthenie* (2nd ed.). Paris: Bailliere.

Jenike, M., Baer, L., Minichiello, W., Schwartz, C., & Carey, R. (1986). Concomitant obsessive–compulsive disorder and schizotypal personality disorder. *American Journal of Psychiatry, 143*, 530–532.

Jenike, M. A., Buttolph, L., Baer, L., Ricciardi, J., & Holland, A. (1989). Open trial of fluoxetine in obsessive–compulsive disorder. *American Journal of Psychiatry, 146*, 909–911.

Joffe, R. T., & Swinson, R. P. (1991). *Biological aspects of obsessive–compulsive disorder.* Paper prepared for the DSM-IV committee on obsessive–compulsive disorder.

Karno, M. G., Golding, J. M., Sorensen, S. B., & Burnam, A. (1988). The epidemiology of OCD in five U.S. communities. *Archives of General Psychiatry, 45*, 1094–1099.

Kasvikis, Y. G., Tsakiris, F., Marks, I. M., Basoglu, M., & Noshirvani, H. F. (1986). Past history of anorexia nervosa in women with obsessive–compulsive disorder. *International Journal of Eating Disorders, 5*, 1069–1075.

Kazarian, S. S., Evans, D. R., & Lefave, K. (1977). Modification and factorial analysis of the Leyton Obsessional Inventory. *Journal of Clinical Psychology, 33*, 422–425.

Kearney, C. A., & Silverman, W. K. (1990). Treatment of an adolescent with obsessive–compulsive disorder by alternating response prevention and cognitive therapy: An empirical analysis. *Journal of Behavior Therapy and Experimental Psychiatry, 21*(1), 39–47.

Kenny, F. T., Mowbray, R. M., & Lalani, S. (1978). Faradic disruption of obsessive ideation in the treatment of obsessive neurosis: A controlled study. *Behavior Therapy, 9*, 209–221.

Kenny, F. T., Solyom, L., & Solyom, C. (1973). Faradic disruption of obsessive ideation in the treatment of obsessive neurosis. *Behavior Therapy, 4*, 448–451.

Kozak, M. J., & Foa, E. B. (1994). Obsessions, overvalued ideas, and delusions in obsessive–compulsive disorder. *Behaviour Research and Therapy, 3*, 343–353.

Kozak, M. J., Foa, E. B., & Steketee, G. (1988). Process and outcome of exposure treatment with obsessive–compulsives: Psychophysiological indicators of emotional processing. *Behavior Therapy, 19*, 157–169.

Laessle, R. G., Kittl, S., Fichter, M. M., Wittehen, H., & Pirke, K. M. (1987). Major affective disorder in anorexia nervosa and bulimia: A descriptive diagnostic study. *British Journal of Psychiatry, 151*, 785–789.

Lang, P. J. (1979). A bio-informational theory of emotional imagery. *Psychophysiology, 6*, 495–511.

Leckman, J. F., & Chittenden, E. H. (1990). Gilles de La Tourette's syndrome and some forms of obsessive–compulsive disorder may share a common genetic diathesis. *L'Encephale, XVI*, 321–323.

Lelliott, P. T., Noshirvani, H. F., Basoglu, M., Marks, I. M., & Monterio, W. O. (1988). Obsessive–compulsive beliefs and treatment outcome. *Psychological Medicine, 18*, 697–702.

Lewis, A. J. (1935). Problems of obsessional illness. *Proceedings of the Royal Society of Medicine, 29*, 325–336.

Lucey, J. V., Butcher, G., Claire, A. W., & Dinan, T. G. (1993). The anterior pituitary responds normally to protirelin in obsessive–compulsive disorders: Evidence to support a neuroendocrine serotonergic deficit. *Acta Psychiatrica Scandinavica, 87*, 384–388.

Mallya, G. K., White, K., Waternaux, D., & Quay, S. (1992). Short- and long-term treatment of obsessive–compulsive disorder with fluvoxamine. *Annals of Clinical Psychiatry, 4*, 77–80.

Marks, I. M. (1977). Recent results of behavioral treatments of phobias and obsessions. *Journal of Internal Medicine Research, 5*, 16–21.

Marks, I. M., Hallam, R. S., Connelly, J., & Philpott, R. (1977). *Nursing in behavioral psychotherapy*. London: Royal College of Nursing of the United Kingdom.

Marks, I. M., Lelliott, P., Basoglu, M., Noshirvami, H., Monteiro, W., Cohen, D., & Kasvikis, Y. (1988). Clomipramine self-exposure, and therapist-aided exposure for obsessive–compulsive rituals. *British Journal of Psychiatry, 152*, 522–534.

Marks, I. M., Stern, R. S., Mawson, D., Cobb, J., & McDonald, R. (1980). Clomipramine and exposure for obsessive–compulsive rituals—I. *British Journal of Psychiatry, 136*, 1–25.

McCarthy, P., & Foa, E. B. (1990). Treatment interventions for obsessive–compulsive disorder. In M. Thase, B. Edelstein, & M. Hersen (Eds.), *Handbook of outpatient treatment of adults* (pp. 209–232). New York: Plenum Press.

McFall, M. E., & Wollersheim, J. P. (1979). Obsessive–compulsive neurosis: A cognitive behavioral formulation and approach to treatment. *Cognitive Therapy and Research, 3*, 333–348.

Meyer, V. (1966). Modification of expectations in cases with obsessional rituals. *Behaviour Research and Therapy, 4*, 273–280.

Meyer, V., & Levy, R. (1973). Modification of behavior in obsessive–compulsive disorders. In H. E. Adams & P. Unikel (Eds.), *Issues and trends in behavior therapy* (pp. 77–138). Springfield IL: Thomas.

Meyer, V., Levy, R., & Schnurer, A. (1974). A behavioral treatment of obsessive–compulsive disorders. In H. R. Beech (Ed.), *Obsessional states*. London: Methuen.

Minichiello, W. E., Baer, L., & Jenike, M. A. (1987). Schizotypal personality disorder: A poor prognostic indicator for behavior therapy in the treatment of obsessive–compulsive disorder. *Journal of Anxiety Disorders, 1*, 273–276.

Montgomery, S. A., & Maneezux, A. (1992). Fluvoxamine in the treatment of obsessive–compulsive disorder. *7*(Suppl. 1), 5–9.

Montgomery, S. A., McIntyre, A., Osterheider, M., Sarteschi, P., Zitterl, W., Zohar, J., Birkett, M., Wood, A. J., & The Lilly European OCD Study Group (1993). A double-blind, placebo-controlled study of fluoxetine in patients with DSM-III-R obsessive–compulsive disorder. *European Neuropsychopharmacology, 3*, 143–152.

Mowrer, O. A. (1939). A stimulus–response analysis of anxiety and its role as a reinforcing agent. *Psychological Review, 46*, 553–565.

Mowrer, O. A. (1960). *Learning theory and behavior*. New York: Wiley.

Öst, L. A., Salkovskis, P. M., & Hellstrom, K. (1991). One-session therapist-directed exposure vs. self-exposure in the treatment of spider phobia. *Behavior Therapy, 22*(3), 407–422.

O'Sullivan, G., Noshirvani, H., Marks, I., Monteiro, W., & Lelliott, P. (1991). Six-year follow-up after exposure and clomipramine therapy for obsessive–compulsive disorder. *Journal of Clinical Psychiatry, 52*, 150–155.

Pato, M. T., Zohar-Kadouch, R., Zohar, J., & Murphy, D. L. (1988). Return of symptoms after desensitization of clomipramine and patients with obsessive–compulsive disorder. *American Journal of Psychiatry, 1145,* 1521–1525.

Pauls, D. L. (1989). *The inheritance and expression of obsessive–compulsive behaviors.* Proceedings of the American Psychiatric Association, San Francisco, CA.

Pauls, D. L., Towbin, K. E., Leckman, J. F., Zahner, G. E., & Cohen, D. J. (1986). Gilles de la Tourette's syndrome and obsessive–compulsive disorder. *Archives of General Psychiatry, 43,* 1180–1182.

Perse, T. (1988). Obsessive–compulsive disorder: A treatment review. *Journal of Clinical Psychiatry, 49,* 48–55.

Perse, T., Griest, J. H., Jefferson, J. W., Rosenfeld, R., & Dar, R. (1987). Fluvoxamine treatment of obsessive–compulsive disorder. *American Journal of Psychiatry, 144,* 1543–1548.

Philpott, R. (1975). Recent advances in the behavioral measurement of obsessional illness: Difficulties common to these and other instruments. *Scottish Medical Journal, 20,* 33–40.

Price, L. H., Goodman, W. K., Charney, D. S., & Heninger, G. R. (1987). Treatment of severe obsessive–compulsive disorder with fluvoxamine. *American Journal of Psychiatry, 144,* 1059–1061.

Rabavilas, A. D., & Boulougouris, J. C. (1974). Physiological accompaniments of ruminations, flooding and thought-stopping in obsessive patients. *Behaviour Research and Therapy, 12,* 239–243.

Rabavilas, A. D., Boulougouris, J. C., & Perissaki, C. (1979). Therapist qualities related to outcome with exposure *in vivo* in neurotic patients. *Journal of Behavior Therapy and Experimental Psychiatry, 10,* 293–299.

Rabavilas, A. D., Boulougouris, J. C., & Stefanis, C. (1976). Duration of flooding sessions in the treatment of obsessive–compulsive patients. *Behaviour Research and Therapy, 14,* 349–355.

Rachman, S., & DeSilva, P. (1978). Abnormal and normal obsessions. *Behaviour Research and Therapy, 16,* 233–248.

Rachman, S., DeSilva, P., & Roper, G. (1976). The spontaneous decay of compulsive urges. *Behaviour Research and Therapy, 14,* 445–453.

Rachman, S., & Hodgson, R. (1980). *Obsessions and compulsions.* Englewood Cliffs, NJ: Prentice-Hall.

Rachman, S., Marks, I. M., & Hodgson, R. (1973). The treatment of obsessive–compulsive neurotics by modelling. *Behaviour Research and Therapy, 8,* 383–392.

Rachman, S. J., & Wilson, G. T. (1980). *The effects of psychological therapy.* Oxford: Pergamon Press.

Rapoport, J. L. (1991). Recent advances in obsessive–compulsive disorder. *Neuropsychopharmacology, 5,* 1–10.

Rapoport, J. L., & Wise, S. P. (1988). Obsessive–compulsive disorder: Evidence for basal ganglia dysfunction. *Psychopharmacology Bulletin, 24,* 380–384.

Rasmussen, S. A., & Eisen, J. L. (1989). Clinical features and phenomenology of obsessive–compulsive disorder. *Psychiatric Annals, 19,* 67–73.

Rasmussen, S. A., & Eisen, J. L. (1990). Epidemiology of obsessive–compulsive disorder. *Journal of Clinical Psychiatry, 51,* 10–14.

Rasmussen, S. A., & Tsuang, M. T. (1986). Clinical characteristics and family history in DSM-III obsessive–compulsive disorder. *American Journal of Psychiatry, 1943,* 317–382.

Reed, G. E. (1985). *Obsessional experience and compulsive behavior: A cognitive structural approach.* Orlando, Florida: Academic Press.

Riggs, D. S., Hiss, H., & Foa, E. B. (1992). Marital distress and the treatment of obsessive–compulsive disorder. *Behavior Therapy, 23,* 585–597.

Roper, G., & Rachman, S. (1976). Obsessional–compulsive checking: Experimental replication and development. *Behaviour Research and Therapy, 14,* 25–32.

Roper, G., Rachman, S., & Hodgson, R. (1973). An experiment on obsessional checking. *Behaviour Research and Therapy, 11,* 271–277.

Salkovskis, P. M. (1985). Obsessive–compulsive problems: A cognitive–behavioral analysis. *Behaviour Research and Therapy, 23,* 571–583.

Salkovskis, P. M., & Warwick, H. M. C. (1985). Cognitive therapy of obsessive–compulsive disorder: Treating treatment failures. *Behavioral Psychotherapy, 13,* 243–255.

Scarone, S., Columbo, C., Livian, S., Abbruzzese, M., Ronchi, P., Cocatetti, M., Scotti, G., & Smeraldi, E. (1992). Increased right caudate nucleus size in obsessive–compulsive disorder: Detection with magnetic resonance imaging. *Psychiatry Research, 45,* 115–121.

Schilder, P. (1938). The organic background of obsessions and compulsions. *American Journal of Psychiatry, 94,* 1397.

Schneider, K. (1925). Schwangs zustände in schizophrenie. *Archives für Psychiatrie und Nerven Krankheislen, 74,* 93–107.

Sher, K. J., Frost, R. O., Kushner, M., Crews, T. M., & Alexander, J. E. (1989). Memory deficits in compulsive checkers: A replication and extension in a clinical sample. *Behaviour Research and Therapy, 27,* 65–69.

Sher, K. J., Frost, R. O., & Otto, R. (1983). Cognitive deficits in compulsive checkers: An exploratory study. *Behaviour Research and Therapy, 21*, 357–364.

Solyom, L., Sookman, D., Solyom, C., & Morton, L. (1985). *Behavior therapy vs. drug therapy in the treatment of obsessional illness.* Unpublished manuscript.

Stanley, M. A., Turner, S. M., & Borden, J. W. (1990). Schizotypal features in obsessive–compulsive disorder. *Comprehensive Psychiatry, 31*, 511–518.

Stebeteo, G. S. (1992). *Treatment of obsessive–compulsive disorder.* New York: Guilford.

Steketee, G. S., Foa, E. B., & Grayson, J. B. (1982). Recent advances in the treatment of obsessive–compulsives. *Archives of General Psychiatry, 39*, 1365–1371.

Stern, R. S. (1978). Obsessive thoughts: The problem of therapy. *British Journal of Psychiatry, 132*, 200–205.

Stern, R. S., Lipsedge, M. S., & Marks, I. M. (1975). Obsessive ruminations: A controlled trial of thought-stopping technique. *Behaviour Research and Therapy, 11*, 650–662.

Stern, R. S., Marks, I. M., Wright, J., & Luscombe, D. K. (1980). Clomipramine: Plasma levels, side effects and outcome in obsessive–compulsive neurosis. *Postgraduate Medical Journal, 56*, 134–139.

Swedo, S. E., Rapoport, J. L., Cheslow, D. L., Leonard, H. L., Ayoub, E. M., Hosier, D. M., & Wald, E. R. (1989). High prevalence of obsessive–compulsive symptoms in patients with Sydenham's chorea. *American Journal of Psychiatry, 146*, 246–249.

Thoren, P., Asberg, M., Bertilsson, L., Melstrom, B., Sjoqvist, F., & Traskman, L. (1980). Clomipramine treatment of obsessive–compulsive disorder: II. Biochemical aspects. *Archives of General Psychiatry, 37*, 1289–1294.

Thoren, P., Asberg, M., Cronholm, B., Jornestedt, L., & Traskman, L. (1980). Clomipramine treatment of obsessive–compulsive disorder. I. A controlled clinical trial. *Archives of General Psychiatry, 37*, 1281–1285.

Tynes, L. L., White, K., & Steketee, G. S. (1990). Toward a new nosology of obsessive–compulsive disorder. *Comprehensive Psychiatry, 31*, 465–480.

Weizman, A., Carmi, M., Hermesh, H., Shahar, A., Apter, A., Tyano, S., & Rehavi, M. (1985). High-affinity imipramine binding and serotonin uptake platelets of adolescent and adult obsessive–compulsive patients. [Summary]. *Abstract, 4th International Congress of Biological Psychiatry*, Philadelphia, PA.

Zohar, J., & Insel, T. (1987). Obsessive–compulsive disorder: Psychobiological approach to diagnoses treatment and pathophysiology. *Biological Psychiatry, 22*, 667–687.

Zohar, J., Mueller, E. A., Insel, T. R., Zohar-Kadouch, R., & Murphy, D. L. (1987). Serotonergic responsivity in obsessive–compulsive disorder: Comparison of patients and healthy controls. *Archives of General Psychiatry, 44*, 946–951.

4

Cognitive–Behavioral Treatment of Social Phobia

Agnes Scholing, Paul M. G. Emmelkamp,
and Patricia Van Oppen

INTRODUCTION

Description of the Disorder

Many people are familiar with temporary feelings of apprehension in certain social situations, such as having to speak to an audience, to perform in public, or to talk to authority persons. When such feelings become so prominent that social situations are avoided or life is dominated by a constantly present anticipatory fear, a diagnosis of social phobia can be justified. Criteria in the fourth edition of the *Diagnostic and Statistical Manual of Mental Disorders* (DSM-IV; American Psychiatric Association, 1994) for social phobia (alternatively labeled as Social Anxiety Disorder) are provided in Table 4.1.

If the fears are present in most social situations, the disorder is specified as "generalized type," and for those patients an additional diagnosis of Avoidant Personality Disorder (Axis II) must be considered.

Comparing criteria with the manual's third revised edition (DSM-III-R; American Psychiatric Association, 1987) three differences are striking. The first is the explicit inclusion of the fear of showing (visible) symptoms of anxiety (e.g., blushing, trembling, or sweating) in the diagnosis. With DSM-III-R criteria, some patients with this fear were difficult to classify, namely, those who are preoccupied with the symptoms themselves and the experience of losing control of the symptoms. Generally, these patients are caught in a vicious cycle of anticipatory anxiety (resembling patients with panic disorder), whereas

Agnes Scholing and Paul M. G. Emmelkamp • Department of Clinical Psychology, University of Groningen, Oostersingel 59, 9713 EZ Groningen, The Netherlands.   **Patricia Van Oppen** • Department of Psychiatry, Free University of Amsterdam, Valeriusplein 9, 1075 BG Amsterdam, The Netherlands.

Sourcebook of Psychological Treatment Manuals for Adult Disorders, edited by Vincent B. Van Hasselt and Michel Hersen. Plenum Press, New York, 1996.

Table 4.1. Diagnostic Criteria for Social Phobia

A. A marked and persistent fear of one or more social or performance situations in which the person is exposed to unfamiliar people or to possible scrutiny by others. The individual fears that he or she will act in a way—or show anxiety symptoms—that will be humiliating or embarrassing.

B. Exposure to the feared social situation almost invariably provokes anxiety, which may take the form of a situationally bound or situationally predisposed panic attack.

C. The person recognizes that the fear is excessive or unreasonable.

D. The feared social or performance situations are avoided, or else are endured with intense anxiety or distress.

E. The avoidance, anxious anticipation, or distress in the feared social or performance situation(s) interferes significantly with the person's normal routine, occupation (academic) functioning, or with social activities or relationships with others, or there is marked distress about having the phobia.

F. In individuals under age 18 years, the duration is at least 6 months.

G. The fear or avoidance is not due to the direct effects of a substance (such as drugs, medication) or a general medical condition, and is not better accounted for by another mental disorder, such as Panic Disorder with or without agoraphobia, Separation Anxiety Disorder, Body Dysmorphic Disorder, a Pervasive Developmental Disorder, or Schizoid Personality Disorder.

H. If a general medical condition or other mental disorder is present, the fear in A is unrelated to it.

Note: Reprinted by permission from the *Diagnostic and Statistical Manual of Mental Disorders*, Fourth Edition. Copyright 1994 American Psychiatric Association.

scrutiny by others or behaving in an embarrassing way is feared in the second instance. A second, and related, disparity is implied in the notion that the fear may take the form of a situationally bound or predisposed panic attack. This addition seems highly useful in view of the problems that have been reported in distinguishing social phobia and panic disorder with or without agoraphobia. In fact, many social phobics report that they had at least one panic attack in the past and have received both diagnoses (e.g., Andersch & Hanson, 1993). Finally, DSM-IV differs from DSM-III-R in providing additional comments for diagnosing social phobia in children (e.g., criterion A is amplified with the notion that "in children, there must be evidence of capacity for social relationships with familiar people and the anxiety must occur in peer settings, not just in interactions with adults ..." [pp. 416–417]). The section on assessment methods (to be discussed) provides more details about differential diagnostic considerations.

Characteristics of Social Phobics

The central fear of social phobics concerns negative evaluation by other people. This fear is expressed in characteristic cognitions, behavior, and physiological symptoms.

Cognitions can be distinguished in positive and negative self-statements, irrational beliefs, attributions, dysfunctional schemas, expectancies, and self-focused attention. Several studies have compared social phobics with normals on such cognitive aspects. The use of different instruments precludes definite conclusions, but more or less solid evidence has shown that social phobics differ from normals on all of these features (e.g., Gormally et al., 1981; Sanderman et al., 1987). In short, social phobics report a high frequency of negative self-statements (e.g., "I will make a fool of myself"); are characterized by anxious self-preoccupation (e.g., continuously monitoring what they say, and whether they start blushing, trembling, or sweating); negatively evaluate the quality of their social performance (being more demanding to themselves than to other people); notice what went wrong instead of what went right; remember unpleasant events and situations in which they "failed," forgetting what went well; ascribe unpleasant social interactions and events to themselves and pleasant ones to others; and are preoccupied with the evaluation of others and practice thought reading (i.e., thinking that other people continuously observe them and judge them negatively).

With respect to social phobic behavior, two aspects are important: social skills and avoidance of social situations. In the past, it has been suggested that inadequate social skills are characteristic of patients with an avoidant personality disorder and not for social phobics (e.g., Greenberg & Stravynski, 1983). However, recent studies on generalized social phobia versus avoidant personality disorder, discussed later in this chapter, have not corroborated this notion. Apart from that, it is doubtful whether social skills are important in the etiology and maintenance of social fears. First, it is often difficult to determine objectively the adequacy of social behavior. Second, many people with "inadequate" social behavior seem to experience surprisingly little social anxiety. On the other hand, some patients show adequate social skills but report considerable anxiety.

The degree of avoidant behavior differs largely across patients. In a strict sense, avoidance of social situations is not a prerequisite for a diagnosis of social phobia; endurance of social situations with a significant level of anxiety is sufficient. Some patients report that they always urge themselves to enter the feared situations. However, detailed information gathering usually reveals more subtle forms of avoidance in the situation (e.g., avoidance of eye contact, lack of participation in discussions, no use of coffee or other drinks). Such behavior can be viewed as passive avoidance, intended to prevent becoming the center of attention. Other patients show active avoidance, such as increased talking in an attempt to keep the interaction under control, and preventing silences in which other persons could pose difficult questions.

Studies of somatic symptoms have found differences between social phobics and patients with panic disorder, and patients with generalized anxiety disorder (Amies, Gelder, & Shaw, 1983; Reich, Noyes, & Yates, 1988). The latter investigation demonstrated that most symptom differences were in the category of autonomic hyperactivity. Patients with social phobia reported more "visible" symptoms, such as blushing, trembling, or sweating, than both other groups of patients.

Impairment in Daily Life

According to criteria in the third edition of the *Diagnostic and Statistical Manual of Mental Disorders* (DSM-III; American Psychiatric Association, 1980), social phobia was conceptualized as a kind of a simple phobia, being only rarely incapacitating in daily life. The diagnosis was reserved for patients who feared one specific social situation, whereas patients with more generalized fears received a diagnosis of avoidant personality disorder. Subsequently, research has demonstrated that social phobia is a much more distressing and debilitating disorder than was initially assumed. Many social phobics fear and avoid multiple situations (Holt, Heimberg, Hope, & Liebowitz, 1992b; Turner, Beidel, Dancu, & Keyss, 1986). They also report significant problems in educational, occupational, social, and marital functioning (Liebowitz, Gorman, Fyer, & Klein, 1985). The broad impact of the impairment seems to be caused partly by the early onset of the disorder (late childhood or early adolescence), which implies that it often strongly affects important and more or less irreversible decisions, such as which school or job to choose.

A subject that is still under debate is the distinction of subtypes. It has been repeatedly observed that social phobics constitute a heterogenous group. This observation has led to attempts to divide patients into more homogeneous subgroups. DSM-III-R defined a generalized type (patients with fear in most social situations), thereby suggesting (but not explicitly mentioning) a "nongeneralized" type (i.e., patients with more circumscribed fears). Previously, these patients have been referred to as specific, circumscribed, discrete, or limited social phobics, without further specification. As a result, studies have used different definitions for the nongeneralized social phobics, e.g., public speaking phobics (Heimberg, Hope, Dodge, & Becker, 1990), patients with fear in circumscribed situations (Turner, Beidel, & Townsley, 1992b), and patients with fear of displaying anxiety symptoms (Scholing & Emmelkamp, 1993a). In the DSM-IV options book, it was suggested (on the basis of existing literature) that social phobia can be subdivided along two dimensions: (1) the degree of generalization of fear and avoidance, ranging from one situation to all or most situations and (2) the focus of concern, ranging from performance in front of others versus social interactions. Based on these extremes, a subtyping scheme was proposed, including the performance type, the limited-situational type, and the generalized type. Heimberg and Holt (1989; cited in Heimberg et al., 1993) proposed a distinction in generalized, nongeneralized, and circumscribed social phobia. In spite of the fact that such distinctions may be useful in predicting differential treatment response, they are not maintained in DSM-IV criteria. To date, some empirical studies (reviewed by Heimberg, Holt, Schneier, Spitzer, & Liebowitz, 1993) have compared some subtypes and have pointed to several differences (e.g., in age, severity of complaints, education, familial and social background). An interesting finding was reported by Heimberg et al. (1990), who found that public-speaking phobics performed objectively well but were characterized by a greater tendency toward negative bias, whereas the generalized social phobics were characterized by objectively poorer performance. In addition, both groups showed distinct patterns of physiological arousal.

Holt et al. (1992b) examined which situations are avoided by social phobics and distinguished the following four domains: (1) formal speaking and interaction (e.g., public speaking, speaking to an authority figure), (2) informal speaking and interaction (casual and more intimate relationships with same and opposite-sex partners, social interactions at school and work), (3) being observed by others (e.g., eating or writing in public), and (4) assertion. The percentages of patients who reported problems in these domains were 70%, 46%, 31%, and 22%, respectively. It appeared that the domains could be more or less hierarchically ordered: If patients reported fears in only one situation, it was most likely in the domain of formal speaking and interaction. Patients who feared observation of their behavior generally also feared situations in all other domains. Patients who feared assertive interaction usually also feared situations in the first two domains, but not observation of behavior, and so on.

Social Phobia and Avoidant Personality Disorder

In DSM-III-R, three of the seven criteria for avoidant personality disorder (APD) are equivalent to the criteria for social phobia, generalized type, namely (1) avoidance of social or occupational activities that involve interpersonal contact, (2) reticence in social situations because of a fear of saying something inappropriate or foolish, and (3) fear of being embarrassed by blushing, crying, or showing signs of anxiety in front of other people.

Three other criteria of APD also refer to avoidance of social interactions. Recently, three studies addressed the question of whether both disorders are qualitatively different (Herbert, Hope, & Bellack, 1992; Holt, Heimberg, & Hope, 1992a; Turner, Beidel, & Townsley, 1992b), producing largely consistent results. Most patients with APD also fulfilled criteria for generalized social phobia; however, the reverse was not true, suggesting that APD can be considered as an extreme variant of generalized social phobia, not as a qualitatively different disorder. Although all three studies demonstrated some (quantitative) differences between both disorders, the similarities were more prominent. Widiger (1992), in a commentary on the three studies, concluded,

> It is then inaccurate and misleading to provide both diagnoses to the same patient, because such dual diagnosis suggests that the patient is suffering from two distinct and comorbid mental disorders ... instead of simply one disorder that meets the criteria for different diagnoses ..." (p. 341).

In DSM-IV, the demarcation of APD and generalized social phobia is even more difficult, due to the fact that all APD criteria are referring to social inhibition, feelings of (social) inadequacy, and hypersensitivity to negative evaluation. In fact, the reported age of onset of social phobia (late childhood to early adolescence) and the course of the disorder seem more characteristic for a personality disorder than for an Axis I disorder. Empirical studies have shown a high degree of overlap between both disorders, with 21.4% to 90% of the social phobics also diagnosed with avoidant personality disorder.

Social Phobia and Shyness

Social phobia and shyness seem to have much in common, such as anxiety in social situations, lack of adequate social behavior, and avoidance of social situations. The results of (scarce) epidemiological studies suggest that shyness is much more common than social phobia; Zimbardo (1977) reported that 40% of 5,000 "normal" Americans considered themselves currently shy, whereas 90% of the respondents answered that they had felt shy at least once in their life. In contrast, the prevalence of social phobia in the general population is about 2% (Pollard & Henderson, 1988; Robins et al., 1984). It must be noted that the epidemiological data on social phobia have been collected according to the (restricted) criteria of DSM-III, and, in fact, refer to more circumscribed social phobics. With application of DSM-III-R or DSM-IV criteria, much higher prevalence rates have been found (e.g., Kessler et al., 1994). Turner, Beidel, and Townsley (1990) reviewed the literature on social phobia versus shyness. They tentatively concluded that both syndromes might be differentiated on social and occupational functioning, course, overt behavioral characteristics, and onset, but not on somatic and cognitive features.

ASSESSMENT METHODS

It is important to distinguish various goals of assessment. Assessment may be (1) directed at establishing a formal diagnosis of social phobia, (2) aimed at a broader analysis of the problem in order to enable the selection of a specific treatment strategy, (3) focused on the evaluation of treatment, or (4) directed at the processes involved in a particular treatment method. These goals will be discussed consecutively, with emphasis on the first and the second. For some purposes, the use of specific assessment instruments may be desirable; they are described later in this chapter.

Establishing a Formal Diagnosis of Social Phobia

One goal of the first intake session is to collect sufficient information for making a formal diagnosis according to DSM-IV. Research has demonstrated considerable comorbidity among different anxiety disorders, especially social phobia, panic disorder with or without agoraphobia, and generalized anxiety (Mannuzza, Fyer, Liebowitz, & Klein, 1990; Sanderson, DiNardo, Rapee, & Barlow, 1990; for a review, see Montego & Liebowitz, 1994). Rather than being considered as distinct categories (as is done in DSM-IV), anxiety symptoms are better viewed as lying in a number of different continua, fear of negative evaluation being one of them. The actual primary diagnosis depends on the predominant features in a particular patient. As soon as it becomes clear that anxiety is the main reason for a patient's seeking professional help, it is useful to employ a semistructured interview for establishing the formal diagnosis. One example is the Anxiety Disorders Interview Schedule, described later in this chapter.

DSM-IV offers a clear improvement in the distinction between social phobia and panic disorder, in the notion that the fear may take the form of a situationally bound panic attack. Following Hope and Heimberg (1993), the following questions must be answered to distinguish social phobia from panic disorder: (1) Is the individual afraid of the symptoms themselves, even when he or she is alone? (2) Do panic attacks (also) occur in nonsocial situations? (3) Is the onset of the disorder more typical of panic disorder or social phobia? Affirmative responses to the first two questions suggest a diagnosis of panic disorder instead of social phobia. With respect to the third question, it has been reported that panic-disorder patients generally remember their first panic attack quite well, having experienced the attack as suddenly "coming out of the blue," whereas social phobics often report a more gradual development of the fear, or a sudden panic attack in a social-evaluation situation.

Some patients present a fear of incapacitating or extremely embarrassing panic-like symptoms or limited symptom attacks, but have never experienced "full-blown," unexpected panic attacks. Examples of such symptoms are loss of bladder control, dizziness, fainting, or vomiting. This fear typically occurs in situations where other people are present (e.g., in a busy street, in shops, during a meeting, when traveling by bus or train), not when they are alone at home. Although resembling social phobics (who also often complain about sickness, gastrointestinal discomfort, and diarrhea), these patients receive a diagnosis of agoraphobia without a history of panic attacks.

The differentiation from obsessive–compulsive disorder usually does not pose problems, although some patients initially present themselves as obsessive–compulsives, but in fact must be diagnosed as social phobic. For example, one of our patients had to clean her house very often. Further questioning revealed that the reason for doing so was anxiety of being criticized by visitors rather than fear of contamination. In the same way, patients may try to prevent criticism by other people by compulsive-like checking their work.

In children, social phobia must be differentiated from separation disorder. Children with separation anxiety disorder may avoid social settings due to concerns about being separated from their caretaker and concerns about being embarrassed by needing to leave situations prematurely to return to home.

In some patients, fear of negative evaluation may be related to body dysmorphic disorder. Patients qualify for this diagnosis when they are preoccupied with a presumed physical anomaly of their body, with no objective basis. The distinction is sometimes difficult because most dysmorphophobics experience anxiety in social contacts and tend to avoid these situations.

The distinction from avoidant personality disorder was previously discussed. Other disorders that must be considered before giving a diagnosis of social phobia are schizoid personality disorder (Axis II) and a pervasive developmental disorder (Axis I). Patients with these disorders differ from social phobics either in their lack of interest in other people, or their incapacity to perceive and handle social signals adequately.

There is little confusion between the diagnoses social phobia and substance dependence, but the comorbidity between social phobia and substance abuse or dependence is substantial (Van Ameringen, Mancini, Styan, & Donison, 1991). Data concerning the prevalence of substance abuse problems in social phobia as compared to panic disorder are discrepant (Amies et al., 1983; Himle & Hill, 1991). Social phobics with concurrent alcohol abuse are more anxious than social phobics without an alcohol problem (Schneier, Martin, Liebowitz, Gorman, & Fyer, 1989).

Assessment Aimed at Choosing a Specific Treatment Plan

Whereas a semistructured interview is particularly helpful in establishing the diagnosis, a more open-ended interview is required to gain information on the development of the social phobia, associated problems (if any), and on factors associated with the maintenance of the problem. Since it is necessary to go into detail about the conditions that provoke the anxiety and the consequences in different situations, neither questionnaires nor behavioral observation by themselves will provide the necessary information. In the initial interview(s), the therapist tries to establish the degree of anxiety and avoidance in a variety of social situations. It can be helpful to adhere to the different social domains of social phobia that were distinguished by Holt et al. (1992b).

Although most social phobics suffer from somatic symptoms, it is important to determine whether fear of sweating, trembling, and blushing is their main problem, because this generally has implications for the content of the treatment. Special attention should be directed to more subtle avoidance behavior such as making excuses, not looking in the eyes of persons when speaking, wearing inconspicuous clothes, not starting conversations or breaking them off abruptly, drinking alcohol to reduce anxiety, or smoking cigarettes to give oneself airs. Patients with fear of blushing may wear long hair, use makeup, wear sunglasses, or sit in dark places to prevent others from seeing them blushing. Similar subtle avoidance is found for patients with fear of trembling or sweating.

It is also important to assess the patient's social skills. Given the situational specificity of social behavior, the therapist impression during the interview might not be an accurate reflection of the actual behavior in a variety of social situation. Although a formal behavioral test of social skills can provide useful information, such a test is usually difficult to administer in a clinician's office. An alternative is detailed discussion of frequently occurring daily-life interactions, eventually amplified with a demonstration of the skills in role play.

Finally, it is important to focus on the irrational and negative thoughts patients may have in (anticipation on) social situations. Whereas there are a number of measures available (to be discussed), many of them are not specifically directed to social phobic cognitions. The way patients discuss their problems during the initial interview may provide important cues with respect to underlying "schemas" and "core beliefs" (e.g., "It's terrible to make a mistake, because then I am vulnerable"). A diary in which patients record daily social situations, their behavior, their thoughts, and their anxiety level is often indispensable to obtain a more accurate picture of the problem (see Sidebar 4–1).

Sidebar 4–1

Diary for Social Situations

Date:

Situation	My behavior	My thoughts	Feeling (0–10)

Situation	My behavior	My thoughts	Feeling (0–10)

It was already noted that a formal diagnosis according to DSM-IV does not automatically yield a treatment plan. This is especially true for social phobia, because research (discussed later in this chapter) has demonstrated that different strategies can be helpful in decreasing the fear of negative evaluation. If patients also present other problems, formulation of a macroanalysis (Emmelkamp, 1982; Emmelkamp, Bouman, & Scholing, 1992) is useful to decide which problem should be treated first. For example, one of our social phobic patients was also quite depressed and her marital relationship was poor. Detailed assessment revealed that, before she married, she was quite outgoing and hardly socially anxious. The social phobia developed after her marriage with an overcritical husband who often criticized and ridiculed her. In this case, treatment focusing on the relationship rather than on the social fears seemed to be more appropriate. In another case, a social phobic female suffered also from a post-traumatic stress disorder as a result of sexual abuse in the past by her stepfather. It was highly unlikely that anxiety in social interactions would subside without dealing with the painful emotional experiences related to the abuse. In consultation with the patient, it was decided to focus the treatment on the sexual abuse first, while treatment for the social phobia was postponed.

Before going into the evaluation of treatment effects and the process of treatment, we discuss instruments that are useful for assessment of social phobic aspects.

Behavioral Interview

For establishing a formal diagnosis of social phobia, the Anxiety Disorders Interview Schedule–Revised (ADIS-R), a structured interview developed by DiNardo and Barlow (1988), was particularly suitable under the DSM-III-R criteria. A revised version, adapted to DSM-IV, is available (Brown, DiNardo, & Barlow, 1995). With this interview, information is obtained about the various anxiety disorders as well as depression, somatoform disorders, and substance abuse. The interrater reliability for most anxiety disorders, including social phobia, is satisfactory.

Self-Report Questionnaires

In the last decade, a number of self-report questionnaires have been developed or evaluated that are particularly suited to assess more specific aspects of the anxiety, avoidance, and cognitions of social phobics. The most important instruments are briefly reviewed. Some of them are directed at specific features (e.g., avoidance behavior); others cover several aspects of social phobia. Recently, more attention has been directed to the construction of measures for assessment of cognitive aspects of social phobia. These measures are discussed separately.

Fear Questionnaire (FQ; Arrindell, Emmelkamp, & Van der Ende, 1984; Marks & Mathews, 1979). This questionnaire measures the extent to which a patient avoids feared situations. After one open question regarding the patient's most important phobia, the FQ consists of 15 questions assessing the avoidance associated with agoraphobia, social phobia, and blood and injury phobia, respectively. In addition, it contains five questions assessing the degree of anxiety and depression that patients experienced the last week. The FQ has been used in almost all treatment studies of social phobia, so many data are available. It is particularly useful as a first-screening device. The scale is less suitable for treatment evaluation in clinical practice due to its limited range of social situations and their global circumscription.

Anxiety and Avoidance Scale (AAS). This measure is an adapted and amplified version of the Watson and Marks (1971) scales. It contains five idiosyncratic situations, determined in consultation with the patient. It attempts to choose situations that (1) are most fear provoking for the patient, (2) preferably occur regularly, and (3) have a certain diversity. Patients rate each situation on fear (from zero = *No Fear at All*, to 8 = *Extreme Fear*), and subsequently on avoidance behavior (from zero = *No Avoidance at All*, to 8 = *Always Avoided*). Because it contains personally relevant situations for the patient, the AAS is a suitable outcome measure, especially if it is combined with other, more objective measures.

Social Avoidance and Distress Scale (SADS) and *Fear of Negative Evaluation Scale* (FNE; Watson & Friend, 1969). Although the FNE is a more cognitive measure, we discuss it together with the SADS because both questionnaires are generally applied together. They have been used extensively over the past decades, both for research and clinical purposes, and have been found to be sensitive to treatment changes. Recently, the scales were criticized because they were developed on a student population (Heimberg, Mueller, Holt, Hope, & Liebowitz, 1992) and presumably assess general emotional distress more than social anxiety (Turner, McCanna, & Beidel, 1987).

Social Interaction Anxiety Scale and the *Social Phobia Scale* (SIAS and SPS; Mattick & Clarke, 1989; Heimberg, Mueller, Holt, Hope, & Liebowitz, 1992). The SIAS assesses anxiety in direct social interactions, whereas the SPS evaluates anxiety in situations in which the individual may be observed by others. Both scales (consisting of 19 and 20 items, respectively) discriminate social phobics from community volunteers, and there is some evidence for their convergent validity (Heimberg et al., 1992).

Social Phobia and Anxiety Inventory (SPAI; Turner, Beidel, Dancu, & Stanley, 1989). The SPAI was designed to assess somatic symptoms and cognitions characteristic of social phobia and to measure anxiety, avoidance, and escape behaviors across a range of social situations. Internal consistency and temporal stability are satisfactory (Turner et al., 1989). The SPAI successfully discriminates social phobics and nonsocial phobics, and there is some evidence for its concurrent validity (Beidel, Borden, Turner, & Jacob, 1989; Beidel, Turner, Stanley, & Dancu, 1989). Furthermore, the SPAI has been found capable of assessing reliable and clinically significant change after therapy (Beidel, Turner, & Cooley, 1993).

Cognitive Measures

There are a number of questionnaires available that measure more general irrational beliefs (e.g., the Rational Behavior Inventory; Shorkey & Whiteman, 1977; the Irrational Beliefs Inventory; Koopmans, Sanderman, Timmerman, & Emmelkamp, 1994), but they are of limited use for assessment of social phobia. Apart from the FNE scale (discussed earlier), no cognitive measures are available that contain separate (sub)scales for specific social phobic cognitions and beliefs, with the exception of the Social Cognition Inventory (SCI; Van Kamp & Klip, 1981).

A number of methods have been used to assess the self-statements of social phobic patients, including thought listing, think-aloud tasks, and self-statement questionnaires (see review by Arnkoff & Glass, 1989). For clinical practice, the Social Interaction Self-

Statement Test (SISST; Glass, Merluzzi, Biever, & Larsen, 1982) is the most promising. The SISST is capable of discriminating socially anxious from non-socially anxious subjects and there is also some evidence for its concurrent validity (Arnkoff & Glass, 1989).

Assessment of Social Skills

Although there are a number of questionnaires that evaluate the self-reported frequency of positive and negative social behaviors (see Glass & Arnkoff, 1989), their clinical utility is problematic, since these measures actually may reflect patients' cognitions about their social behavior rather than their *actual* social behavior. Furthermore, these measures may be influenced by accuracy of recall and awareness of the problematic behavior. We regularly found that patients judged themselves as less skilled at the posttest of social skills training than at the pretest. In the course of social skills training, they had become aware of a number of negative social behaviors and deficits that they had failed to recognize as such at the pretest. Self-monitoring of specific social situations on a daily basis may provide the clinician with more relevant information with respect to behavior of patients in specific social situations; however, some of the problems associated with the social skills questionnaires are also relevant here.

While *in vivo* observation in a variety of social situations would obviously be the best strategy for assessing social skills, this is for practical and ethical reasons precluded in clinical practice. Having the patient role-play social situations in the therapist's office is a cost-effective alternative that can be easily administered in routine clinical practice. Role-play scenes are based on specific problems in social interactions that the patient has had in the past. If the clinician has access to confederates, a number of other observational measures can be employed. One of them is the Social Interaction Test (SIT; Trower, Bryant, & Argyle, 1978), in which social phobics have to interact for 12 minutes with a male and a female confederate. Confederates and judges rate the behavior and physical appearance of patients on a rating scale. Even more easily arranged is an impromptu speech task. For example, Beidel, Turner, and Jacob (1989) asked social phobics to speak for 10 minutes to a small audience, consisting of three members of the staff. Test–retest reliability for physiological, cognitive, and behavioral variables was satisfactory. Another promising behavioral observation instrument is the Simulated Social Interaction Test (SSIT; Curran, 1982). The advantage of this measure over the SIT and an impromptu speech task is that behavior in eight different role-played situations is assessed. Each of the situations is initiated by a series of prompts from a male or female confederate. The patient's behavior is rated by confederates and judges. Interrater reliability and concurrent validity of this measure are satisfactory (Mersch, Breukers, & Emmelkamp, 1992).

Treatment Evaluation

If treatment evaluation is conducted in the scope of a controlled outcome study, the choice of assessment instruments is largely dependent on the hypotheses. In that case, self-report instruments may be supplemented with behavioral tests. For clinical practice, such assessment may be too time consuming; however, the use of some of the instruments described earlier is desirable. The AAS is significant because it contains situations that are most relevant for the patient. In addition, the SPAI or the combination of SPS and SIAS may be used for broader assessment of social phobic phenomena. These measures can be employed in a qualitative fashion. Inspection of the questionnaires may reveal characteristics of the patients' fear that might be useful in the development of a treatment strategy. A Symptom Checklist (SCL-90; Derogatis, 1977), can be added for assessment of other complaints (e.g., depression).

Treatment Process

Objective assessment of the treatment process is not usual in clinical practice. However, diaries can be very helpful in treatment, for example, to get a more objective picture of the frequency and duration of social contacts, the frequency of feared situations (e.g., being criticized, starting to blush or tremble), or to monitor the use of medication or alcohol. Obviously, it is not possible to include all elements in a diary, because that would cost patients too much time and therefore would be discouraging. If it is relevant to obtain information about all those aspects, it is often better to modify the content of the diary after some weeks, depending on the information that is desired in the specific phase of treatment.

TREATMENT PROCEDURES

Research Findings on the Treatment of Social Phobia

Several reviews have been published about the efficacy of (cognitive) behavioral treatments for social phobia (Emmelkamp & Scholing, 1990; Heimberg, 1989; Turner, Beidel, & Townsley, 1992a), and the main findings are summarized here.

The last decades have demonstrated a gradual shift in the strategies used. In the 1970s, treatments for social anxiety or social failure (at that time, social phobia was not acknowledged as a separate anxiety disorder) consisted largely of social skills training, although some studies used systematic desensitization or flooding. Over the last 10 years, investigations of treatment outcome with social phobics concentrated almost exclusively on exposure *in vivo*, cognitive strategies, or treatments in which cognitive and behavioral strategies were integrated (Butler, Cullington, Munby, Amies, & Gelder, 1984; Emmelkamp, Mersch, Vissia, & Van der Helm, 1985; Heimberg, Becker, Goldfinger, & Vermilyea, 1985; Mattick & Peters, 1988; Mattick, Peters, & Clarke, 1989; Scholing & Emmelkamp, 1993a,b). The general conclusion is that all complaint-directed strategies that included some kind of *in vivo* exposure to difficult situations appeared to be effective. Although some studies reported that integrated packages were more effective than single treatments, the differences were not consistent, and their clinical relevance was limited.

In accordance with the reported heterogeneity of social phobics, several attempts have been made to divide patients into more homogenous subgroups and to match treatment strategies to specific patient characteristics. The general conclusion is that matched and standardized treatments both lead to improvement and are equally efficacious.

Chambless and Gillis (1993), reviewing the literature on cognitive–behavioral therapy for anxiety disorders, concluded that cognitive change may be a strong predictor of treatment outcome (consistent with findings by Mattick, Peters, & Clarke, 1989), but that such change can be produced by a number of therapeutic approaches.

The observed equivalence of the disparate strategies suggests that they share a large amount of identical ingredients. It seems that almost all interventions, except the pure cognitive treatments (without behavioral experiments or exposure *in vivo*), include exposure to difficult situations, whether included to practice newly learned social or relaxation skills or to test anxiety-provoking cognitions. Traditionally, it was assumed that exposure is a passive process of physiological habituation to fearful stimuli. However, it is increasingly recognized that cognitive factors play an important role (e.g., Davey, 1992).

Taken together these findings indicate that treatment protocols for social phobia should include behavioral and cognitive elements. Although it is not evident that an integrated package must be preferred above "single" treatments, it seems plausible that an integrated package will be applicable for a larger group of patients than a single treatment. Therefore, it is not surprising that there has been a recent trend towards the development of integrated treatments, consisting of different strategies (e.g., Turner, Beidel, Cooley, Woody, & Messer, 1994).

On the following pages, the practical application of treatment is described. We present an integrated cognitive–behavioral treatment protocol, because we believe that such an approach has the broadest scope in clinical practice. Nevertheless, there may be reasons to start with a single strategy, for example, when treatment has to be completed in a limited number of sessions, or when (on the basis of assessment data) there is reason to believe that a particular patient will benefit most from a specific strategy. For example, some patients avoid so many situations that they have hardly any opportunity to check their expectations about social interactions. With them, we prefer to start with "classical" (repeated, prolonged) exposure *in vivo*. An example of such treatment with a relatively large emphasis on exposure *in vivo* is described in the case illustration near the end of this chapter. Patients who clearly display social skills deficits might benefit from separate social skills training. For that reason, we also devote some attention to the application of these strategies.

Irrespective of strategy, several aspects deserve special emphasis in each treatment for social phobia, and we start with a discussion of these points.

General Aspects of Treatment

Nonspecific Factors

Research has isolated several nonspecific treatment factors that explain a large amount of treatment progress: a warm, emotional relationship with the therapist, a recognizable treatment context, presentation of a credible rationale for treatment, and specific procedures (Frank, 1984; Lambert, 1986). (The relationship with the therapist is discussed later.) Each treatment should contain a clear explanation of the model for treatment, how it relates to the problems of the individual patient, and the strategies that will be used to ameliorate these difficulties. It is advisable to have this rationale written on a handout, so that patients can read it at home. The same applies for the treatment procedures. For example, in our exposure treatments, we use forms with examples of exposure exercises and directives for working out personal exposure assignments. For giving accounts of assignments that were practiced as homework in cognitive–behavioral treatment, we employ standard forms to (1) inventory and challenge irrational thoughts, and (2) report about the results of behavioral experiments.

The Therapeutic Relationship

Social phobics' fear of negative evaluation is not limited to situations outside the sessions. More than other patients, they may perceive the therapist as a source of possible rejection, which has consequences for the therapeutic relationship, for patients' ability to concentrate during the session, and for the preparation and discussion of homework exercises. The therapist has to be alert for signals that patients perceive the treatment as just another situation in which they are judged. This is accomplished by paying attention to anxiety symptoms, such as blushing or sweating, avoidance of eye contact, difficulties in the retrieval of anxiety-provoking cognitions and self-statements, or failure to make analyses of irrational cognitions at home. It is not always desirable to discuss such observations immediately. Opening the discussion about the therapeutic relationship can be very threatening for patients, especially during the first sessions, and in this stage, therapists should mention the signals shortly, in an accepting manner (e.g., "I can imagine that it is not easy to tell such personal things to a complete stranger"). Later in treatment, the patient can discuss opportunities that the therapeutic relationship offers to practice new behavior (e.g., maintaining eye contact, asking for explanation in an earlier stage than they usually do, discussing difficult topics) or check assumptions about supposed critical judgments by the therapist on the patient's reality. Some individuals are most anxious in the first sessions; however, most patients only gradually develop this fear through the sessions, just as in daily life they often feel increasingly anxious when people get to know them better, and when they think they have raised expectations that they cannot fulfill. As a consequence of their fear and anxious self-preoccupation, patients may have difficulty concentrating on the conversation with the therapist. For that reason, it is suggested that therapists (1) use written handouts and blackboards, (2) ask patients to write down important topics in the session (at least, the homework agreements), and (3) ask patients to listen to audiotapes of the sessions at home.

Agreement about Treatment Goals

Irrespective of the treatment strategy selected, agreement concerning the goal of treatment is important in the first phase of the treatment. Some patients enter treatment with the assumption that they will learn to feel always comfortable in the presence of other people, always being able to respond in a relaxed, quick-witted way. Assuming that treatment will consist of 10 to 20 sessions, conducted over a few months, and considering the fact that complaints often have existed since late childhood or early adolescence, it cannot be expected that patients will have conquered their fears completely by the end of treatment (although the result is also dependent on the severity of the complaints). Even if treatment were prolonged, attainment of such a goal would be highly unrealistic, simply because most "normal" people occasionally experience feelings of uncertainty in social interactions.

Many social phobics expect that treatment will provide clear rules as to how they should behave in social situations. Although treatment can certainly provide them some direction (e.g., training in specific social skills), it is important to emphasize from the start that it is very difficult to give such clear rules, partly because social situations are unpredictable, and because people may have different opinions about what reactions are most adequate. Instead of searching for rules, patients could better learn to accept and handle their uncertainty, for example, by observing how other people behave, by asking other people for help, by sharing their fears with other people, or by learning to see the relativity of consequences.

Agreement on a realistic treatment goal applies especially to those patients who are preoccupied with the occurrence of somatic symptoms (blushing, trembling, sweating) in social situations. These patients usually enter treatment with the conviction that their problems would be completely solved if only they would never blush, tremble, or sweat again. In our treatments, we emphasize that many people experience somatic symptoms, such as heart palpitations or getting warm, when they feel distressed. We also point out that in some persons these somatic symptoms are more visible than in others. Furthermore, we state that this is partly dependent on individual characteristics such as a sensitive nerve system or a thin, light-colored skin. In the goal-setting phase of treatment, we explain that treatment should be primarily aimed at decreasing the fear of the symptoms, although it can be expected that their frequency and intensity will decrease when the fear is lessened and patients are no longer caught in vicious circles. Many patients are initially disappointed by this treatment goal. It is our experience that this topic has to be discussed several times in subsequent sessions before patients start to assume a more accepting attitude.

Treatment progress can be impeded when therapists have more ambitions than patients. Patients with other complaints are often sufficiently assertive to resist high demands from the therapist; social phobics are often more inclined to blame the failure to carry out homework on their own incapacity and, becoming depressed, will drop out.

Pharmacotherapy in Combination with Cognitive–Behavioral Strategies

Some patients use medication when they enter our treatments, generally anxiolytics, antidepressants, or beta blockers. Although research on the effects of drugs in the treatment of social phobia has demonstrated some favorable effects in the short term, most patients relapsed to pretreatment levels when medication was tapered off (see reviews by Emmelkamp, Bouman, & Scholing, 1992; Welkowitz & Liebowitz, 1990). The aim of all cognitive–behavioral techniques described here is for patients to learn strategies that will enable them to gradually conquer their anxiety and not just to suppress it temporarily. Various opinions have been proffered about the risk of state-dependent learning (e.g., Bouton, Kennedy, & Rosengard, 1990; Bouton & Swartzentruber, 1991; Eysenck, 1992). Theoretically, it is preferable to extinguish anxiety in the "state" (and situation) in which it was acquired (mostly without the use of medication), and to learn new behavior in the "state" that is desired in the future (without medication). For that reason, our policy with regard to the use of medication is that (in consultation with the physician) we ask patients to taper the medication before they start treatment and, at any rate, to stop incidental use of medication. The importance of preparing patients for the fact that initially they will become more anxious is self-evident. If patients are too anxious to taper off medication, we arrange that they first keep a fixed dose at fixed times, preferably before bedtime and never immediately before they carry out exposure or behavioral experiments. Otherwise, patients will remain dependent on the medication and will not build more self-confidence.

Cognitive–Behavioral Therapy for Social Phobia

On the following pages, a detailed treatment protocol is presented. It includes cognitive and behavioral interventions and is based on the assumption that treatment will be optimally effective when (1) both elements are integrated as much as possible, and (2) the protocol allows for adjustment to individual patients' characteristics. The first aspect refers to the fact that clarification and discussion of irrational cognitions are used to motivate patients to carry out *in vivo* exposure behavioral assignments, whereas the results of exposure or behavioral assignments are used to change cognitions. The second aspect implies that the basic strategies are equally relevant for all patients, but that for some of them specific elements may be included in the protocol (e.g., prolonged exposure *in vivo* for patients who show extensive avoidant behavior; relaxation strategies for patients who report that they often suffer from bodily tension, both in social situations and when alone). In practice, we encourage patients from the start of treatment to change their behavior, to take more initiatives with other people to find out whether the disasters they fear do indeed occur.

The protocol is primarily based on the cognitive model of anxiety disorders expounded by Beck and Emery (1985), which focuses on a short-term, structured, and problem-oriented treatment. A good therapeutic relationship is regarded as prerequisite to successful patient cooperation. The Socratic-like dialogue is used if possible, but only if it fits with the style of the patient. It is important to the credibility of the treatment that the therapist be confident about the principles of the cognitive model.

Some topics are part of each session, and they are discussed before the description of the individual sessions. Such recurrent topics include (1) setting an agenda, (2) discussing homework assignments from the previous week, (3) agreeing on new homework assignments, and (4) evaluating the session.

Setting the Agenda

Each session begins with setting an agenda. An agenda ensures that session time is used efficiently and that important topics are not overlooked. It is advisable to write the agenda on the blackboard, with therapist and patient both providing input. The agenda includes elements of treatment that require further discussion or explanation (e.g., discussion of behavioral experiments, challenge of a specific cognition, presentation of new homework assignments, discussion of medication issues, if necessary). Other important topics can be included as long as they are related to the social–phobic problems. Points on the agenda that are not covered during one session are placed on the agenda for the next session. Topics that appear important during the session can also be listed for the next session. For example, during the preparation of new behavioral experiments, it repeatedly appears that the patient is inclined to avoid even small risks, which impedes treatment progress. The therapist, reflecting on previous sessions, decides that it may be helpful to confront the patient's hesitation more directly by making a cost–benefit analysis, and proposes this topic for the agenda of the next session. Although the agenda is explored as a guideline for a structured approach to problem solving, it should be used flexibly. In some instances, it is sensible to deviate from the agenda (e.g., when patients have experienced significant events during the previous week that cannot be ignored, or when there are clear reasons for discussing the therapeutic relationship); however, when this occurs, it must always be explicitly agreed on by patient and therapist.

Discussion of Assigned Homework.   Another recurring point is the discussion of homework assignments from the previous session. Therapists must always pay attention to this topic by asking, in detail, how the assignments went, and by reading reports of patients about their homework. Even when other topics seem more important, agreed-on homework should not be overlooked. The therapist must encourage and reinforce all attempts by patients that are in the desired direction, and also should empathically and seriously deal with those aspects that were (too) difficult.

Discussion of New Homework.   Homework for the next week can be given partly throughout the session and at the end of the session. For example, if the discussion of homework of the previous week reveals that certain aspects should be repeated, this should be agreed on immediately. During the session, a list of such agreements is kept so that patient and therapist maintain a survey. At the start of the session, the therapist includes those assignments that are given in the protocol (e.g., reading the written explanation of behavioral experiments, making a list of exposure assignments). With regard to new homework, it is important that (1) the assignments are completely understood and accepted by the patient, (2) all assignments are written out in detail, (3) the patient is asked to make written reports of assignments, and (4) the list with new homework is rehearsed at the end of the session.

Session Evaluation.   The session evaluation is particularly important during the first few sessions, and therapists must take enough time for this part. The evaluation is one sided: Only patients provide feedback. They are asked to express, in their own words, what they learned from the session, what they found useful, and whether there are issues that are still unclear. If time permits, the therapist tries to explain such obscurities immediately. If not, they are placed on the agenda for the next session.

Phases of Treatment

Treatment generally consists of the following phases:

1. Presenting goals and method of treatment.
2. Identifying automatic thoughts.
3. Challenging the automatic thoughts and formulating rational thoughts, if possible, on the basis of behavioral experiments.
4. Detecting dysfunctional assumptions.
5. Challenging and altering dysfunctional assumptions, again, with the help of behavioral experiments.

In the early stages, it is important to keep rational analyses simple and direct, remaining somewhat superficial, conceding if necessary that the more deep-seated thoughts underlying them will be discussed later.

Techniques of challenge that are frequently used with social phobics include the following:

1. Determining the probabilities that feared situations will come true (e.g., by asking patients to list the occasions when their fears came true, but also the occasions when they did not).
2. Pointing out the contrast between black-and-white thinking versus subtle and multidimensional thought (e.g., distinguishing different factors that determine a person's capability, instead of the patients' tendency to use global judgments of capable versus incapable).
3. Revealing the double standard (i.e., making fewer demands of other people than of themselves).
4. Investigating the "worst of the worst" ("So, the worst you think that will happen is that you blush, don't know anything to say, and are laughed at. And then what?").
5. Role reversal ("How would you react if you saw other people blushing?").
6. Conducting a cost–benefit analysis ("What has it cost you to go on this way, and what could it cause if you take this risk?)

- Setting the agenda
- Discussion of the practical "rules" of treatment:
  - ○ Frequency of sessions (once a week)
  - ○ Evaluation after a fixed number of sessions (12)
  - ○ Importance of homework (about one hour each day)
  - ○ Cooperative relationship between therapist and patient
- Explanation of rationale behind treatment. The theoretical model is described. On the blackboard is written:

Events–Interpretation–Emotions–Behavior

This is used to discuss several aspects of treatment. The therapist explains the difference between thoughts and feelings, and between irrational and rational thoughts. He or she discusses the link between events, thoughts, emotions, and behavior, underscoring that there often are numerous ways to interpret events. He or she points out that fear-provoking thoughts have become automatic in the course of many years, and that it is difficult and time consuming, but possible to trace and change such automatic thoughts.

- The therapist explains the last point by using an example that is not related to the problem at hand: "Suppose that somebody is lying in bed late at night and suddenly hears a noise. The person thinks: 'There is a burglar in the house.' What would this person feel, and what would he or she do?" After the patient has answered, the therapist goes on: "Suppose that the same person were to think, 'The cat must have knocked a vase over.' What would the person feel and do then?"
- Next, a problem-related example is presented: "You have made a date with a new acquaintance to go have a drink in town. At the appointed time, there is no sign of him. In the 20 minutes that follow, you are sitting waiting and all sorts of thoughts go through your mind, such as: "I bet he doesn't really like me, or he would be here already. This goes to show that nobody likes me at all." You lose your self-confidence and become depressed. The same thing happens to a friend of yours, but as she sits waiting she thinks: "Something must have delayed him to make him late," or "Maybe we misunderstood each other when we made our appointment, or perhaps he has forgotten our appointment. I'll wait a few minutes more, and then go and ring him to see if there has been some misunderstanding." She is a little disappointed, perhaps, but has not immediately begun to doubt herself, and she doesn't feel depressed. Now, the same event has happened to both persons, but one person is depressed and the other is not. This shows that your thoughts influence your emotions about the situation. In treatment, we will pay attention to thoughts that you have about other people and their judgments about you. It may be that many of your thoughts are not very realistic and, in fact, lead you to feel more anxious in social interactions than is necessary."
- The patient is asked to provide an example from his or her own life, in which the anxiety-provoking role of negative cognitions is identified.
- The importance of identifying automatic thoughts is discussed. "In time, it becomes a habit to respond to events with certain thoughts. You no longer notice that you have them. The same applies to this type of thinking. It becomes so automatic that you don't notice it anymore. It may, therefore, seem as though a particular situation

Sidebar 4–2

Daily Record of Dysfunctional Thoughts

Situation	Emotion(s)	Automatic thought(s)	Challenge	Rational response	Outcome
Describe the actual event, or the stream of thoughts, the daydream, or the recollection leading to the unpleasant emotion.	Specify your emotion (anxious/angry etc.) Rate the degree of the emotion. (1—100)	Write the automatic thought(s) that preceded the emotion(s). Rate the belief in (each of) the automatic thoughts. (1—100)	Ask questions about the automatic thought(s). Write answers on these questions.	Write a rational response to the automatic thought(s). Rate the belief in the rational response. (0—100)	Rerate the belief in the automatic thought(s). (0—100) Specify and rate the subsequent emotion. (0—100)
Telephoning in room full of people (at my work).	Anxiety (70)	Everybody will look at me. (75) I will flounder and people will think me stupid. (85)			

Explanation: If you have an unpleasant emotion, describe the situation in which it occurs. If you felt this while you are thinking or daydreaming etc., make a note of it. Then describe the automatic thoughts that were associated with this emotion. Assess the degree of certainty on the next scale: completely unlikely (= 0) to absolutely certain (= 100).

Create challenges by asking yourself questions about your automatic thoughts. You might, for example, ask yourself: What evidence do I have for this? How can I understand what others are thinking? How can I predict the future? Am I forgetting to look at the positive side? How would I react if the roles were reversed? etc.

Next, note down a rational thought which can serve as an alternative to the original automatic thought. Then indicate how likely you find this thought (these thoughts): completely unlikely (= 0) to absolutely certain (= 100). Finally, the result of this approach is scored. What degree of certainty do you now attach to the original automatic thought: completely unlikely (= 0) to absolutely certain (= 100). Make a final note of the feeling which this prompts to and how strong this feeling is.

Note: Adapted from Beck, Rush, Shaw, and Emery (1979).

prompts certain behavior, but actually there is an important intermediate step, composed of these automatic thoughts." It is important that patients learn to distinguish between thoughts and emotions from the onset of the therapy.

- The example provided by the patient is used to complete the first three columns of the "thought diary" (see Sidebar 4–2).
- The therapist asks the patient to describe the cognitive model in his or her own words. If the patient is unable to do this, the model is explained again. Aspects that are still unclear are elaborated further. The patient is asked to read the rationale as homework.
- In discussion of new homework for the next session, the patient is asked to read the written explanation of the treatment and to complete the first three columns of the "thought diary" (for about 30 minutes per day). The therapist stresses that the purpose of this stage is only to identify the link between events, thoughts, and emotions; no effort is to be made to change them yet.
- Session evaluation.

Session 2

- Setting the agenda.
- Discussion of the homework assignment in detail. Especially in the first sessions, the therapist must be alert to teach the patient to describe situations objectively and to write interpretations and thoughts about that situation in the next column. The patient should be asked about any cognitive responses to the events described. Patients must be able to determine to what extent they believe that the automatic thoughts are true (from zero% = "I don't believe it at all," to 100% = "I am absolutely convinced"). For that purpose, the therapist writes the automatic thoughts down verbatim, formulating them positively, with elimination of such words as *perhaps*, *probably*, and *possibly*. Thereafter, the therapist asks the patient to rate each thought as to its credibility (e.g., "I believe that for 80%").
- In challenging the automatic thoughts, the therapist chooses an automatic thought that is relatively easy to challenge. It is more didactic to challenge one single thought comprehensively than to list a large number of automatic thoughts and challenge them generally. The irrational thought is written on the blackboard.
- Before starting the challenge, the therapist categorizes the thought under one of the following headings: (1) The situation might not be observed accurately (e.g., "Everybody looks at me when I start to tremble," or (2) False logic was used (e.g., "If I start to tremble, then I am weak and worthless"). This is important because both categories require different challenge techniques. In discussing thoughts from the first category, emphasis is placed on teaching patients to observe reality more accurately and in different situations. With thoughts from the second category, patients are challenged to scrutinize the validity and the origin of their beliefs with questions such as, "What makes a person worthless?" Depending on the kind of reasoning error, questions are directed to allow patients to discover for themselves that the automatic thought might not be the most appropriate response to the situation. For example, suppose you are invited for a dinner with colleagues, and even the prospect of it makes you feel tense and miserable. You continue to worry and fret yourself, and get negative about it. These emotions are the result of a series of thoughts that go through your mind, such as "It will be a waste of time" or

"Everybody thinks that I'm an idiot because I blush." Now, the next step in treatment will be to investigate the negative automatic thoughts and to change them into more rational or realistic thoughts. You can do this by asking yourself one or more of the following questions: What is the evidence for this reasoning? What evidence is there to support it or refute it? Are there alternative points of view? What would other people think about it? Is my reasoning correct? Specific questions in this situation might be: "How do I know beforehand what will happen?" "What exactly is a waste of time? In whose eyes?" "What determines whether time is wasted?" "Would they have invited me if they see it as a waste of time?" "How do I know that people find me an idiot? Has everybody ever told me that I'm an idiot?" "Has anybody told me other opinions about myself?" "What reasons can there be for getting a red color on my cheeks?" and so on.

- In formulating rational thoughts, the therapist encourages the patient, reinforcing each alternative thought that the patient might have, and particularly those that are more rational. Again, several questions can be presented, such as: "What effect do these thoughts have on me?" "How does it make me feel and how will I react?" "What are the advantages and disadvantages of this way of thinking?" "Is there another way to think about it which would have a more positive (or less negative) effect?"

- The therapist inquires about the credibility of these rational thoughts. After the challenge, the therapist notes for each automatic thought the degree of confidence for this thinking, as the patient perceives it at this time. The emotions that arise after the introduction of rational thoughts should also be noted and scored. Original thoughts and emotions in response to the situation are compared and reassessed.

- The therapist assigns new homework. If automatic thoughts have been challenged successfully, the patient is asked to practice the challenge technique in relevant situations concerned, whenever they occur. For example, when rational thoughts are formulated about making telephone calls, the assignment is as follows: "Before you make a telephone call, try to think in the rational thought mode. Instead of just allowing the automatic thought to take over, ask yourself these challenging questions and formulate rational thoughts." To allow the patient to practice, it is desirable that the situation occurs several times a week. For that purpose, some time is spent discussing how this can be accomplished (e.g., by making a list of telephone calls).

- The second homework assignment involves maintaining a "thought diary" (all columns) for a half-hour each day.

- Session evaluation.

Session 3

- Setting the agenda.
- Detailed discussion of homework of the previous week. Especially in the first session, considerable time must be spent on homework completion. Patients are asked about any problems encountered, and these are discussed. Based on homework, new challenges are presented in the session.
- The therapist explains the use of behavioral experiments to the patient. This explanation is given in Sidebar 4–3.

Sidebar 4–3

Explanation of Behavioral Experiments

One way to challenge your automatic thoughts in daily life is the execution of behavioral experiments. Behavioral experiments are conducted in order to indicate (1) whether the expected results really occur, and if so, how frequently and (2) how great the catastrophe is, if the worst expectations are true. They are based on the rule "seeing is believing." Just as in scientific research, the aim is to collect information and see if it is possible to draw certain conclusions. Experience shows that conducting experiments to discover whether your thoughts concur with reality is helpful in challenging automatic thoughts, and in uncovering more realistic, alternative thinking. In order to provide a better idea of what a behavioral experiment really means, I'll give you an example.

A woman who is shopping for clothes is frightened to ask the assistant to help her. Her automatic thought is that the shop assistant will find her bothersome and annoying if she asks for help or time, especially if she eventually decides not to buy anything. So, her hypothesis is: "If I tell shop assistants that I will not buy anything, after they have helped me for at least 5 minutes, they will find me bothersome and annoying, and will react in an unfriendly manner." Her confidence (or degree of belief) in this assumption is 70%. Consequently, she is already nervous when she goes into a shop; she sometimes leaves the store quickly without looking properly or noticing whether there is something nice there, and sometimes buys clothing that does not fit exactly or which she ends up not really liking. Now, by discussing this situation in a session she may recognize that the expectation that she will be seen as bothersome and annoying is without any evidence. In challenging the thoughts, the following arguments are discussed: "It is a shop assistant's job to help customers properly. If an assistant gets irritated, then you could wonder whether she does her work well, and it says more about her than it does about me. As a customer I have the right to say "no" if I don't want to buy. I don't have to apologize. Capable shop assistants know that clients don't come back if they react irritated." As a result, she may come to a (possibly more

---

- Assignment of new homework: reading the explanation about behavioral experiments, filling in the "thought diary," practicing rational thoughts that have been agreed on in the session (from the diary).
- Session evaluation.

Session 4

- Setting the agenda.
- Discussion of homework assignments of past week.
- Development of a behavioral experiment. In designing behavioral experiments, it is important to consider several points. First, for purposes of the behavioral experiment, automatic thoughts are viewed as hypotheses that must be checked against reality. As in a scientific experiment, predictions are distilled and compared against experimental results (zero hypothesis = "if A then B"; alternative hypothesis = "if

realistic) alternative thought, such as: "If I tell shop assistants that I will buy nothing, after they have helped me for at least 5 minutes, they will accept that without further discussion. They may be a little disappointed, but will not change their attitude and will be friendly." She rates the credibility of this thought at 50%; however, she still does not know for sure, and in many cases it may be important to know whether your expectations are realistic. So, she agrees with her therapist to go to as many shops as possible, allowing herself to be helped extensively, but never buying anything. Her original idea has been that all shop assistants are irritated and unfriendly if a customer asks for time and attention. The alternative hypothesis is that shop assistants will accept her refusal and will stay friendly. Now, the proof of the pudding is in the eating. It is agreed that she will visit at least eight shops (as many as are necessary to convince her) and collect information about both outcomes. She will watch how shop assistants react and what aspects of their behavior she interprets as signs of irritation. After that, she can rate with more confidence the credibility of both assumptions.

It is important to bear the following points in mind when conducting behavioral experiments:

1. Experiments often create tension, but that is inevitable. The only way to test the validity of your thoughts is by entering situations that you fear, so that you can observe whether your predictions come true. However, there is no reason to start with the most difficult situation, so don't make it too difficult in the beginning.

2. It is wise to investigate a range of situations (the more the better) before your draw your conclusions. You may find that your predictions come true in one situation but not in others.

3. Once you have drawn conclusions on the basis of the experiments, then adopt your behavior (e.g., If you have come to the conclusion that people don't laugh when you ask a question, then go on with asking questions).

4. If the automatic thought reoccurs, then stop and indicate its significance.

5. An experiment always provides some information, irrespective of outcome. It may be that your anxious expectations prove to be right one or more times, but then you can find out whether that is really as catastrophical as you thought it would be.

Throughout the rest of your treatment we will strive to investigate your own automatic thoughts and to test them with behavioral experiments.

A then not B"). Second, it is important that patients view behavioral experiments as credible; otherwise, the result will have little or no significance for the patient. Finally, it is important to ensure that the design of the experiment contains clear and observable criteria in advance; also, it should be possible to determine which hypothesis is supported (i.e., not "If I ring Y, then Y will think …").

The following is an example of a behavioral experiment: Knocking over a cup of coffee in a restaurant, the patient's expectation is "If I knock over a cup of coffee then I will get a reprimand." The formulation of the alternative expectation is "If I do that, I won't be reprimanded." Before this experiment can be carried out, the patient has to specify exactly (in terms of observable behavior) what he or she means by "get a reprimand." A second example of a behavioral experiment might be attending a meeting at work, and saying something that is not pertinent to the topic. The patient's expectation is "If I do that, then I'll be laughed at in the meeting and be put on the spot by my boss." The alternative thought is "If I do that, then nobody will laugh and my boss won't bring it up again." A final example of a (more complex) behavioral experiment is looking at people on the train. The patient's expectation is "If I do that, then I'll find out that everybody is looking at me; then I will start to blush, and everybody will laugh at me." The alternative expectation is, "If I do that, then I'll find out that no one stares at me. I will not blush and nobody will laugh at me," or, "I will blush, but nobody will laugh." The ultimate intention is that the degree of belief ascribed to the automatic thoughts decreases gradually by conducting experiments. When starting behavioral experiments, it is important to begin with a relatively easy situation. Moreover, it is also important that, having completed such an experiment successfully, patients continue to put the experiment into practice in order to ensure that they rehearse the new thoughts.

- Homework consists of completing the thought diary, conducting the assigned behavioral experiments, and filling in the behavioral experiments report form.
- Session evaluation.

Sessions 5–7

- Setting the agenda.
- Discussion of homework assignments. The diary forms and behavior experiments are discussed.
- Discussion of the challenges made at home, on the basis of the diary. If sufficient progress has been made in creating challenges to catastrophic expectations and developing alternative thoughts, but the patient continues to find it difficult to challenge such catastrophic expectations in the actual, fear-evoking situation, then use can be made of the "flashcard." On one side, the patient writes his catastrophic expectation; on the other side, the challenges and alternative thinking are described. The patient is instructed to use the card as an aid in the actual situation.
- New behavioral experiments are developed in these sessions.
- Homework consists of completing the "thought diary," conducting the assigned behavioral experiments, and filling in the behavioral experiments report form.
- Session evaluation.

Sessions 8–12

- Setting the agenda.
- Discussion of homework assignments.
- Uncovering dysfunctional assumptions. In this final phase of treatment, attention is directed to more basic dysfunctional thoughts (i.e., assumptions such as, "I have to be perfect in all counts to be a valuable person", "People will always try to hurt you when you are vulnerable"). Most of the work consists of analyzing the material from previous sessions with the patient. Are there themes that can be identified in the examples the patient provides? A theme can be any grouping, title, or association that relates to a range of similar behaviors. These become clear through the course of therapy. It is preferable not to lead patients too strongly, but to let them try to formulate the assumption for themselves.
- Formulating dysfunctional assumptions. Whenever one or more dysfunctional assumptions are detected, they are presented to the patient in a tentative manner. The patient gives his or her opinion about the validity of this assumption. The patient

must be able to rate the credibility of the assumption; therefore, it must be formulated positively and unambiguously. Underlying assumptions can be detected by:

○ Examining the list of automatic thoughts expressed by the patient during the course of therapy.

○ Examining frequently used words such as *guilt*, *perfect*, and *vulnerable*. Ask what they really mean to the patient.

○ Allowing the patient to associate (about childhood, memories, etc.)

○ Noting the patient's resistance to alternative behaviors: "Yes, but that's not the way I think, because ..." (assumption).

The formulated assumption must correlate closely with the implicit regimen of the patient. The often-extreme nature of the regimen must be clearly expressed and for that aim, it can be helpful to use absolute words like *always* and *never*, even if patients insist that their thoughts are not that extreme. The thought errors in the assumption must be clearly indicated. An assumption is preferably stated as follows: "If A, then B," where B is something negative. The absoluteness of the statement makes it easier to formulate the alternative thought. The following basic assumptions are commonly observed in social phobics: "If I don't do everything perfectly, then it is a disaster", "If somebody doesn't like me, then it's terrible", "If things don't go according to my plan, then it's a catastrophe."

- Challenging dysfunctional assumptions. After the assumption has been formulated, it is important to show empathy: "Now I see why you have a problem with social insecurity. If you think like that ..."). The patient must be provided with the insight that it is not so much about a single thought, but more about an attitude that is applied uncritically, without consideration of the reality to which it relates. The link between this assumption and the way in which events are interpreted (selective abstraction), their self-fulfilling nature, and the consequences thereof for both emotions and behavior must be made clear to the patient. Once a basic assumption is recognized by the patient, then it can be challenged in the sessions and at home. In this process, it is not up to therapists to prove that the assumption is incorrect. Rather, patients should provide evidence for their assumptions and for alternative rules. In principal, this occurs by using the same method of challenges for dysfunctional thinking that were discussed in previous sessions. In addition, the following methods can be employed: (1) Demonstration of false logic in the assumption, (2) Establishing the arbitrary nature of such assumptions. Often they are perceived as unalterable facts, a type of natural law against which everybody must struggle. The assumptions determine what patients perceive—what they see as reality. The inevitable nature of these assumptions is countered by the observation that different people have disparate assumptions. (3) Making a list of advantages and disadvantages that are the consequences of keeping such assumptions.
- Testing assumptions. This (once again) occurs through behavioral experiments. Agree, for example, that something will be said in a meeting on 10 different occasions to determine which hypothesis is correct.
- Homework involves the investigation of old and new assumptions.
- Session evaluation.

After the 12th session, treatment progress is formally evaluated, although more informal evaluations generally have occurred over the course of treatment. A small number of patients appear to have (almost) completely overcome their fear. In those cases, it is sensible to make one or two follow-up appointments and finish treatment. Most patients report considerable progress but still feel more or less anxious in some situations. For them, it is often sensible to continue the treatment and to fade out sessions in a gradual fashion. If, after the 12th session, patients have not noticed any beneficial effects, there is no reason to continue with this kind of treatment.

Exposure in Vivo

For patients who avoid many social situations, treatment may start with an emphasis on prolonged exposure *in vivo*. The following sections contain a brief description of important aspects of exposure treatment. For further details the reader is referred to Butler (1985, 1989).

Although direct comparative studies between imaginal and *in vivo* exposure have not been conducted with social phobic patients, *in vivo* exposure is preferred. Indeed, this strategy has proven its efficacy for this population, and studies on other anxiety disorders have demonstrated that *in vivo* exposure is much more effective than imaginal exposure (Emmelkamp, 1982; Marks, 1987). It was also found that exposure is most successful when carried out using a prolonged, uninterrupted period of time, while escape and avoidance are prevented.

Exposure *in vivo* for social phobia is often hindered by disorder-specific problems (see discussion by Butler, 1985); for example, (1) many social interactions are time-limited and, therefore, not suitable to practice long enough, (2) exposure for social phobia often provides no direct information about the reality of the social fears (negative judgment by other people), whereas exposure with other complaints mostly demonstrates that the feared events do not occur—often leading to cognitive changes, and (3) the unpredictability of social situations is an obstacle to the gradual practice of increasingly difficult situations.

In addition, a large part of the exposure program for social phobias must be applied via self-controlled homework assignments. Because of the nature of the feared situations, many assignments cannot be practiced in the treatment session (e.g., visits to or from certain people or situations at work). A disadvantage of a self-controlled homework program is that the therapist has no opportunity to observe how the patient behaves during assignments, and in some cases such information is very relevant. On the other hand, self-controlled exposure has the advantage that patients practice from the start in naturalistic situations; therefore, there is little risk that improvements are limited to the treatment setting. Practically, we sometimes accompany patients during exposure assignments, especially when the assignment has proven to be difficult.

Conducting Exposure Treatment

Explanation of Treatment Rationale. The verbatim explanation of treatment to a patient with fear of criticism is provided in Sidebar 4–4.

It is important that patients understand the rationale and become aware of their (often subtle) forms of avoidance behavior, as well as the relationship between avoidance and the endurance of fear. For social phobics, this is the more important, because patients will often have to adapt assignments while practicing. It is often useful to have patients rephrase the rationale in their own words before the start of actual exposure sessions. Possible misunderstandings can then be corrected. At the end of the session, patients are asked to read the written explanation of the rationale at home.

Sidebar 4–4

Explanation of Exposure Rationale

Because you are afraid of being criticized, you avoid many situations, such as speaking in public, saying what you really think, taking initiatives with other people, and so on. In the past, you have been subjected to these tendencies because you have observed that the tension decreases when you escape from such situations. Now you have learned that by avoiding such situations, you can prevent becoming anxious. In the short term, this avoidance is an effective strategy, because you don't have to face your fears. In the longer term, however, the result is not beneficial. As you have noticed, your fear has become more and more inhibiting over the years.

Now, through your strategy to avoid, you can't observe what happens when you don't subject yourself to this inclination to avoid. If you don't avoid, anxiety will increase initially, and that, of course, is what you try to prevent. However, if you persist, you will find that the anxiety will decrease after some time. How soon that will be depends on the specific situation and on the degree of anxiety that you feel. Sometimes it is only after you have persisted a number of times that you get more comfortable, but generally, once you have endured a difficult situation, the next time you face it will be a little less frightening. Now, in treatment you will practice situations that are difficult for you. It is important to note that we start easy, with situations that are successful every now and then and invoke little tension. Only after these assignments are mastered, that is to say, when you can endure the situation without too much tension and you have noticed that your anxiety decreases, we move to the next situation, which is a bit more difficult. You'll notice that during treatment you'll gradually develop more and more self-confidence. To achieve that, you practice gradually; we start with the construction of a hierarchy of assignments. For that purpose, we use a so-called fear thermometer: a scale from zero = *No Fear at All* to 100 = *Panic*. We make a number of exposure assignments (at least about 20) and then you rate each assignment on this scale. We purposely choose assignments in such a way that their ratings gradually increase from zero to 100, without large gaps. However, we will see that sometimes it is very difficult to determine the difficulty of an assignment in advance, because social situations are unpredictable.

Hierarchy Construction.   Before carrying out an exposure program, it is essential that the therapist have all relevant information about the cues that trigger anxiety and understand the exact nature of avoidance behavior. This is accomplished by a detailed discussion of situations that the patient fears. Sometimes patients feel ashamed to admit that they feel anxious in what they see as relatively "easy" situations (e.g., walking in the street, sitting in a bus). From that point of view, the therapist should routinely inventory a number of such situations. As for the construction of the hierarchy, it is helpful to list factors that influence the assignment difficulty. Some examples include the number of other people present (some patients have problems in groups; others are anxious in more personal interactions), familiarity of other people (some have fear with complete strangers, whereas others become increasingly anxious when others become more familiar), and the sex, age, status, and so on, of other people. For patients with fear of blushing, the following aspects may be influential: location (inside or outside), temperature, degree of light (daylight or evening light), clothes, makeup, presence of beards, or wearing sunglasses. For patients with fear of trembling, it is important what kind of cups they use, or what course they have to eat (e.g., bouillon). Detailed discussion of difficult situations can bring other factors to the fore.

After these factors are inventoried, extremes of the fear thermometer are established for the patient. This involves formulating one assignment that provokes no anxiety and another that causes extreme anxiety. Consequently, a number of personally relevant exposure assignments are developed. Because patients should carry out the exposure program on their own, this is a very important phase. The hierarchy that is established at the beginning of therapy has to be flexible. In many cases, circumstances will make it necessary to adapt the assignments, to adjust their difficulty, or to add new ones.

It is important that assignments are made as specific as possible, with clear specification of behavior to be emitted (or not carried out, in the case of response prevention). It is better to formulate an assignment as specific as "Go tomorrow morning at 10 o'clock to the mall and ask at least 20 attractive passengers of the opposite sex what time it is," than "If you do some shopping, ask passengers what time it is." In the latter case, it is much easier to postpone the assignment and to avoid real exposure. The following is another example of a suitable exposure assignment: "Friday morning, at work, practice making telephone calls from 9:00 to 10:00 A.M. with your colleague in the same room. Have a list with telephone numbers ready so that you can call one after another. Start each call with the same introduction, tell that you want some information, and ask for the right person. Then, take your time to ask for all the information you want. Don't turn your face away when calling, and look at your colleague every now and then. If he or she happens to be absent, repeat the assignment another morning, when he or she is present." In preparation for such an assignment, a list of possible telephone calls and relevant questions is made in the session.

During formulation of assignments, patients often are startled when they hear what kinds of exercises can be constructed. It is important that the therapist informs them that (1) they are not forced to do assignments that are too difficult, (2) the pace of practicing is self-determined, and (3) assignments higher in the hierarchy will be less difficult once easier assignments have been successfully practiced repeatedly.

Many patients find some exposure exercises that we propose "overdone." For example, they object that "no one will set off alarm clocks in a shop." It must be explained that the assignments may help them to overcome their anxiety, but are not meant as a standard for their future lives, and that overlearning is useful in order to prevent relapse. Examples of situations that can be employed in exposure assignments are shown in Sidebar 4–5.

After determining hierarchical elements along some examples, patients are asked to extend the list of assignments at home; this will increase their concern for the assignment. Most patients will be more strongly motivated to carry out self-formulated assignments than those made by the therapist.

Although there are no strict rules with respect to the number of situations included in a hierarchy, we strive for at least 20 assignments of gradually increasing difficulty, without large gaps in between.

Exposure Sessions. Social phobic patients are often unsystematically exposed to the daily-life situations they fear, without showing definitive improvement. There are a

Sidebar 4–5

Examples of Situations That Can Be Worked Out as Exposure Assignments

- Walking through busy streets and asking passersby what time it is, the way to the station, or for a light.
- Asking precedence at the checkout counter in a supermarket with the exact money.
- Asking for information on articles without buying them.
- Returning or exchanging articles.
- Forgetting your money and asking whether the articles could be put aside and collected later without your having to wait in line.
- Trying on clothes or shoes without buying any.
- Asking for information at a travel agency.
- Giving compliments and criticisms.
- Listening in an established record shop to a number of compact disks without buying any of them.
- Asking a number of people in the street where they bought their coat, bag, tie, and so on.
- Starting and finishing conversations with familiar people.
- Starting and finishing conversations with unfamiliar people.
- Participating in conversations of other people.
- Making mistakes.
- Making telephone calls (formal and informal) to different people, whether or not observed by other people.

number of reasons why such unsystematic exposure does not lead to habituation. First, exposure to a specific situation is often short. A patient may continue to be present at two hour-long meetings at work, but may prevent the situation he really fears (i.e., being the center of attention). In case it does occur (e.g., someone asks for his or her opinion), he or she will give a brief answer. Thus, in this particular case, real exposure may occur just a few minutes per week, which is much too brief a time for habituation to occur. Therefore, agreements must be made that the patient engages more actively in the meeting and for a longer period of time. A related reason, as noted by Butler (1985), is the intrinsic time limit of many social situations. Although conversations with other people may last up to 2 hours, many other social situations are time-limited (e.g., shaking hands, asking a question in an audience, being criticized). Therapeutically, it is useful to prolong exposure until anxiety decreases. In situations where prolonged exposure is not possible, frequently repeated exposure is recommended.

Finally, "daily-life exposure" does not lead to habituation if the encountered situations are too difficult, which implies that more time is needed for habituation. In terms of the exposure principle, one could say that the assignment is too high in the hierarchy. Patients, often quite unexpectedly, are confronted with situations that would be rated 90 or 100, and which they are unable to handle. In practice, they often escape from the situation without having experienced that feelings of anxiety decrease after some time. In light of these problems, patients have to practice various assignments of the same sort and of the same subjective anxiety level without any break until they feel better. In a typical exposure session in our treatments, patients go to the town center and practice a number of successive assignments, all of which can be performed nearby. Such a quick succession of assignments enables habituation to occur and precludes patients from leaving the stage with a feeling of relief that they have escaped another time.

In exposure *in vivo*, patients generally are encouraged to take a more active attitude in all social contacts, to stop avoiding and postponing social interactions, and to take more initiative with other people. An important argument for assuming a more active attitude is that patients maintain more control of the situation if they take initiative. Because they normally expend all energy to avoid situations, patients often are startled and feel vulnerable and helpless when they suddenly become the center of attention.

Patients are encouraged to confront the feared situation until the anxiety has eased. It may be useful to have patients rate their anxiety level at regular intervals throughout the exposure session, for example, on a 10-point scale. The session will not be completed until the anxiety level has diminished substantially. This also implies that patients should not start with more demanding assignments a few minutes before the end of the exposure session.

The therapeutic relationship is essential for the implementation of exposure therapy. Generally, the therapist's style should be empathic, but firm. If patients disregard certain items or have "rational" objections (e.g., "I don't have to buy my clothes in a shop, I always buy them by mail order"), the therapist must not give in too easily. Objections to certain assignments are often motivated by patients' fears. For that reason it is sensible to emphasize that patients will be able to make a free (and possibly better) decision once they are not hindered by their fear.

If the therapist accompanies the patient during exposure *in vivo*, a discussion of other problems is postponed until the exposure is completed, as are negotiations about the necessity of carrying out one or more assignments (provided that it was agreed in the session to practice these assignments).

No general guidelines can be offered with respect to the number of situations per homework session. It depends on the patient and the difficulty of the assignments. Some patients quickly perceive the basic principles and apply them in other situations as well. Other patients are more reluctant and may need more encouragement to rehearse the exercises in every situation again. More important than the number of assignments is that patients practice as often as possible, and that they continue to practice once assignments are successfully mastered.

Some problems are difficult to deal with in exposure treatment. For example, exposure to criticism and aggression is not easy to arrange in the homework assignments. Systematic exposure to situations involving conflict or aggression in the therapist's office may be necessary. This can be done either imaginally or *in vivo* through role play. In the latter case, the therapist should clearly explain the "as if" character of the situation.

When patients are afraid of blushing, trembling, or sweating, it is essential that they be exposed to situations in which these symptoms occur. In such cases, it is generally necessary to include explicit instructions about response prevention. The rationale should stress that frequent and prolonged confrontation with the feared stimulus without trying to escape or hide symptoms will lead to anxiety reduction. Examples of exercises are talking about difficult topics while maintaining eye contact, wearing blouses with open necks, drinking coffee out of small cups in the company of others, and talking with others about fear of symptoms. Exposure to sweating can be conducted by wearing warm pullovers, by heating the room with the windows closed, and by having the patient do physical exercises (without washing) before meeting people. Response prevention should target behaviors such as bending down, wearing sunglasses or makeup, escaping to the toilet, looking in the mirror, coughing, sitting in dark places, avoiding artificial light, putting a glass down, signing checks at home rather than in the company of others, and holding cups or glasses with two hands.

Social Skills Training

Social skills training has proven to be effective in decreasing fear of negative evaluation, but the exact process of treatment is unclear. In any case, the relationship between quality of social skills and degree of social anxiety is far from perfect.

In the treatment of social phobia, social skills training can be implemented in two ways: (1) as a separate module, with emphasis on the acquisition of various social skills *per se*, or (2) on a more limited basis, in which the skills training is integrated into the cognitive–behavioral treatment that was described previously. Both applications are discussed below.

Inclusion of a separate social skills training module is indicated for patients who display deficits in basic social skills during the first session (e.g., they avoid eye contact with the therapist, keep very silent and passive, have problems in adequate listening and responding to questions, or talk with a low voice). A social skills training module provides the opportunity to spend enough time and effort for (1) discussion of social skills, (2) observation of other people in daily life, (3) modeling by the therapist, and (4) repeated behavioral rehearsal through role play. Each session focuses on one or two specific skills and includes assignments to practice newly acquired skills in daily life. Besides the training of social skills *per se*, this module serves two additional goals: (1) to enhance the self-confidence of the patient to start with exposure *in vivo* or behavioral experiments, and (2) to increase the likelihood that behavioral assignments will have encouraging results, because other people will react positively. For that reason it is wise to include this module early in the treatment. In our experience, it is sufficient to devote 6 to 10 sessions to skills training, although more time is necessary to consolidate gains in daily-life situations. For elaborate manuals on social skills training, the reader is referred to more specialized publications (e.g., Curran & Monti, 1982).

Other patients demonstrate adequate social skills in the session (e.g., maintain adequate eye contact, ask questions appropriately or talk about themselves) so that skills training seems superfluous; however, during the course of treatment, it may become apparent that they lack the required skills in specific social situations. Some of them have problems expressing criticism or presenting themselves in applications or oral examinations. Patients who are preoccupied with fear of blushing, trembling, or sweating often seem socially skilled until they experience the symptoms. At those moments they become silent, avoid eye contact, and do not know how to react. For these patients, limited skills training may be indicated, depending on the specific skills deficits, and it is advisable to integrate such training in discussions of irrational thoughts and practice of exposure *in vivo* or in behavioral assignments. For example, a behavioral experiment revealed that classmates made few initiatives to talk to the patient. Several explanations were proposed for this finding, one of them being that the patient's attitude generally did not encourage other people to say something. It was predicted that another attitude would gradually lead to other reactions from classmates. In that context, an "inviting attitude" (eye contact, asking questions, nonverbal encouragements) was repeatedly practiced in role play before it was used in a behavioral experiment.

It is our experience that such implementation of social skills training is sufficient for a large number of patients.

Group versus Individual Treatment

Especially for social phobics, group therapy may have clear advantages. First, group treatment provides a continuous exposure to a group—for many social phobics a highly anxiety-provoking situation. Second, group treatment offers the opportunity to share fears with partners in distress. Most social phobics, convinced that their fears are uncommon and strange, are inclined to hide their fears from other people. Discovering that others have the same difficulties is often a revelation and a relief. Group intervention also requires less of a therapist's time than individual treatment; therefore, more patients can benefit from treatment. Finally, specific treatment effects, regardless of whether treatment consists of exposure *in vivo*, cognitive therapy, or social skills training, can be enhanced by assistance from other group members. Furthermore, certain feared situations can be arranged more easily in a group setting. For example, making telephone calls, writing, or drinking coffee while being observed by others is easier to carry out in a group format than in individual treatment. Patients who are afraid of blushing have to sit in front of others while wearing an open-necked blouse until anxiety subsides. Others who fear that their hands may tremble have to write at the blackboard and serve tea to the group. For most patients, reading and giving an impromptu speech for the group are important exercises. In our exposure groups for social phobias, an important part of treatment is actual exposure *in vivo* in the center of the city. Patients and therapist go to the town center, where patients have to perform a number of difficult tasks. In some cases, patients may carry out exposure assignments with one or two other patients before trying them on their own. When patients succeed in overcoming their anxiety during the exposure session, they frequently devise even more difficult tasks for themselves and their group members than those suggested by the therapist. A friendly competitiveness is common in exposure groups. In social skills training, group members provide different models of social skills that can be observed and imitated. In cognitive treatment, it is possible for patients to check whether their fear of negative evaluation is realistic.

Group treatment also has some disadvantages. Most important is the inability of the therapist to direct much attention to individual problems. For that reason, it is important that patients have no other significant difficulties that require much attention. For example, one of our patients, who had a business of his own, had financial problems that rapidly increased because he was too afraid to ask for help in an early stage. Although group treatment helped him to take some necessary steps, he was so obsessed with the threat of bankruptcy that he could not concentrate in the group. In fact, he required individual sessions, in which all time could be spent on his specific situation.

MAINTENANCE STRATEGIES/RELAPSE PREVENTION

Five studies have reported on the long-term effects of treatment of social phobics (Heimberg, Salzman, Holt, & Blendell, 1993; Mersch, Emmelkamp & Lips, 1991; Scholing & Emmelkamp, 1995a, b; Wlazlo, Schroder-Hartwig, Hand, Kaiser, & Munchau, 1990) and only three of them provided data about patients who relapsed and needed additional treatment. Mersch et al. (1991) found that lack of social skills predicted need for additional treatment during follow-up. These results suggested that anxiety reduction alone is not sufficient, but that a number of social phobics may need additional social skills training in order to prevent relapse. In the Scholing and Emmelkamp (1995a) study, several patients reported a temporal relapse in the interval between the termination of treatment and long-term follow-up (after 18 months). Most of them had conquered their fears without professional help, whereas some had reentered treatment. In all, we have only a limited understanding of the problem of relapse in social phobics. Although several strategies are considered useful to prevent relapse, future research should provide more information about which patients are vulnerable to relapse, and which interventions should be applied to prevent relapse.

The most common form of relapse prevention is the implementation of booster sessions (i.e., additional sessions at regular intervals posttherapy). This strategy has been found to prevent (some of the) relapses in such diverse areas as depression, headache, hypertension, smoking, and obesity (see Wilson, 1992). Essential to booster sessions is that therapists concentrate on why patients did not succeed by themselves, and that they teach patients problem-solving strategies that will enable them to cope more effectively with potential relapse the next time. For that purpose, a list can be made of the steps patients should take (e.g., filling in "thought diaries," carrying out systematic exposure, behavioral experiments).

Furthermore, it seems therapeutically useful to emphasize techniques that patients can apply without the help of a therapist. For that reason, therapists should supply patients with written or audiotaped material as much as possible (e.g., explanation of treatment strategies and behavioral experiments, directives for making exposure assignments), and patients are advised from the start to keep this information. During treatment, diaries or homework reports are returned to patients after each session.

There is some evidence that, irrespective of the particular treatment method employed, relapse is more likely when cognitions did not change during treatment (Butler et al., 1984; Chambless & Gillis, 1993; Mattick & Peters, 1988; Mattick et al., 1989). If these results are confirmed in future studies, an important relapse-prevention strategy would be to continue treatment not only until avoidance behavior is decreased, but also until negative cognitions (e.g., fear of evaluation) have been transformed into more neutral ones.

Another important strategy to prevent relapse is the implementation of more structural changes in the lifestyle of the patient (e.g., expanding the social network, doing volunteer work), especially in case a regular job is unavailable.

If depression is associated with social phobia and the patient is still depressed at the end of treatment, he or she is particularly vulnerable for relapse. In such cases, additional interventions are indicated. These would consist of cognitive–behavioral therapy directed at the depression, drug treatment, or a combination of both.

Problems in Implementation

Problems may arise in several phases in the treatment. We will not dwell on more general problems that can occur in every treatment. Rather, we will limit our discussion to obstacles that are often reported in the treatment of social phobic patients. The following areas are distinguished: the therapeutic relationship, homework, cognitive strategies, and exposure *in vivo*.

Therapeutic Relationship

As stated earlier, the therapist must take into account that social phobic patients can be anxious during sessions. Their fear of negative evaluation by the therapist may have different consequences (e.g., patients falling silent, not being able to report thoughts, and forgetting what has been said in the session). Some general strategies were described to help patients to overcome their fear and their problems in concentration (e.g., an accepting and empathic therapist, writing down all agreements about homework and other important aspects of treatment, giving patients audiotapes of the session to listen to at home). If the fear seriously disrupts the proceedings of treatment, it can be desirable to confront this problem directly, for example, by discussing fear-provoking thoughts in detail at the moment at hand, or by including exposure assignments in the contact with the therapist (e.g., maintaining eye contact, telling personal matters for a gradually longer time). The "cognitive dialogue" of patients is discussed, and the fact that patients have to divide their attention between talking and listening to the therapist and focusing on their own fearful cognitions. It is often helpful for patients to practice concentrating more on the discussion (e.g., asking questions, making short paraphrases, or observing other people more accurately). All of these strategies are designed to divert the attention away from the patients themselves to their surroundings.

In addition, therapists should be aware that social phobics may become more anxious once treatment proceeds. Some patients seem relatively at ease in the first sessions. They are often relieved that the therapist is aware of their fears, and that there is no reason to hide them. However, just as in the "real world," their fear of negative evaluation often increases after a number of sessions, partly because they start to build up thoughts about the therapist's expectations of them. As a consequence, they can become anxious about disappointing the therapist by, for example, protesting against homework assignments they find useless or too difficult, admitting that they could not fulfill their homework assignment, or expressing their disappointment with the results of treatment. For that reason, therapists have to be alert about subtle signs of patients trying to please the therapist, instead of expressing their own wishes and feelings, because this tendency can eventually stimulate early dropout. This is all the more important because social phobics, more than other patients, are inclined to ascribe treatment failure to themselves, and not to the therapist or the specific strategy utilized.

Homework

If homework has not been completed, it is important to find out why. The approach may be a little different when this problem is encountered immediately in the second session than when it is reported in the 10th session, after patients have carried out all previous assignments in the prescribed fashion. However, by ignoring such events, therapists undermine the credibility of the treatment and themselves. From the first session, it must be clear that treatment success depends to a large extent on the completion of homework. In questioning the patient, the therapist tries to determine why it has not been done. Was it too difficult? Has anything important happened in the last few days? Is the patient not convinced of the effectiveness of the treatment or disappointed in it or in the therapist? For example, some social phobics fear making incorrect analyses at home, and would, therefore, rather not engage in such a project at all. It is important to address this concern and the cognitive reasoning behind it. It may be sufficient to explain that the patient is not required to make perfect analyses, and that cognitive therapy is difficult for everybody. It can also be useful to deal more comprehensively with the situation (i.e., sitting at home and making an analysis) by taking such behavior as the subject for analysis. Only if patients insist that they had no clear reason for not completing the assignment, or had no time, or were "just not in the mood," should therapists ask how they want to proceed with the treatment, given the fact that assignments form an essential part of it, and that therapy sessions are of little value if patients come unprepared. More specific problems with homework assignments are discussed in the next section.

Problems during Cognitive Strategies

One of the problems most frequently reported by patients is that they still feel anxious, in spite of the fact that they now think more rationally. Several interventions can be helpful. First, the therapist has to emphasize that patients have trained themselves in nonrealistic thinking for many years and in many different situations. It cannot be expected that such thought patterns can be changed within a few weeks. Furthermore, patients can be asked to self-monitor how often they still engage in negative thinking. Although the ultimate treatment goal is for patients to permanently change their irrational thoughts into more realistic ones, in the beginning they are only able to do so when concentrating on their thoughts; at other times, they continue their usual thinking patterns. Therefore, it may be that the time spent on realistic thinking is marginal compared with that for negative thoughts and that, in fact, they still think irrationally when feeling anxious. This problem can be eradicated partially by asking patients to examine their thoughts more frequently (e.g., 5 minutes every hour) or before entering a social interaction. Especially for patients who are caught in vicious circles (e.g., patients with fear of bodily symptoms), it can be beneficial to discuss their cognitive dialogue and to teach them to concentrate on the task at hand, as described earlier in the section on problems in the therapeutic relationship.

If patients continue to report difficulty in thinking more realistically, rational imagination (RI) may be helpful. In RI, patients imagine the difficult situation as vividly as possible (as in imaginary exposure), and then try to feel less anxious by rehearsing realistic thoughts. The therapist can assist them by describing the situation. RI is only suitable for patients who can imagine the situations so realistically that they experience the same feelings; after some training, many patients are able to do so.

Cognitive Therapy Is Too Difficult.   The therapist has to adapt his or her style to the patient. It is usually sensible to start with a Socratic-like dialogue, but not always. Although this technique may be a very effective strategy for more intelligent people or for people who are comfortable with this approach, some patients find this style frustrating. They react better to a more persuasive or directive style (e.g., with therapists suggesting thoughts that would be more helpful to them). One of our patients became considerably less anxious after the therapist suggested that he think the following before entering social situations: "And so what if they don't like me? I'm as good as everybody else, and if they are unkind to me, they can go to hell" (which he also had a on a flash card). Although they may sound rather aggressive, these thoughts gave him the courage he needed to behave more self-confidently.

Other signs may indicate that the cognitive strategy is too difficult (e.g., when patients keep confusing objective situations and their interpretations, or when their challenges remain very stereotyped, with the same superficial questions). Sometimes it helps when patients repeat challenges at home with the use of an audiotape of the session. Furthermore, therapists may provide patients with lists of questions that they can ask themselves, or with some completed examples of diaries (from themselves or from other patients).

Patient Is Too Afraid to Carry Out a Behavioral Experiment. If a patient fails to conduct a particular experiment (e.g., to knock over a cup of coffee in a restaurant) because he or she is afraid of being thrown out, the experiment can first be attempted in a situation that is less threatening (e.g., not knocking over a complete cup of coffee, but spilling only a little coffee). Another possibility is to discuss whether the patient has a friend or family member who is willing to complete the experiment while the patient observes. The primary goal of a behavioral experiment is to collect information about the hypotheses, not habituation (as with exposure *in vivo*) or behavioral rehearsal (as in skills training). In this example, the essential point is the reaction of staff to people who knock over a cup of coffee; it is of minor importance who knocks over the coffee. Even when the patient is convinced that staff will react differently to him or her than to friends or family members, observing others can lower the threshold. In addition, it is useful to discuss why the patient thinks that staff will react differently (e.g., by questioning what factors determine the reaction of others, what evidence the patient has for his or her conviction, etc.). However, the belief that people react differently to the patient than to others is, in fact, another theme that can be tested in other (and easier) behavioral experiments as well.

Cognitive Interventions Have an Antitherapeutic Effect. In some instances, we discovered that cognitive strategies worked out the wrong way. In the first session, patients are often enthusiastic about cognitive therapy. Some of them feel that they have finally found a strategy that will help them to control themselves under all circumstances, so that they will never feel vulnerable. This applies especially to patients with fear of blushing, trembling, or sweating, who hope that controlling their thoughts will guarantee that symptoms will no longer occur. If therapists ignore this wish for absolute control, treatment will often fail. Therapists must emphasize that absolute control may not be feasible and discuss why it is so catastrophic not to have everything under control (basic assumption: "If I don't have everything under control at every moment, then …").

In the same vein, behavioral experiments may be carried out with the "wrong" motives, as was demonstrated by one of our patients who was afraid of blushing. One of the behavioral experiments in his treatment was collecting information about the opinion of colleagues and friends about his blushing (he thought that they saw him blushing almost daily, and judged him weak, vulnerable, and pitiful when blushing). In letters to these people, he explained his fears. He was very reassured by the answers he received; few of the responders them had ever seen him blush, and they hardly thought about it. It had by no means influenced their opinion about him, and they were pleased with his openness. In general, the letters were very complimentary. At first, this behavioral experiment was considered very successful. However, as the patient continued telling more people about his blushing, the therapist realized that this strategy was potentially antitherapeutic. In fact, the patient avoided consideration of his more basic assumption (i.e., his conviction that his worth as a person was dependent on other people's opinion of him). This was discussed with the patient, and he admitted that he would be very upset if one person would indeed confirm his anxious expectations, despite all of the positive feedback he had received. The focus of the next treatment sessions shifted to this basic assumption.

Problems with Exposure in Vivo

Patients Report That They Stay Anxious, in Spite of Practicing. The response of the therapist depends on the hypothesized reason for the patient's remaining anxious. If the problem is that the patient has only just started to practice, the therapist uses the same intervention as was described earlier, emphasizing that the patient should not expect to eliminate a habit that he or she has had for years within just a few days; it simply means that the patient needs more practice before mastering it completely. The most important point at this stage is for patients to notice that the fear decreases during prolonged exposure, even if this change is only slight. In the same vein, some patients report that anxiety subsides during exposure assignments, without any effect on their anxious cognitions. They keep anticipating the situation, and the next time they practice, they are as anxious as they were before. In such cases, the following feedback may be helpful: "With a number of social phobics, such thoughts change over the course of treatment. The first step is that the anxiety subsides during practice, and in that respect you can be satisfied. Should it appear after several weeks that your thoughts still don't change, we will examine them more closely."

If patients have practiced frequently and still report no change in feelings, it is likely that the situation they really fear has not yet occurred; therefore, strictly speaking, exposure has not occurred. This was the case with one of our patients, who was very afraid that her voice would start to tremble when having to read aloud a few pages in the classroom, and that she would become so anxious that she would not be able to read on. Although she had practiced a number of times, her fear did not decrease. In the discussion, it appeared that, until now, she had had to read only about 10 lines, and every time she had stopped with a sigh of relief because she had just escaped another time. It was decided that first she would practice reading a number of pages in front of several groups of students in our department; then, she would stop after a few sentences with the announcement that she could not read further. Consequently, she would read three lines in her own classroom, and stop with the words that she could not read further because she did not feel well. When she had finished all the steps, her fear had considerably decreased. At the same time, it can be very helpful to ask patients to practice making "mistakes," especially for those patients who "spasmodically" try to avoid mistakes and strive for perfection under all circumstances. Some examples are calling wrong telephone numbers with other people observing them, spilling coffee, trembling, buying articles and returning them one day later, asking "stupid" questions, and responding "I don't know" to questions. It is useful to agree upon the reaction of patients in case other people notice their "mistakes." Some patients are habitual "excusers"; they apologize even for very minor mistakes in order to prevent people from criticizing them. Response prevention may be necessary for exposure to occur.

Patients Demonstrate Active Avoidance Behavior during Exposure (e.g., Coughing, Bending Down, Talking Fast, Asking for Reassurance).   Asking for reassurance is a frequently occurring phenomenon with obsessive–compulsives, but may occur with some social phobics as well. For example, during a therapist-assisted exposure session, one of our social phobics asked after every assignment whether anyone could see her trembling. Although some reassurance during the initial assignments can be helpful, such interventions may be countertherapeutic when given repeatedly. By such reassurance, the therapist may actually reinforce the patient's anxiety. If the anxiety subsides, it may not be a result of habituation, but rather a function of the reassurance received from the therapist, which may result in a lack of generalization to other situations. If patients keep asking for reassurance, it is important that the therapist explain the principles of active avoidance behavior and response prevention, and inform patients that reassurance often has adverse effects.

Patients Are Particularly Afraid of Unexpected Situations.   Examples of such situations are meeting specific "difficult" persons (e.g., on the street or in a shop), being asked something in a meeting, being called while other people are observing, being addressed in a shop, and suddenly becoming the center of attention with other people around. The problem with these kinds of situations is that they occur with low frequency, and are therefore difficult to arrange. Similar problems arise in exposure with patients who fear bodily symptoms. These individuals should practice while blushing, trembling, or sweating, but these symptoms are difficult to provoke deliberately. In such cases, the patient's essential fear must be ascertained. Often, it appears that it is not the unexpectedness of the situation *per se* that is problematic, but the fact that the situation cannot be avoided or controlled. It also appears that many patients would avoid the situation if they could foresee it (e.g., they would avoid calling up other people when observed, or take a roundabout way if they saw people they did not want to meet). These patients can practice by taking initiatives (e.g., asking people in a shop for information, starting a chat, deliberately trembling while drinking coffee, writing checks or eating soup). It is our experience that the unexpected situations become less problematic once such "expected" situations have been frequently practiced and have become less difficult. In addition, patients eventually regain a greater sense of control if they take an active attitude.

CASE ILLUSTRATION

Joyce is a 24-year-old female. Her general practitioner referred her to our clinic after Joyce consulted him for her social fears and depression. Two intake sessions were conducted, the first (with the ADIS) for establishing the formal diagnosis, the second for obtaining detailed information about the social-phobic complaints in order to formulate a behavioral analysis and treatment plan. Information from the first two sessions is summarized in Sidebar 4–6.

Treatment Considerations

After the intake sessions, Joyce was offered treatment for the social-phobic complaints. For the choice of the specific treatment plan, the following considerations were made. Although Joyce lacked some specific social skills, her extensive avoidance of social situations and her maladaptive cognitions seemed to be more central in the maintenance of the complaints. Her fear was not limited to social-interaction situations; she feared and avoided situations in all four domains distinguished by Holt et al. (1992b). Situations such as walking on the street, waiting in her car for a traffic light, and traveling by bus or train were difficult, because Joyce felt anxious when observed by other people. In such situations, she avoided eye contact. In addition, she complained about depressive feelings and little self-confidence. Although social skills training would have been helpful to enhance her self-confidence before starting with exposure, the same goal could probably be reached by starting with daily practice of relatively easy exposure assignments. Such exposure might help to change Joyce's passive attitude into a more active one, which might have a favorable effect on her depressed mood and feelings of demoralization. There was no reason to expect that basic exposure assignments (e.g., keeping eye contact) would fail because Joyce lacked the required skills. After these considerations, it was decided to start with the cognitive–behavioral treatment protocol, with an emphasis on prolonged exposure *in vivo* during the first sessions.

Selected phases of Joyce's treatment are described in order to illustrate the use of the treatment protocol.

Session 1

First, the AAS was employed to evaluate the effects of treatment. Joyce decided that the following situations were most relevant for her (her ratings on fear and avoidance are given in parentheses):

1. Starting a conversation with an unknown, "interesting" person at a party. (8,8)
2. Active participation in conversations with colleagues during coffee breaks and lunches at work. (8,8)
3. Making telephone calls at work while observed by colleagues. (6,4)
4. Having an interesting person for a drink at my home. (6,6)
5. Joining a team sport club (rowing, volleyball) and participating in trainings and matches. (6,6)

The rationale of the cognitive–behavioral treatment was explained, and it was agreed that the first sessions would emphasize self-controlled exposure *in vivo*, in order to acquire a more active attitude in social situations and to create the conditions for behavioral experiments in later sessions. The principle of the fear thermometer was clarified with personal examples from Joyce (zero = talking with my sister about my work today; 100 = being the center of attention while telling personal things about myself in a group of colleagues). Before devising assignments, the factors that influenced the difficulty of assignments were established. For Joyce, talking with men (especially with men she found attractive) was more difficult than talking with women; talking in a group was more difficult than talking with one person; on the other hand, situations in which no direct conversation was required were easier (more anonymous) when many people were around. In the last part of the session, the first exposure assignment was prepared. The therapist proposed to Joyce that she start with learning to maintain eye contact in different situations. This assignment had several advantages. First, it could be rehearsed frequently each day. Second, it could be easily varied in difficulty by lengthening the duration and frequency of eye contact, or by choosing more difficult people (e.g., first with younger and older people, then with people of the same age, and finally, with people in authority), or by choosing more difficult situations (e.g., discussing more difficult/personal topics). In this manner, the principles of repeated and prolonged exposure would soon become evident. It was agreed that Joyce would start with making eye contact with unknown people in the street or on the

Sidebar 4-6

Information about the Complaints after Two Intake Sessions

Observation

Joyce is a friendly-looking, well-groomed young woman. In spite of the fact that she seems to talk about her fears rather easily, she makes a timid impression due to her low, monotonous voice and an uneasy way of keeping eye contact. Although she looks at the therapist occasionally, she almost immediately looks away. Her red cheeks and light trembling hands give away that she feels nervous.

General Information

Joyce is the third child from a family of four children. She has two brothers (3 and 5 years older) and a sister 3 years younger. Her mother died 4 years ago from cancer. Joyce has a close relationship with her father, who suffers from multiple sclerosis and is dependent on a wheelchair. Joyce feels very responsible for his well-being and visits him almost daily. She calls him the most important person in her life and almost always asks his advice when she has to make decisions. She lives in a small house in a village, near her parental home. She has no friends, except an ex-colleague and her husband. She meets them infrequently, about once every 2 months, mostly at their initiative. At the time of the intake, she has worked in the clerical staff of a bank for 4 weeks. Before she started in this job, she was unemployed for 6 months, after she had lost her previous job at a state hospital through a reorganization. Outside of her work she has few pursuits, despite the fact that she has many ideas about hobbies she would like to pursue, such as rowing, swimming, taking photographs, or studying a foreign language. She passes the time by reading, watching television, and visiting her father or her brothers (who live about 3 and 8 kilometers from her house).

Description of Complaints

Fear and Anxiety

Main fears/main reason to seek help:
Joyce's main complaint is that she often feels anxious in the company of other people. She is afraid to look foolish or to say the wrong things, leading to unkind reactions from others. In anticipation of such reactions, she seldom takes initiatives toward other people. She is afraid of being criticized for her behavior. She is convinced that other people see her as a slow, uninteresting person, less capable and intelligent than other people. She is, however, convinced that her fears are not realistic. In some situations, the fear developed into a panic attack. She never had panic attacks outside of social situations.

Behavior

Joyce avoids many social situations, especially more informal gatherings. Business talk is less difficult. She can make some short telephone calls at her work, as long as they are meant to exchange business information and nobody observes her when calling. She seldom takes the initiative to contact other people unless she is almost certain that they are interested in her. She avoids all parties except family parties, which she feels obliged to attend. In company of other people, she is mostly silent, trying to avoid becoming the center of attention. Calling people by telephone or meeting people in the street is difficult. She fears entering small shops in the village where she lives, mainly because she is afraid to meet acquaintances. She prefers to do her shopping in a large "anonymous" supermarket in the city where she works. Warehouses are not difficult as long as no sellers are bothering her. She often buys her clothes via mail-order services. At first sight, no clear skills deficits are noticed during the intake sessions, apart from the initial avoidance of eye contact. Joyce seems to listen carefully and her responses to questions are adequate.

Detailed discussion of various social situations reveals that Joyce lacks some specific social skills. When she is criticized or if she suddenly becomes the center of attention, she usually falls silent. In real-life situations, carefully listening to other people is difficult, partly because she is caught in anxious self-preoccupation.

Cognitions

The next cognitions, with minor variations, recur in many situations:

"They will not like me," "I'll make a fool of myself," "They won't listen," "I've nothing interesting to tell," "They'll think that I'm stupid," "They'll see that I'm nervous and will take advantage of that."

Characteristic Physiological Symptoms

The anxiety is expressed in symptoms, such as heart palpitations, trembling, sweating, and blushing, both in difficult situations and in anticipation of such situations. Although Joyce feels hindered by the bodily symptoms, they are not her main concern; she views them as annoying consequences of her anxiety.

Development of Complaints

Joyce remembers that she was badgered in elementary school because of her red hair and glasses. On such occasions, she became angry and abusive. Looking back, she feels that she gradually learned to be on guard with other people and to attract as little attention as possible. At secondary school, she was not badgered, but felt more or less ignored. She avoided social events as much as possible. After secondary school, she followed a specialized correspondence course on clerical work (after she had decided that she no longer wanted classroom education), and when she was 20, she started a job in a state hospital. She worked there for 3 years, until her job was terminated through reorganization. She functioned well in this job as far as the content of the job was concerned. Contacts with colleagues were found to be difficult.

Other Information

Apart from the social fears, Joyce reports no other anxiety complaints. Two years ago, she had a depressive episode, partly due to a conflict with Joan, a female colleague, whom she felt unable to handle. She was treated with antidepressants and had some treatment sessions at a psychiatric clinic. Although the severe depression has dissipated, Joyce is still frequently depressed and fulfills the diagnostic criteria for a dysthymic disorder.

bus. For that purpose, it was decided that she would take the bus to work daily so that she could practice at least twice a day for 30 minutes. In addition, she would utilize lunchtime by walking through the streets of the city and looking people in the eyes.

Homework for the next session was:

- Expand the list with assignments, trying to get at least 20 assignments for different situations of increasing difficulty.
- Practice daily (in the bus and during lunchtime) maintaining eye contact with unknown people.
- Change the old habit of looking away into a new habit of looking people straight in the eyes.
- Write experiences down on the report forms.

Session 2

First, the execution of the exposure assignment was discussed. Joyce appeared to have practiced daily. She was surprised and enthusiastic about the results. Initially, she felt nervous before entering the bus. She chose a single seat in the back of the bus, so that nobody could sit next to her and only a few people could sit behind her (and observe her). At first, it was difficult for her to look every entering passenger in the eyes; however, she noticed that most of them averted their eyes before she did so. She also noticed that many people did not even look at her. With each successive bus ride, she shifted one or two rows toward the front of the bus. During the week, she gradually became less nervous and more self-confident. Walking through the street during lunchtime was less difficult because eye contact was shorter and she felt less "trapped" than in the bus. The therapist reinforced Joyce's efforts and emphasized that successfully mastered assignments must be sustained so that they could become "second nature." For the next session, it was agreed that Joyce would extend the assignment to people at her work. In this context, it was also agreed that Joyce would practice in treatment sessions by maintaining longer eye contact with the therapist. Next, the second homework assignment (making a list with exposure tasks) was discussed. After some hesitation, Joyce confessed that she had left the list at home. She stated that she had spent much time on this assignment but could not think of more tasks. After further discussion, it appeared that, for each assignment, she doubted whether this was the best formulation, and whether other assignments would not be more useful. The therapist explained that, in general, it is better to have several assignments that must be expanded than having no assignments at all, and that it is very difficult to determine which one is best. The remainder of the session was spent making a number of assignments together (after which it was agreed that Joyce would again try to complete the list at home), and agreeing about the second exposure assignment: making telephone calls for information.

Homework for the next session included the following:

- Practicing eye contact with more familiar people.
- Making telephone calls to ask for information (bus, train, advertisements, etc.).
- Finishing the exposure list.

Session 3

The first topic on the agenda was discussion of the exposure assignment. Maintaining eye contact with people at work had been more difficult than Joyce had expected, and she was disappointed. She practiced with colleagues, but felt rather nervous, and this feeling got worse instead of better. In this session, the importance of detailed discussion of the homework became clear. The therapist reacted empathically to Joyce's disappointment and proposed to start a detailed discussion of the assignment. It appeared that Joyce also practiced with her brothers and a neighbor of her father, which had gone well. The first days that she practiced at work also passed without problems. However, she gradually became increasingly nervous because she was convinced that her colleagues noticed that she was practicing eye contact. She was afraid that one of them would say something about that and, as a consequence, she stopped practicing. Joyce thought that the assignment was too difficult and proposed that she first continue with less familiar people. The therapist pointed out that most of the assignment was successful; he confronted Joyce about her tendency to recall only the less successful aspects. He resolved to return to Joyce's inhibiting thoughts, if still necessary, after the cognitive principles had been explained. When it appeared that Joyce's fear related to only 2 of her 12 colleagues, it was agreed that she would practice only with "easy" colleagues. Furthermore, it was decided that Joyce would also practice looking around her when waiting in her car for the traffic lights. Calling for information had posed little difficulty, although occasionally Joyce finished the telephone call without having obtained the exact information she wanted. It was agreed that she would repeat this assignment and attempt to make it more difficult by calling people back for some additional questions 2 minutes after she hung up the telephone, and by calling while observed by her father or brothers. The exposure hierarchy appeared to be finished; it was agreed that Joyce would practice asking information from unknown people (e.g., in the bus, on the street). In the last part of the session, the principles of cognitive treatment and the use of the cognitive diary were explained.

The homework for the next session included the following:

- Asking for information (e.g., time, directions) from people on the street.
- Making telephone calls, some of them while being observed.
- Maintaining eye contact at work, but only with "easy" colleagues.
- Reading the explanation of the cognitive treatment.

Session 4

This week Joyce had continued to maintain eye contact, first with the "easy" colleagues, and the last 2 days with the two difficult colleagues. To her relief, nobody made remarks, and she noticed that the fear gradually decreased.

Before asking for information from unknown people Joyce felt more anxious than she had anticipated. She approached 15 people, and all but one had reacted in a friendly manner. In the discussion, it appeared that she had restricted herself to "easy" people, mainly women, and most of them older than she. It was agreed that next time she would start with the same assignment, and only when she felt more self-confident would she expand to men and to younger people, and that she would try to make the question "more difficult" (e.g., shopping at the market and asking how she has to prepare fish, meat, or unknown vegetables). The explanation of cognitive therapy had not raised questions. Much time was spent on the cognitive diary as the basis for the next exposure assignment: starting informal conversations. Joyce mentioned some situations in which she would like to speak to someone (e.g., in the bus), but until now she had not had the courage. It appeared that it was not so much that Joyce did not know what to say, but that she judged all sentences as dull and nonsense. She was afraid that other people would not react, would look at her with disdain, or would respond with one sentence and then look away. A "thought diary" was filled in about this situation. The following questions were discussed: What makes a topic dull or nonsense? How do you know that people will not react? How often has that happened? If they did not react, what reasons could they have for that? Could your own attitude have influenced their reaction? The results of this discussion are provided in Sidebar 4–7.

Homework for the next session included the following:

- Using her diary at least 30 minutes per day to describe difficult social situations using the "thought diary." Trying to fill in the first three columns.
- Asking for information from other people at least twice during the week, starting with the same information as last week, but with younger people and men; when this has proceeded well, asking for information at the market.

Session 5

First, results of the exposure assignments were discussed. Joyce again practiced a number of times, according to the exposure rules. She proceeded until the anxiety decreased. The first time she did the same assignment as the previous week. Again she felt anxious before she started, but noticed that the fear diminished more quickly on prior occasions. Next, she went to the market. This assignment was completed successfully. She had chosen a relatively quiet moment (early Friday morning), so that the people would have time for her and she would not feel hurried by other customers.

Much time was spent discussing the "thought diaries." Joyce described four different situations. They were all reviewed briefly, after which one of them was chosen to discuss in more detail (asking for information at the market).

Two of the diaries referred to starting conversations. Joyce stated that several times in the past week she had been on the verge of starting such a conversation, but each time she hesitated. The rational thoughts that were formulated in the last session (e.g., "Many topics can be chosen for a conversation," "Topics in themselves are not dull," "People differ largely as to which topics they find interesting," etc.) did not help her very much. She was still convinced that some topics, such as the weather or what she saw yesterday evening on television, were dull. In this context, the principles of behavioral experiments were explained. It was concluded that, before Joyce would start such an experiment, she would benefit with more information about how "normal" people start conversations, and what subjects they talk about. For that purpose she was to observe other people's conversations as often as possible. She was asked to monitor the topics they discussed and the reactions of both participants.

Homework included the following:

- Read the explanation of behavioral experiments.
- Fill in the thought diaries (all columns).
- Monitor conversations of other people in different situations
  - ○ Who started, and how.
  - ○ Topics
  - ○ What was said about these topics.
  - ○ Reactions of the participants in the discussion.

Joyce observed conversations of other people in the bus, at her coffee break at work, in village shops, and in the library. She noticed that the topics discussed were diverse. People talked about their families, children, the weather, work, school, books, and television programs. In many cases, she missed the beginning of the conversation, so she could not observe who initiated them. She did observe, however, how the conversations ended. She noticed that the contribution of both partners differed across the various conversations: Sometimes one partner talked as much as the other; in other cases, it was more a monologue by one of them. In all, the reactions of the participants were very different. She also noticed that whether a conversation was absorbing was more dependent on the style of talking than on the subject, and that the duration of the conversations varied. Based on her experiences, a behavioral experiment was formulated. It was agreed that Joyce would address at least 10 people during the week, starting with those who were not too difficult (e.g., older women). She was to try to choose a simple topic, depending on the situation (saying something about the surroundings, the weather, etc.). Her expectation was that most of them would look annoyed, would give only a short answer, and would look in another direction. The alternative hypothesis was that most of them would be friendly and say something in return. To prepare, initiation of conversations was practiced several times in the session via role play.

The remainder of the session was spent on challenging thoughts about asking information in shops, such as asking about different kinds of floor lacquers and paints (Joyce wanted to redecorate her living room). It was discussed which information was required and how Joyce would try to get it (e.g., assume a self-confident attitude, make eye contact, talk with a clear and cheerful voice). In addition, it was agreed that Joyce would practice this situation several times, both to collect information about her expectations and to allow her anxiety to decrease. Homework included the following:

- Fill in "thought diaries" (all columns).
- Behavioral experiment: starting conversations with 10 relatively unknown people, recording results in terms of her hypotheses.
- Behavioral assignment: asking for extensive information in shops in the city (e.g., in a travel agency, a do-it-yourself shop, a stereo shop) a number of times, recording her experiences, and trying to evaluate to what extent they corroborated or refuted her expectations.

Session 7

Starting conversations provided some useful experiences. On many occasions, Joyce recoiled from the assignment; however, on four occasions she managed to say something, once at work, once to her neighbor, and twice on the bus. To her surprise, everyone reacted kindly. No one showed annoyance, and with her neighbor and one woman in the bus, she talked for about 5 minutes. Although she had not succeeded in talking to 10 people, the preliminary results suggested a refutation of her original expectations. It was agreed that she would continue this assignment (and self-monitoring) to collect more information.

Asking for information in shops in the city had been a difficult but instructive task, not only for decreasing her social anxiety, but also for increasing her knowledge about floor lacquers and paints. It was agreed that she would extend this assignment to her work: She

Sidebar 4-7

Daily Record of Dysfunctional Thoughts

Situation	Emotion(s)	Automatic thought(s)	Challenge	Rational response	Outcome
Describe the actual event leading to the emotion; or the stream of thoughts, the daydream, or the recollection leading to the unpleasant emotion.	Specify your emotion (anxious/ angry etc.) Rate the degree of the emotion. (0—100)	Write the automatic thought(s) that preceded the emotion(s). Rate the belief in (each of) the automatic thoughts. (0—100)	Ask questions about the automatic thought(s). Write answers on these questions.	Write a rational response to the automatic thought(s). Rate the belief in the rational response. (0—100)	Rerate the belief in the automatic thought(s). (0—100) Specify and rate the subsequent emotion. (0—100)
I sit in the bus next to somebody I would like to talk with.	Anxiety (75)	I don't know how to begin. (90) I will say something stupid. (90) She will not give an answer. (75) She will tell me to keep my mouth shut. (50)	• How do I know that I will not know any subject to talk about? • What subjects do people talk about in such situations? • Who determines which subjects are interesting? Who determines what is stupid? • What topics could I broach? • How bad is it when I say something stupid? • If somebody does not want to talk to me, what reasons could they have for that?	It is not that I don't know a topic, but that I judge all topics as dull. (50) I don't know whether I'll say something stupid. Besides, what some people find stupid other people find interesting. (50) It is very unlikely	I don't know how to begin. (60) I will say something stupid. (40) She will not give an answer. (20) She will tell me to keep my mouth shut. (10) Anxiety. (35)

• persons would be pleased if I try to start a conversation? • How do I feel if somebody addresses me? • If I would feel less anxious, how would I feel then if somebody starts to talk to me? • Has it ever happened that I said someting to another person and that the other did not respond? • Has it ever happened that somebody told me to keep my mouth shut in such circumstances? • What is the worst that can happen? • How big is the chance that that will happen? • If that happens, what can I do then? • If that happens, how strongly will that affect my life?	will not give any answer or will tell me to keep my mouth shut. Even if they are not in the mood, they will say something. (80)

Explanation: If you have an unpleasant emotion, describe the situation in which it occurs. If you felt this while you are thinking or daydreaming, etc., make a note of it. Then describe the automatic thoughts that were associated with this emotion. Assess the degree of certainty on the next scale: completely unlikely (= 0) to absolutely certain (= 100).

Create challenges by asking yourself questions about your automatic thoughts. You might, for example, ask yourself: What evidence do I have for this? How can I understand what others are thinking? How can I predict the future? Am I forgetting to look at the positive side? How would I react if the roles were reversed? etc.

Next, note down a rational thought which can serve as an alternative to the original automatic thought. Then indicate how likely you find this thought (these thoughts): completely unlikely (= 0) to absolutely certain (= 100). Finally, the result of this approach is scored. What degree of certainty do you now attach to the original automatic thought: completely unlikely (= 0) to absolutely certain (= 100). Make a final note of the feeling which this prompts to and how strong this feeling is.

would ask "easy" colleagues whether they knew something about floor lacquers, paints, and holiday destinations. Again, this assignment was prepared by writing down her expectations about their reactions (she expected different reactions from the disparate colleagues) and formulating alternatives, and by doing one role play. In this session, the list of assignments that had been practiced already were reviewed to check whether they were still maintained and to determine how difficult they were now.

Homework included the following:

- Filling in "thought diaries" about difficult situations daily, at least one situation each day.
- After filling in the diaries: try to formulate behavioral assignments that might be suitable to test expectations.
- Behavioral experiment: asking colleagues for information about floor lacquers, paints, and holiday destinations.
- Exposure experiment: going to different shops with shoes and clothes (self-service) and trying on shoes or clothes in each of them; leaving the fitting room each time she tried on something else, and judging herself extensively in the mirror.

Session 8

Joyce entered the room with a depressed look on her face. She said that she had a very difficult week, and that she felt bad for several days. It appeared that the day after the last treatment session, she had an argument with a colleague. This man smoked a cigarette while sitting in a no-smoking area in the canteen. Joyce had taken offense toward him before, because the man was often inconsiderate of colleagues who did not smoke. This time Joyce criticized the man and told him to smoke somewhere else. The colleague reacted rather sarcastically (with two other colleagues watching), and Joyce left the situation with embarrassment and shame. Since that moment, she had felt her self-confidence diminish rapidly, which also affected the assignments she had already mastered, especially those at work. Joyce appeared dejected while relating her experiences. Further inquiry by the therapist revealed that Joyce had also lost confidence in treatment. Until this time, she had been satisfied with her progress, gradually cherishing the hope that this treatment, finally, would help her to overcome her fears. Now she felt that she was back at zero, with even less hope than she had had before she started. The therapist considered which situation to choose for the discussion (the situation with the colleague or Joyce's evaluation of the treatment progress). In view of the severity of Joyce's depressive feelings, he proposed to add a new point at the agenda, namely Joyce's thoughts and feelings in case an assignment fails. This included such thoughts as "See, I'll never learn to feel more self-confident," "This proves that I have made no progress at all," "I'm a lost case," and so on. In the challenge, much attention was spent on Joyce's "black-and-white" thinking; her selective memory, neglecting all other assignments; and her more basic assumption that improvement was reached in a linear fashion without setbacks. Comparisons were made with the acquisition of other skills, such as driving a car. Furthermore, the consequences of these thoughts (self-fulfilling prophecy) and of alternative thoughts were examined. It was concluded that setbacks can provide important information, that it can be sensible to take a step back, and that more practice is the only way to overcome the fears. Only after this challenge was the situation with the colleague further analyzed.

Homework included the following:

- Filling in "thought diaries."
- Behavioral experiment: starting conversations with "easy" colleagues at work (only in one-to-one situations; e.g., at the copier, while standing at their desks because she wants to ask them something)
- Behavioral experiment: collecting extensive information about clubs you would like to join.

Session 9

This week was more successful than the previous one. Joyce realized how often she avoided meeting people in one-to-one situations. Now that she had forced herself to take initiatives, she had noticed that, in fact, many opportunities were available to start a short conversation. On one occasion, a colleague asked her to have lunch with her, which had been very pleasant.

Collecting information had been an amusing occupation. Three times she had promised to attend a club activity meeting (volleyball, singing in a choir, and bridge) in the following weeks. The "thought diaries" that she filled in about these assignments were discussed. Joyce's expectations about attending the club activities were listed and after some hesitation, she agreed that next week she would visit the choir and the volleyball club. To help her control her nerves, flash cards were developed in the session.

Homework included the following:

- Behavioral experiment: attending volleyball and the choir.
- Behavioral experiment: continue starting conversations. Practice different ways of stopping the conversation (e.g., break off yourself, wait until the other person breaks off)
- Filling in "thought diaries" about inviting somebody to her home for a cup of coffee.

Session 10

Joyce was moderately satisfied about the homework. Although she had practiced all assignments, she was somewhat disappointed that on some occasions she felt considerably nervous. Fortunately, the flashcards had been a valuable tool. At the choir meeting, she had felt very anxious, especially when she was asked to sing aloud in order to have her voice judged. Before she attended the choir, Joyce decided that this first time she would only listen. She felt browbeaten by being asked to sing and had not dared to refuse. Although her voice had trembled, in all, the singing went well. In the evaluation, the positive and negative aspects of her visit to the choir were weighed and Joyce concluded that, overall, it was an important step forward.

It was agreed that she would again visit the choir and attempt to join. She anticipated that she would be more anxious than the first time. Her anxiety was partly caused by thoughts such as "Now this is my chance to make new acquaintances. I must take care not to spoil this chance. All eyes will be on me." After these thoughts were discussed and replaced by less demanding ones, the emphasis was gradually shifted to more basic assumptions, by having Joyce visualize the situation that her voice would fail, and that they would tell her that she was not good enough to join the choir. Joyce's assumption was "If

I fail in one aspect, I'm a worthless person" and "If I fail in one aspect, people will ignore me."

Homework included the following:

- Filling in "thought diaries" about the assumptions.
- Judging other people in different respects and rating how competent they were in each of these respects.
- Behavioral experiment: asking a neighbor to have a cup of tea in the garden.
- Visiting the choir and telling them she would like to join; starting informal conversations with at least two people.
- Visiting the volleyball club.

Session 11

Joyce asked her neighbor to drink coffee with her, but after a short hesitation, he responded that he had no time. Fortunately, he spontaneously proposed to have a drink another time, because the first thought that came to Joyce's mind was: "You see, he thinks I'm a dull person, not interesting to talk with." They made an appointment for the next Tuesday afternoon. In thinking it over, she had already concluded that her thoughts were unreasonable. In fact, she felt relieved when her neighbor refused, and this feeling was analyzed in more detail. Joyce stated that she was almost sure that her neighbor liked her, but also admitted that this made the situation worse. Instead of feeling reassured and less anxious, she assumed that he had high expectations of her that she would not be able to fulfill. She was afraid to disappoint him, and was inclined to sever the contact in an early stage to prevent embarrassing situations. The situations she had in mind were discussed in detail. Their probability of occurrence was rated. It was considered that new social contacts always carry a certain risk, but that they can also be the first step toward new friendships. Different ways to cope with the feared situations were discussed, and topics were listed that she could broach into the conversation.

Homework included the following:

- Filling in "thought diaries" about conversations at work and about asking Janet (a friendly colleague) to have lunch.
- Designing behavioral experiments for these situations, specifying which outcomes she expected.
- Carrying out both assignments.

Session 12

After reviewing homework, the progress of treatment to date was discussed. Joyce felt that she had improved about 75%. Overall, she was satisfied with her progress. Many situations were much less difficult than at the start of treatment. She was confident that those situations would become easier the more she practiced them. On the other hand, several situations had not yet been practiced and she was not sure whether she would be able to master them without the assistance of the therapist. For that reason, she wished to continue treatment for a number of sessions. It was agreed that five more sessions would be scheduled, followed by another evaluation. Joyce completed the AAS. Her ratings on the five situations were as follows:

1. Starting a conversation with an unknown "interesting" person at a party. (4,2)

2. Active participation in conversations with colleagues during coffee breaks and lunches at work. (2,2)
3. Making telephone calls at work while observed by colleagues. (2,0)
4. Having an interesting person for a drink at my home. (3,4)
5. Joining a team sport club (rowing, volleyball) and participating in trainings and matches. (2,1)

Commentary

Joyce was a patient with a severe, generalized social phobia. For that reason, it was not surprising that after 12 sessions (over 3 months), she still experienced significant fear in certain social interactions. In fact, several situations, such as speaking in formal group interactions or dealing with more intimate interactions, had not yet been the focus of treatment. The reason for this is simply that the pace of the treatment is set by the patient. Nevertheless, we always emphasize that treatment is not infinite, and that progress will be evaluated regularly. As described earlier, we do not continue treatment until patients *never* experience feelings of anxiety in social situations. With such fears (that have existed for years), patients generally need considerable time to alter their negative expectations and their habits of avoiding social situations more definitely. One important goal of treatment is to give patients hope that they will be able to proceed independently with practicing new social behavior. Again, the importance of goal setting in the first phase of treatment must be stressed. At the start of treatment, Joyce had indicated her personal goals on the AAS. At the evaluation, she was reasonably satisfied with her progress with respect to these goals; however, she had gradually shifted her aims to goals that were too distant at the start of treatment. For that reason, new goals were agreed on in the evaluation. Ten more sessions were held on a weekly basis to work on her new goals, and then the frequency of sessions was faded gradually. Treatment was terminated 5 months later, after another eight sessions.

SUMMARY

This chapter dealt with the cognitive–behavioral treatment of social phobia. The definition of social phobia according to DSM-IV and characteristic qualities of social phobic patients were discussed. Assessment of social phobia was described in four areas: (1) establishing a formal diagnosis, (2) more detailed assessment in order to develop a treatment plan, (3) treatment evaluation and (4) assessment during the course of treatment. Instruments that are useful for assessment of one or more aspects of social phobia were described. A review was presented of the results that have been reported in studies of the effectiveness of different strategies, with emphasis on social skills training, exposure *in vivo*, and cognitive strategies. Next, the practical implementation of the treatment was provided. First, some general aspects, important in every treatment of social phobia, were discussed (e.g., the therapeutic relationship, the goal of treatment, and the fact that social phobics often are in search of rigid rules about "normal" behavior). Then, a cognitive–behavioral treatment protocol (12 sessions) was presented, consisting of cognitive interventions (e.g., challenging automatic thoughts by means of "thought diaries"), and behavioral assignments (behavioral experiments to test the automatic and alternative thoughts as to their rationality). Finally, application of single approaches, such as prolonged exposure *in vivo* or social skills training, was discussed. Strategies that can be used to maintain treatment results and to prevent relapse were summarized. Some of these included providing the patient with written materials of the treatment strategy (explanations, diaries), use of booster sessions, and trying to expand the range of patients' social commitments. Next, problems common to the treatment of social phobics were described, and suggestions were offered on how to deal with them. For example, patients fear negative evaluation by the therapist, are more inclined to please the therapist than to express their own wishes and feelings; do not do their homework; consider behavioral assignments too difficult. In the last section of the chapter, the use of the treatment protocol was illustrated in a case study. In this treatment, the flexibility of the protocol was utilized by starting with a relatively large emphasis on "classical" exposure *in vivo*, while the cognitive strategies were introduced after a few sessions.

REFERENCES

American Psychiatric Association (1980). *Diagnostic and statistical manual of mental disorders* (3rd ed.). Washington, DC: Author.

American Psychiatric Association (1987). *Diagnostic and statistical manual of mental disorders* (3rd ed., rev.). Washington, DC: Author.

American Psychiatric Association (1994). *Diagnostic and statistical manual of mental disorders* (4th ed.). Washington, DC: Author.

Amies, P. L., Gelder, M. G., & Shaw, P. M. (1983). Social phobia: A comparative clinical study. *British Journal of Psychiatry, 142,* 174–179.

Andersch, S. E., & Hanson, L. C. (1993). Comorbidity of panic disorder and social phobia. *European Journal of Psychiatry, 7,* 59–64.

Arrindell, W. A., Emmelkamp, P. M. G., & Van der Ende, J. (1984). Phobic dimensions: I. Reliability and generalizability across samples, gender and nations. *Advances in Behaviour Research and Therapy, 6,* 207–254.

Beck, A. T., & Emery, G. (1985). *Anxiety disorders and phobias: A cognitive perspective.* New York: Basic Books.

Beck, A. T., Rush, A. J., Shaw, B. F., & Emery, G. (1979). *Cognitive therapy of depression* (pp. 403). New York: Guilford.

Beidel, D. C., Borden, J. W., Turner, S. M., & Jacob, G. (1989). The Social Phobia and Anxiety Inventory: Concurrent validity with a clinic sample. *Behaviour Research and Therapy, 27,* 573–576.

Beidel, D. C., Turner, S. M., & Cooley, M. R. (1993). Assessing reliable and clinically significant change in social phobia: Validity of the Social Phobia and Anxiety Inventory. *Behaviour Research and Therapy, 31,* 331–337.

Beidel, D. C., Turner, S. M., & Jacob, R. G. (1989). Assessment of social phobia: Reliability of an impromptu speech task. *Journal of Anxiety Disorders, 3,* 149–158.

Beidel, D. C., Turner, S. M., Stanley, M. A., & Dancu, C. V. (1989). The Social Phobia and Anxiety Inventory: Concurrent and external validity. *Behavior Therapy, 20,* 417–427.

Bouton, M. E., Kennedy, F. A., & Rosengard, C. (1990). State-dependent fear-extinction with two benzodiazepine tranquilizers. *Behavioral Neuroscience, 104,* 44–55.

Bouton, M. E., & Schwartzentruber, D. (1991). Sources of relapse after extinction in Pavlovian an instrumental learning. *Clinical Psychology Review, 11,* 123–140.

Brown, T. A., DiNardo, P. A., & Barlow, D. A. (1995). *Anxiety disorders interview schedule—IV.* New York: Graywind Publications, Inc.

Butler, G. (1985). Exposure as a treatment for social phobia: Some instructive difficulties. *Behaviour Research and Therapy, 23,* 651–657.

Butler, G. (1989). Issues in the application of cognitive and behavioral strategies to the treatment of social phobia. *Clinical Psychology Review, 9,* 91–106.

Butler, G., Cullington, A., Munby, M., Amies, P., & Gelder, M. (1984). Exposure and anxiety management in the treatment of social phobia. *Journal of Consulting and Clinical Psychology, 52,* 642–650.

Cameron, O. G., Thyer, B. A., Nesse, R., & Curtis, G. C. (1986). Symptom profiles of patients with DSM-III Anxiety Disorders. *American Journal of Psychiatry, 143,* 1132–1137.

Chambless, D., & Gillis, M. M. (1993). Cognitive therapy of anxiety disorders. *Journal of Consulting and Clinical Psychology, 61,* 248–260.

Curran, J. P. (1982). A procedure for the assessment of social skills: The Simulated Social Interaction Test. In J. P. Curran & P. M. Monti (Eds.), *Social skills training: A practical handbook for assessment and treatment* (pp. 348–373). New York: Guilford Press.

Curran, J. P., & Monti, P. M. (Eds.). (1982). *Social skills training: A practical handbook for assessment and treatment.* New York: Guilford.

Davey, G. L. (1992). Classical conditioning and the acquisition of human fears and phobias: A review and synthesis of the literature. *Advances in Behaviour Research and Therapy, 14,* 29–66.

Derogatis, L. R. (1977). *SCL-90 administration, scoring and procedures manual for the R(evised) version and other instruments of the psychopathology rating scale series.* Baltimore, MD: John Hopkins University School of Medicine.

DiNardo, P. A., & Barlow, D. H. (1988). *Anxiety Disorders Interview Schedule Revised (ADIS-R).* Albany, NY: Center for Stress and Anxiety Disorders.

Emmelkamp, P. M. G. (1982). *Phobic and obsessive–compulsive disorders: Theory, research and practice.* New York: Plenum Press.

Emmelkamp, P. M. G., Bouman, T. K., & Scholing, A. (1992). *Anxiety disorders: A practitioners guide.* New York: Wiley.

Emmelkamp, P. M. G., Mersch, P. P. A., Vissia, E., & Van der Helm, M. (1985). Social phobia: A comparative evaluation of cognitive and behavioral interventions. *Behaviour Research and Therapy, 23,* 365–369.

Emmelkamp, P. M. G., & Scholing, A. (1990). Behavioral treatment for simple and social phobics. In G. D. Burrows, R. Noyes, & M. Roth (Eds.), *Handbook of Anxiety, Vol. 4: The treatment of anxiety* (pp. 327–361). Amsterdam: Elsevier.

Eysenck, J. (1992). *Anxiety: The cognitive perspective.* Hillsdale, NJ: Erlbaum.

Glass, C. R., & Arnkoff, D. B. (1989). Behavioral assessment of social anxiety and social phobia. *Clinical Psychology Review, 9,* 75–90.

Glass, C. R., Merluzzi, T. V., Biever, J. L., & Larsen, K. H. (1982). Cognitive assessment of social anxiety: Development and validation of a self-statement questionnaire. *Cognitive Therapy and Research, 6,* 37–55.

Gormally, G., Sipps, G., Raphael, R., Edwin, D., & Varvil-Weld, A. (1981). The relationship between maladaptive cognitions and social anxiety. *Journal of Consulting and Clinical Psychology, 39,* 300–301.

Greenberg, D., & Stravynski, A. (1983). Social phobia: A letter. *British Journal of Psychiatry, 143,* 526–527.

Heimberg, R. G. (1989). Cognitive and behavioral treatments for social phobia: A critical analysis. *Clinical Psychology Review, 9,* 107–128.

Heimberg, R. G., Becker, R. E., Goldfinger, K., & Vermilyea, A. J. (1985). Treatment of social phobia by exposure, cognitive restructuring and homework assignments. *Journal of Nervous and Mental Disease, 173,* 235–245.

Heimberg, R. G., Holt, C. S., Schneier, F. R., Spitzer, R. L., & Liebowitz, M. R. (1993). The issue of subtypes in the diagnosis of social phobia. *Journal of Anxiety Disorders, 7,* 249–269.

Heimberg, R. G., Hope, D. A., Dodge, C. S., & Becker, R. E. (1990). DSM-III-R subtypes of social phobia: Comparison of generalized social phobics and public speaking phobics. *Journal of Nervous and Mental Disease, 178,* 172–179.

Heimberg, R. G., Mueller, G. P., Holt, C. S., Hope, D. A. & Liebowitz, M. R. (1992). Assessment of anxiety in social interaction and being observed by others: The Social Interaction Anxiety Scale and the Social Phobia Scale. *Behavior Therapy, 23,* 53–73.

Heimberg, R. G., Salzman, D. G., Holt, C. S., & Blendell, K. A. (1992). Cognitive–behavioral group treatment for social phobia: Effectiveness at five-year follow-up. *Cognitive Therapy and Research, 17,* 325–339.

Herbert, J. D., Hope, D. A., & Bellack, A. S. (1992). Validity of the distinction between generalized social phobia and avoidant personality disorder. *Journal of Abnormal Psychology, 101,* 332–339.

Himle, J. A., & Hill, E. M. (1991). Alcohol abuse and the anxiety disorders: Evidence from the Epidemiologic Catchment Area survey. *Journal of Anxiety Disorders, 5,* 237–245.

Holt, C. S., Heimberg, R. G., & Hope, D. A. (1992a). Avoidant personality disorder and the generalized subtype of social phobia. *Journal of Abnormal Psychology, 101,* 318–325.

Holt, C. S., Heimberg, R. G., Hope, D. A., & Liebowitz, M. R. (1992b). Situational domains of social phobia. *Journal of Anxiety Disorders, 6,* 63–77.

Hope, D. A., & Heimberg, R. G. (1993). Social phobia and social anxiety. In D. H. Barlow (Ed.), *Clinical handbook of psychological disorders: A step-by-step treatment manual (2nd ed.),* pp. 99–136. New York: Guilford Press.

Kessler, R. C., McGonagle, U. A., Zhao, S., Nelson, C. B., Hughes, M., Eshleman, S., Witchen, H., & Kendler, K. S. (1994). Life-time and 12-month prevalence of DSM-III-R psychiatric disorders in the United States. *Archives of General Psychiatry, 51,* 8–19.

Koopmans, P. C., Sanderman, R., Timmerman, I., & Emmelkamp, P. M. G. (1994). The Irrational Beliefs Inventory (IBI): Development and psychometric evaluation. *European Journal of Psychological Assessment, 10*, 15–27.

Liebowitz, M. R., Gorman, J. M., Fyer, A. J., & Klein, D. F. (1985). Social phobia: Review of a neglected anxiety disorder. *Archives of General Psychiatry, 42*, 729–736.

Mannuzza, S., Fyer, A. J., Liebowitz, M. R., & Klein, D. F. (1990). Delineating the boundaries of social phobia: Its relationship to panic disorder and agoraphobia. *Journal of Anxiety Disorders, 4*, 41–59.

Marks, I. M. (1987). *Fears, phobias and rituals.* Oxford, UK: University Press.

Marks, I. M., & Mathews, A. M. (1979). Brief standard self-rating for phobic patients. *Behaviour Research and Therapy, 17*, 59–68.

Mattick, R. P., & Clarke, J. C. (1988). *Development and validation of measures of social phobia scrutiny fear and social interaction anxiety.* Unpublished manuscript, University of New South Wales, Sydney, Australia.

Mattick, R. P., & Peters, L. (1988). Treatment of severe social phobia: Effects of guided exposure with and without cognitive restructuring. *Journal of Consulting and Clinical Psychology, 56*, 251–260.

Mattick, R. P., Peters, L., & Clarke, J. D. (1989). Exposure and cognitive restructuring for social phobia: A controlled study. *Behavior Therapy, 20*, 3–23.

Mersch, P. P. A., Breukers, P., & Emmelkamp, P. M. G. (1992). The Simulated Social Interaction Test: A psychometric evaluation with Dutch social phobic patients. *Behavioral Assessment, 14*, 133–151.

Mersch, P. P. A., Emmelkamp, P. M. G., Bögels, S. M., & Van der Sleen, J. (1989). Social phobia: Individual response pattern and the effects of behavioral and cognitive interventions. *Behaviour Research and Therapy, 27*, 421–434.

Mersch, P. P. A., Emmelkamp, P. M. G., & Lips, C. (1991). Social phobia: Individual response patterns and the long-term effects of behavioral and cognitive interventions. A follow-up study. *Behaviour Research and Therapy, 29*, 357–362.

Montego, J., & Liebowitz, M. R. (1994). Social phobia: Anxiety disorder comorbidity. *Bulletin of the Menninger Clinic, 58*, A21–A42.

Pollard, C. A., & Henderson, J. G. (1988). Four types of social phobia in a community sample. *Journal of Nervous and Mental Disease, 176*, 440–445.

Reich, J. H., Noyes, R., & Yates, W. (1988). Anxiety symptoms distinguishing social phobia from panic and generalized anxiety disorders. *Journal of Nervous and Mental Disease, 176*, 510–513.

Robins, R. N., Helzer, J. E., Weissman, M. M., Orvaschel, H., Gruenberg, E., Burke, J. D., & Regier, D. A. (1984). Lifetime prevalence of specific psychiatric disorders in three sites. *Archives of General Psychiatry, 41*, 949–958.

Sanderson, W. C., DiNardo, P. A., Rapee, R. M., & Barlow, D. H. (1990). Syndrome comorbidity in patients diagnosed with a DSM-III-R anxiety disorder. *Journal of Abnormal Psychology, 99*, 308–312.

Sanderman, R., Mersch, P. P., van der Stern, J., Emmelkamp, P. M. G., & Ormel, J. (1987). The Rational Behavior Inventory (R.B.I.): A psychometric evaluation. *Personality and Individual Differences, 8*, 561–569.

Schneier, R., Martin, L. Y., Liebowitz, M. R., Gorman, J. M., & Fyer, A. J. (1989). Alcohol abuse in social phobia. *Journal of Anxiety Disorders, 3*, 15–23.

Scholing, A., & Emmelkamp, P. M. G. (1990). Social phobia: Nature and treatment. In H. Leitenberg (Ed.), *Handbook of social and evaluation anxiety* (pp. 269–324). New York: Plenum Press.

Scholing, A., & Emmelkamp, P. M. G. (1993a). Cognitive and behavioural treatments of fear of blushing, trembling or sweating. *Behaviour Research and Therapy, 31*, 155–170.

Scholing, A., & Emmelkamp, P. M. G. (1993b). Exposure with and without cognitive therapy for generalized social phobia: Effects of individual and group treatment. *Behaviour Research and Therapy, 31*, 667–681.

Scholing, A., & Emmelkamp, P. M. G. (1995a). *Cognitive and behavioural treatments of fear of blushing, trembling or sweating: Effects at long-term follow-up.* Submitted.

Scholing, A., & Emmelkamp, P. M. G. (1995b). *Treatments of generalized social phobia: Effects at long-term follow-up.* Submitted.

Shorkey, C. T., & Whiteman, V. L. (1977). Development of the Rational Behavior Inventory: Initial validity and reliability. *Educational and Psychological Measurement, 37*, 527–534.

Trower, P., Bryant, B., & Argyle, M. (1978). *Social skills and mental health.* Pittsburgh: University of Pittsburgh Press.

Turner, S. M., Beidel, D. C., Cooley, M. R., Woody, S. R., & Messer, S. C. (1994). A multicomponent behavioral treatment for social phobia: Social effectiveness therapy. *Behaviour Research and Therapy, 32*, 381–390.

Turner, S. M., Beidel, D. C., Dancu, C. V., & Keys, D. J. (1986). Psychopathology of social phobia and comparison to avoidant personality disorder. *Journal of Abnormal Psychology, 95*(4), 389–394.

Turner, S. M., Beidel, D. C., Dancu, C. V., & Stanley, M. A. (1989). An empirically derived inventory to measure social fears and anxiety: The Social Phobia and Anxiety Inventory. *Psychological Assessment, 1,* 35–40.

Turner, S. M., Beidel, D. C., & Townsley, R. M. (1990). Social phobia: Relationship to shyness. *Behaviour Research and Therapy, 28,* 497–505.

Turner, S. M., Beidel, D. C., & Townsley, R. M. (1992a). Behavioral treatment of social phobia. In S. M. Turner, K. S. Calhoun, & H. E. Adams (Eds.), *Handbook of clinical behavior therapy (2nd ed., pp. 13–37).* New York: Wiley.

Turner, S. M., Beidel, D. C., & Townsley, R. M. (1992b). Social phobia: A comparison of specific and generalized subtypes and avoidant personality disorder. *Journal of Abnormal Psychology, 101,* 326–331.

Turner, S. M., McCanna, M., & Beidel, D. C. (1987). Validity of the Social Avoidance and Distress and Fear of Negative Evaluation scales. *Behaviour Research and Therapy, 25,* 113–115.

van Ameringen, M., Mancini, C., Styan, G., & Donison, D. (1991). Relationship of social phobia with other psychiatric illness. *Journal of Affective Disorders, 21,* 93–99.

van Kamp, I., & Klip, E. (1981). Cognitive aspecten van subassertief gedrag. *Gedragstherapeutisch Bulletin, 14,* 45–56.

Watson, D., & Friend, R. (1969). Measurement of social evaluative anxiety. *Journal of Consulting and Clinical Psychology, 33,* 448–457.

Watson, J. P., & Marks, I. M. (1971). Relevant and irrelevant fear in flooding. A crossover study of phobic patients. *Behavior Therapy, 2,* 275–293.

Welkowitz, L. A., & Liebowitz, M. (1990). Pharmacological treatment of social phobia and performance anxiety. In R. Noyes, M. Roth, & G. D. Burrows (Eds.), *Handbook of anxiety, Volume 4: The treatment of anxiety* (pp. 233–253). Amsterdam: Elsevier.

Widiger, T. A. (1992). Generalized social phobia versus avoidant personality disorder: A commentary on three studies. *Journal of Abnormal Psychology, 101,* 340–343.

Wilson, P. H. (Ed.). (1992). *Principles and practice of relapse prevention.* New York: Guilford Press.

Wlazlo, Z., Schroeder-Hartwig, K., Hand, I., Kaiser, G., & Munchau, N. (1990). Exposure in vivo vs social skills training for social phobia: Long-term outcome and differential effects. *Behaviour Research and Therapy, 28,* 181–193.

Zimbardo, P. G. (1977). *Shyness: What it is and what to do about it.* Reading, MA: Addison-Wesley.

5

Social Skills Training for Depression

A Treatment Manual

Alan S. Bellack, Michel Hersen,
and Jonathan M. Himmelhoch

INTRODUCTION

Since the late 1970s, behavior therapists have turned their attention to the assessment (Hersen, 1981; Rehm, 1976) and treatment of unipolar depression (cf. Craighead, 1980; Hersen, Bellack, & Himmelhoch, 1982; Kovacs, 1979; Lewinsohn, 1975; Lewinsohn & Hoberman, 1982; Rehm, 1977; Rehm & Kornblith, 1979; Wolpe, 1979). The word *unipolar* here refers to an affective disorder of nonpsychotic proportions. During the long history of changing diagnostic labels, such depression has alternatively been referred to as *reactive*, *neurotic*, or *unipolar*. Some authorities in the field (e.g., Wolpe, 1979) still continue to speak of "neurotic depression" in spite of the *fourth edition* of the *Diagnostic and Statistical Manual of Mental Disorders* (DSM-IV; American Psychiatric Association, 1994), which refers to it as a Major Depressive Episode.

In any event, with respect to our discussion of the behavioral treatment of depression, we follow the guidelines of DSM-IV, that is, the diagnostic label of Major Depressive Episode is given if five or more of the following symptoms have been present for at least 14 consecutive days, and the mood disturbance must result in impairment in social or occupational functioning.

Alan S. Bellack • Department of Psychiatry, Medical College of Pennsylvania, Philadelphia, Pennsylvania 19129; *present address*: Department of Psychiatry, University of Maryland School of Medicine, Baltimore, Maryland 21201-1549.   **Michel Hersen** • Center for Psychological Studies, Nova Southeastern University, Fort Lauderdale, Florida 33314.   **Jonathan M. Himmelhoch** • Department of Psychiatry, Western Psychiatric Institute and Clinic, University of Pittsburgh School of Medicine, Pittsburgh, Pennsylvania 15213.

Sourcebook of Psychological Treatment Manuals for Adult Disorders, edited by Vincent B. Van Hasselt and Michel Hersen. Plenum Press, New York, 1996.

1. Depressed mood most of the day, almost every day.
2. Decreased interest or pleasure in most daily activities.
3. Decreased appetite and/or significant weight loss if not dieting, or weight gain.
4. Insomnia or hypersomnia almost every day.
5. Psychomotor agitation or retardation almost every day.
6. Fatigue or anergia almost every day.
7. Feelings of worthlessness or inappropriate guilt almost every day.
8. Diminished ability to concentrate.
9. Suicidal ideation.

The large preponderance of behavioral treatments has been given to depressed patients evincing several or most of the aforementioned symptoms (cf. Rehm & Kornblith, 1979).

In reviewing the extant behavioral treatments for depression, Rehm and Kornblith (1979) have placed them into five principal categories: (1) contingency management, (2) social skills training, (3) imagery-based procedures, (4) cognitive therapy approaches, and (5) self-control techniques. In the outcome studies conducted to date, some of the behavioral strategies have been pitted against one another (e.g., Zeiss, Lewinsohn, & Munoz, 1979) or against pharmacological techniques (e.g., Rush, Beck, Kovacs, & Hollon, 1977). In other clinical trials behavioral approaches have been contrasted to psychotherapy, drug therapy, and placebo-control conditions (Elkin et al., 1989; McLean & Hakistan, 1979).

In evaluating the emerging data, it is clear that the behavioral treatments for depression do result in beneficial outcomes (cf. DeRubeis & Hollon, 1981; Kovacs, 1979). However, from a "beauty-contest perspective," it is unclear as to which of the treatments "leads the field." Indeed, in the Zeiss et al. (1979) study, there was a failure to differentiate among those behavioral strategies applied, although each proved effective in alleviating depression.

On the basis of these results, Zeiss et al. (1979) concluded that any therapy that meets the following four criteria should yield positive results in treating depression:

1. Therapy should begin with an elaborated, well-planned rationale. This rationale should provide initial structure that guides the patient to the belief that he or she can control his or her own behavior and, thereby, his or her depression.
2. Therapy should provide training in skills that the patient can utilize to feel more effective in handling his or her daily life. These skills must be of some significance to the patient and must fit with the rationale that has been presented.
3. Therapy should emphasize the independent use of these skills by the patient outside of the therapy context and must provide enough structure so that the attainment of independent skill is possible for the patient.
4. Therapy should encourage the patient's attribution that improvement in mood is caused by the patient's increased skillfulness, not by the therapist's skillfulness. (pp. 437–438)

Generally, the proponents of each behavioral strategy find support in the research literature on behalf of their cherished techniques. However, as already noted, at this point in time we cannot unequivocally state that any one strategy is truly superior. Indeed, when we consider that even among homogeneous depressives, there appear to be diverse causes for similar symptom patterns. We agree with Wolpe (1979) that "depression … is a symptom complex that has many causes" (p. 555). Craighead (1980) echoed this position, arguing that "each of the problem areas characteristic of depression should be assessed, and the treatment procedure(s) should be matched to the problem area(s)" (p. 122). In essence, then, it may very well turn out that aspects of each of the behavioral strategies need to be combined for a given case. For example, in a given depressive, social skills deficits may require remediation through skills training in addition to dealing with the apparent cognitive distortions, which would be dealt with using cognitive therapy.

Unfortunately, the field has not advanced to the point at which the salient features of each approach can be best tailored to the unique needs of each patient. Rather, of the behavioral techniques currently being applied, three tend to stand out in their usage: (1) social skills training, (2) cognitive therapy, and (3) self-control techniques. The purpose of this chapter, then, is to describe how we apply social skills training to our depressed patients. Before describing the specific procedures, we briefly present some of the background that led to the establishment of our protocol.

Social skills training for depressed patients, as described herein, is based on the work of Wolpe (1973, 1979) in assertiveness training, on Lewinsohn's (1975) work with depressed clients, and our own work in social skills training (Bellack & Hersen, 1979; Hersen et al., 1982; Wells, Hersen, Bellack, & Himmelhoch, 1979). Lewinsohn's (1975) approach to depression follows Ferster's (1965) notion that the depressed person is on an extinction schedule. According to Lewinsohn's (1975) theoretical notions, the depressed patient is under a schedule whereby response-contingent positive reinforcement is diminished as a result of specific skills deficits, and the depressed person is unable to obtain the kind of gratification needed from the environment. However, he or she does obtain attention for complaints of depression in the form of sympathetic social response, usually forced and maintained. As depressed behavior is reinforced and maintained, it then tends to alienate *others* in the environment. This often results in the depressed individual being deserted by such others, leading to further loss of reinforcement, social isolation, and increased depression.

As noted by Hersen et al. (1981), Lewinsohn's "notions suggest that depressed individuals will emit fewer behaviors, elicit more behaviors from others than they emit, interact with fewer numbers of individuals, emit fewer positive reactions to others' behaviors, and have longer action latencies than nondepressed individuals." Several of these hypotheses have been investigated by Lewinsohn and his colleagues (Lewinsohn & Shaffer, 1971; Libet & Lewinsohn, 1973) and confirmed. In another study, Sanchez and Lewinsohn (1980) provided additional experimental data in support of Lewinsohn's theoretical stance. Specifically, they found a $-.50$ correlation between assertiveness and depression over a 12-week period in 12 depressed patients. Moreover, on those days when assertiveness was more evident, level of depression was decreased. Quite interestingly, "rate of emitted assertive behavior predicted subsequent (next day) level of depression at statistically significant levels, whereas level of depression did not reliably predict subsequent rate of emitted assertive behavior" (Sanchez & Lewinsohn, 1980, p. 119).

Lewinsohn's (1975) treatment for depression centers on having the patient (1) engage in pleasant activities, and (2) improve his or her social skills. This is done in a 3-month time-limited approach that first is concerned with establishing the diagnosis, the depth of the depression, and the potential for suicide. A functional analysis of depressed and other critical behaviors is conducted. Behaviors that need to be increased or decreased are clearly identified and targeted for modification. At times the depressed patient's behavior is evaluated in a group setting or in the presence of a family member.

Although Lewinsohn's theoretical approach to depression appears to be basically sound, the actual treatment package he used is not as sophisticated as the assessment strategy carried out. Furthermore, its sophistication does not equal that of its theoretical foundation. Nonetheless, portions of Lewinsohn's skills training package have received positive confirmation in outcome studies conducted by McLean, Ogston, and Grauer (1973) and Mclean and Hakistan (1979). However, it should be recognized that social skills training, in these studies, comprised only a portion of the total behavioral strategy.

A perhaps more sophisticated approach to the treatment of depression has been formulated by Wolpe (1979) on the basis of his clinical experience of some three decades. In reviewing 25 created cases, they were classified into four distinct categories on the basis of etiology: (1) depression due to prolonged anxiety that is conditioned, (2) depression due to anxiety based on cognitive distortions, (3) depression due to anxiety in interpersonal situations leading to poor control, and (4) depression due to an excessive bereavement response. Each of the four types of depression requires a somewhat different treatment approach. The third category, of course, is the one in which a social skills approach would seem most appropriate. According to Wolpe (1979),

> As might be expected, assertive training figures largely in the treatment of depressions of this kind. This achieves weakening of the anxiety response habits through inhibiting anxiety by the expression of anger or other appropriate responses, and simultaneously provides conditions for the reinforcement of effective motor behavior. (p. 562)

As already mentioned, our social skills approach to the treatment of depression incorporates features described by Lewinsohn (1975) and Wolpe (1979). However, we should underscore the fact that our program is considerably more didactic in nature than Lewinsohn's approach. There is more emphasis on directly teaching patients how to respond; thus, our therapists are more likely to use techniques of modeling and guided practice. Also, we tend to deal with a much wider range of interpersonal issues, considering as well the nonverbal, paralinguistic, and verbal aspects of communications. In addition, we have our own unique blend of treatment foci. We are concerned with the expression of both positive and negative feelings in a socially appropriate manner. Interpersonal expression is evaluated in the context of role-played interaction with strangers, friends, family members, and school or work encounters. The treatment itself has four components: (1) skills training, (2) social-perception training, (3) practice (including homework assignments), and (4) self-evaluation and self-reinforcement. Finally, our program involves a period of maintenance therapy following original treatment in order to consolidate initial gains.

TRAINING FOCUS

Social skills training is one of several structured learning therapies. It is designed to teach the specific skills necessary for a given patient to perform effectively in a variety of interpersonal situations. By *performing effectively* we refer to the patient's obtaining maximum positive reinforcement from the environment. Social punishment should be kept to a minimum. This conception, of course, assumes that the individual may, at times, reap some negative consequences from others in the process of standing up for his or her rights; however, it is expected that a healthy adjustment will be maintained. Such balance appears to be quite important for depressed patients, who often are either overdemanding of others or oversubmissive. Being oversubmissive seems to be due to the patient's effort to avoid punishment at all costs. This may result in the absence of positive reinforcement from significant others.

Social skills require the coordinated delivery of a variety of verbal and nonverbal response components. The person's social impact depends upon what is said, how it is said, when it is said, and how the person appears while speaking. The various response elements intermesh to form a gestalt. At times, the elements can compensate for one another, overcoming specific deficits or imperfections. It is also possible for certain elements to completely outweigh or counter the effects of others. For example, variations of speech intonation can make the words "I love you" communicate great affection, a statement of fact, or deceit. Unfortunately, there are no objective rules for determining the critical weightings or balance of the elements in different situations. The therapist must use clinical judgment and his or her own social skills to assess the patient's impact, determine which behavior(s) is (are) at fault, and select appropriate targets for treatment. This requires a judgment about how others would react to the patient's communication. It is important that the therapist be sensitive to and tolerant of different interpersonal styles. The therapist's task is not to teach the patient to act as he or she does, but to teach him or her how to be effective in his or her own environment.

The beginning social skills therapist may sense that the patient is doing something "wrong," but not know precisely where the problem lies. The major components of social skills are presented in Table 5.1. The therapist should become familiar with these elements and appraise the patient's performance on each. The reader is referred to Harper, Wiens, and Matarrazzo (1978) for a more detailed analysis. The first category, *Expressive Features*, includes all of the response characteristics that determine how the person comes across in social situations. The most important feature generally is *Speech Content*: what the person says. *Paralinguistic Features* refer to voice quality: the way in which the person speaks. They give emphasis and clarification to the speech content, allowing the listener to translate the words into a meaningful communication. Paralinguistic aspects of speech appear to be critical in communicating emotion, perhaps more important than the words spoken. Tone, or information, is probably the most central factor in this regard.

Nonverbal Behavior refers to the variety of things people do with their bodies while speaking. *Proxemics* entails the physical relationship of the people in the interaction, such as interpersonal distance and forward and backward leaning. These factors affect comfort in the interaction, the degree of formality, and patterns of dominance. *Kinesics* refers to body movements, including hand gestures. Two important categories are *illustrators*, which provide emphasis, and *autistic gestures* (e.g., hand rubbing, foot tapping), which signal anxiety and discomfort. *Eye contact* (or gaze) and *Facial Expression* have been given extensive attention in the literature, and their significance is self-evident. *Interactive Balance*, often referred to as *response timing*, is not a particular response, but we have included it here to underscore its importance. Social interchange is a dynamic process, and the appropriate timing of responses is critical. The patient must know when to take various responses, how long a response latency is required between responses, and when to continue or shift the topic of conversation, and so on.

Receptive Features are discussed in the context of social-perception training. This category underscores the fact that the patient must attend to interpersonal cues in order to determine which instrumental responses (e.g., speech content) will be appropriate and effective. The *Special Repertoires* category reflects the fact that social skills are situationally specific. Different interpersonal situations and social tasks require distinct configurations of response skills. Our program places special emphasis on positive and negative assertion and conversational skills to be discussed.

Associated Factors are diverse cognitive and affective factors that affect performance

Table 5.1. Components of Social Skill

A. Expressive features
   1. Speech content
   2. Paralinguistic elements
      a. Voice volume
      b. Pace
      c. Pitch
      d. Tone
   3. Nonverbal behavior
      a. Proxemics
      b. Kinesics
      c. "Eye contact"
      d. Facial expression
   4. Interactive balance (response timing)
B. Receptive features (response timing)
   1. Attention
   2. Decoding
   3. Knowledge of context factors and cultural mores
C. Special repertoires
   1. Assertiveness
   2. Heterosocial skill
   3. Job interview skill
   4. Etc.
D. Associated factors
   1. Reinforcement history/Cognitive factors
      a. Goals
      b. Expectancies
      c. Values
      d. Etc.
   2. Affect
      a. Anxiety
      b. Depression
      c. Anger
      d. Etc.

in social situations. Social skills responses do not occur in a vacuum. The therapist must be aware of these other issues and plan accordingly if treatment is to be effective. Expectancies play an important role in work with depressed patients. As will be discussed, such patients often expect to fail and frequently are reluctant to stand up for their rights for fear of retaliation or of hurting other peoples' feelings. In regard to affect, anxiety can inhibit the occurrence of newly learned responses or reduce the quality of responses mastered under the safe conditions of the therapist's office. Of course, anhedonia associated with depression can make it difficult for the patient to initiate social activity. Dysphoric mood can produce a monotonic speech and make it difficult for the patient to learn proper intonation. In general, the therapist should not presume that patients come to treatment with the "proper" values, goals, or expectancies, or that they will be able to respond easily to his or her instigation. Rectifying these problems can sometimes be among the most difficult and time-consuming aspects of the treatment program.

Social skills training primarily deals with three types of social skills, each of which has special relevance for depressed women: positive assertion, negative assertion, and conversational skills. *Positive assertion* refers to the expression of positive feelings to others.

There are four major subcategories of positive assertion: (1) giving compliments, (2) expressing affection, (3) offering approval and praise, and (4) making apologies. These responses are each powerful social reinforcers. Their use reflects consideration of others and reciprocation of positive responses. They play an important role in maintaining casual relationships and are critical for the development of more intense relationships.

Several guidelines should be followed in training any compound behavior. Each response must be broken down into components, representing the major elements of the response. For example, in offering an apology, (1) make an "I" statement of regret (e.g., "I'm really sorry!"), (2) given an explanation (e.g., "I didn't know you would be coming"), and (3) comment on the person's feelings or discomfort (e.g., "I hope you didn't have too much trouble"). Verbal content is usually taught first, followed by paralinguistic features and then nonverbal behavior. Of course, the amount that can be covered at once depends upon the skills level of the patient and the complexity of the particular target behavior. But, there generally is a tendency to present too much material or focus on too many issues at once. It is always easier to start out simply and then speed up, than to start out at too high a level and have to backtrack.

Depressed patients generally do not spontaneously make positive assertion responses to others. They often have the requisite verbal content in their repertoire or can easily learn what to say, but they often are too preoccupied with themselves to think about the feelings of others, or they respond blandly, without enthusiasm. The major training tasks are (1) to teach the patient the appropriate times to make these responses, (2) to shape the appropriate paralinguistic components, and (3) to stimulate the patients to actually make the responses. Because of their dysphoric mood, these patients have great difficulty with voice intonation and inflection. Consequently, their responses generally lack a sense of warmth, enthusiasm, and the positive feeling tone necessary to make these responses effectively.

Negative assertion the second target area, refers to the expression of displeasure and standing up for one's rights. This is a significant problem for many depressed women and seems to play a critical role in their dysphoric mood (Sanchez & Lewinsohn, 1980). Four categories of negative assertion are included in our training program:

1. *Refusing unreasonable requests.* This is the most basic task in resisting mistreatment by others. It is most effectively accomplished by a clear yet sympathetic statement, coupled with an explanation (e.g., "I'm sorry, but I just can't help you out. I have another appointment and have to leave")
2. *Requesting new behavior from others.* Standing up for one's rights often entails getting other people to change their unacceptable behavior. Here again, an "I" statement followed by a reason is effective: "I really can't concentrate with the TV so loud. Please turn it down a little!"
3. *Compromise and negotiation.* Being "assertive" does not require always getting one's own way. Frequently, reinforcement is maximized by cooperation and compromise. The task here involves (a) stating one's feelings or desires, (b) reflecting the partner's feelings or desires, and (c) suggesting a mutually acceptable resolution: "I know you want to eat out, but I'm trying to diet. How about if we go to a movie and then get a snack. That way I won't eat so much."
4. *Expressing disapproval and annoyance.* At times, an undesirable situation is concluded, or cannot be changed. Nevertheless, it is often appropriate to express discontent. Such a communication may prevent future mistreatment. Also, unexpressed annoyance can have a variety of maladaptive consequences, not the least of

which is depression. The goal of training is to facilitate productive complaints rather than an angry outburst or passive–aggressive "bitching." An appropriate response contains (a) an "I" statement followed by (b) a description of the stimulus, and (c) a request or suggestion for future behavior (e.g., "I'm really angry at you. I told you I was planning a special meal. If you can't be on time, call me so I know in advance")

Considerable time in training is devoted to development of the coordinated delivery of verbal, paralinguistic, and nonverbal components of each category. Once again, para-linguistic features are especially difficulty to train. However, the verbal content of these responses also presents problems. The stressful nature of negative–assertion situations has a disruptive effect. It interferes with concentration and makes it difficult for the person to generate appropriate statements. Many depressed patients also are reluctant to make these responses, fearing a negative reaction from the interpersonal partner. They often fail to distinguish assertion (which is nonhostile) from aggression. Modification of these faulty cognitions is a central part of the training. The depressed person must be taught that the reactions from others will generally be less negative than expected, and that they will be less painful than continued passivity and submission.

The third target area is *conversational skill*. This includes the ability to initiate, maintain, and gracefully end conversations. Depressed patients often do not interact enough, and they often fail to have pleasant interactions. This segment of the program is designed to correct the difficulty and, as a result, increase the receipt of social reinforcement. The major elements of conversational skills training are presented in Table 5.2. The particular behaviors covered depend on the individual patient's repertoire. Frequently, one of the most important aspects of this training is to teach the patient how to be more positively reinforcing to others. Patients are taught to use social reinforcement (e.g., head nods, "um hmm") to express agreement and provide encouragement. They are also taught to inhibit "sick talk," and to avoid complaining and whining.

As stated earlier, social skills are situationally specific. Training the patient to be assertive or conversant in one situation will not necessarily generalize to other people or situations. Thus, we provide training on each target behavior in each of four social contexts:

Table 5.2.   Conversational Skills

A. Initiating conversations
    1. Initiating a conversation with an acquaintance
    2. Meeting someone new
    3. Social phone calls
B. 1. Asking questions
      a. Open-ended versus closed-ended questions
      b. Prying versus response facilitation
    2. Providing information
      a. Expressing opinions
      b. Talking about yourself
      c. What not to say
    3. Social reinforcement
C. Ending conversations
    1. Timing your goodbye
    2. Arranging future contact
    3. Judging when the partner wants to leave

---

1. *Interactions with strangers.* Two issues predominate here. The first involves negative assertion: standing up for rights and avoiding mistreatment by store clerks, waiters, craftsmen (e.g., plumbers, painters, auto mechanics) and the like. The second issue involves initiating interactions with strangers and increasing the range of social contacts. A frequent topic is starting interactions with casual acquaintances or people who are recognized by sight but whom the patient has never actually met (e.g., positive and negative assertion, *with friends*). All three skills repertoires (e.g., positive and negative assertion, conversational skill) may be covered in this context. There is considerable variability in the types of difficulties patients have with friends.

2. *Interactions with family members.* This context can include parents, spouse, or children. We also include nonmarital, heterosocial relationships here, although they could be covered under the friendship category. The predominant focus with parents and husbands is negative assertion. Many patients feel bullied and must be taught how to express their opinions and avoid being manipulated. There often is a sense of resentment and unexpressed anger toward these significant figures. Patients must sometimes be persuaded that the goal of training is to eliminate the causes of hostile feelings, not simply to express old complaints. Some patients have too little trouble expressing dissatisfaction and becoming angered. They have a demanding quality to their requests, stimulate hostility, and respond in kind. They must be taught how to make requests in a more tempered fashion, and try to compromise when they face disagreement. Whether patients are too assertive or too unassertive, they frequently expect the environment to make quick and dramatic changes in response to their new skills. They must be prepared for the fact that established relationships will only change slowly, and sometimes not at all. When new responses are being tried out, they often will be imperfect and inconsistent, and the partner may not notice the change for some time. The value of new behaviors for the patient must be emphasized, independent of the short-term effects on parents, husband, or others. In fact, the patient may sometimes face a negative reaction. After all, her increased assertion may well mean a loss of power on the part of the significant other. The therapist should make certain that the patient also is positively assertive, and not simply teach her to suddenly clamp down on the other person.

3. *Interactions at work or school.* Many patients seem to lack positive social relationships in these important settings. They remain distant even from people they see regularly. Many unmarried patients need training in responding to sexual and heterosocial interactions: both turning off the undesired advances and facilitating or stimulating desired interactions. The most common problem at work seems to be a negative assertion with employers. Issues here run the gamut from resisting unfair assignments and excessive demands, to securing promotions and salary increments. Issues also arise in regard to beginning school or finding a job; however, selecting a career or learning how to act on a job interview are specialized topics that could require extensive work. The therapist should not allow such topics to dominate training. It is impossible to cover all areas of difficulty in a circumscribed therapy program.

The four social contexts must be appraised as to their significance for the patient. Generally, one or two present no problem or have little relevance for her. These can be ignored. The remaining areas are treated in order of increasing significance. This arrangement is followed in order to develop basic skills and achieve some success before tackling the most difficult issues.

Once the relevant contexts are identified, an assessment is conducted to determine precisely *who* the person has difficulty with, in *what* particular types of interactions, and in *which* of the four social contexts. For example, a patient might have difficulty initiating conversations with attractive males (e.g., potential dating partners), but have little problem in maintaining a conversation. She might be unable to refuse unreasonable requests from her employer but be able to resist such requests from her mother. Conversely, she may be unable to express positive feelings toward her mother. These specific deficits are ordered hierarchically and trained in order of increasing difficulty as each social context is confronted.

COMPONENTS OF TRAINING

The training program consists of four separate components: (1) skills training, (2) social-perception training, (3) practice, and (4) self-evaluation and self-reinforcement. Each is applied to each of the social contexts selected for treatment.

Skills Training

This component involves the set of procedures that have typically been called "social skills training" in the literature (cf. Bellack & Hersen, 1977, 1978, 1979). It is the basic strategy for training each of the specific response skills. The three training components are designed to reinforce preliminary changes produced by skills training, and ensure that the newly learned behaviors are appropriately applied *in vivo* and maintained.

Before beginning skills training, it is necessary to conduct a careful assessment. As indicated earlier, it is necessary to determine the specific targets: which interpersonal partners in what social contexts. The first step in this process is for the therapist to review the pretreatment assessment battery. We administer a multifaceted battery, including psychiatric ratings, self-report inventories, behavioral observation, and ratings by significant others. The battery is described in Table 5.3. The most important elements are the role play test, the Hamilton interview, and the Katz Adjustment Scale.

The role-play test consists of 16 items, covering each of the general target areas, each social context, and a variety of interpersonal partners. Representative items are presented in

Table 5.3. Assessment Battery

Type	Description
Self-report	Beck Depression Inventory
	Lubin Depression Adjective Checklist
	Hopkins Symptom Checklist
	Wolpe–Lazarus Assertiveness Scale
	Eysenck Personality Inventory
Observer ratings	Raskin Eligibility Depression Scale
	Hamilton's Rating Scale for Depression
	Paykel et al.'s Assessment of Social Adjustment
Behavioral	16-Item Role-Play Test
	(Extended interaction)
Significant other	Katz Adjustment Scale–Relative

Table 5.4.   Representative Scenes from the Role-Play Test   **189**

Friends (Negative)

Narrator:	Some friends have asked you to join them for a picnic in the country. You tell them you don't feel like going today. One of them (she) says:
Role model prompt:	I think you stay in the house too much. Why don't you come along?
Subject response:	
Second Prompt:	We were counting on you coming along—we won't take "no" for an answer.
Subject response:	

Work (Positive)

Narrator:	You've been working on a different job all week. Your boss comes over to you with a very pleased smile on his face. She says:
Role model prompt:	That's a very good job you've done; I'm going to give you a raise next week.
Subject response:	
Second prompt:	I don't say this very often, but I wanted you to know I appreciate your work.
Second response:	

Work (Negative)

Narrator:	You have had a very busy day at work and are tired. Your boss comes in and asks you to stay late for the third time this week. You really feel you would like to go home tonight. She says:
Role model prompt:	I'm leaving now. Would you mind staying late again and finishing this work for me?
Subject response:	
Second prompt:	There's a deadline for this job and we need to get it done.
Subject response:	

Family (Positive)

Narrator:	You've been working hard all day cleaning the house and preparing a delicious meal. Your (husband) comes home from work, looks around and says:
Role model place:	The house looks great. Dinner sure smells good.
Subject response:	
Second prompt:	It looks like you've been busy all day.
Subject response:	

Table 5.4. The therapist forms preliminary hypotheses about areas of deficit by observing a videotape of the role-play performance. These impressions are supplemented by studying a videotape of the Hamilton Rating Scale for Depression interview. The focus here is not symptom reports, but interpersonal style. Finally, the significant-other report on the Katz Adjustment Scale–Relative identifies additional potential problem areas.

The patient is the best source of data about her own distress, and she can identify the situations that are most painful for her. She can also indicate sources of difficulty and the relevance of various issues. However, the patient can only provide a biased and limited report. She often does not know how she comes across to others, why she fails in social interactions, and precisely which response elements she performs poorly. Consequently, it is necessary to observe the patient in action. This is accomplished by having her *role-play* various interactions. This last step allows the therapist to determine the precise verbal, nonverbal, and paralinguistic elements that must be trained. Role-play scenes are developed by having the patient describe specific problem interactions she has had in the past. The more accurately the role-play scene represents a real experience, the more valid will be the patient's enactment. It is desirable to have her describe the way the interpersonal partner responded, as well as her own reaction.

Once the assessment is completed, the therapist can develop a tentative treatment plan, including a hierarchy of contexts, behaviors, and interpersonal partners. Of course, assessment is a continuing process throughout the course of treatment. Frequent modifications are made in the plan as the therapist gathers more information, as the patient develops new skills, as problems and roadblocks appear, and as the patient's life situation changes.

Training proper begins once the final assessment step is completed and the therapist identifies a precise starting point (e.g., a specific behavior in a specific context). The first step is to describe the target to the patient and provide a rationale for its use in the designated manner. The rationale is critical if the patient is to appreciate the importance of the behavior and work diligently. It should emphasize the social value of performing the response in the desired fashion. It should also be brief and straightforward, not an extensive lecture. For example,

> **T:** The next thing we need to work on is eye contact. It is important that you look straight at people when you tell them that you are displeased. If you do, they'll know you are serious and you will not be taken lightly. If you don't, they'll think that you are unsure of yourself and can be bullied. Okay? Do you understand why it is so important? Good.

The therapist should be certain that the patient's assent is based on understanding and agreement, not lip service. Usually, the patient will be able to relate the behavior to a problem interaction in the past.

Once the patient agrees to the importance of the behavior, *instructions* are provided as to how the response should be performed. Instructions should be specific and succinct. For example,

> **T:** I want you to look at my face for the entire time you speak. You don't need to look directly at my eyes. Let your gaze shift slowly from my forehead, to my nose, to my mouth, and back to my forehead. But keep looking at my face. O.K.? Good.

Vague instructions, such as "Look at me when you talk," will not produce the requisite response. Extended instructions with convoluted rationales and if–then clauses are confusing, and the patient will typically recall only a small portion. The therapist must be careful to avoid overcomplicating the task by attempting to give too much qualification or dealing with exceptions to the rule. These special cases should be covered only after the basic skill is mastered. Whenever possible, instructions should specify what the patient *should* do, not what she *should not* do.

Social skills are much like motor skills (e.g., bicycle riding, swimming). They cannot be learned solely by didactic instruction. Proper performance must be observed and performed. The bulk of skills training is devoted to serial trials of observation and performance. Often, instructions will not be sufficient to convey how the response is to be performed. The therapist then *models* appropriate performance. The modeling display is presented in a role-play format. The therapist portrays the patient and the patient enacts the relevant interpersonal partner. The scenario to be enacted should be developed with the patient's input. As with the assessment role plays described earlier, the more detail provided, the more life-like the response.

Before role playing begins, the therapist should clearly specify the aspect of his or her response to which the patient should attend. If not, the patient is likely to attend to an irrelevant component. The interaction should be kept very brief. One or two sentences are ample. Longer interactions at this preliminary stage result in distraction and confusion. For example,

> **T:** Okay, the situation is the one with your husband we just discussed. You play your husband and tell me you don't want me to go out. I'll play you. Listen to the way I first tell him I understand and then insist anyway. All right, you start.

The patient responds, and the therapist replies: "Gee, I understand that you don't like me to go out at night, but I really have to go." *Simplicity* is the guiding word whenever new behaviors are presented. After the modeling display, the therapist should question the patient to be sure she attended to the proper element and understands how it is to be performed. Repeated modeling displays are sometimes required.

The next step is the most important: *role playing*. Here, the patient attempts to perform the target response in a simulated interpersonal scenario. The parameters of the scenario are first carefully specified if they have not been explicated previously. For example,

> **T:** I'll play your boss. It's about 4:30 and you're getting ready to leave. You have a date tonight and you're in a hurry. I'm going to ask you to stay late to get some work done and you're going to refuse.

The therapist then reviews how the response is to be performed. "Remember, you indicate that you understand the problem and that you would like to help, but that you have a prior commitment and can't stay." This instruction should be relatively simple and cover *only the immediate target*. The patient can only be expected to master one response element at a time. The various response parameters must be taught sequentially. The therapist and patient then role-play the interaction. Initial trials should be kept brief, and the therapist should portray a cooperative partner. Resistance and complications can be added in subsequent trials.

> **T:** Susan, I'd like you to stay late tonight to finish that report.
> **P:** I'm sorry Mr. Smith. I know it has to be done right away, but I have a date tonight and I can't stay.
> **T:** Oh, all right.

Following the role play, the therapist provides *feedback* and *positive* reinforcement. Feedback should be specific and limited to the behavior under focus. Problems with other response components should be ignored. Moreover, feedback should be couched in positive terms. It should emphasize positive aspects of the response and how it could be improved. The patient and the response should never be criticized! Also, feedback should always contain some positive reinforcement. The therapist *must* point out some positive aspect of the response. Effort or improvement can be reinforced, even if the response is of poor quality. An appropriate feedback response is as follows:

> **T:** That was a good try. I liked the way you looked at me when you spoke. You really looked as if you meant what you said. Let's try it again, and this time let's work some more on your volume. I'd like you to try and speak a little louder. It will make you even more convincing.

Repetition is a fundamental feature of skills training. No response is adequately mastered after a single trial. Even a successful role play must be repeated. The patient sometimes covertly rehearses a response and performs well on the initial trial, but response quality breaks down when the response is varied on repetition. We require our therapists to perform at least two or three repetitions of each scenario (the more the better). Slight variations can be used to avoid boredom. Feedback and reinforcement are supplied for each repetition. When difficulties are encountered, further instructions and modeling can also be provided. If the patient does not master the response after five trials, some modification in the procedure is required. In some cases, simpler versions of the response can be presented or the target can be broken down into elements. The patient need not make the most eloquent response. These procedures are especially useful in training verbal content. The patient may teach herself by listening to a tape recording of the previous role-play interaction. This type of feedback seems to be more informative than verbal descriptions of intonation or voice volume. However, some patients are especially self-critical when hearing their responses on tape. Tape replay may be punishing rather than helpful.

The therapist should recognize that some patients will never achieve mastery of certain responses. It is counterproductive to continue "hammering" away after a plateau is reached. The goal of training is to have the patient produce the *minimum acceptable response*. This is the least that must be done to achieve a goal. Once this point is reached, the therapist should consider moving on to the next response. Continued attempts to push the patient beyond her ability will be highly punishing to the patient, as well as frustrating for the therapist. It is more likely to result in termination than in a breakthrough. The patient should not to be encouraged to memorize specific verbal content. She should be taught the major elements of effective responses, and practice alternative phrasings.

Social Perception Training

Current approaches to social skills assessment and training have placed almost exclusive emphasis on motoric response components. It generally has been presumed that the quality of interpersonal performance depends (almost) entirely on the response skills in the repertoire; however, this conception only accounts for part of the variance in social skills. Whereas the individual cannot perform effectively without the requisite response capability, the mere presence of such skills in the repertoire does not ensure effective performance. More specifically, the individual must know *when* and *where* to make various responses, as well as *how* to make them. This aspect of interpersonal skill has been referred to as *social* or *interpersonal perception* (Morrison, Bellack, & Bashore, 1988). It includes (1) knowledge about the meaning of various response cues and familiarity with social mores; (2) attention to the relevant aspects of the interaction, including the context and the interpersonal response cues provided by the partner; (3) information-processing capability; and (4) the ability to accurately predict interpersonal consequences (Bellack, 1979).

Social-perception training is a vital component of social skills training, although it is the last formalized component. It does not consist of a series of specific strategies that are implemented in a prescribed fashion. Rather, there are a number of general techniques that are intermittently applied throughout training. The foremost and most consistently employed technique is *information giving*. The therapist is a teacher. He or she teaches the patient about social interactions: what to expect from others, what various responses mean, when responses can be made, and so on. Every response skill that is trained is placed in the context of when, where, and why it should be made. This information can be imparted while giving the rationale for responses, in the context of feedback, during general discussions about how the responses can be utilized, when planning homework assignments (see section entitled Practice), and in the course of reviewing reports of how homework was carried out. The patient is not simply given factual information, but is taught to attend to the social environment and the interpersonal partner. Consider the following example:

> T: If you're going to ask your husband to do something disagreeable, you'll have to find the right time and place. If he starts out being irritable as he comes home from work, how about during dinner? He should be relaxed by then and more receptive. People also tend to be more cooperative when you give them a lead in or advance warning. So, we don't want to simply come down hard out of the blue.

A second vehicle for the development of social-perception skills is the therapist's role-play performance. As training progresses and basic skills are mastered, the therapist gradually presents more and more difficult responses. For example, he or she may resist the patient's attempts to compromise, or insist on an unfair request. These variations give the patient practice in interpreting and responding to different social cues. The therapist specifically points out the cues that were varied and illustrates how they are discriminative for different counterresponses. During the latter stages of training, the therapist can prompt the patient for the same type of analyses: "What would you do if I hesitated and gave a weak response to your question?" or "How would you know if I was angry but didn't say so?" A related strategy is for the therapist to model a range of responses around a common theme and have the patient provide an appropriate counter to each variation. For example, in the context of requesting a raise, the therapist could portray an employer who was ambivalent, hostile, understanding but not complying, too busy to discuss the issues, and so on. Of course, the therapist would attempt to vary paralinguistic and nonverbal response elements as well as verbal content.

Practice

The gains made in sessions have a low probability of being maintained if they are not overlearned. There is ample evidence demonstrating that newly learned responses drop out under stress, replaced by well-established patterns (Bellack, 1980). Therefore, it is vital to ensure extensive practice of new social skills. Repeated role-play trials in sessions serve this purpose. However, it is also critical for the patient to practice newly learned responses in the natural environment. *In vivo* practice facilitates generalization, as well as contributing to overlearning.

First, beginning with the second session, the patient is given a homework assignment at the conclusion of every session. The assignment is based on the skills learned during that particular session. It is worked out jointly with the patient to help ensure compliance. She must agree on its relevance and feasibility. There are several vital guidelines to be used in generating assignments. First, the instructions must be specific or the task will not be performed in the desired manner. "Try to meet some new people this week" is not adequate. An appropriate task is as follows:

> T: The homework for this week is to start conversations with three different people at work whom you know by sight, but have never met. The best place would be the employee cafeteria or the elevator. I want you to do at least one by Tuesday and the second by Thursday. Remember, you can keep it brief. Smile and say something about the situation. Okay? Any questions? Good luck.

It is helpful to give the patient written instructions to ensure that she remembers the details.

Second, the patient must be able to perform the assignment adequately. Of course, she should have the opportunity to do it. It also should be geared to her skills level; she should already have achieved a degree of competence on the response. Homework is designed to overtrain, not to provide basic instruction. Finally, the assignment should be in keeping with the patient's overall level of functioning and state of depression. She will not be able to make quick and drastic changes in a long-standing behavior, even if she has learned the specific social skills responses needed. For example, a woman who has not dated in several years might be instructed to initiate a conversation with an attractive male, but not to invite him out.

The third guideline is that the homework assignment should lead to reinforcement. There should be high probability that the patient will be successful. The therapist must consider the likelihood that the interpersonal partner will respond favorably. This often is independent of the patient's skills level. For example, a long-standing pattern of maladaptive communication with a husband is not likely to be quickly changed. Such difficult problems must be reserved for later in the course of treatment, when the depression is somewhat abated, skills are more refined, and the patient is better able to accept only partial success.

One final note on homework needs to be mentioned. The patient should monitor homework performance and keep a diary or record form. The therapist should teach her what and how to monitor. The previous assignment is briefly discussed at the beginning of each therapy session. The patient should be heartily reinforced for *effort*. Problems should be identified and targeted for further training. Discussion of the assignment often leads to identification of new targets and relevant role-play scenarios. Reports of noncompliance should be followed by a reminder of the importance of completing assignments and a quick shift to the next topic in training. The patient should not be scolded, preached at, or given support and sympathy for failure to comply.

Self-Evaluation and Self-Reinforcement

Depressed individuals tend to make inappropriately negative evaluations of their behavior (Rehm, 1977). Either their standards are too high or they selectively attend to negative feedback. In either case, patients are liable to perceive their efforts as inadequate. They may also fail to perceive environmental reinforcement of their homework performance, and view partial success as failure. Either occurrence could mitigate the effects of treatment. To prevent this, individuals are trained to evaluate their responses more positively and to provide self-reinforcement (cf. Bellack, 1976; Bellack, Glanz, & Simon, 1976; Fuchs, & Rehm, 1977). Beginning with the second content area the therapist assigns a letter grade to the response (i.e., A, B, C, D, F). Following grades of A or B, patients are instructed to make a positive self-statement such as, "I did that pretty well. I'm really learning."

Initially, patients tend to grade themselves quite negatively. The therapist should correct inappropriately low evaluations by providing more appropriate and objective criteria. The correction should be presented in a warm, encouraging tone of voice, not as a critique. The patient should be made aware that she really did all right, not criticized for a faulty grade. For example, "I think that was a strong 3. We were focusing only on verbal content that time, and you made a clear statement of your feelings. It was a really good response." The therapist also prompts for and models appropriate, positive self-statements.

Patients are instructed to perform similar self-evaluative and self-reinforcing operations for homework responses. Specific criteria are supplied when the assignment is given (e.g., "Give yourself an A if you state your preference and have a firm tone of voice, a B if your tone is only moderately firm. ... Don't worry about his response when you grade yourself. Just focus on how you presented yourself.")

STRUCTURE OF TRAINING

Our training program is divided into two parts: (1) primary treatment and (2) maintenance. The primary phase consists of 12 weekly individual sessions of 60-minutes duration. An overview of the session-by-session course of training is presented in Table 5.5. The first session is devoted to introducing the patient to treatment, developing rapport, and preliminary assessment and treatment planning. It is important to provide the patient with a clear and cogent rationale for the treatment. Most patient expect therapy to entail open-ended discussion of their symptoms and some critical life issues. They generally must be persuaded of the logic of the social skills model, as well as the structured aspect of the training program. This must be accomplished right at the beginning of treatment. It is difficult to establish or reinstate the structured approach if the patient is reinforced over several sessions for self-exploration and bemoaning his or her fate. The rationale for treatment must be tailored so as to explain the distress experienced by the patient. It should not be an impersonal, textbook explanation of depression.

Skills training begins in the second week. The schema presented in Table 5.5 projects two sessions for each of the first two problem areas and three sessions each for the third and fourth areas. In practice, training generally covers only two or three areas. Moreover, there often is one area or issue (e.g., a particular work or marital problem) that requires as much as half of all training sessions.

The pace and breadth of coverage are subjectively determined. The therapist must spend enough time on any critical issues to ensure some change. But, he or she must also cover enough relevant problem areas to ensure a broad-based impact. Training in social perception skills and self-evaluation and self-reinforcement begin at about Session 4, although this is somewhat flexible. The final session must contain a summary of accomplishments and plans for dealing with problems that seem likely to crop up in the future.

Table 5.5. Session by Session Plan of Treatment

Session 1	Overview and rationale
	Assessment
	Preliminary treatment planning
Sessions 2, 3	Train on first problem area
Sessions 4, 5	Train on second problem area
	Introduce social perception training
	Introduce self-evaluation and self reinforcement
Sessions 6, 7, 8	Train on third problem area
Sessions 9, 10, 11	Train on fourth problem area
Session 12	Summarize accomplishment
	Plan for future problems
Sessions 13–18	Problem solve and review

New response categories should not be introduced in this session unless they are likely to be mastered without further training. Plans should also be made for the maintenance phase of treatment.

The structure activity within sessions is depicted in Tables 5.6 and 5.7.

The basic elements of training and the sequence of their application are presented in Table 5.6. The specific procedures have already been described more fully. The sequence of steps from A to H illustrates the process of training a single behavior, in a single context, with a single interpersonal partner. This sequence is repeated many times throughout the course of the program. Table 5.7 shows the manner in which the sequence is applied to successive targets within each session. The three 15-minute training blocks represent the application of A to H sequences to three distinct targets or interpersonal partners. The time limits are flexible and can be varied according to the pace of progress. However, they are useful guidelines that help ensure breadth of coverage and a sufficient number of role-play trials. Without such guidelines, sessions often evolve into rambling discussions (see section on Problems in Training).

Twelve weeks is a relatively brief period of time in which to produce durable changes. Aside from the comparatively small amount of therapist–patient contact in this period, it does not afford an opportunity to try out new skills in the face of a diversity of real-life problems. Consequently, we administer six to eight booster sessions over the following 6 months. These sessions follow a *prn* schedule, averaging about one per month. The first few often are scheduled at shorter intervals than those at the end of this period. In this way, therapist contact is gradually faded out. New material is not presented in these sessions. Rather, the focus is on review and problem solving. The patient is given further role-play practice on difficult issues, and established skills are translated to new problems. The goal is to reestablish skills that have begun to fade and to help the patient in her own efforts to use her skills to handle new problems.

INTERPERSONAL STYLE

One of the most important aspects of our training program is the interpersonal style or tone of the therapy. The procedure is didactic and highly structured, but it does not follow a lockstep sequence. It is presented in a conversational manner, and there is considerable discussion between therapist and patient throughout. The patient's feelings and thoughts are not ignored. However, the discussion is focused on the training tasks, not simply on self-exploration and catharsis. Consider a woman who has long-standing feelings of anger and

Table 5.6. Training Format

A. Role play to assess response style
B. Rationale for modification
C. Instructions
D. Modeling
E. Role play
F. Feedback and positive reinforcement
G. Repeat role play
H. Self-evaluation and self reinforcement

Table 5.7. Flow within Sessions

First 10 minutes	Review homework and reinforce effort.
Next 15 minutes[a]	Train on the least difficult interaction.
Next 15 minutes[a]	Train on a second interaction.
Next 15 minutes[a]	Repeat on a third interaction.
Next 5 minutes	Summarize and assign homework.

[a]Conduct at least 2–3 role-play repetitions for each interaction.

resentment toward her husband, who has dominated her for years. In the course of identifying target behaviors and role-play scenarios, these feelings are apt to surface. The woman might well begin to shift the focus of the discussion from skills to her feelings. Frequently, this will be accompanied by crying. The therapist's task here is to be empathic and supportive, but shift the discussion back to training tasks:

> **T:** I can see that you are really upset about your marriage. It sounds like you've been angry for years, but didn't know what to do. I would like for us to use these feelings in planning our treatment. We can work on developing skills that will keep you from being bullied in the future. We can't change your husband's past behavior, but by your learning new skills, we can insure that you are not dominated anymore.

An exception to the general rule concerning refocusing of the discussion occurs when there is a crisis situation. The therapist never lets the protocol interfere with the dictates of good clinical judgment. Occasionally, an entire session may be devoted to handling a crisis. However, the therapist must not interpret every crying episode as a crisis, or as an excuse to deviate from the protocol.

The atmosphere of therapy is definitely not cold or harsh. The therapist must be warm and express high personal regard for the patient. He or she actively and continuously works at maintaining a positive therapeutic atmosphere. The therapist is directive, but he or she should not be dictatorial. The patient should be made to feel that the therapist understands her and is working toward alleviating her distress, even when the focus of the interaction shifts away from direct discussion of her most prominent concerns. Operationally, the therapist provides extensive positive reinforcement; he or she must express honest enthusiasm over patient progress. The therapist secures patient input on the content of treatment and expresses understanding of patient concerns. Conversely, the therapist is not critical of the patient, does not ignore her complaints, and does impose values or force her into directions she does not with to pursue.

PROBLEMS IN TRAINING

We have described a relatively smooth course for training. Some cases actually progress at a steady and uneventful rate. But, as with any therapy, exceptions to the rule seem to occur as often as the rule. Nothing can replace good clinical skill in keeping problems to a minimum. The therapist must be a keen observer, sensitive to subtle interpersonal messages and cues signaling distress or dissatisfaction. Failure to sense such cues can have severe, disruptive consequences. A sense of confidence in oneself and one's ability to handle problems also is essential. All too often, the inexperienced therapist overreacts to modest problems or conflicts. Given the dysphoric mood of depressed patients and their low threshold for crying, it is difficult to judge the momentary depth of their distress and decide whether they are able to continue or need to be supported. Our sense is that brief periods of silence followed by gentle prodding often are more "therapeutic" and productive than oversolicitiousness. Unfortunately, there are no clear-cut guidelines for choosing a course of action.

The most characteristic problem in training lies with the therapist, not the patient: failure to follow the protocol. Even committed behavioral therapists regularly drift from the structure and provide too few role-play repetitions. In its place, there is a gradual increase in didactic lecturing and abstract discussion of issues. Conversation and verbal instruction replace demonstration and practice as the medium for training. We have found it helpful to provide our therapists with checklists for each session. Each session is divided into segments as displayed in Table 5.7. A criterion number of role-play repetitions should be completed in each segment. The therapist keeps a running tally *during the session* in order to guide his or her activity. Without such overt structure, the urge to "talk" seems to be overwhelming.

Patient-produced problems often revolve around role playing. Many patients are initially embarrassed by the prospect of role playing and attempt to avoid it. Instead of responding to prompts as if they were actually in the situation, many patients offer an explanation, such as "I would do ... ," or "I would say ..." The therapist should not accept such avoidance behavior. An effective response is, "Okay, but I would like you to imagine that you are really in the situation. Don't tell me that you would say such and such, but actually say it as if we were there." Positive insistence without chastisement generally is effective when coupled with the therapist as a model of appropriate role-play behavior. If the patient is still too self-conscious, she should be asked to close her eyes and visualize the situation. The enactment is then carried out with her eyes still closed. After a few trials with her eyes closed, she should be sufficiently comfortable to follow the regular procedure.

Patients also attempt to avoid role playing in order to talk about their problems. Some patients report a new crisis or "terrible" experience each week. Others simply like to complain about how bad they feel or how impossible their husband, mother, or boss is. The most appropriate strategy for handling such diversions is extinction. The therapist gently but firmly steers the discussion back to the training procedure. An empathic statement is helpful here: "I can understand that was painful and you would like to talk about it, but I'd like for us to get back to our role play. The quickest way to get you to feel better is to work on your ability to stand up for yourself." We recognize that catharsis may have some value for some patients. However, it is important to remember that the therapist cannot deal with all problems in 12 weeks. The primary focus must be on improving social skills. The more therapy time is diluted by attention to diverse issues, the less effect training will have.

SUMMARY

In this chapter we describe our social skills training package for the treatment of women diagnosed as having a major depressive episode of the nonpsychotic variety. The rationale for the social skills approach is first presented. The current treatment approach owes its heritage to the work of Wolpe and Lewinsohn, but is more didactic and wider in scope than previously described. There is more emphasis on directly teaching patients how to respond. Thus, our therapists are more likely to use techniques of modeling and guided practice. Also, we tend to deal with a much wider range of interpersonal issues, considering as well the nonverbal, paralinguistic, and verbal aspects of communications. In addition, we have our own unique blend of treatment foci. We are concerned with the expression of both positive and negative feelings in a socially appropriate manner. Interpersonal expression is evaluated in the context of role-played interactions with strangers, friends, family members, and school or work encounters. The treatment itself has four components: (1) skills training, (2) social-perception training, (3) practice (including homework assignments), and (4) self-evaluation and self-reinforcement. Finally, our program involves a period of maintenance therapy following original treatment in order to consolidate initial gains. Instructions are provided for implementing each aspect of the treatment program. Frequently encountered problems are described, and solutions are discussed.

REFERENCES

American Psychiatric Association. (1994). *Diagnostic and statistical manual of mental disorders* (4th ed.). Washington, DC: Author.

Bellack, A. S. (1976). A comparison of self-monitoring and self-reinforcement in weight reduction. *Behavior Therapy, 7,* 68–75.

Bellack, A. S. (1979). Behavioral assessment of social skills. In A. S. Bellack & M. Hersen (Eds.), *Research and practice in social skills training* (pp. 75–106). New York: Plenum Press.

Bellack, A. S. (1980). Anxiety and neurotic disorders. In A. E. Kazdin, A. S. Bellack, & M. Hersen (Eds.), *New perspectives in abnormal psychology* (pp. 175–203). New York: Oxford University Press.

Bellack, A. S., Glanz, L. M., & Simon, R. (1976). Self-reinforcement style and covert imagery in the treatment of obesity. *Journal of Consulting and Clinical Psychology, 44,* 490–491.

Bellack, A. S., & Hersen, M. (1977). *Behavior modification: An introductory textbook.* Baltimore: Williams & Wilkins.

Bellack, A. S., & Hersen, M. (1978). Chronic psychiatric patients: Social skills training. In M. Hersen & A. S. Bellack (Eds.), *Behavior therapy in the psychiatric setting* (pp. 169–195). Baltimore: Williams & Wilkins.

Bellack, A. S. & Hersen, M. (Eds.). (1979). *Research and practice in social skills training.* New York: Plenum Press.

Craighead, W. C. (1980). Away from a unitary model of depression. *Behavior Therapy, 11,* 122–218.

DeRubeis, R. J., & Hollon, S. D. (1981). Behavioral treatment of affective disorders. In L. Michelson, M. Hersen, & S. M. Turner (Eds.), *Future perspectives in behavior therapy* (pp. 103–129). New York: Plenum Press.

Elkin, I, Shea, M. T., Imber, S. T., Sotsky, S. M., Collins, J. F., Glass, D. R., Pilkonis, P. A., Leber, W. R., Docherty, J. P., Fiester, S. J., & Parloff, M. B. (1989). National Institute of Mental Health treatment of depression collaborative research program: General effectiveness of treatments. *Archieves of Sexual Psychiatry, 46,* 971–982.

Ferster, C. B. (1965). Classification of behavioral pathology. In L. Krasner & L. P. Ullmann (Eds.), *Research in behavior modification* (pp. 6–26). New York: Holt, Rinehart & Winston.

Fuchs, C. Z., & Rehm, L. P. (1977). A self-control behavior therapy program for depression. *Journal of Consulting and Clinical Psychology, 45,* 206–215.

Harper, R. G., Wiens, A. N., & Matarazzo, J. D. (1978). *Nonverbal communication: The state of the art.* New York: Wiley.

Hersen, M. (1981). Assessment of deficits and outcomes. In L. P. Rehm (Ed.), *Behavior therapy for depression: Present status and future directions* (pp. 301–316). New York: Academic Press.

Hersen, M., Bellack, A. S., & Himmelhoch, J. M. (1982). Social skills training with unipolar depressed women. In J. P. Curran & P. M. Monti (Eds.), *Social competence and psychiatric disorders: Theory and practice* (pp. 159–184). New York: Guilford Press.

Kovacs, M. (1979). Treating depressive disorders: The efficacy of behavior and cognitive therapies. *Behavior Modification, 3,* 496–517.

Lewinsohn, P. M. (1975). The behavioral study and treatment of depression. In M. Hersen, R. M. Eisler, & P. M. Miller (Eds.), *Progress in behavior modification* (Vol. 1, pp. 19–64). New York: Academic Press.

Lewinsohn, P. M. & Hoberman, H. M. (1982). Depression. In A. S. Bellack, M. Hersen, & A. E. Kazdin, (Eds.), *International handbook of behavior modification and therapy* (pp. 397–431). New York: Plenum Press.

Lewinsohn, P. M., & Shaffer, M. (1971). Use of home observations as integral part of the treatment of depression: Preliminary report and case studies. *Journal of Consulting and Clinical Psychology, 37*, 87–94.

Libet, J., & Lewinsohn, P. M. (1973). Concept of social skill with special reference to the behavior of depressed persons. *Journal of Consulting and Clinical Psychology, 40*, 304–312.

McLean, P. D., & Hakistan, A. R. (1979). Clinical depression: Comparative efficacy of outpatient treatments. *Journal of Consulting and Clinical Psychology, 47*, 818–836.

McLean, P. D., Ogston, K., & Grauer, L. (1973). A behavioral approach to the treatment of depression. *Journal of Behavior Therapy and Experimental Psychiatry, 4*, 323–330.

Morrison, R. L., Bellack, A. S., & Bashore, T. R. (1988). Perception of emotion by schizophrenic patients. *Journal of Psychopathology and Behavioral Assessment, 10*, 319–332.

Rehm, L. P. (1976). Assessment of depression. In M. Hersen & A. S. Bellack (Eds.), *Behavioral assessment: A practical handbook*. New York: Pergamon Press.

Rehm, L. P. (1977). A self-control model of depression. *Behavior Therapy, 8*, 787–804.

Rehm, L. P., & Kornblith, S. J. (1979). Behavior therapy for depression: A review of recent developments. In M. Hersen, R. M. Eisler, & P. M. Miller (Eds.), *Progress in behavior modification* (Vol. 7, pp. 277–318). New York: Academic Press.

Rush, A. J., Beck, A. T., Kovacs, M., & Hollon, S. (1977). Comparative efficacy of cognitive therapy and pharmacotherapy in the treatment of depressed outpatients. *Cognitive Therapy and Research, 1*, 17–37.

Sanchez, V., & Lewinsohn, P. M. (1980). Assertive behavior and depression. *Journal of Consulting and Clinical Psychology, 48*, 119–120.

Wells, K. C., Hersen, M., Bellack, A. S., Himmelhoch, J. (1979). Social skills training in unipolar nonpsychotic depression. *American Journal of Psychiatry, 136*, 1331–1332.

Wolpe, J. (1973). *The practice of behavior therapy*. New York: Pergamon Press.

Wolpe, J. (1979). The experimental model and treatment of neurotic depression. *Behaviour Research and Therapy, 17*, 555–565.

Zeiss, A. M., Lewinsohn, P. M., & Munoz, R. F. (1979). Nonspecific improvement effects in depression using interpersonal skills training, pleasant activity schedules, or cognitive training. *Journal of Consulting and Clinical Psychology, 47*, 427–439.

6

Cognitive Behavior Therapy Manual for Treatment of Depressed Inpatients

Michael E. Thase

INTRODUCTION

Although most inpatient psychiatric programs incorporate psychotherapeutic principles, surprisingly little attention has been devoted to development of specific models of treatments for hospitalized depressed individuals (Markowitz, 1989). Beck's model of cognitive therapy (Beck, 1976; Beck, Rush, Shaw, & Emery, 1979) or, as more broadly conceived, cognitive behavior therapy (CBT) is well-suited for this purpose (Bowers, 1989; Scott, 1988; Shaw, 1981; Thase, 1994a; Thase & Wright, 1991; Wright, Thase, Beck, & Ludgate, 1993). In this chapter, the most recent version of our inpatient CBT of depression is described.

BACKGROUND

CBT is distinguishable from dynamic or interpersonally oriented therapies in a number of important ways. First, CBT is almost always viewed as time limited. Second, the therapist plays a very active role, often approaching the activity level of a teacher or coach. Third, case formulations and treatment strategies are specifically guided by the cognitive model of psychopathology (Beck, 1976; Persons, 1989). Thus, specific treatment strategies are chosen to address dysfunctional patterns of thoughts, feelings, and behaviors associated

Michael E. Thase • Department of Psychiatry, Western Psychiatric Institute and Clinic, University of Pittsburgh School of Medicine, Pittsburgh, Pennsylvania 15213.

Sourcebook of Psychological Treatment Manuals for Adult Disorders, edited by Vincent B. Van Hasselt and Michel Hersen. Plenum Press, New York, 1996.

with Axis I syndromes and/or personality pathology are measured objectively. And fourth, the effects of treatment on dysfunctional thoughts, feelings, and behaviors are monitored throughout the course of therapy.

Cognitive Model of Depression

The cognitive model of depression is understood in terms of the interaction between selected vulnerabilities in information processing and changes in affect, behavior, and cognition. *Cognitive primacy* refers to the hypothesis that changes in thinking (e.g., in response to a loss or some other stressor) trigger or "drive" the affective and behavioral correlates of depression (e.g., Beck, 1976). Alternatively, the hierarchical and interactive relationships between cognitive, behavioral, and affective processes associated with depression suggests that changes in cognition may be either a cause or a result of states of emotional distress (Thase & Beck, 1993). Thus, a neurochemical disturbance underlying diurnal mood variation may predispose an individual to function poorly in the morning which, in turn, results in both behavioral deficits and self-critical commentary about such underperformance. Contemporary applications of the cognitive model (e.g., Persons, 1989; Wright & Thase, 1992) incorporate such complexity, while still retaining an emphasis on intervention via cognitive and behavioral strategies. With respect to cognitive interventions, the targets of interest may be termed *disturbances* of the process, structure, and content of cognition.

The term *cognitive process* describes the acquisition, storage, and retrieval of information, including recall of affectively laden memories. Considerable evidence documents mood-dependent changes in information processing in depression, as well as other states of affective distress (e.g., Coyne & Gotlib, 1983; Haaga, Dyck, & Ernst, 1991; Robins & Hayes, 1993). Changes in information processing associated with depression include selective abstraction, selective recall, overgeneralization, personalization, "mind reading," "fortune-telling," and arbitrary inference (see Table 6.1). It appears that such mood-dependent changes in information processing serve to clarify or intensify the depressive state. For example, recall of memories about past adverse events, negative interpretations of current events, and pessimistic predictions about the future increase the valance of the predominant affect (Thase & Beck, 1993). Controversy persists whether disturbances of information processing have specific, etiologic significance (e.g., Beck, 1976) or are simply correlates of depression (Coyne & Gotlib 1983).

The structure of cognition in Beck's model incorporates three categories of mental activity: (1) automatic thoughts, (2) attitude and beliefs, and (3) schema or basic assumptions (Beck, 1976; Dobson & Shaw, 1986). From the cognitivist vantage point, disturbances of cognitive structure in depression deviate from normal by matter of degree or excess. For example, automatic thoughts are more frequent and negatively valanced during depressive episodes. Similarly, depressive attitudes and beliefs are considered to be dysfunctional because of their more extreme and rigid nature.

Automatic thoughts intrusively enter consciousness effortlessly and their content typically reflects the depressed person's mood state. The more intrusive cognitions associated with dysphoric affects are referred to as *automatic negative thoughts* (ANTs). Automatic negative thoughts are readily observed in the mental dialogue of depressed individuals, as well as in their daydreams and other visual images. The term *cognitive triad* is used to describe the organization of thoughts into themes about one's self, the larger world, and the future (Beck, 1976). At times of emotional distress, the percentage of automatic

Table 6.1. Common Examples of Distorted Information Processing in Anxiety and Depression[a]

1. *Emotional reasoning*: A conclusion or inference is based upon an emotional state (i.e., "I *feel* this way, therefore I *am* this way).

2. *Overgeneralization*: Evidence is drawn from one experience or a small set of experiences to reach an unwarranted conclusion with far-reaching implications.

3. *Catastrophic thinking*: An extreme example of overgeneralization, in which the impact of a clearly negative event or experience is amplified to extreme proportions (e.g., "If I have a panic attack I will lose *all* control and go crazy [or die]").

4. *All-or-none (black or white; absolutistic) thinking*: An unnecessary division of complex or continuous outcomes into a polarized extreme (e.g., "Either I am a success at this, or I'm a total failure").

5. *Shoulds and musts*: Imperative statements about self that dictate rigid standards or reflect an unrealistic degree of presumed control over external events.

6. *Negative predictions*: Premature or inappropriate use of pessimism or previous experiences of failure to predict failure in a new situation. Also known as "fortune-telling."

7. *Mind reading*: Negatively toned inferences about the thoughts, intentions, or motives of another person.

8. *Labeling*: An undesirable characteristic of a person or event is made definitive of that person or event (e.g., "Because I *failed* to be selected for the ballet, I am a *failure*").

9. *Personalization*: Interpretation of an event, situation, or behavior as salient or personally indicative of a negative aspect of self.

10. *Selective negative focus*: Undesirable or negative events, memories, or implications are focused on at the expense of recalling or identifying other, more neutral or positive information. In fact, positive information may be ignored *or* disqualified as irrelevant, atypical, or trivial.

11. *Cognitive avoidance*: Unpleasant thoughts, feelings, or events are misperceived as overwhelming and/or insurmountable and are actively suppressed or avoided.

12. *Somatic (mis)focus*: The predisposition to interpret internal stimuli (e.g., heart rate, palpitations, shortness of breath, dizziness, or tingling) as *definite* indications of impending catastrophic events (e.g., heart attack, suffocation, collapse).

[a]Adapted from Thase and Beck (1993).

negative thoughts may shift from the normal "golden zone" (i.e., about 20%) to 60% to 80% of even higher (Garamoni et al., 1991; Schwartz & Garamoni, 1986). In states of suicidal despair, the depressed person is often stuck in a negative monologue, in which 90% or even 100% of cognitions are negatively valanced (Schwartz & Garamoni, 1986). The term *cognitive triad* is used to reflect the fact that automatic negative thoughts are usually organizable into thematic areas pertaining to self, the larger world, and the future (Beck, 1976).

Attitudes and beliefs represent a "deeper" level of cognition, providing rules for conduct or behavior to help maintain the illusion of consistency. Dysfunctional attitudes characteristic of depression typically reflect unrealistic standards of performance (e.g., perfectionism) and/or excessive interpersonal dependence. Attributional style (i.e., a characteristic or habitual tendency to ascribe causality and meaning to events) also is pertinent to many cases of depression (Abramson, Seligman, & Teasdale, 1978; Spangler et al., 1993). In depression, a pattern is often observed in which events are attributed to personal weakness (i.e., internality), have far-reaching effects (i.e., globality), and/or exert an enduring impact (i.e., stability). Thus, the depression-prone person's attributional style may be described as internal/global/stable (namely, the cognitive triad: self/world/future).

The cognitive model of psychopathology suggests that dysfunctional attitudes and attributional style are persistent sources of vulnerability. However, dysfunctional attitudes and depressogenic attributional style have both been shown to be, at least partially, state dependent (see Haaga et al., 1991). Thus, these presumed trait-like parameters are, at least to some extent, inflated by the illness itself. This observation is also reflected by reductions in ratings of dysfunctional attitudes in response to various antidepressant treatments (e.g., Hamilton & Abramson, 1983; Miranda & Persons, 1988; Simons, Garfield, & Murphy, 1984). Nevertheless, depressions characterized by persistent elevations of dysfunctional attitudes tend to be more chronic or treatment resistant in nature (Miller & Norman, 1986; Thase & Howland, 1994). Moreover, high residual levels of dysfunctional attitudes have been related to an increased risk of relapse after termination of therapy (Eaves & Rush, 1984; Thase et al., 1992).

The deepest level of cognition incorporated in Beck's model is that of silent assumptions or schemas. The term *schema*, as derived from Piagetian theory (Rosen, 1989), is used to describe a particular type of preverbal mental structure, hypothesized to guide cognition and conduct implicitly. One example of a schema would be the mechanism that organizes one's knowledge about how to tie a shoe or water-ski. Schemas more central to the cognitive model of depression include fundamentally negative, unspoken beliefs about important domains such as competence, attractiveness, lovability, and the dependability of caregivers (see Table 6.2). Although pathological schemas are presumed to result from early adversity or harsh developmental experiences, they also are proposed to remain modifiable throughout adult life (Beck et al., 1990).

The episodic nature of most depressive disorders suggests that pathological schemas may be clinically "silent" for years at a time. Cognitive theory posits that acute depression results from the interactions between schematic vulnerability and "matching" life events (e.g., Hammen, Ellicott, Gitlin, & Jamison, 1989). For example, the onset of major depression would be more likely to follow divorce or the end of a love affair if an individual has a pathological schema pertaining to lovability (e.g., "Without a lover, I'm nothing") than one about competence. By contrast, the latter individual would be more likely to become depressed following a vocational or professional setback. Fully integrative models incorporate cognitive vulnerability within a broader framework of risk factors, including potential genetic and neurobiological correlates, as well as potential "buffering" or offsetting factors such as social support (e.g., Monroe & Simons, 1991, Thase & Beck, 1993). In therapy, schemas are inferred from repetitive patterns or themes revealed in ANTs and dysfunctional attitudes. Alternatively, attitudinal inventories (e.g., the Dysfunctional Attitude Scale (DAS); Weissman & Beck, 1978) or the Sociotropy Autonomy Scale (Hammen et al., 1989) may be used to help "identify" pathological schemas.

Behavioral changes associated with depression may sometimes appear to be given short shrift in Beck's written manuals (e.g., Beck, 1976, Beck et al., 1979; Beck et al., 1990). Like the cognitive changes associated with depression, behavioral difficulties may be subcategorized into state-dependent or state-independent (i.e., trait-like) forms. Examples of more enduring behavioral problems associated with an increased risk for depression include poor social skills (e.g., underassertiveness) and decreased social problem-solving ability (Hersen et al., 1984; Nezu, 1986). Conversely, behavioral difficulties apparent during episodes of depression include aversive interpersonal behavior (i.e., complaining,

Table 6.2. Proposed Maladaptive Schema[a]

Autonomy

1. *Dependence.* The belief that one is unable to function without the constant support of others.

2. *Subjugation/Lack of Individuation.* The voluntary or involuntary sacrifice of one's own needs to satisfy others' needs.

3. *Vulnerability to Harm or Illness.* The fear that disaster (i.e., natural, criminal, medical, or financial) is about to strike at any time.

4. *Fear of Losing Self-Control.* The fear that one will involuntarily lose control of one's own impulses, behavior, emotions, mind, and so on.

Connectedness

5. *Emotional Deprivation.* The expectation that one's needs for nurturance, empathy, or affection will never be adequately met by others.

6. *Abandonment/Loss.* Fear that one will imminently lose significant others and/or be emotionally isolated forever.

7. *Mistrust.* The expectation that others will hurt, abuse, cheat, lie, or manipulate.

8. *Social Isolation/Alienation.* The belief that one is isolated from the rest of the world, different from other people, and/or doesn't belong to any group or community.

Worthiness

9. *Defectiveness/Unlovability.* The assumption that one is *inwardly* defective or that, if the flaw is exposed, one is fundamentally unlovable.

10. *Social Undesirability.* The belief that one is outwardly undesirable to others (e.g., ugly, sexually undesirable, low in status, dull, or boring).

11. *Incompetence/Failure.* The assumption that one cannot perform competently in areas of achievement, daily responsibilities, or decision making.

12. *Guilt/Punishment.* The conclusion that one is morally bad or irresponsible and deserving of criticism or punishment.

13. *Shame/Embarrassment.* Recurrent feelings of shame or self-consciousness, experienced because one believes that one's inadequacies (as reflected in schemas 9 to 12) are totally unacceptable to others.

Limits and standards

14. *Unrelenting Standards.* The relentless striving to meet extremely high expectation of oneself, at all costs (i.e., at the expense of happiness, pleasure, health, or satisfying relationships).

15. *Entitlement.* Insistence that one should be able to do, say, or have whatever one wants immediately.

[a]Adapted from Thase and Beck (1993).

clinging, rejecting help and/or crying), decreased involvement in reinforcing activities, procrastination, and insomnia.

The emotional reactions characteristic of loss or withdrawal of reinforcement are a hallmark of behavioral models of depression (e.g., Ferster, 1973). Of note, neurochemical changes in limbic–forebrain structures may interact with such behavioral changes to further dampen the depressed patient's response to any particular loss (Costello, 1972). Thus, the depressed person may require more than encouragement in order to resume participation in pleasant events; often it is necessary to expose the depressed patient to a higher grade of reinforcers in order to compensate for such anhedonia.

Adaptation of Cognitive Behavior Therapy for Inpatients

The characteristics of hospitalized depressed patients, the nature of contemporary inpatient psychiatric practice, and an interest in developing CBT as an alternative to pharmacotherapy were the essential reasons that we chose to modify the original outpatient treatment manual of Beck et al. (1979). With respect to patient variables, important factors that must be taken into account include a high likelihood of suicidal ideations, increased clinical severity, more disturbed neurocognitive function (i.e., greater magnitude of memory and concentration disturbances, as well as a loss of abstract capabilities), a greater probability of prior nonresponse to standard therapies, and a less supportive social network (Freeman & Reinecke, 1993; Thase 1993a; Thase & Wright, 1991). Inpatients are also more likely to have comorbid personality disorders, although this may not necessitate significant changes in CBT (Beck et al., 1990; Thase, 1994a).

In order to address these challenges, an increased frequency of therapy sessions is a key difference between outpatient and inpatient CBT. Declining lengths of stay currently limit the hospitalization of depressed patients to 10 to 18 days, virtually necessitating the use of daily sessions. Frequent sessions are particularly valuable in order to provide greater continuity and repetition of materials that help to offset hopelessness, clinical severity, and/ or difficulties with learning and memory (Scott, 1988; Thase, 1993a). Furthermore, therapists are able to promptly modify therapeutic tasks when they have not achieved the desired results. Thus, more frequent sessions reduced the likelihood that patients will "flounder" between therapy sessions.

The therapist's choice of treatment strategies also may differ for inpatient therapy, particularly early in the course of treatment. For example, inpatient therapists generally make greater use of behavioral strategies and more explicit methods to make cognitive tasks more understandable, such as the use of "coping cards" and written summaries of within-session materials (Scott 1988; Thase, 1993a; Thase & Wright, 1991). The coping card, typically written on a 3×5-inch index card, provides a predetermined list of rational responses to a recurrent, negative automatic thought. Patients also are encouraged to keep a therapy notebook to facilitate recall of therapy material. The notebook is used to record the rationale for assignments, collect activity schedules, keep a running account of progress of therapy (i.e., Beck Depression Inventory (BDI) and DAS forms), and write down homework assignments.

Common behavioral strategies include activity schedules, graded task assignments, and mastery and pleasure exercises (e.g., Scott, 1988; Thase & Wright, 1991). Other less common behavioral strategies, such as thought stopping (Beck et al., 1979), relaxation training (Bernstein & Borkovec, 1973), behavioral rehearsal (Bellack et al., 1981), problem-solving (Nezu, 1986), and scheduled exercise (Simons, Epstein, McGowan, Kupfer, & Robertson, 1985), may be added to the treatment plan when indicated. Although novice therapists may mistakenly overlook such methods (i.e., in preference to more technically sophisticated cognitive interventions), the value of these focused tasks to help more severely impaired patients cope with otherwise overwhelming symptoms should not be discounted.

Unfortunately, the brevity of most inpatient admissions limits what can be accomplished. Even with daily sessions, most patients receive an average of only 8 to 12 sessions of therapy during the hospitalization (Thase, 1993a). Thus, it is important that inpatient

CBT programs emphasize psychoeducation, enculturation into the CBT model of therapy, and basic skills acquisition; continued outpatient treatment to address schema and relapse prevention can be pursued following discharge (Thase, 1993b). Indeed, in the study of Miller, Norman, Keitner, Bishop, and Dow (1989b), the major benefits of a combined CBT–pharmacotherapy regimen emerged during outpatient continuation therapy. In the Pittsburgh group's experience, inpatient CBT should not be used as the principal treatment (i.e., in lieu of pharmacotherapy) *unless* continued outpatient therapy is available (Thase, 1993b; Thase, Bowler, & Harden, 1991).

Types of Inpatient Cognitive Behavior Therapy Programs

The existing structure and orientation of the inpatient unit's milieu also is an important consideration. Only a handful of inpatient programs is conceptually organized around CBT principles; more often than not, CBT is an "add-on" component to a more conventional model of treatment focused on a more electric biopsychosocial model of intervention (Wright et al., 1993). In an eclectic milieu, it is important for the therapist to be able to integrate CBT with other models of psychopathology and treatment. Accordingly, it is suggested that the CBT therapist take responsibility in order to ensure that therapy is fully integrated within the overall treatment plan (Thase & Wright 1991). Thus, the CBT therapist attends multidisciplinary treatment team meetings and works with nurses, ancillary staff, and social workers to implement the treatment plan. The importance of unit-wide support for a CBT treatment program must be emphasized (Wright, Thase, & Sensky, 1993).

Detailed discussions of ways to incorporate the efforts of treatment team members are provided elsewhere (Scott, 1988; Wright, Thase, & Sensky, 1993). Particularly early in the course of treatment, it is useful for the therapist to "sign off" each homework assignment to a specific member of the nursing staff. Beyond issues of communication, nurses and ancillary staff provide a unique resource to help patients complete homework assignments. Moreover, after a modest amount of training, ward staff may assist with *in vivo* application of therapy strategies (Bowler, Moonis, & Thase, 1993; Scott, 1988). Psychiatric nurses also may be invited to "sit in" on individual therapy sessions to gain a better understanding of the methods of CBT. Similarly, the social worker's contacts with family assessments provide a natural opportunity to educate the patient's family about CBT and to engage the patient's significant others within the therapeutic alliance (Thase & Wright, 1991).

Group CBT is a particularly cost-efficient means of delivering treatment to a larger number inpatients (Ludgate, Wright, Bowers, & Camp, 1993). The utility of group CBT is suggested by several outpatient studies (e.g., Covi & Lippman, 1987; de Jong, Treiber, & Henrich, 1986; Ross & Scott, 1985). The rapid turnover of patients mitigates against use of conventional closed groups. Rather, a "revolving" curriculum of 6 to 10 sessions covering key topics seems to provide the most flexibility (Thase, 1993a). As noted earlier, involvement of psychiatric nurses and ancillary staff as cotherapists may facilitate completion of homework assignments and exert an important positive effect on the unit morale.

Selection of Therapists

The vast majority of CBT therapists practice in outpatient venues. Accordingly, the "add-on" model of treatment, in which an experienced therapist is recruited to join an existing inpatient treatment team, has proven to be the easiest model implement (Wright, Thase, & Sensky, 1993). Despite its feasibility, the value of the add-on model is inherently limited if the knowledge and skill of the therapist remain peripheral to the zeitgeist of the treatment team. Moreover, the longevity of such collaborations also may leave much to be desired. In the long run, it is desirable to obtain CBT training for existing inpatient staff (Wright et al., 1993).

Psychiatric inpatient units provide an excellent place for training in CBT (Padesky, 1993; Thase, 1993a). There is never a shortage of patients to work with and the "case mix" is varied in terms of severity, acuity, and complexity. Selection of candidates is ideally based on three factors: (1) core psychotherapeutic qualities (i.e., accurate empathy, understanding, and genuineness); (2) willingness to learn; and (3) the ability to use more active, interventionistic methods. Appropriate candidate therapists range from staff and resident psychiatrists, psychologists, clinical social workers, and more experienced nursing staff.

Ideally, all trainees receive on-site supervision by an experienced CBT therapist. Without such supervision, CBT (like other skill-based behaviors) may be compromised as the therapist repeats "bad habits" over and over again. Unfortunately, on-site supervision is not widely available, and most therapists learn from other modes of supervision (Padesky, 1993).

First, the therapist–trainee needs to develop a sound working understanding of the cognitive model of psychopathology and the basic tenets of therapy. In addition to our own work, we use Beck et al. (1979), Burns (1980), and Persons (1989) as core readings. When a relatively large number of trainees is available at a single site, didactic material can be covered in a 6- to 12-session orientation seminar. After a sufficient orientation period, trainees begin clinical work. Second, it is desirable to begin clinical training with group therapy, providing the trainee the opportunity to observe an experienced therapist. Again, this method is limited by the availability of an experienced therapist. Third, relatively straightforward cases of major depression are selected for the first individual-training cases. If resources are available, sessions may be video- or audio-taped for use in supervision. More difficult patients can be selected as the trainee gains confidence and skills. Generally, it is not a good idea for trainees to treat unmedicated patients.

Although, training and supervision are expensive and time consuming, some evidence suggests that the therapist's competence probably improves the chances of a favorable outcome (DeRubeis & Feeley, 1990; Thase, 1994b). Programs may minimize the expense of training by sending candidates away to attend brief, intensive, off-site programs (Padesky, 1993). Conversely, when an on-site CBT supervisor is available, group supervision may be used as a cost-efficient training strategy.

There is no professional organization to establish standards for credentialing CBT therapists. The most widely utilized method was developed by Shaw (1984) to train therapists for the National Institutes of Mental Health Treatment of Depression Collaborative Research Program (e.g., Elkin et al., 1989). This method of "certification" includes (1) professional licensure and at least 2 years of posttraining experience (i.e., as a psychologist, psychiatrist, social worker, or nurse–clinical specialist); (2) completion of at least 1 year of supervised treatment of depressed outpatients; and (3) confirmation of technical skill and adherence as rated by the Cognitive Therapy Scale (Vallis, Shaw, & Dobson, 1986): Ratings are typically based on either videotape (preferred) or audiotape, although direct observation also could be utilized. In practice, consistent scores greater than or equal to 40 (i.e., the "red line"; Shaw, 1984) for at least two consecutive cases are used as the minimum criterion for competence. For work with hospitalized individuals, it would seem that an even higher standard of competence should be adopted. At the Pittsburgh program, we require supervised experience treating at least 10 moderately to severely depressed inpatients before therapists are "certified" to treat unmedicated patients.

Combining Inpatient Cognitive Behavior Therapy and Medication

209

Cognitive Behavior
Therapy for
Treatment of
Depressed Inpatients

Aside from research, virtually all hospitalized depressed patients are treated with antidepressant medication or electroconvulsive therapy. Thus, it is likely that CBT's major use will be in combination with pharmacotherapy. Both philosophically and pragmatically, CBT and pharmacotherapy are quite compatible (Wright, Thase, & Sensky, 1993). Moreover, as reviewed subsequently, the results of several inpatient studies suggest that additive effects can be expected for more chronically or complicated patients (Bowers, 1990; Miller, Norman, & Keitner, 1990; Scott, 1992; Whisman, Miller, Norman, & Keitner, 1991). An additive effect may be gleaned from several levels. At the most superficial level, the combined strategy offers a broader spectrum of "coverage" for a heterogeneous patient population. Synergy or additive effects may also operate at a deeper, theoretically meaningful level. For example, CBT may be used to target dysfunctional thoughts and "residual" clinical symptoms (e.g., anxiety) that are sometimes not fully responsive to pharmacotherapy. CBT also may be used to address problems such as medication noncompliance, in order to increase the chances of pharmacotherapy response (Wright et al., 1993). Conversely, antidepressant medication may help "turn down" state-dependent pathological arousal that would otherwise impair acquisition or generalization of therapy material, or "turn on" prefrontal cortical function and restore working memory and abstraction capabilities (Thase & Howland, 1994; Wright & Thase, 1992).

Indications for Inpatient Cognitive Behavior Therapy

A number of studies (Bowers, 1990; Miller et al., 1989a, 1989b, 1990; Whisman et al., 1991; Scott, 1988, 1992) suggest that the combination of CBT and pharmacotherapy is more effective than standard treatment alone. Research to date suggests several potentially responsive subgroups. Miller et al. (1990) found that the CBT–pharmacotherapy combination was significantly more effective than standard treatment in patients with high levels of pretreatment dysfunctional attitudes. In fact, the combination of CBT and standard inpatient treatment plan did not improve the outcome of patients with more normal (i.e., not elevated) scores on the DAS. Rather, the high-DAS subgroup had an extremely *poor* response to standard treatment. Prior studies have found an association between high DAS scores and chronicity, "neuroticism," and comorbidity (see Thase & Howland, 1994). Thus, the combination of CBT and standard treatment would appear to improve the course of patients with more chronic or complicated depressive disorders. Although not yet the topic of specific research, suicidal individuals also may receive particular benefits from combined treatment via CBT's utility for reduction of hopelessness and related cognitive symptoms (Whisman et al., 1991).

There are virtually no absolute contraindications for use of CBT in combination with pharmacotherapy. Even delusionally depressed patients may benefit from the use structure and selected behavioral techniques (e.g., Bishop, Miller, Norman, Buda, & Foulke, 1986). Continuing CBT during a course of electroconvulsive therapy may be somewhat inefficient (i.e., because of the latter treatment's effects on memory), but certainly would not be contraindicated (Wright, Thase, & Sensky, 1993). Depressed elders showing signs of early dementia also may have a more difficult time with therapy; however, CBT would not be contraindicated if allowances were made for the patient's memory difficulties. Finally, the use of CBT as an acute-phase therapy for bipolar affective disorder has not yet been evaluated; however, some evidence suggests that CBT may help improve treatment adherence and the overall outcome of bipolar patients during maintenance pharmacotherapy (Cochran, 1984).

Tentative selection criteria for use of CBT as the primary treatment for unmedicated depressed patients have recently been proposed (Stuart & Thase, 1994; Thase & Wright, 1991) for the following: (1) nonpsychotic patients who are adamantly opposed to taking antidepressant medication; (2) patients who have not been able to tolerate a number of antidepressants; and (3) patients who manifest one or more relative contraindications for antidepressant medication, such as women during the first trimester of pregnancy or nursing mothers. In our group's experience (Stuart & Thase, 1994; Thase, 1993a; Thase et al., 1991), depressed patients with acute, relatively uncomplicated major depressive disorders have the best responses to inpatient CBT. This is an inherently "good-prognosis" group and, in the absence of studies utilizing appropriate control groups, it cannot be stated that CBT's efficacy as a primary treatment is any better (or worse) than other psychosocial inpatient intervention.

We also have found that inpatient CBT has a valuable secondary role in support of research studies in which patients must remain off psychotropic medications for 7 to 14 days (e.g., Dubé, Dobkin, Bowler, Thase, & Kupfer, 1993; Malone et al., 1993). In this context, inpatient CBT has provided a useful form of nonpharmacological treatment during a required antidepressant taper or washout period. Furthermore, when effective as the primary treatment, CBT offers a unique opportunity to study the biological correlates of depression across the remission process without the potentially confounding effects of somatic treatments of brain functions (Thase & Simons, 1992).

Not all depressed inpatients are responsive to CBT, even in its intensive form. In our group's experience, depressions complicated by another DSM-III-R (American Psychiatric Association, 1987) Axis I mental disorder or a severe Axis II disorder have relatively poorer responses to CBT (Thase, Simons, & Reynolds, 1993), as do patients who have failed other antidepressant treatments (Thase & Howland, 1994). Clinical severity also plays a significant role: Inpatients in the highest quartile of severity (i.e., Hamilton Rating Scale for Depression [HRSD] scores ≥ 25) have typically had poorer responses to CBT alone (Thase, 1994). Similarly, perhaps the best studied neurobiological correlate of severe depression, hypercortisolism (i.e., mean urinary free cortisol excretion values greater than 90 mcg/24 hours) has been associated with poor response to inpatient CBT (Thase et al., 1993). Finally, ethical concerns have led the Pittsburgh group to refrain from treating any patients with psychotic or bipolar depressions without concomitant pharmacotherapy.

An additional caveat concerns an apparent dose–response relationship for inpatient CBT. The Pittsburgh group's experience is based on a treatment protocol designed to provide up to 4 weeks or 20 sessions of treatment (e.g., Thase & Wright, 1991). Between the program's inception in 1989 and early 1994, average length of stay on our depression units dropped by more than a week, with the average course of therapy dropping from about 15 to only 10 sessions. As the number of sessions has decreased, so has our confidence in the "durability" of therapeutic gains resulting from CBT (Stuart & Thase, 1994). Thus, in our program, inpatient CBT is no longer offered as the principal treatment unless outpatient continuation therapy is feasible.

Overview of the Treatment Protocol

Declining lengths of stay have necessitated condensation of our initial inpatient-treatment protocol (Thase & Wright, 1991) to three phases, with each phase lasting from several days to up to a week. As before, therapists are encouraged to pace the introduction of new material in relation to the patient's clinical state and length of time available for inpatient treatment. As will be described, Phase 1 consists of orientation, psychoeducation, and introduction of basic therapy concepts. Phase 2 emphasizes acquisition, practice, and mastery of cognitive and behavioral coping skills. Phase 3 principally centers around *in vivo* application of therapy skills and preparation for discharge. The BDI and the Beck Hopelessness Scale are administered at the beginning of treatment and weekly thereafter in order to monitor progress.

INDIVIDUAL COGNITIVE BEHAVIOR THERAPY PROTOCOL FOR TREATMENT OF DEPRESSED INPATIENTS

Phase One: Sessions 1–5

The major goals of Phase 1 are to (1) establish a collaborative treatment alliance; (2) identify a problem list and areas of individual strength, including "reasons for living"; (3) psychoeducation about CBT; and (4) reduction of hopelessness and suicidal risk. The recommended approach for the first five sessions is described here.

Session 1

The first session introduces the therapist, the model of therapy, and the process by which the therapy is conducted. The first goal is development of a collaborative alliance. To help achieve this, the therapist simultaneously calls on the "core skills" of accurate empathy and genuineness while also modeling the more active stance of collaborative empiricism. Explicit use of questions that elicit feedback help illustrate the latter style. For example, the therapist may periodically ask the patient about potential areas of confusion. In working with hospitalized depressed patients, it is also essential in the first session to identify factors leading to and/or maintaining hopelessness and/or suicidality. Initial targets for therapeutic intervention are thus identified, and at least one intervention to lessen hopelessness is introduced. The following outline is used to guide the session:

1. *Patient and Therapist Introduction.* The therapist greets the patient in a warm yet professional manner. Initial discussion may include a description of the therapist's level of experience and/or professional background. The therapist also asks about the patient's past treatment experiences and his or her knowledge about depression and CBT.

2. *Setting the Agenda.* The agenda is an essential characteristic of CBT, exemplifying the relatively structured approach to therapy. The therapist introduces the use of an agenda within the first few minutes of the session. The following statement demonstrates the agenda's importance: "I'd like to set an agenda to guide what we are going to work on today. We've found that therapy is better organized and more productive when each session follows an agenda. It is kind of like using a map to guide a trip." The first item on the agenda for Session 1 is usually a concise review of the patient's history.

3. *Brief Review of the Patient's History.* No matter how good the medical record, it is still useful for the therapist to have the chance to listen to the patient tell his or her own story. This "recap" of the patient's history gives the therapist the opportunity to begin to understand the patient's narrative in terms of a history of presenting complaints, current difficulties, and background issues. For suicidal individuals, this approach also helps to

clarify the phenomenology or "justifying" personal logic underpinning hopelessness and life-threatening behavior.

4. *Developing a Problem List.* Development of a well-specified problem list is typically the second agenda item. The problem list includes both pressing life problems and distressing symptoms (i.e., can't sleep, can't concentrate, nervousness, or can't stop crying). The specificity of the problem list serves to teach patients another aspect of the process and methods of CBT: The therapist helps to "translate" vague, overgeneralized, or global problem statements into operationalized or more precisely defined targets. Constructing the problem list also provides the opportunity for the therapist to listen for ANTs and to use Socratic questioning, solicit feedback, and summarize key points (i.e., early illustrations of the collaborative–empirical approach to the therapeutic relationship).

If necessary, the problem list may be organized into a hierarchy, ranking problems from most distressing to least. The problem list is then supplemented by collecting a parallel list of assets and strengths. A chalkboard or notepad is then used to construct a grid, matching problems with areas of strengths. Upon completion of these tasks, the therapist elicits feedback about their accuracy to ensure that the problem list clearly reflects patients' perceptions about their condition and need for hospitalization. The problem list thus serves as a "master" agenda for the entire course of therapy, guiding selection of therapeutic "targets" during subsequent sessions.

5. *Clarifying the Phenomenology of Suicidal Ideations and Hopelessness.* When pertinent, the problem list also helps to operationalize the patient's logical basis for contemplating suicide (i.e., in essence, the "reasons for dying"): Hopelessness, in turn, reflects the degree of certainty that these problems cannot change (Kovacs, Beck, & Weissman, 1975). Alternatively, characterization of the patient's strengths, resources, and assets provides a foundation on which therapy is based. Important areas for assessment include education, employment history, social support (i.e., family, friendships, and romantic relationships, both current and historical), and any past history of overcoming adversity. A "Reasons for Living List" is sometimes used to help suicidal patients objectively consider the future in relation to their strengths, hopes, aspirations, and goals (Linehan, Goodstein, Nielsen, & Chiles, 1983). The probabilities of future successes or satisfaction in areas such as romantic love, parenting or grandparenting, vocational/professional achievement, and leisure are examined from a more neutral vantage point (i.e., "If you are able to recover from this depression …"). Often, constructing the Reasons for Living List has a mood-lifting effect, making it an ideal strategy for the first session of therapy (Thase, 1994a). Patients frequently verbalize ANTs during this exercise, permitting a natural transition to psychoeducation about CBT, as described subsequently.

The cognitive model of psychopathology postulates that suicidal patients have an unrealistically negative appraisal of their situation, due in part to cognitive errors such as selective recall and overgeneralization. It is the therapist's task to help the patient view these difficulties from a less devastating perspective (see Table 6.3). Nevertheless, the phenomenon of depressive realism (i.e., the ability of a depressed person to perceive a negative event more accurately than a nondepressed person; Alloy & Abramson, 1988) should not be overlooked: *Bona fide* deficits in coping skills, interpersonal relationships, leisure-time activities, and vocational/professional spheres are commonplace and typically require therapeutic attention. However, depressive realism does not explain obviously distorted statements such as a college graduate's assertion that "I have failed at everything I've tried" or a parent's complaint that "No one has ever loved me."

During the first session, it is useful to encourage the patient take a more objective,

Table 6.3. Cognitive Formulations of Risk Factors Associated with Suicidal Behavior

Associated risk factor	Cognitive formulation
Physical Illness	Illnesses may sap energy, affect mood, and force inactivity. Some illnesses (e.g., malignancies or endocrinopathies) are associated with higher than expected rates of depression. Loss of well-being may activate schema pertaining to control, unfairness, or vulnerability. People overreliant on active methods of coping may be less able to tolerate distress. Life-threatening illnesses may trigger thoughts about mortality. Chronic or degenerative illnesses engender thoughts about declining abilities, disfigurement, unendurable pain, and so on.
Loss of a loved one	Grief may be accompanied by thoughts of death and, in extreme cases, fantasies to join the deceased. Divorce, separation, or romatic rejection may combine grief with feelings of humiliation. Both may activate schema related to lovability and intolerance of aloneness.
Poor social support	Disharmony in relationships increases the likelihood of conflict and reduces one's ability to tolerate other stresses. Conflict in key relationships provides situational context for automatic negative thoughts about self, world, and future. Lack of a confidante may prevent obtaining a neutral appraisal of an event.
Substance abuse	Acute or withdrawal effects of drugs or alcohol may lower mood and/or trigger mood-dependent cognitions. Most intoxicants decrease inhibitions, increasing the likelihood of impulsive behavior. Shame about substance abuse may trigger self-denigrating cognitions. Cravings or withdrawal symptoms may intensify feelings of being out of control.
Family history of suicide	Beyond neurobiology (see below), attitudes or superstitious beliefs about familial curses or predispositions may create a self-fulfilling prophecy.
Neurobiological correlates	Suicidal behavior is associated with low levels of serotonin metabolites in the central nervous system and hypercortisolism. The former may reflect a trait-like predisposition, the latter is a severity-linked correlate of the depressive state. Trait or state vulnerabilities require special attention in therapy (i.e., use of behavioral strategies or more frequent sessions to offset severity).
Older male status	Older men have the highest suicide rates. Choice of more violent means represents one reason, but declining productivity, loss of health, and related cognitions point to an evidence base underpinning perceptions of powerlessness and/or hopelessness.
Economic adversity	A major potential source of stress. Financial means are often considered an objective measure of one's worth. Loss of means is usually the result of bad luck, poor decision making, loss of employment, and/or poor money management. All may activate competence-based schema. Severe adversity may compromise and even abrogate long-term goals, negating plans for the future.

external view of situations. The therapist may ask questions such as, "What would you have said about that (i.e., attribute, situation, relationship, and so on), when you weren't so depressed?" or "What would your best friend (or boss or spouse) say about that?" By helping the depressed person shift perspective from a more biased point of view to a more objective one, a tangible improvement in mood is often achieved. Moreover, demonstration that the relationship between perception or meaning and mood is modifiable helps to establish another one of the fundamental concepts of CBT in the first hour of therapy.

6. *Explanation of the Cognitive Model and CBT Procedures*. The cognitive model of depression is introduced to the therapist with a brief statement, such as: "I'd like to take a few moments to explain the basic approach we use to understand and treat some of the active ingredients of depression." The interactions between moods (affects), actions (behaviors), and thoughts (cognitions) are illustrated using a simple diagram, such as the A-B-C triangle (see Figure 6.1). Next, the therapist uses several events from the patient's life over the several days to illustrate the model. The goal of this exercise is to make obvious the interdependence of affect, behavior, and cognition, underscoring the conclusion that there are several different avenues by which to effect change.

7. *Obtain Feedback*. The therapist may use this point of the session to "break" for feedback, such as the patient's impressions about the therapy so far. If there has been a major shift in mood at any point in the session, the therapist may inquire if the patient noticed this change. More often than not, recognition of a shift upwards will offer the opportunity for the patient to make a genuinely optimistic statement.

8. *Homework*. The use of homework is introduced at the end of the first session. The usual initial homework assignment is to request that the patient view a videotape describing cognitive therapy and/or read of the pamphlet *Coping With Depression* (Beck & Greenberg, 1974). The patient is also asked to write down his or her impressions and questions. Other individualized homework assignments may be recommended if indicated by the material addressed in the first session. Some patients feel demeaned by having to do homework. We have generally had success by emphasizing that the depression is manifest all day long, whereas the amount of time spent in therapy is much more limited. Similarly, the notion that CBT involves *learning* new methods with which to cope and master longstanding

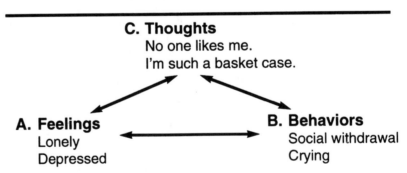

Figure 6.1. A-B-C Triangle illustrating the interrelationship of feelings (affects), actions (behaviors), and thoughts (cognitions) in depression.

problems provides a compelling rationale for the need to *practice*. It is important to make certain that (a) the general rationale for use of homework assignments is understood, and (b) the patient agrees to complete the assignment.

9. *Feedback*. The session ends with eliciting feedback about the patient's impressions, including worries or negative opinions about the first session of therapy. When questions or concerns arise, a nondefensive response will help to strengthen the treatment alliance. It is important for the therapist to express a genuine respect for the patient's skepticism and/or pessimism and not to convey an unrealistically positive view of the patient's condition.

Assessment of Level of Intervention

Following the first session, it is useful to assess the patient's functional capacity for therapy. This assessment includes consideration of symptomatic severity, level of hopelessness, sense of humor, mood reactivity, ability to concentrate and use abstract thought, and degree of behavior impairment, as well as impressions about the patient's level of motivation and capacity to collaborate. A high level of motivation and/or a more active coping style may offset, to some extent, a higher level of clinical severity (Burns, Rude, Simons, Bates, & Thase, 1994).

Patients may be grouped into one of three levels for supervisory and research purposes:

1. *Low level*: severe psychomotor retardation, anhedonia (e.g., virtually no involvement in meaningful or pleasurable activities), lack of mood reactivity (i.e., little sense of humor, few spontaneous mood shifts), markedly impaired concentration or attention, and/or significant difficulties engaging in the collaboration.
2. *Mid level*: moderate psychomotor retardation, impaired concentration, limited mood reactivity, some reduction of goal-directed behavior and/or overt skepticism or detachment from collaboration that lessens during the course of the session.
3. *High level*: mild or no psychomotor retardation, minimal or no problems with concentration, good range of mood reactivity, mild to moderate behavioral impairment and/or enthusiastic engagement in the session.

Most hospitalized patients meet criteria for the lower two levels of capacity for therapy. The remainder of the first treatment phase is tailored for such patients. These patients tend to do better when behavioral procedures and relatively simple cognitive techniques are emphasized in Phase 1. When patients with a high functional capacity are admitted, it is usually because of suicidal risk or nonresponse to somatic therapies. After Session 2, less severely impaired patients are typically able to proceed to the second treatment phase. Regardless of level of intervention, subsequent inpatient sessions are organized around a structured, coherent framework, including (1) setting an agenda; (2) reviewing homework; (3) working on selected agenda items, (4) eliciting feedback, and (5) assigning new homework.

Session 2

1. *Setting an Agenda*. The first agenda item is for the therapist to obtain feedback about the initial session. Questions might include "Have additional questions or 'second

thoughts' about CBT arisen?" "Are revisions of the problems list necessary?" A second agenda item is to inquire about the patient's well-being since the previous session. Thereafter, the remaining agenda items are noted, beginning with a review of the homework assignment.

2. *Reviewing the Homework.* Homework review is an important part of every session. The therapist needs to provide sincere verbal reinforcement of the patient's efforts to complete assignments. As in other forms of structured learning, overlooking assignments devalues homework and may decrease the likelihood of further compliance. Therapists too busy or overextended to have 100% spontaneous recall of particular homework assignments need to write down the assignment.

If the homework has not been completed, time within the session is allotted in order to finish the assignment. For example, the therapist may produce another copy of *Coping with Depression* for review during the session. Use of therapy time to make up unfinished homework is not intended to be punishment. Rather, it helps to establish the importance of the assignment and explicitly demonstrates the therapist's commitment that assignments are to be completed. The therapist should, *under no circumstances*, criticize the patient for not completing an assignment. It also is not helpful to attribute the noncompletion to some construct such as low motivation or "acting out."

3. *Activity Scheduling.* Daily-activity scheduling assignments are typically begun in the second session. The activity schedule provided in the *Coping with Depression* pamphlet is used during the session and completed for the past 24 to 36 hours (see Table 6.4). Most patients readily grasp the significance of the association between symptomatic worsening and inactivity, and demonstrating this relationship *in vivo* provides a powerful vehicle to teach about the downward spiral (see Figure 6.2). The downward spiral subsequently becomes a central model to examine changes in mood as a function of cognitions and/or behavior.

Table 6.4. Sample Activity Schedule for One Hospital Day

Time period	Activity[a]
0600	Woke up, showered (M_0, P_0, S)
0700	Went to breakfast (M_0, P_2)
0800	Attended morning focus group (M_2, P_0)
0900	Waiting for Drs.' rounds (M_0, P_0, S)
1000	Saw Drs. (M_0, P_0, S)
1100	Attended therapy group (M_3, P_2)
1200	Lunch (M_0, P_4)
1300	Attended relaxation group (M_4, P_5)
1400	"Quiet Time" in room (M_0, P_4, S)
1500	Met with therapist (M_4 P_2)
1600	Skipped exercise group (M_0, P_2, S)
1700	Dinner (M_0, P_4)
1800	Spoke with wife on phone (M_2, P_2, S)
1900	Watched televsion (M_0, P_2)
2000	Tried to read pamphlet (M_0, P_0, S)
2100	Went to bed—slept poorly (S)

[a]M = Mastery (competence), 0 (none)—10 (maximum)
P = Pleasure (enjoyment), 0 (none)—10 (maximum)
S = Suicidal ideation

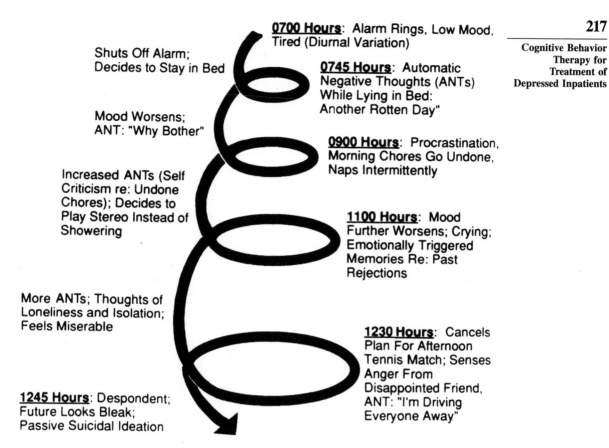

0700 Hours: Alarm Rings, Low Mood, Tired (Diurnal Variation)

0745 Hours: Automatic Negative Thoughts (ANTs) While Lying in Bed: Another Rotten Day"

Shuts Off Alarm; Decides to Stay in Bed

0900 Hours: Procrastination, Morning Chores Go Undone, Naps Intermittently

Mood Worsens; ANT: "Why Bother"

Increased ANTs (Self Criticism re: Undone Chores); Decides to Play Stereo Instead of Showering

1100 Hours: Mood Further Worsens; Crying; Emotionally Triggered Memories Re: Past Rejections

More ANTs; Thoughts of Loneliness and Isolation; Feels Miserable

1230 Hours: Cancels Plan For Afternoon Tennis Match; Senses Anger From Disappointed Friend, ANT: "I'm Driving Everyone Away"

1245 Hours: Despondent; Future Looks Bleak; Passive Suicidal Ideation

Figure 6.2. The downward spiral illustrating the interaction of affect, behavior, and cognition in triggering a worsening mood state.

The activity schedule is expanded in later sessions to include hour-by-hour ratings of mood, suicidal ideations, or particular patterns of negative thought. For most patients, a zero–10 scale is used to rate moods, with zero defined as *As Bad as Possible* and 10 defined as *Not at All Depressed*. Variability in mood ratings thus helps to establish functional relationships (among situations, behaviors, and particular cognitions). Alternate mood rating scales (i.e., zero–100) may be necessary for more severely depressed patients in order to establish mood variability.

Beyond its use for assessment, the activity schedule is typically the first behavioral method used to address depressive signs and symptoms. After identification of particular times of day in which mood is predictably worse (e.g., early morning, following "process" group, after visiting hours), preselected activities are scheduled to fill those time slots. Scheduled behaviors are drawn from a list or menu of highly reinforcing and/or distracting activities, including activities previously enjoyed by the patient and leisure-time activities on the unit. A distracting or pleasurable activity thus is used to build a floor or foundation to "block" a downward spiral.

Although activity scheduling is almost always helpful, its use is sometimes trivialized by higher functioning patients (e.g., "I can just run off and use the Nordic Track every time I get down!"). The therapist may use this opportunity to elicit "hotter" automatic negative thoughts (e.g., "This Mickey Mouse therapy won't work—my problems are too deep"), or may simply agree that activity scheduling is not, in and of itself, a complete treatment of severe depression. Rather, activity scheduling is viewed as a basic *starting* point to help improve coping.

Activity scheduling is next expanded to include mastery and pleasure (M and P) ratings (see Figure 6.2). M and P ratings are used to categorize reinforcing activities into domains of competence (Ms) and hedonic capacity (Ps). The patient is helped to rate Ms and Ps on the previous 24-hour activity schedule, again using a 10-part scale. Subsequently, scheduled activities may be used to increase the number and breadth of P activities. Conversely, deficits in M ratings typically provide the opportunity for cognitive interventions, as described subsequently.

4. *Other Agenda Items*. Other agenda items are selected from the problem list on an "as-needed" basis, as gauged by the patient's level of functioning and progress. For example, stimulus-control procedures and relaxation training (e.g., Bernstein & Borkovec, 1973) may be introduced to help patients cope with anxiety and insomnia. For less symptomatic patients, an introductory "lesson" on identification of cognitive distortions and automatic negative thoughts may be added to the agenda. Typically, the thought-recording technique is introduced at this time (see Table 6.5). The therapist begins the thought-recording exercise using a three-column sheet to write down the situation, the patient's mood, and the patient's thoughts. A question such as "What went through your mind just a moment ago?" helps to elicit automatic thoughts *in vivo*. Afterwards, the therapist may provide a wrist counter to help the patient keep track of selected types of negative thoughts. Alternatively, preprinted three-column forms may be provided to outline key situations, moods, and thoughts. Additional reading (e.g., Burns's [1980] self-help book, *Feeling Good*) also may be assigned.

5. *Feedback*. The therapist again uses each transition point in the session as an opportunity to ask for specific feedback and to clarify any misunderstandings or points of confusion that have arisen. Patients who remain markedly pessimistic about the potential value of therapy after two sessions may have a particularly poor prognosis (Whisman, 1993). As such, extra efforts on the part of the therapist are warranted to enhance engagement and collaboration.

6. *Homework*. The second session's homework assignment typically is to complete an activity log for the next 24 hours, with concomitant ratings of mood, mastery, and pleasure.

Table 6.5. Use of a Three-Column Sheet to Record Automatic Negative Thoughts in Relation to Situations and Moods

Date	Situation	Mood intensity (0–100%)	Automatic thoughts
5/29/94	Sitting in my room after doctors' rounds	Depressed (80%)	This new medicine won't work, just like the others. They just don't understand.
		Anxious (60%)	If I don't get better soon, I'll lose my job.
		Angry (40%)	Don't these guys know anything? Picking medicines is like guess work—where's the coin to flip?

Most patients also are able to begin thought recording using three-column sheets. More severely depressed patients may, instead, be assigned completion of a behavioral task. For example, 15 minutes of light exercise may be assigned each morning to help offset diurnal mood variation. More specific homework assignments to help patients manage suicidal ideation may include use of a distraction technique (e.g., positive imagery, talking to someone else, thought stopping). Similarly, a coping card may be filled out during the session for use afterwards (see Figure 6.3).

Session 3

1. *Setting the Agenda.* An agenda is collaboratively determined, including obtaining feedback about the previous session, reexamination of the problem list, review of homework, and identification of one or two topics for emphasis within the session. As appropriate, the therapist also may introduce specific behavioral strategies to help the patient cope with anxiety, ruminations, and/or insomnia.

2. *Homework.* Homework is reviewed in a supportive manner, reinforcing approximations of success. Noncompletion of homework is dealt with in a decisive fashion. For example, it may be useful to have the patient verbalize his or her thoughts about not doing the assignment. It is likely that the patient tried to initiate the assignment or at least thought about starting, only to encounter automatic negative thoughts (e.g., "Why bother—this won't really help"). This provides an excellent opportunity to begin cognitive interventions *in vivo.* As before, the assignment is determined within the session.

Review of the previous 24-hour activity log will almost always point to periods of dysphoria, particularly during times when the patient has been thinking about his or her problems, has felt alone, or has thought about family or loved ones. Periods of inactivity also are correlated with ratings of suicidal ideation, and mastery and pleasure.

3. *Illustration of the Cognitive Model.* The therapist begins this segment by again describing the reciprocal and interactive nature of thoughts, feelings, and behaviors. The

---

Coping Card

1. I'm in the hospital for treatment of an illness, depression, *not* because I'm weak.

2. It's normal to feel embarassed; most people do because of the stigma.

3. I can't control what people think about me. I can control how much I work on getting better.

4. This treatment is likely to help. The doctors are experts and they've helped many others.

Figure 6.3. An example of a Coping Card, to be used PRN to help manage automatic negative thoughts about hospitalization.

role of ANTs and distorted cognitive processes as mediators of behavior and affect is illustrated using several examples from the patient's activity schedule. The patient is encouraged to test the functional relationships between these domains.

Next, a recent three-column sheet is expanded in fuller form as the Daily Record of Dysfunctional Thoughts (DRDT; Young & Beck, 1982; see Table 6.6). In addition to columns for recording the situation, mood, and thoughts, the DRDT includes columns for "rational responses" and assessing changes in mood in response to the cognitive intervention. The therapist models generation of rational responses using one of the patient's recent three-column sheets.

New behavioral assignments intended to counteract periods of inactivity might include the patient's use of preferred hobbies as M and P activities during scheduled leisure-time periods. The patient is enlisted to help to identify novel ways in which these activities can be incorporated within the inpatient milieu, including recreational and occupational therapies. Family members also may be asked to bring in materials for pleasure (e.g., video games, crossword puzzles, needlework) and mastery (e.g., paperwork, income tax material) assignments.

It is important to caution patients not to expect a "normal" amount of pleasure to result from P activities. This is because of depressive anhedonia. In fact, depressive illness may be invoked as a mediating construct in order to explain the reduced salience of reinforcers. One method of coping with anhedonia is to set relatively low goals for performance. For example, the therapist may ask, "What if this gave you only a 20% pleasure rating? Is that an acceptable first goal?" Metaphors such as "priming the pump" may be used to help the patient to conceptualize the progressive nature of therapeutic interventions. Again, patients' thoughts and feelings about their activities provide a useful opportunity to elicit cognitive distortions.

Although behavioral interventions often still predominate at this point in therapy for more severely depressed patients, it is still useful for the therapist to introduce the concept of ANTs. When appropriate, the therapist helps the patient identify ANTs linked to feelings and behaviors. As noted earlier, shifts in mood observed *in vivo* provide invaluable opportunities to elucidate such relationships. It may be helpful to use a type of guided discovery, referred to as the downward-arrow technique (Burns, 1980), to help the patient better recognize more emotionally laden or "hot" ANTs (see Table 6.5).

4. *Symptom-Reduction Procedures.* At least half of each session with severely depressed patients typically is devoted to practicing behavioral strategies. A supplementary tape for relaxation training or a workbook assignment (e.g., Howell & Thase, 1991) also may be provided for the use between sessions.

5. *Other Agenda Items.* Incorporated as described in Session 2.

6. *Feedback.* The therapist obtains feedback about the session and helps to summarize what has been accomplished so far. Areas of ongoing difficulty are identified for emphasis in future sessions.

7. *Homework.* Homework assignments following the third session generally include continued use of the activity scheduling and M and P ratings. Graded task assignments may be assigned to increase participation in more demanding or complex activities. Thought recording and DRDT exercises also might be assigned. If relaxation training has been included in the treatment plan, time needs to be allotted for practice. Conditions conducive for mastering relaxation skills also need to be specified. Ancillary therapists (e.g., expressive arts therapists or nursing staff) may be enlisted to help patients practice relaxation skills. At least 1 hour each day is recommended for practice.

Table 6.6. Daily Record of Dysfunctional Thoughts (DRDT)

Situation	Emotion(s)	Automatic thought(s)	Rational response	Outcome
Describe: 1. Actual event leading to unpleasant emotion, or 2. Stream of thoughts, daydreams, or recollection leading to unpleasant emotion.	1. Specify sad/anxious/angry, etc. 2. Rate degree of emotion, 1–100%.	1. Write automatic thought(s) that preceded emotion(s). 2. Rate beliefs in automatic thought(s), 0–100%.	1. Write rational response to automatic thought(s). 2. Rate belief in rational response 0–100%.	1. Rerate belief in automatic thought(s), 0–100%. 2. Specify and rate subsequent emotions, 0–100%.
Date: 5/30/94				
Sitting in room during "quiet time"	Depressed, crying	I feel so bad. (100%)	I feel bad because I'm ill. My illness, depression, almost always responds to treatment.	I feel so bad. (80%)
		Why isn't the medicine working? (50%) (It won't work.)	I've gotten better before, and it will probably happen again.	Why isn't the medicine working? (It won't work.) (20%)
		I'll never get better (80%)	The new medicine takes time to get up to a therapeutic level—at lest, so far, I don't have bad side effects. I'm learning new skills to cope better with my illness.	I'll never get better. (20%)

Explanation: When you experience an unpleasant emotion, note the situation that seemed to stimulate the emotion. (If the emotion occurred while you were thinking, daydreaming, etc., please note this.) Then note the automatic thought associated with the emotion. Record the degree to which you believe this thought: 0% = *Not at All*; 100% = *Completely*. In rating degree of emotion: 1 = *A Trace*; 100 = *The Most Intense Possible*.

1. *Agenda*. The agenda is developed collaboratively for the fourth session, including obtaining feedback about the last session.

2. *Homework Review*. As in previous sessions. Successfully completed assignments are verbally reinforced and problems with the assignments are immediately dealt with, as described for Session 3.

3. *Relaxation Training (Optional)*. If relaxation training is being utilized, a major allocation of time within this session (i.e., 20 minutes) is devoted to practicing this skill and troubleshooting any difficulties. It should be recalled that some patients feel more anxious when trying to relax. For these individuals, alternate methods may need to be considered (see Bernstein & Borkovec, 1973)

4. *Applying a Cognitive Strategy to an Issue from the Problem List*. Virtually all hospitalized patients will have interpersonal conflicts, vocational problems, or other stressful issues on their problem lists that need to be addressed in therapy. The therapist helps the patient select an item from the problem list and the cognitive model is applied to the difficulty. The DRDT technique is well suited for this purpose. The patient is asked to visualize a recent *situation* related to the problem. The patient is then asked to describe his or her *mood* at the time and to verbalize, aloud, his or her *thoughts*. The patient's appraisal of the accuracy of these thoughts is obtained using a zero% to 100% rating. Socratic questioning is used to help the patient test out the validity of each thought in terms of the evidence, for and against, the "proposition" invoked by the ANT. Rational responses are then generated based on the evidence summary. Some patients may have difficulty using the DRDT method because they cannot generate more adaptive alternatives to the ANTs. In such cases, the therapist actively coaches and shapes verbalization of rational alternatives. The validity of the rational responses is similarly tested.

Some patients have an easier time testing the validity of ANTs using the analogy of a legal trial (Thase & Beck, 1993). From this perspective, each ANT is viewed as a charge or accusation. The patient's inherent belief in the ANTs and his or her disbelief in rational responses is viewed as analogous to the prosecution. It may be pointed out that, like the prosecution in a criminal trial, depressive information processing results in presentation of the "evidence" in the most convincingly skewed manner. This includes, on occasion, outright distortion of facts and suppression of evidence to the contrary. Moreover, just as the prosecution gets the opportunity to present their case first, the ANTs and dysfunctional attitudes in depression are similarly manifest *before* the patient is able to respond rationally.

The therapist–patient alliance represents the "defense" team. It is the defense's responsibility to examine the evidence in favor of the prosecution's case, rebut any "facts" based on cognitive distortions, and point out logical fallacies. Often, especially early in therapy, the prosecution has an advantage because of the patient's relative inexperience applying the rational-response method. However, with the therapist acting as the equivalent of a senior counsel, helping to guide the defense, the DRDT exercise proceeds by evaluating whether the patient is guilty of the charge. If there is evidence in support of a guilty charge, it is important to determine if there are any extenuating circumstances that might mitigate guilt or lessen the associated consequences.

Another useful exercise addresses depressive attributional style. The patient is asked to make the distinction between the uncontrollability of an event and the relative controllability of one's responses. As noted earlier, patients prone to develop depression in response to stressful events tend to attribute their problems to an internal (i.e., personal) cause, with global consequences of an enduring impact (Abramson, Metalsky, & Alloy, 1989). Questions, such as "How much are you *really* responsible for this problem?" and "What you can do to cope better with this problem?" are posed to help the patient develop a more objective perspective and more effective responses.

5. *Feedback.* As before, the patient's understanding of the session's material is reviewed, as is his or her overall sense of progress.

6. *Homework.* A relevant homework assignment is developed from the session's material. Homework assignments include continued use of targeted behavioral assignments and the DRDT. Building on initial successes, the therapist and patient may identify a new activity that demands an even greater level of mastery. The impact that depression, as an illness, has on energy, concentration, and motivation is invoked to account for decreased productivity, shifting the attribution away from internal causal constructs (e.g., weakness, laziness, incompetence). Particularly large tasks that are perceived as overwhelming may be approached using the graded task assignments. This method subdivides large tasks into well-defined and more readily manageable "chunks." Initially, completion of a certain amount of time "on task" may be used as the criterion for success rather than completion of the entire task. It is important to define what constitutes a success beforehand, with explicit recognition that goals must take into account that the patient is unable to perform at his or her usual level. For example, spending 30 minutes on the task "paying the bills" would be the agreed-on criterion for success, not the number of checks written.

Session 5

1. *Agenda.* The agenda incorporates any new developments. This is particularly true for patients who made impulsive, low-lethality suicide attempts, for whom discharge may be imminent. As this is the end of the first phase of therapy, the agenda also includes discussion of the patient's evaluation of the treatments progress. The BDI and Hopelessness Scale are repeated to help quantify degree of improvement.

2. *Homework Review.* Each session provides the opportunity for the therapist to continually reinforce successes and shape close approximations.

3. *Therapy Topics.* At least two agenda topics are identified to work on (e.g., graded task assignments, identification of automatic thoughts, or a DRDT exercise pertaining to a situation eliciting suicidal ideation or feelings of hopelessness). At least 20 minutes are devoted to each topic.

3. *Feedback.* Obtain feedback about the session.

4. *Homework and Weekend Planning.* With the weekend in mind, the patient is encouraged to anticipate difficulties and plan for managing the "down" times that inevitably characterizes a weekend in the hospital. Appropriate homework tasks are identified, typically drawing on the material covered in this session. An activity schedule is developed for Saturday and Sunday, incorporating pleasurable activities and therapeutic tasks for both days. Goals for the weekend generally should be modest.

6. *Treatment-Team Update.* A conference between the therapist and the remainder of the inpatient treatment team is planned to coincide with the end of the first phase of therapy.

7. *Family Update.* The first phase of therapy also includes at least one session with the patient's spouse or significant other. The purpose of this meeting is to gather additional history, educate the family about CBT, and answer any questions about CBT. The family session also may be used to engage the significant other in conjoint CBT sessions if marital disorder has been included on the problem list.

Michael E. Thase

1. *Overview.* Therapy is necessarily individualized during the second phase of treatment, although each session continues to follow the consistent structure established during the first phase of treatment. This includes (a) agenda, feedback, and homework review; (b) focused attention to two or three specific problem areas; and (c) summary of session, feedback, and homework assignments.

The second phase begins with a review of the problem list and, if appropriate, revisions based on progress to date. The pace of therapy is dictated by the symptomatic progress made during the preceding phase, particularly with respect to symptomatic improvement. Suggested therapeutic approaches for patients who have achieved significant symptomatic improvements, a more modest level of improvement, or virtually no improvement are outlined later.

2. *Significant Improvements.* Patients who have improved after only three to five sessions undoubtedly had the best prognoses to begin with, perhaps facilitated by the structure and support of inpatient CBT. These patients are typically ready for more intensive work using the cognitive component of the therapy. Most of these patients will already be planning a pass home. Activity scheduling, relaxation training, and other behavioral strategies are faded or continued, with decreased emphasis. More specific attention is now devoted to: (a) identification of ANTs and use of the DRDT technique; (b) identification of specific cognitive errors, using the labels described by Burns (1980) to define them (see Table 6.1); (c) organization of automatic thoughts into themes in order to facilitate identification of schema; and (d) preparation for discharge.

A small number of rapidly improving patients may claim that their suicide attempt was a "mistake" and minimize their need for therapy. Relieved family members or loved ones also may endorse this view, perhaps in part because of their discomfort with the stigma of hospitalization. The long-term course of such individuals is not well documented and it is conceivable that they are correct. Thus, the therapist bases any subsequent intervention on explicit respect for the patient's viewpoint. In the spirit of collaboration, the therapist asks if the patient has considered the possibility that the problems that led to the suicide attempt may resurface after discharge. It is useful to help the patient recreate the time leading up to the suicide attempt, in order to better understand the thoughts and feelings that, however transiently, justified dying. Patients who are unwilling to engage in such an exercise may still be provided psychoeducation about depression and the risks of relapse and recurrence.

3. *Modest Improvement.* Patients who have achieved a more modest degree of improvement usually benefit from more practice using cognitive interventions, although their level of symptomatology typically warrants continued use of activity scheduling and graded task assignments. Despite a slower pace, DRDT sheets should be used in every session. Thoughts elicited within-session often provide the best targets for these interventions.

Depending on the patient's overall progress and the available family support, weekend passes also may be considered. The focus of the passes is often quite structured (e.g., going to a movie or a restaurant with a friend or with a significant other).

4. *No Improvement.* Management of patients who have experienced little reduction in symptoms requires special attention. This includes detailed review of the problem list, short-term goals, expectations, and collaboration. It is important to establish that the patient's low level of symptomatic improvement is not a rational basis for discouragement. Specific psychoeducation about average hospital length of stay for patients receiving

various types of antidepressant therapy is usually helpful. Impatience for quicker improvement (on the part of the patient, family, or a team member) is addressed in a nondefensive manner, using the cognitive model to understand discouragement as a consequence of ANTs and distorted information processing. It is also important for therapists to be aware of their own demoralization, as illustrated by ANTs such as the following: (a) "This patient doesn't have depression—it's a personality disorder"; (b) "I can't treat this patient with CBT, he (or she) has a biological depressive syndrome"; or (c) "This patient doesn't want to get better."

It is similarly essential to deal with developing impatience or frustration from treatment team members. An empirical stance is always preferred. Data from our group suggests that only a minority of nonpsychotic, nonbipolar patients have depressions that respond poorly to CBT alone (Thase et al., 1993; Thase, 1994a) and concomitant use of antidepressant medication further mitigates this concern.

A therapist's creativity is called upon to identify possible missing ingredients in the treatment plan. This process may draw liberally from the methods outlined in more recent writings (e.g., Beck et al., 1990; Persons, 1989; Wright, Thase, & Sensky, 1993). Particular attention is given to persistent suicidal ideation and explicit understanding of the patient's phenomenological field: What is it that still makes suicide a logical solution? Finite, even molecular, steps away from this position are identified and appropriate interventions are implemented. Planned activities may need to be reduced and focused more specifically on events that are highly reinforcing. The daily exercise schedule may be intensified and shifted to morning, when diurnal mood variation is at its worst. Conversely, the therapy appointment may be shifted to the late afternoon, or even early evening, for the same purpose. An evening staff member may need to be identified to provide more intensive coaching to ensure that specific assignments are completed.

For those patients who are not well enough to take a weekend pass, detailed weekend-activity schedules are developed, along with carefully specified homework assignments. Weekend plans are reviewed with the nursing staff, and shift-by-shift assignments are delegated. Phase 2 concludes with a treatment-team meeting and discussion of plans for the following week.

Phase 3—Sessions 11–15

1. *Overview.* The individualized approach utilized during the second phase of therapy continues, with sessions following the structure and pace as described earlier. The third phase begins with a review of the problem list and progress made to date. New goals for the coming week are established. Common issues for this phase of therapy are summarized here.

2. *Treatment Strategies.* The therapist and patient collaboratively identify treatment methods that have been helpful and those that have been relatively ineffective. Ineffective strategies may have been mistimed, misguided, or indifferently applied. Next, the treatment plan is revised with input from the remainder of the treatment team.

Generally, attention is now focused on the successful application of the DRDT and other cognitive techniques. Generalization of interventions from within-session to *in vivo* application of the rational-response technique is critical to the ultimate success of this method. Review of audiotapes of several previous sessions can be particularly helpful. Attention also may be paid to long-standing schematic or attitudinal issues, such as those related to excessive interpersonal dependence or perfectionism.

Alternate interventions may include (a) use of other "active" behavioral interventions (i.e., role playing, assertiveness training, therapist's modeling of behaviors, and behavioral rehearsal); (b) increasing the focus on developing solutions to ongoing or anticipated life problems that may be helping to maintain hopelessness; (c) increasing the use of strategies to enhance emotional experiences within sessions, such as imagery or guided recall of relevant upsetting events; or (d) increased attention to the role of anger in maintaining the patient's dysphoria, such as by capitalizing on the coincidental emergence of anger during a session state or rehearsing methods to control inappropriate anger.

As the end of the third phase of treatment approaches, attention is always given to anticipated difficulties following discharge. Passes are planned whenever possible; most patients will be discharged the following week, even if only partially remitted. Weekend passes address improvement in psychosocial functioning, stability of mood outside of the hospital, and ability to use CBT skills in the natural environment (Thase, 1993b). Expectations again need to be tempered, whereas discouraging areas of difficulty revealed during passes may point to important revisions in the treatment plan.

A major reevaluation of the treatment plan should be considered for patients who have not benefited following 3 weeks of CBT. The expense and associated family burden resulting from a prolonged hospitalization warrant such intensive management. If appropriate, changes in pharmacotherapy or a trial of electroconvulsive therapy also should be considered.

Therapy during the final phase of inpatient treatment also includes some preparation for anticipated difficulties after discharge. It is useful to begin by identifying longer term goals. A frank assessment of vocational and interpersonal deficits is performed to identify factors that may interfere with goal attainment. Long-term plans to address these deficits may thus be developed. For example, dissatisfaction and/or poor performance in the workplace often result from inadequate training or education. In such cases, retraining in another line of work might be considered. If appropriate, the hospital's neuropsychological assessment service may be consulted to help facilitate a plan for vocational retraining. Often, there are very real and understandable situations that have led to underemployment, such as an unplanned pregnancy, family difficulties, attention-deficit disorder or learning disability, or an unrecognized episode of depression in adolescence or during college. Clarifying the impact of such factors on one's career path may have a powerful effect on attributions about the "cause" of underachievement. Alternatively, the individual may have unrealistically high expectations for success (i.e., outstripping his or her talents and capabilities). Interventions in this latter scenario include exploration of dysfunctional attitudes and schemas that may underpin such unrealistic appraisals.

With respect to predischarge preparation, the narrower focus of the final week of therapy specifically deals with the following questions pertinent to the patient: (a) "What problems will I encounter when I leave the hospital? What will stress me?" (b) "What am I likely to feel when stressed?" (c) "What are the likely automatic negative thoughts accompanying my reaction to stress?" (d) "What are my warning signs for worsening depression?" (e) "What have I learned in the hospital to help me cope with these reactions? What are my likely rational responses?"; and (f) "What can I do if my coping strategies aren't working?"

These questions need to be addressed during the final two sessions, providing the basis for at least several homework assignments. The remaining issues, of course, can be examined in continuation therapy.

Another predischarge task is termination with the inpatient unit's staff and patients.

The intensity of the inpatient experience may make termination difficult and, at times, ANTs regarding issues of friendship, dependency, desertion, and responsibility for the well-being of others are activated. Such reactions are readily addressed by cognitive techniques such as the DRDT.

AFTERCARE

Discharge from psychiatric hospitalization is seldom the end point of treatment; perhaps it should never be. Most patients are discharged in partial remissions and have only tenuously restabilized social supports. Moreover, the first several months following discharge are times of high risk for relapse (Thase, 1993b). Clinical correlates of relapse include high residual depression ratings, inadequate social support, and significant, ongoing life stress (Belsher & Costello, 1988; Hooley & Teasdale, 1989; Thase, 1993b). Careful attention to continuity of care and discharge planning are the therapist's principal strategies to help offset such vulnerability.

Outpatient continuation therapy is recommended for all patients who have been treated as inpatients (Thase, 1993b). In our experience, such continuation treatment provides additional support during the time of transition from inpatient to outpatient status, facilitates consolidation and guided practice of new skills learned, and promotes further work on relapse prevention. As Miller et al. (1989a, 1989b) have demonstrated, such extra efforts may have notable results.

We have found the outpatient treatment manual of Beck et al. (1979) must be modified somewhat for continuation (posthospitalization) treatment (Thase, 1993b). For example, we have extended the average course of outpatient therapy from 4 months up to 6 months (Thase, 1993b). Most patients should be seen initially twice weekly and, when justified by marked symptomatic worsening, even more frequent sessions may be indicated. We have observed minor symptomatic worsening, as defined by up to a 25% increase in HRSD or BDI scores, in up to half of unmedicated patients during the month after discharge (Thase, 1993b). It is likely, although not empirically established, that patients receiving concomitant pharmacotherapy would have had a more stable posthospital course (e.g. Miller et al. 1989b). Termination of outpatient CBT should *not* be considered until patients have achieved and maintained a complete remission (Thase et al. 1992).

ACKNOWLEDGMENT. Completion of this manual was supported in part by grants MH-41884 and MH-30915 (MHCRC) from the National Institutes of Mental Health. We thank Ms. Lisa Stupar for her assistance in preparation of the manuscript.

REFERENCES

Abramson, L., Metalsky, G., & Alloy, L. (1989). Hopelessness depression: A theory-based subtype of depression. *Psychological Review, 96,* 358–372.

Abramson, L., Seligman, M., & Teasdale, J. D. (1978). Learned hopelessness in humans: Critique and reformulation. *Journal of Abnormal Psychology, 87,* 49–74.

Alloy, L., & Abramson, L. (1988). Depressive realism: Four theoretical perspectives. In L. Alloy (Ed.), *Cognitive processes in depression* (pp. 223–265). New York: Guilford Press.

American Psychiatric Association. (1987). *Diagnostic and statistical manual of mental disorders* (3rd ed., rev.). Washington, DC: Author.

Barker, W. A., Scott, J., & Eccleston, D. (1987). The Newcastle Chronic Depression Study: Results of a treatment regime. *International Clinical Psychopharmacology, 2,* 261–272.

Beck, A. T. (1976). *Cognitive therapy and the emotional disorders.* New York: International Universities Press.

Beck, A. T., Freeman, A., Pretzer, J., Davis, D., Fleming, B., Ottaviani, R., Beck, J., Simon, K., Padesky, C., Meyer, J., & Trexler, L. (1990). *Cognitive therapy of personality disorders.* New York: Guilford Press.

Beck, A. T., & Greenberg, R. L. (1974). *Coping with depression (a booklet).* New York: Institute for Rational Living.

Beck, A. T., Kovacs, M., & Weissman, A. (1975). Hopelessness and suicidal behavior: An overview. *Journal of the American Medical Association, 234,* 1146–1149.

Beck, A. T., Rush, A. J., Shaw, B. G., & Emery, C. (1979). *Cognitive therapy of depression.* New York: Guilford Press.

Beck, A. T., Steer, R., Kovacs, M., & Garrison, B. (1985). Hopelessness and eventual suicide: A 10-year prospective study of patients hospitalized with suicide ideation. *American Journal of Psychiatry, 142,* 559–563.

Beck, A. T., Weissman, A., Lester, D., & Trexler, L. (1974). The measurement of pessimism: The Hopelessness Scale. *Journal of Consulting and Clinical Psychology, 42,* 861–865.

Bellack, A. S., Hersen, M., and Himmelhoch, J. (1981). Social skills training compared with pharmacotherapy and psychotherapy in the treatment of unipolar depression. *American Journal of Psychiatry, 138,* 1562–1567.

Belsher, G., & Costello, C. G. (1988). Relapse after recovery from unipolar depression: A critical review. *Psychological Bulletin, 104,* 84–96.

Bernstein, D. A., & Borkovec, T. C. (1973). *Progressive relaxation training: A manual for the helping professions.* Champaign, IL: Research Press.

Bishop, S., Miller, I. V., Norman, W., Buda, M., & Foulke, M. (1986). Cognitive therapy of psychotic depression: A case report. *Psychotherapy, 23,* 167–173.

Bowers, W. A. (1989). Cognitive therapy with inpatients. In A. Freeman, K. M. Simon, L. E. Beutler, & H. Arkowitz (Eds.), *Comprehensive handbook of cognitive therapy* (pp. 583–596). New York: Plenum Press.

Bowers, W. A. (1990). Treatment of depressed inpatients. Cognitive therapy plus medication, relaxation plus medication, and medication alone. *British Journal of Psychiatry, 156,* 73–78.

Bowler, K. A., Moonis, L. J., & Thase, M. E. (1993). The role of the nurse in the cognitive milieu. In J. H. Wright, M. E. Thase, A. T. Beck, & J. W. Ludgate (Eds.), *The cognitive milieu: Inpatient applications of cognitive therapy* (pp. 247–270). New York: Guilford Press.

Burns, D. (1980). *Feeling good: The new mood therapy.* New York: Morrow.

Burns, D. D., Rude, S. T., Simons, A. D., Bates, M. A., & Thase, M. E. (1994). Does learned resourcefulness predict the response to cognitive behavioral therapy for depression? *Cognitive Therapy and Research, 18,* 277–291.

Coccaro, E., Siever, L., Klar, H., Maurer, G., Cochrane, K., Cooper, T., Mohs, R. R., & Davis, K. (1989). Serotonergic studies in patients with affective and personality disorders: Correlates with suicidal and impulsive aggressive behavior. *Archives of General Psychiatry, 46,* 587–599.

Cochran, S. D. (1984). Preventing medical noncompliance in the outpatient treatment of bipolar affective disorders. *Journal of Consulting and Clinical Psychiatry, 52,* 873–878.

Costello, C. G. (1972). Depression: Loss of reinforcers or loss of reinforcer effectiveness. *Behavior Therapy, 3,* 340–347.

Covi, L., & Lipman, R. S. (1987). Cognitive–behavioral group psychotherapy combined with imipramine in major depression. *Psychopharmacological Bulletin, 23,* 173–177.

Coyne, J. C., & Gotlib, I. H. (1983). The role of cognition in depression: A critical appraisal. *Psychology Bulletin, 94,* 472–505.

de Jong, J. A., & Roy, A. (1990). Relationship of cognitive factors to CSF corticotropin-releasing hormone in depression. *American Journal of Psychiatry, 147,* 350–352.

de Jong, J. A., Treiber, R., & Henrich, G. (1986). Effectiveness of two psychological treatments for inpatients with severe and chronic depressions. *Cognitive Therapy Research, 10,* 645–663.

DeRubeis, R. J., & Feeley, M. (1990). Determinants of change in cognitive therapy for depression. *Cognitive Therapy Research, 14,* 469–482.

Dobson, K., & Shaw, B. (1986). Cognitive assessment with major depressive disorders. *Cognitive Therapy and Research, 10,* 13–29.

Dubé, S., Dobkin, J. A., Bowler, K. A., Thase, M. E., & Kupfer, D. J. (1993). Cerebral perfusion changes with antidepressant treatment in depression. *Biological Psychiatry, 33,* 47A.

Eaves, G., & Rush, A. (1984). Cognitive patterns in symptomatic and remitted unipolar major depression. *Journal of Abnormal Psychology, 93,* 31–40.

Elkin, I., Shea, M. T., Watkins, J. T., Imber, S. D., Sotsky, S. M., Collins, J. F., Glass, D. R., Pilkonis, P. A., Leber, W. R., Docherty, J. P., Fiester, S. J., & Parloff, M. B. (1989). National Institutes of Mental Health Treatment of Depression Collaborative Research program: General effectiveness of treatments. *Archives of General Psychiatry, 46,* 971–982.

Fawcett, J., Scheftner, W., Clark, D., Hedeker, D., Gibbons, R., & Corywell, W. (1987). Clinical predictors of suicide in patients with major affective disorders: A controlled prospective study. *American Journal of Psychiatry, 144,* 35–40.

Ferster, C. B. (1973). A functional analysis of depression. *American Psychologist, 28,* 857–870.

Freeman, A., & Reinecke, M. A. (1993). *Cognitive therapy of suicidal behavior: A manual for treatment.* New York: Springer.

Garamoni, G. L., Reynolds, C. F. III, Thase, M. E., Frank, E., Berman, S. R., & Fasiczka, A. L. (1991). The balance of positive and negative affects in major depression: A further test of the states of mind model. *Psychiatry Research, 39,* 99–108.

Haaga, D. A. F., Dyck, M. J., & Ernst, D. (1991). Empirical status of cognitive theory of depression. *Psychology Bulletin, 110,* 215–236.

Hamilton, E., & Abramson, L. (1983). Cognitive patterns and major depressive disorders: A longitudinal study in a hospital setting. *Journal of Abnormal Psychology, 92,* 173–184.

Hammen, C., Ellicott, A., Gitlin, M., & Jamison, K. R. (1989). Sociotropy/autonomy and vulnerability to specific life events in patients with unipolar depression and bipolar disorders. *Journal of Abnormal Psychology, 98,* 154–160.

Hersen, M., Bellack, A. S., Himmelhoch, J. M., and Thase, M. E. (1984). Effects of social skill training, amitriptyline, and psychotherapy in unipolar depressed women. *Behavior Therapy, 15,* 21–40.

Hooley, J. M., & Teasdale, J. D. (1989). Predictors of relapse in unipolar depressives: Expressed emotion, marital distress, and perceived criticism. *Journal of Abnormal Psychology, 98,* 229–235.

Howell, J. R., & Thase, M. E. (1991). Beating the blues: Recovery from depression. In D. C. Daley (Ed.), *Insight to recovery: A practical workbook series for mental health disorders* (pp. 1–27). Skokie, IL: G. T. Rogers Production.

Kovacs, M., Beck, A., & Weissman, A. (1975). The use of suicidal motives in the psychotherapy practice of attempted suicides. *American Journal of Psychotherapy, 29,* 368–383.

Liberman, R., & Eckman, T. (1981). Behavior therapy vs. insight-oriented therapy for repeated suicide attempters. *Archives of General Psychiatry, 38,* 1126–1130.

Linehan, M. M., Armstrong, H. E., Suarez, A., Allmon, D., & Heard, H. L. (1991). Cognitive–behavioral treatment of chronically parasuicidal borderline patients. *Archives of General Psychiatry, 48,* 1060–1064.

Linehan, M., Goodstein, J., Neilsen, S., & Chiles, J. (1983). Reasons for staying alive when you are thinking of killing yourself: The Reasons for Living Inventory. *Journal of Consulting and Clinical Psychology, 51,* 276–286.

Ludgate, J. W., Wright, J. H., Bowers, W., & Camp, G. F. (1993). Individual cognitive therapy with inpatients. In J. H. Wright, M. E. Thase, A. T. Beck, & J. W. Ludgate (Eds.), *Cognitive therapy with inpatients. Developing a cognitive milieu* (pp. 91–120). New York: Guilford Press.

Malone, K. M., Thase, M. E., Mieczkowski, T., Myers, J. E., Stull, S. D., Cooper, T. B., & Mann, J. J. (1993). Fenfluramine challenge test as a predictor of outcome in major depression. *Psychopharmacology Bulletin, 29,* 155–161.

Markowitz, J. C. (1989). "Meat-and-potatoes" inpatient psychotherapy. *Hospital Community Psychiatry, 40,* 877.

Miller, I., & Norman, W. (1986). Persistence of depressive cognitions within a subgroup of depressed inpatients. *Cognitive Therapy and Research, 10,* 211–224.

Miller, I. W., Norman, W. H., & Keitner, G. I. (1989a). Cognitive–behavioral treatment of depressed inpatients: Six- and twelve-month follow-ups. *American Journal of Psychiatry, 146,* 1274–1279.

Miller, I. W., Norman, W. H., & Keitner, G. I. (1990). Treatment response of high cognitive dysfunction depressed inpatients. *Comprehensive Psychiatry, 31,* 62–71.

Miller, I. W., Norman, W. H., Keitner, G. I., Bishop, S. T., & Dow, M. G. (1989b). Cognitive–behavioral treatment of depressed inpatients. *Behavior Therapy, 20,* 25–47.

Miranda, J., & Persons, J. (1988). Dysfunctional attitudes are mood-state dependent. *Journal of Abnormal Psychology, 97,* 76–79.

Monroe, S. M., & Simons, A. D. (1991). Diathesis–stress theories in the context of life stress research: Implications for the depressive disorders. *Psychology Bulletin, 110,* 406–425.

Nezu, A. M. (1986). Efficacy of a social problem-solving therapy approach for unipolar depression. *Journal of Consulting Clinical Psychology, 54,* 196–202.

Padesky, C. A. (1993). Staff and patient education. In J. H. Wright, M. E. Thase, A. T. Beck, & J. W. Ludgate (Eds.), *Cognitive therapy with inpatients: Developing a cognitive milieu* (pp. 393–413). New York: Guilford Press.

Persons, J. B. (1989). *Cognitive therapy in practice: A case formulation approach.* New York: Norton.

Robins, C. J., & Hayes, A. M. (1993). An appraisal of cognitive therapy. *Journal of Consulting and Clinical Psychology, 61,* 205–214.

Rosen, H. (1989). Piagetian theory and cognitive therapy. In A. Freeman, K. Simon, L. Beutler, & H. Arkowitz (Eds.), *Comprehensive handbook of cognitive therapy* (pp. 189–212). New York: Plenum Press.

Ross, M., & Scott, M. (1985). An evaluation of the effectiveness of individual and group cognitive therapy in the treatment of depressed patients in an inner city health centre. *Journal Royal College of General Practitioners, 35,* 239–242.

Roy, A., Agren, H., Pickar, D., Linnoila, M., Doran, A., Cutler, A., Cutler, N., & Paul, S. (1986). Reduced cerebrospinal fluid homovanillic acid and lower ratio of homovanillic acid to 5-hydroxyindolacetic acid in depressed patients: Relationship to suicidal behavior and dexamethasone nonsuppression. *American Journal of Psychiatry, 143,* 1539–1545.

Roy, A., & Linnoila, M. (1988). Suicidal behavior, impulsiveness, and serotonin. *Acta Psychiatrica Scandinavica, 78,* 529–535.

Salkovskis, P. M., Atha, C., & Storer, D. (1990). Cognitive–behavioral problem solving in the treatment of patients who repeatedly attempt suicide: A controlled trial. *British Journal of Psychiatry, 157,* 871–876.

Samson, J. A., Mirin, S. M., Hauser, S. T., Fenton, B. T., & Schildkraut, J. J. (1992). Learned helplessness and urinary MHPG levels in unipolar depression. *American Journal of Psychiatry, 149,* 806–809.

Schotte, D., & Clum, G. (1987). Problem–solving skills in suicidal psychiatric patients. *Journal of Consulting and Clinical Psychology, 55,* 49–54.

Schwartz, R. M., & Garamoni, G. L. (1986). A structural model of positive and negative states of mind: Asymmetry in the internal dialogue. In P. C. Kendall (Ed.) *Advances in cognitive–behavioral research and therapy* (Vol. 5, pp. 1–62). New York: Academic Press.

Scott, J. (1988). Cognitive therapy with depressed inpatients. In W. Dryden, P. & Trower, *Developments in cognitive psychotherapy* (pp. 177–189). London: Sage.

Scott, J. (1992). Chronic depression: Can cognitive therapy succeed when other treatments fail? *Behavioral Psychotherapy, 20,* 25–36.

Shaw, B. F. (1981). Cognitive therapy with an inpatient population. In G. Emery, S. D. Hollon & R. C. Bedrosian (Eds.), *New directions in cognitive therapy* (pp. 29–49). New York: Guilford Press.

Shaw, B. F. (1984). Specification of the training and evaluation of cognitive therapists for outcome studies. In J. B. W. Williams & R. L. Spitzer (Eds.), *Psychotherapy research: Where we are and where we should go?* (pp. 173–189). New York: Guilford Press.

Simons, A. D., Epstein, L. H., McGowan, C. R., Kupfer, D. J., & Robertson, R. J. (1985). Exercise as a treatment for depression: An update. *Clinical Psychology Review, 5,* 553–568.

Simons, A. D., Garfield, S. L., & Murphy, C. E. (1984). The process of change in cognitive therapy and pharmacotherapy for depression. *Archives of General Psychiatry, 41,* 45–51.

Spangler, D. L., Simons, A. D., Monroe, S. M., and Thase, M. E. (1993). Evaluating the hopelessness model of depression: diathesis-stress and symptom components. *Journal of Abnormal Psychology, 102,* 592–600.

Stuart, S., & Thase, M. E. (1994). Inpatient applications of cognitive-behavior therapy: A review of recent developments. *Journal of Psychotherapy Practice and Research, 3,* 284–299.

Thase, M. (1993a) Inpatient cognitive-behavioral therapy of depression. In E. Liebeneuft, A. Tasman, & S. A. Green (Eds.). *Less time to do more: Psychotherapy on the short-term inpatient unit* (pp. 111–140). Washington, DC: American Psychiatric Association Press.

Thase, M. E. (1993b). Transition and aftercare. In J. H. Wright, M. E. Thase, A. T. Beck, & J. W. Ludgate (Eds.), *Cognitive therapy with inpatients: Developing a cognitive milieu* (pp. 414–435). New York: Guilford Press.

Thase, M. E. (1994a). Cognitive-behavior therapy of severe unipolar depression. In L. Grunhaus, & J. Greden, *Severe depressive disorders.* Washington, DC: American Psychiatric Press, *44,* 269–296.

Thase, M. E. (1994b). After the fall: Cognitive behavior therapy of depression in the "post-collaborative" era. *The Behavior Therapist, 17,* 48–52.

Thase, M. E., & Beck, A. T. (1993). An overview of cognitive therapy. In J. H. Wright, M. E. Thase, A. T. Beck, & J. W. Ludgate (Eds.), *Cognitive therapy with inpatients: Developing a cognitive milieu* (pp. 3–34). New York: Guilford Press.

Thase, M. E., Bowler, K., & Harden, T. (1991). Cognitive behavior therapy of endogenous depression: Part 2. Preliminary findings in 16 unmedicated patients. *Behavior Therapy, 22,* 469–477.

Thase, M. E., & Howland, R. (1994). Refractory depression: Relevance of psychosocial factors and therapies. *Psychiatric Annals, 24,* 232–240.

Thase, M. E., & Simons, A. D. (1992). Cognitive behavior therapy and relapse of nonbipolar depression: Parallels with pharmacotherapy. *Psychopharmcology Bulletin, 28,* 117–122.

Thase, M. E., Simons, A. D., McGeary, J., Cahalane, J. F., Hughes, C., Harden, T., & Friedman, E. (1992). Relapse after cognitive behavior therapy of depression: Potential implications for longer courses of treatment? *American Journal of Psychiatry, 149,* 1046–1052.

Thase, M. E., Simons, A. D., & Reynolds, C. F. III (1993). Psychobiological correlates of poor response to cognitive behavior therapy: Potential indications for antidepressant pharmacotherapy. *Psychopharmacology Bulletin, 29,* 293–301.

Thase, M. E., Wright, J. H. (1991). Cognitive behavior therapy manual for depressed inpatients: A treatment protocol outline. *Behavior Therapy, 22,* 579–595.

Vallis, T. M., Shaw, B. F., & Dobson, K. S. (1986). The cognitive therapy scale: Psychometric properties. *Journal of Consulting and Clinical Psychology, 54,* 381–385.

Weissman, A., & Beck, A. T. (1978). *Development and validation of the dysfunctional attitude scale,* Paper presented at the Annual Meeting of the Association for the Advancement of Behavior Therapy, Chicago, IL.

Whisman, M. A. (1993). Mediators and moderators of change in cognitive therapy of depression. *Psychology Bulletin, 114,* 248–265.

Whisman, M. A., Miller, I. W., Norman, W. H., & Keitner, G. I. (1991). Cognitive therapy with depressed inpatients: Specific effects on dysfunctional cognitions. *Journal of Consulting and Clinical Psychology, 59,* 282–288.

Wright, J. H., & Schrodt, G. (1989). Combined cognitive therapy and pharmacotherapy. In A. Freeman, K. Simon, L. Beutler, & H. Arkowitz (Eds.), *Comprehensive handbook of cognitive therapy.* New York: Plenum Press.

Wright, J. H., & Thase, M. E. (1992). Cognitive and biological therapies: A synthesis. *Psychiatric Annals, 22,* 451–458.

Wright, J. H., Thase, M. E., Beck, A. T., & Ludgate, J. W. (1993). *Cognitive therapy with inpatients: Developing a cognitive milieu.* New York: Guilford Press.

Wright, J. H., Thase, M. E., & Sensky, T. (1993). Cognitive and biological therapies: A combined approach. In J. H. Wright, M. E. Thase, A. T. Beck & J. Ludgate (Eds.), *Cognitive therapy with inpatients: Developing a cognitive milieu.* New York: Guilford Press.

Young, J. E., & Beck, A. T. (1982). Cognitive therapy: Clinical applications. In A. J. Rush (Ed.), *Short-term psychotherapies for depression* (pp. 182–214). New York: Guilford Press.

Young, J. E., & Lindemann, M. D. (1992). An integrative schema-focused model for personality disorders. *Journal of Cognitive Psychotherapy, 6,* 11–23.

7

Biobehavioral Treatment and Rehabilitation for Persons with Schizophrenia

Stephen E. Wong and Robert P. Liberman

INTRODUCTION

Unlike other maladies described in this text, schizophrenia is a disorder that pervades all aspects of human functioning (cognitive, affective, instrumental, social interaction) and has protean manifestations. Therefore, a comprehensive approach to treatment must have multiple aims:

1. Amelioration or elimination of positive symptoms (e.g., delusions, hallucinations, thought disorder) and negative symptoms (e.g., apathy, amotivational syndrome, blunted affect) of the disorder.
2. Remediation of functional deficits in social, instrumental, educational, and occupational domains using instructional technology and behavior analysis and therapy.
3. Alleviation or control of deviant and disturbing behaviors that are associated with the symptoms and may be the individual's immature and counterproductive way of meeting his or her instrumental and affiliative needs (e.g., modification of oppositional behavior).
4. Improvement of the personal well-being and subjective quality of life of the afflicted individual.

Stephen E. Wong • School of Social Service Administration, University of Chicago, Chicago, Illinois 60637.   **Robert P. Liberman** • Clinical Research Center for Schizophrenia, Department of Psychiatry, University of California at Los Angeles School of Medicine, Rehabilitation Services, Veterans Affairs Medical Center, Brentwood Division, Los Angeles, California 90073.

Sourcebook of Psychological Treatment Manuals for Adult Disorders, edited by Vincent B. Van Hasselt and Michel Hersen. Plenum Press, New York, 1996.

This chapter describes biobehavioral interventions for the treatment and rehabilitation of these key problem areas. The procedures have evolved from a union of psychiatric rehabilitation (Liberman, 1992) and behavior analysis and therapy techniques (Wong, Massel, Mosk, & Liberman, 1986). Recognizing that social context and physical setting are major determinants in the types of treatment and rehabilitation that can and should be implemented, interventions in this chapter are divided into two sections. The first section reports on two of a series of intensive skills training modules designed by Liberman and associates at the University of California at Los Angeles (UCLA) Clinical Research Centers. The modules discussed here cover topics of Medication and Symptom Management and Skills Training and Cognitive Deficits of Schizophrenia. These modules have a structured format that incorporates didactic techniques and participant exercises to convey clinical information and specific behavioral skills.

The second section of this chapter concerns behavioral programs for residential and community settings derived from contingency-management systems developed in psychiatric hospitals (Allyon & Azrin, 1965, 1968; Liberman, Wallace, Teigen, & Davis, 1974). Contingency-management systems, such as token economies, provided the first dramatic demonstrations that learning principles could be effectively applied in the rehabilitation of chronic mental patients. Given the deinstitutionalization movement and limited resources allocated to community mental health services in this country (Kiesler & Sibulkin, 1987), there is need for efficacious, low-intensity programs that can be applied in outpatient, residential-treatment, and group-home settings. In contrast to hospital programs, community-based approaches should be relatively simple, easy to implement, and closely patterned around individual client capabilities and goals. We discuss and give examples of these programs in the latter half of this chapter.

SELF-MANAGEMENT OF SYMPTOMS AND MEDICATION

Patients with major mental disorders no longer are content to assume a passive role, but now insist on being informed consumers who collaborate with their professional caregivers. The growing consumerism movement has converged with other advances to make the potential for self-management feasible and successful. Building on the high rate of symptomatic remission among individuals with recent-onset schizophrenia, clinical innovations and developments that combine to improve self-directed treatment and positive outcomes include destigmatization of mental illness, improved symptom relief from newer antipsychotic drugs; optimistic follow-up data regarding the course of schizophrenia, the emergence of skills training technology that overcomes the cognitive deficits associated with schizophrenia; the active coping role that helps limit the intrusion of symptoms into everyday life; and the demonstrations of the effectiveness of integrated, comprehensive, and coordinated systems of mental health delivery.

What was formerly viewed as the patient's failure to comply is now seen as faulty communication between patient and clinician, or restricted accessibility (or outreach efforts) to the mental health delivery system. For example, a patient's failure to continue on maintenance antipsychotic medication does not necessarily derive from lack of motivation by the patient, but from inadequate education of the patient about medication benefits and side effects, a rupture in the therapeutic alliance, or failures in the mental health service delivery system. the task for the care provider becomes mobilization of the patient's assets and resources (including the family) to cooperate in a treatment partnership, sharing responsibilities for adherence to mutually agreed treatment prescriptions.

Because of the chronic and relapsing nature of schizophrenia, the patient or his or her family members must understand the stress-related, neurobiological nature of the disorder and develop a close working alliance with their therapists. Failure to educate and engage patients and their caregivers in a long-term, collaborative, and informed therapeutic alliance results in noncompliance with essential antipsychotic medication, psychosocial treatments, and supportive services. The most common barriers to this alliance in treatment can be divided into five domains, as depicted in Table 7.1.

Modules for Training Medication and Symptom Self-Management

A series of user-friendly, highly prescriptive, multimedia programs for training social and independent living skills has been designed by Wallace, Liberman and their associates at the UCLA Clinical Research Center for Schizophrenia and Psychiatric Rehabilitation (Liberman et al., 1993, Wallace et al., 1985). Termed *modules* because they can be readily "plugged into" and implemented by existing treatment programs without wholesale and radical restructuring of the program, the modules in the UCLA Social and Independent Living Skills Program can be reliably used by a wide array of mental health and rehabilitation professionals and paraprofessionals. Two modules have been validated in controlled field trials for their effectiveness in teaching patients to become more responsible and reliable consumers of maintenance antipsychotic medication and psychiatric services—the *Medication and Symptom Management Modules* (Psychiatric Rehabilitation Consultants, 1995).

Each module is a curriculum for teaching a particular area of skills required for survival and adaptation in the community, including instrumental skills, such as medication self-management, symptom self-management, money management, and job finding, as well as affiliative skills (e.g., basic conversation, friendship, dating). Each module is divided into a series of "skills areas," like chapters of a book, that encompass specific educational objectives and desired behaviors. For example, in the fourth skill area of the *Medication Management Module*, "Negotiating Medication Issues with Health-Care Pro-

Table 7.1. Barriers to Patient Collaboration in Treatment and Examples of Corrective Measures

Barrier	Corrective measures
Treatment techniques (side effects)	Educate patients about side effects and their management.
Patient characteristics (cognitive disorganization)	Teach self-monitoring techniques to patient
Family characteristics (unrealistic expectations)	Encourage family participation in psychoeducation and support groups
Clinician–patient relationship	Help patient and family members to set and attain realistic, incremental goals; offer lavish reinforcement when they are achieved and even for effort.
Treatment delivery system (lack of coordination)	Use case managers and continuous-treatment teams with capability for assertive outreach to coordinate services.

viders," patients learn how to describe to their physician their specific side effects with clarity and in sufficient detail, while using assertive and friendly communication skills. The subjects and skills areas for two of the modules produced by the UCLA Clinical Research Center are listed in Table 7.2. Each skills area of each module is taught using the same, highly prescribed sequence of seven structured learning activities, as shown in Table 7.3.

Two other advantages of the modular approach to skills training have enabled the innovators to overcome obstacles to dissemination of this technology, namely, local programmatic constraints in adopting an innovation and difficulty in training the trainers. The modular design of the UCLA skills training program permits any institution or community-based program to literally "plug in" one or more of the modules into existing programs, without having to terminate or radically revamp other elements of the program that are serving patients well. No wholesale renovation of a clinical enterprise is necessary, because the modules are relatively "free-standing" and compatible with a wide range of clinical and theoretical orientations. Previously validated psychosocial and behavioral treatment and rehabilitation programs, such as the Fairweather Lodge, the Fountain House Psychosocial Club, and the Token Economy–Social Learning Program, suffered limited dispersion because they required major restructuring of existing programs (Backer et al., 1986).

Another obstacle that had to be overcome for widespread distribution and use of skills

Table 7.2. Skills Areas and Goals of the Two UCLA Modules for Training Social and Independent Living Skills and Skills Areas for Medication Management

Skills areas	Goals
1. Obtaining information about anti-psychotic medication	To gain an understanding of how these drugs work, why maintenance drug therapy is used, and what benefits result from taking medication.
2. Knowing correct self-administration and evaluation of medication	To learn appropriate procedures in taking medication and how to evaluate responses to medication daily.
3. Identifying side effects of medication	To learn the side effects that sometimes result from taking medication and what can be done to alleviate these problems.
4. Negotiating medication issues with health-care providers	To practice ways of getting assistance when problems occur with medication (e.g., how to call the hospital or doctor, and how to report symptoms and progress).
5. Use long-acting injectable medication	To desensitize fears of injections and learn benefits of biweekly or monthly injectable medication.

Skills areas for symptom management

1. Identify warning signs of relapse	To learn how to identify personal warning signs and monitor them with assistance from others.
2. Managing warning signs	To learn to use specific techniques for managing warning signs and develop an emergency plan.
3. Coping with persistent symptoms	To learn how to recognize persistent symptoms and use techniques for coping with them.
4. Avoiding alcohol and street drugs	To learn about the adverse effects of alcohol and ilicit drugs, and how to avoid them.

1. Introduction to skills area	Introducing the topic and component skills required for managing your medication safely and effectively.
2. Videotape and questions/answers	Viewing the videotape scene and demonstrating assimilation of knowledge of skills, with question-and-answer review
3. Role play	Acting out the skills in behavioral rehearsal.
4. Resource management	Discussing the resources needed to perform the skills.
5. Outcome problems	Solving problems associated with using the skills.
6. *In vivo* exercises	Performing exercises in real-life situations with health-care providers in settings outside training class.
7. Homework assignments	Completing assignments away from the group.

training was the time-consuming requirements for "training the trainers." In over a decade of training psychiatric residents and psychology interns, Liberman and his colleagues were able to graduate only a few dozen competent skills trainers. Competence and confidence in using the more generic approaches to social skills training took apprentices approximately 3 to 5 months of weekly sessions under the tutelage of a mentor and role model. With the skills training encapsulated in a modular format, including a "cookbook" manual for trainers or therapists and a professionally produced videocassette to demonstrate the skills to patients, trainees from all the mental health disciplines could learn effective skills delivery to patients with only 8 to 12 hours of exposure and practice.

Because direct care of chronically mentally ill patients is being increasingly assumed by paraprofessionals who do not have the graduate education necessary to implement complex methods (Graziano & Katz, 1982), the prescriptive form of the module is perforce "user-friendly." Modules are written in a step-by-step manner so that only minimal effort is required to plan and conduct the training sessions for each day. Moreover, the specific prescriptions outlined in each module's trainer's manual make it possible for one trainer to carry out a module on Monday and have a second trainer pick up where the class left off the next day. Moreover, patients can begin the module as inpatients and continue with their learning as outpatients. Modular skills training packages are easily monitored and evaluated, a necessary requirement for quality assurance, treatment-outcome research, and program evaluations.

The UCLA modules specify seven learning activities that trainers use to facilitate patients' skills acquisition. First, an *introductory* learning activity briefly reviews the behaviors that will be taught in the skills area and builds motivation for patients to participate actively in the learning activities that follow. This introductory step serves as an advanced organizer, preparing the patient for *videotape* presentation of the skills area and a subsequent *question-and-answer* period. The videos are professionally produced with actors assuming the roles of patients modeling the skills targeted for training, with clear annotation by a narrator and text subtitles to compensate for patients' cognitive deficits. The question-and-answer segment facilitates both the assessment and the subtle shaping of "receiving" skills or accurate social perception.

Once patients have observed the models demonstrating skills on the video, they have an opportunity to practice the skills in *role plays*. This learning activity assesses both "processing" skills (What different alternatives are possible to address this role play?). and "sending" skills (how successfully did the individual incorporate paralinguistic and non-verbal components in their role play?)."Processing" and "sending" skills are increased to a criterion performance level via trainer's prompts and feedback. Performance feedback and learning can be enhanced by making video recordings of behavior rehearsals and replaying the video to allow the individual, and the group as a whole, to offer performance feedback. Group members are instructed to provide positive comments ("What did you like about the way that John handled that task?") and to avoid the aversive impact of criticisms.

In addition to performance of requisite skills, individuals must learn to garner necessary "resources" to accomplish the targeted instrumental or affectional goal. *Resource management,* the next learning activity, assists patients to (1) understand what is a resource, (2) identify the range of resources necessary to attain a specific goal, and (3) determine how to obtain resources. For example, resources necessary to arrange a doctor's appointment include a phone directory, a telephone, a calendar, and a pad of paper. Individuals who do not have their own phone can overcome this shortcoming with a quarter and use of a public phone.

Despite mastery of targeted skills and the presence of sufficient resources, several unforeseen obstacles may arise as barriers to future performance of learned skills. The *outcome-problems* learning activity introduces the patient to stepwise problem solving necessary to overcome unplanned barriers. For example, what should the patient do when he or she calls the doctor's office for an appointment and gets repeated busy signals, must listen to an automated message from a machine, or is told that the doctor's receptionist is away from her desk? In this learning activity, aspects of the barrier are identified ("receiving" skills) and alternative methods that may remove the barrier are brainstormed ("processing" skills). For example, the patient can call back, ask to make an appointment with someone other than the receptionist, or call another doctor for an appointment. From these alternatives, the patient is instructed to choose a solution with the proviso that one choice is not necessarily superior to another; if this choice later fails, selecting a second choice is a reasonable alternative. The solution is then carried out in role-play fashion for further training of verbal and nonverbal "sending" skills.

A variety of strategies to promote generalization of skills acquired in therapeutic environments has been designed for the modular form of social skills training (Corrigan, Schade, & Liberman, 1992; Liberman, Nuechterlein, & Wallace, 1982; Morrison & Bellack, 1984). These include the problem-solving techniques embedded in the *resource-management* and *outcome-problem* learning activities of each module. Two final learning activities are also directed at improving the transfer of skills to novel, untrained situations. *In vivo* training requires the patient to carry out the newly acquired skills in real-life, individually meaningful situations with the trainer present to aide the person should a barrier become insurmountable (Liberman et al., 1984). After the patient is able to implement the skills without ancillary assistance, *homework* is assigned to independently carry out the newly acquired skills in real-life situations with the trainer present to assist the person, if necessary (Liberman et al., 1984). After the patient is able to implement the skills without ancillary assistance, *homework* is assigned to independently carry out the newly acquired skill in other real-life settings. Patients who are able to implement homework "pass" the learning criteria for the particular skills area of each module and can move on to the next skills area.

The stepwise, procedural instructions for teaching patients with schizophrenia how to identify their warning signs of relapse in preparation for developing a "Relapse Prevention Plan" are provided here as an excerpt from the third learning activity, *Role-play*, from the first skills area ("Identifying Warning Signs of Relapse") of the *Symptom Management Module*.

Remarks to Trainer

The role plays here are designed to reinforce what has been learned in the videotape and questions and answers, and to give patients an opportunity to practice communication skills.

The Role play A for this skills area is a role reversal: Your cotrainer plays the patient and asks questions about how to prevent or minimize relapse; the patient becomes the therapist and answers the cotrainer's questions. In the role-play script, use the patient's personal warning signs.

Although it will seem repetitious, be sure to ask each patient all questions provided in the script. Prompt patients as much as necessary to elicit correct responses.

The purpose of Role play B is to emphasize the importance of involving others in recognizing warning signs. In a later exercise, patients will ask for help in identifying warning signs, probably from the person they choose now. Therefore, this role play is important, because it will enable patients to practice communication skills needed to request help from an appropriate person.

You and your cotrainer should first perform a model role play demonstrating good communication skills. Then, have your cotrainer role-play with patients so you can observe, prompt, and comment on performances.

At first, ask for volunteers to perform role plays. Those who are reluctant may be helped by gentle prompting or positive requests, or by observing others perform. If they continue to refuse, assure them that they will have an opportunity to do the role play later. Emphasize that role plays are actually fun and a good way to learn the material.

It is vital that you praise patients' efforts, no matter how awkward they may be.

Materials needed include the following:

Two chairs
VCR and monitor
Video camera
Blank videotape
Warning Signs Checklist (p. 67 in manual; p. 31 in workbook)
Poster or blackboard listing communication skills
Communication Skills (p. 28 in manual, p. 11 in workbook)

Steps include the following:

1. Read the instructions to group.
2. Set up props and video equipment.
3. Describe role-play scenario; explain five cues.
4. Choose patient to perform role play; ask questions.

5. Perform role play.
6. Review role play; give positive feedback.
7. Complete section of Progress Checklist for this exercise for each patient

Read to Group

I'm glad to see you here and ready to begin practicing some of the skills you saw on the videotape. You did an excellent job answering questions about the video. Now, by role-playing you'll learn more about how to identify warning signs, and you'll have a chance to practice communication skills.

Before we begin, be sure you have your Warning Signs Checklist because (cotrainer) will need to look at it during the role play. Also, let's review Communication Skills on page 11 in your workbook.

You and your cotrainer should perform a model role play.

Do you have any questions?

Set Up Props and Video Equipment; Describe Role-Play Scenario; Explain Five Cues

Now you're going to be the therapist and (cotrainer) will be a patient who is concerned about having a relapse. During the role play, (cotrainer) will come to you and ask for help. So think about what you heard and observed in the videotaped scenes, because you learned the answers to (cotrainer's) questions in those scenes.

As the therapist, there are five things I want you to be sure to do:

1. Explain as best you can how to prevent or minimize a relapse.
2. Explain what warning signs are, and help (cotrainer) decide if the symptoms he or she is experiencing are warning signs.
3. Tell (cotrainer) to go to the doctor when he or she has those symptoms.
4. Tell (cotrainer) to monitor his or her symptoms daily. And,
5. Tell him or her to ask for help from people who are close to him (her).

When it's your turn to do the role-play, give (cotrainer) your Warning Signs Checklist so he or she can use it during the role play.

During the role play, have your cotrainer use the warning signs each patient identified in the Checklist.

Do you have any questions?

Choose First Patient for Role Play; Ask Questions

Ask for a volunteer. If no one volunteers, choose a patient to perform the role-play using his or her Warning Signs Checklist. Provide as much prompting as necessary to ensure that each patient includes the five cues.

Question	Response
What is (cotrainer's) role in this scene?	A patient who's concerned about having a relapse.
What is your role in this scene?	I'm a therapist.

What five things are you supposed to do in this scene?

Explain how to prevent or minimize a relapse.

Explain what warning signs are, and help (cotrainer) decide if he or she is experiencing warning signs.

Tell (cotrainer) to go to the doctor when he or she has those symptoms.

Tell (cotrainer) to monitor his or her symptoms daily.

Tell him or her to ask for help from people who are close to him or her.

Perform role play with each patient

Question	*Response*
I appreciate your seeing me (patient). I'm concerned about having a relapse, and I wonder if there's any way a relapse can be prevented?	Well, you may not be able to prevent a relapse, but the chances can be minimized if you recognize your warning signs in time and do something about them.
What are warning signs?	Those are the symptoms that indicate a relapse may be coming on.
Can you help me find out what my warning signs are?	I'll try. What symptoms did you notice before your last relapse?
Well, I (use patient's warning signs). Is that what you mean?	Yes, those are warning signs.
Is there anything I can do before I have the symptoms?	Yes, if you monitor your symptoms daily, you'll know when they change or get worse. And, take your medication regularly.
That sounds like a good idea. Is there anything else I can do?	You can ask people who are close to you to help you.
How can they help?	They can tell you when they see changes in you behavior that may mean a relapse is coming on.
Talking to people about my illness makes me uncomfortable. Will you help me tell them about my warning signs?	Sure. I'd be glad to help you.
Thank you. I feel much better now.	You're welcome.

Review Role Play; Provide Positive Feedback

Give abundant positive feedback for all efforts. If role play is taped, have group review the performance. Discuss the role play and the content of conversations. Ask each patient what he or she liked about the performance, and what he or she learned from it. Elicit only positive feedback and do not allow patients to criticize one another. Avoid direct statements that anyone is wrong.

Complete Progress Checklist for Each Patient and Determine Whether Additional Training Is Needed

SKILLS TRAINING AND COGNITIVE DEFICITS OF SCHIZOPHRENIA

Formal thought disorder and distractibility can interfere with the patient's participation in skills training modules. Several strategies that can help to overcome these difficulties and thereby improve the patient's learning capacity, are listed in Table 7.4. In general, instructional techniques used in the field of special education for the learning disabled may be an appropriate analogy for psychosocial rehabilitation strategies with incoherent and distractible patients. For example, an attention-focusing approach has been employed to enhance social skills training with cognitively disordered patients (Liberman et al., 1985; Massel et al., 1991). This strategy is characterized by multiple, relatively short, attention-training sessions embedded within more traditional social skills training modules. During these sessions, if the patient provides either no answer or an incorrect response to an "opener" made by a confederate, then the trainer prompts the patient to either repeat the opener or again try to respond. Correct responses are praised and reinforced with suitable material and social rewards. Thought-disordered patients who may be initially ineligible to participate in the classroom format of the modules may achieve "mainstreaming" after intensive training in attention focusing.

Diminishing environmental background noise can improve skills learning as well. Patients are easily distracted by events occurring around them. Thus, training rooms should be relatively quiet and set aside from clinic areas, where traffic, interruptions, or other distractions are frequent. We have found that module sessions should be scheduled on a biweekly basis or more frequently to maximize learning effects and diminish the adverse impact of the short-term memory problems exhibited by schizophrenics (Liberman & Green, 1992). When working with outpatients whose transportation problems impede frequent attendance at a clinic or mental health center, training might be fruitfully "exported" to the patients' residential settings, because modules are portable and require only a VCR and video monitor. Alternatively, transportation by van service can often achieve the desired regularity of attendance that will help to compensate for the cognitive deficits that can impair learning.

Table 7.4. Remedial Strategies for Some Cognitive Deficits of Schizophrenia

Cognitive deficits	Remedial strategy
1. Hyperaroused by overstimulating milieu	Diminish external distractors, ambient noise, likely interruptions.
2. Difficulty sustaining attention over time	Keep training tasks brief and focused. Use frequent prompts to regain attentional focus. Use incentive program and self-management to improve prearranged attention goals.
3. Distracted by irrelevant cues	Keep training site uncluttered of stimuli not germane to modular skill areas.
4. Misinterpret learning points	Post charts that explain skills areas.
5. Difficulty with speeded tasks	Proceed slowly through training steps.
6. Easily overloaded by complex tasks	Conduct task analysis and break tasks down into simpler substeps.
7. Influenced by immediate stimuli in the environment	Avoid accidental pairing of extraneous variables by providing immediate feedback and reinforcement. After overlearning has occurred, gradually fade feedback and reinforcers.
8. Distracted by hallucinations and poor associations	Adopt thought-stopping techniques. Self-monitor disordered thought and hallucinations and avoid stressors that may exacerbate them.

A variety of strategies involving memory aids and devices, the assistance of others, and self-management techniques can help patients compensate for cognitive disorganization. Circumventing this problem might require minimizing the complexity of treatment regimens by using telephone calls, compartmentalized pill boxes, and reminders for patients to take their medications; using cognitive rehabilitation techniques to improve the patient's memory and attention; teaching the patient self-monitoring techniques; and enlisting caregivers' assistance in monitoring compliance.

Evidence is accumulating that deficits in memory and sustained selective attention may be "rate-limiting" factors in the success and efficiency of skills training programs, such as the UCLA Social and Independent Living Skills modules (Bowen, 1988; Corrigan & Storzbach, 1992). Thus, future research should be directed toward answering the question, "Can social skills training, utilizing the modular approach developed at the UCLA Clinical Research Center, be demonstrated to have a salutary effect on the cognitive deficits of persons with schizophrenia?" Whether it is more efficient to overcome cognitive deficits before having a schizophrenic person enter a skills training program (as in the attention-focusing method described earlier) or whether skills training itself can improve cognitive functioning must await further investigation of psychosocial treatment development.

One issue that has been raised questions the utility of a problem-solving emphasis in the UCLA modules (Bellack et al., 1990), because normal individuals do not consciously utilize the step-by-step sequence inherent in the problem-solving training. However, abundant evidence exists showing that schizophrenics lack problem-solving ability (Donahoe et al., 1990) and that episodes of relapse appear to produce a regression in schizophrenics' problem-solving skills (Sullivan et al., 1990). Just as a stroke victim undergoing physical therapy must learn to use a cane or walker in order to resume ambulatory skills, persons with schizophrenia may also need the "cognitive prosthesis" of the deliberate and systematic application of the problem-solving steps to negotiate the sometimes stressful pathways of everyday life in the community. An "artificial" support, such as using the problem-solving steps, may make the difference between community adjustment or institutionalization for persons with cognitive impairments. Evidence from the UCLA Clinical Research Center suggests that schizophrenics can indeed improve their problem-solving ability when exposed to training through the medium of the Interpersonal Problem-Solving Module (Eckman, 1992).

Summary

The preceding pages introduced two components from the UCLA Social and Independent Living Skills Modules. In addition to those mentioned above, modules exist for teaching Basic Conversational Skills, Recreation for Leisure, Grooming and Personal Hygiene, Job Finding, and Community Reentry. Further information on these materials may be obtained from Psychiatric Rehabilitation Consultants, Box 6022, Camarillo, California, 93011-6022.

BEHAVIORAL TREATMENT IN RESIDENTIAL AND COMMUNITY SETTINGS

In this section, we shift our attention to the challenge of assisting clients with schizophrenia to achieve their optimal level of independent functioning with behavioral programs in open settings. Teaching independent living skills to clients with schizophrenia can be a formidable undertaking, but the difficulty is amplified in open settings in which only modest staff and material resources are available for therapeutic purposes. Treatment programs often must be carried out by paraprofessionals, and interventions may be competing with detrimental influences from the nearby community (e.g., illicit drugs, criminal activity, urban social disorganization). On the positive side, almost every community contains the basic resources needed for normal life, and when treating clients within this context, the importance of acquiring functional skills is obvious to staff and clients alike.

Rather than focusing on pathological symptoms, the present programs concentrate on teaching and motivating clients to perform adaptive behaviors. To do this, behavioral programs restructure elements of clients' social and physical environments. Antecedent stimuli, such as staff instructions, actions modeled by others, posted announcements, and other cues in clients' home and work settings are used to prompt desired responses. Consequent stimuli, such as social approval, material goods, privileges, and other forms of positive reinforcement are then administered to strengthen the desired behavior. Behavioral programs build upon clients' existing repertoire by gradually increasing requirements and demands as clients demonstrate competence at a task. When a skill is firmly established, contrived prompts and reinforcers are gradually withdrawn to allow natural consequences to maintain the behavior. Community-based behavioral programs steadily strive for client normalization and are ideally situated to promote use of trained skills in real-life situations.

Behavioral interventions for open settings must be compact and practical. Preferably, they should be part of a community adjustment program that fosters self-reliance in self-care, social, vocational, and recreational domains. Data collection systems, essential feedback mechanisms for behavioral programs, must be streamlined so that the effort they require does not jeopardize the treatment plans that they are designed to monitor. The following pages contain brief treatment plans covering the following problem or skill areas:

Delusional verbalizations
Oppositional behavior
Bizarre stereotypic behavior
Social (conversational) skills
Grooming and hygiene
Prevocational skills
Community/independent leisure skills

These programs are applicable in residential treatment centers, community reentry programs with supervised apartment-living arrangements, and group homes.

PROGRAM TO REDUCE DELUSIONAL VERBALIZATIONS—GEORGE B.

Background

Recently, various staff members have reported that George has been approaching them and making weird and fantastic statements. George has a history of this problem, which periodically emerges and then disappears for unknown reasons. One factor that might be contributing to the increase in George's delusional talk is the presence of new staff and students at the center who are intrigued with George's outlandish claims. We intend to treat this disorder with positive reinforcement for appropriate speech plus redirection and extinction for delusional speech. The plan starts by using staff attention as the reinforcer (Moss & Liberman, 1975), but adds tangible reinforcement if attention alone is ineffective (Patterson & Teigen, 1973; Wincze, Leitenberg, & Agras, 1972). (Note: Staff members considered using a cognitive–behavioral intervention [Chadwick & Lowe, 1990, 1994; Lowe & Chadwick, 1990] to challenge George's delusional beliefs and reshape more appropriate statements; however, it was considered impractical to apply this approach in the group-living situation.)

Data Collection and Analysis

George's delusional verbalizations are defined as false statements that have grandiose or self-persecutory content. Examples include: "I am a professional assassin for the CIA," or "My sperm and parts of my brain have been removed." Because this is a relatively low-frequency behavior, staff should be able to record the number of times it occurs per work shift (i.e., frequency from 7:00 A.M. to 3:00 P.M., 3:00 P.M. to 11:00 P.M., and 11:00 P.M. to 7:00 A.M.).

Treatment Procedures

1. All new staff and interns are notified that delusional verbalization is one of George's targeted problem behaviors and that they should avoid prompting this type of speech or possibly reinforcing it with extra attention. In addition, they are given a copy of this program to refer to.
2. When George begins talking about one of the aforementioned topics, remind him that he is engaging in one of the problem behaviors listed in his treatment plan ("George, Isn't this one of the fantastic stories that you are supposed to stop telling people?").
3. Attempt to *redirect* him to more appropriate behavior ("George, was there anything *else* you would to talk to me about now?" or "What do you think about the movie we saw yesterday?").
4. If George responds to redirection, converse with him in a pleasant manner. When the discussion is over, praise him for speaking appropriately ("See you later. I enjoyed our conversation").
5. If the client does not respond to redirection, tell him that you will not be talking to him about that delusional topic ("George, I am not going to talk with you about your fantasy surgery") and ignore subsequent verbalizations related to that subject. If George persists in trying to get your attention, restate your unwillingness to discuss fantasy topics, but once again offer to talk about realistic subjects.
   Tangible reinforcement: Applied if contingent attention proves ineffective.
6. George will be able to earn one token or one point (Point Store redemption value of approximately 10 cents) for each minute of appropriate speech with staff that is free of delusional content. George must complete the entire conversation without any trace of delusional speech to obtain the reinforcer (e.g., 10 minutes of appropriate speech with one delusional remark at the end of the encounter earns zero points). Utilize all of the procedures listed here and at the end of the conversation with George, tell him how many points he earned for speaking sensibly.

Background

Tom has been mentioned in recent staff meetings concerning his problem in getting up in the morning and his refusals to participate in various therapy groups. On two occasions when staff attempted to get Tom to meet standard expectations, he responded with profanity and aggressive threats. We are addressing these issues by consulting with Tom's psychiatrist to see if his night medications are making him drowsy in the morning, as well as by contacting his family to investigate some apparently unsettling phone calls from home. The present program attempts to reduce the likelihood that the problem behavior will occur by modifying antecedent and consequent events in the residential setting (Mace & Roberts, 1993; Wong, Woolsey, Innocent, & Liberman, 1988b).

Data Collection and Analysis

While this plan was being assembled, staff have been asked to collect data on the frequency of problems in getting up in the morning (defined as requiring more than three prompts to get out of bed) and refusing to participate in therapy groups (defined as verbally refusing to take part in an activity or leaving more than 5 minutes before the activity is finished). The pretreatment/baseline data will be compared to the data obtained while this program is being implemented to evaluate its effectiveness.

Treatment Procedures

Morning Wake-up

Several steps will be taken to prevent Tom from having problems in getting up on time. Tom's case manager will discuss this problem with him and attempt to increase his motivation by rearranging his schedule so that he has more preferred activities occurring in the morning. Tom will also be encouraged to go to bed an hour earlier. Because he enjoys watching late-night movies, he will be allowed to videotape them for viewing during dinner at 6:00 P.M., if he has arisen on time that day. Staff will also use a set routine in waking Tom:

1. The night before, meet with Tom and check to see that he has set his alarm clock for 6:00 A.M. Help him do this, if necessary.
2. At 6:05 A.M. open Tom's bedroom door and give him the first wake-up call.
3. Around 2 minutes later, turn on Tom's bedroom lights and give him a second wake-up call.
4. Around 5 minutes after that, give Tom his third wake-up call and shake him gently on the shoulder to rouse him.
5. If Tom does not wake up after his third wake-up call, allow him to oversleep and experience the natural consequences of his actions.

From now on, Tom will earn a larger proportion of his daily points for getting up on time. The number of points Tom can earn for waking up on time and being civil to staff will be increased from 20 points to *50* points.

247

**Biobehavioral
Treatment of
Schizophrenia**

Refusing Therapy Groups

Although Tom's refusals are not entirely predictable, he often has problems in group community meetings and in group sports activities. We will use different approaches to improve participation in these two group activities.

Since Tom voices a strong dislike of group sports (e.g., baseball, volleyball), and the treatment team is not committed to raising his interest in these activities, Tom will be allowed to earn his evening activity points for a suitable alternate physical activity. Discussions between Tom and staff have identified 20 minutes of walking or bike riding as acceptable alternate activities.

The treatment team feels that Tom *must* attend community meetings to be a member of the group and to stay informed of new residential rules and events. To increase Tom's interest and personal involvement in those meetings, he has agreed to assume responsibility for reading the unit announcements that occur near the end of the meeting. To connect natural consequences to Tom's actions, he will be required to participate in community meetings in order to join in on weekend outings (e.g., shopping trips, restaurant meals), events that he usually looks forward to.

PROGRAM TO REDUCE BIZARRE STEREOTYPIC BEHAVIOR—CARLA R.

Background

Carla has a strange habit of moving her outstretched hands and fingers through the air while walking through the halls. At the same time, she often talks to herself. When asked what she is doing, Carla will reply that she is "touching the ethers and spirits in the room." Carla engages in this behavior during her free hours, and if given an assignment that does not hold her interest, she will exhibit this behavior during a group activity. Although the behavior is harmless, it makes Carla appear very abnormal.

The treatment team has decided to try to ameliorate this problem by involving Carla in a greater variety of leisure and work activities. Efforts will be made to identify appropriate activities that are sufficiently engaging to replace Carla's perseverative behavior (Corrigan, Liberman, & Wong, 1993; Wong, Wright, Terranova, Bowen, & Zarate, 1988c; Wong et al., 1987)

Data Collection and Analysis

Staff will record the occurrence or nonoccurrence of stereotypic behavior during six observation periods, each 5 minutes long, scheduled throughout the day. (This is a crude measure, but the only one feasible given limited availability of staff.) In addition to recording the presence or absence of stereotypic behavior, staff will document Carla's activity at the time, so that the data can be later analyzed to ascertain the correlation between type of activity and stereotypic behavior.

Treatment Procedures

1. *Schedule of daily activities.* To assist Carla in remaining involved in functional behavior throughout the day, staff and Carla have developed an enriched and varied weekly agenda for her (Paul & Lentz, 1977). This schedule is shown in Figure 7.1. We believe this schedule will be helpful because Carla is usually compliant and would respond to verbal reminders to follow her agenda.

2. *Identifying preferred leisure activities.* Staff have been meeting with Carla to identify independent leisure activities that she can choose to occupy her free time. Presently, they have listed knitting, reading magazines while listening to country music, and writing letters to her sister as preferred pastimes.

3. *Redirecting Carla to socially appropriate activity.* This procedure is designed to deal with perseverative behavior that occurs in spite of intensive scheduling or during a scheduled activity. Staff will use response interruption and redirection. For example, if clients and staff are gathered in the dayroom watching television and Carla begins pacing while talking to herself, a staff member should say something to her, such as, "Carla, we're here to watch television, talk, or read the newspaper. Why don't you sit down and find your favorite section of the news?"

PROGRAM TO IMPROVE SOCIAL (CONVERSATIONAL) SKILLS— MARY C.

Background

Mary almost never initiates conversations and sometimes fails to respond when spoken to. Mary has said that she enjoys interacting with others but at times is uncomfortable and does not know what to say or do. The treatment team will attempt to improve Mary's interactions with others through social skills training. To maximize the likelihood that trained skills generalize to real-life encounters, instruction will occur *in situ* or in the residential setting (Wong et al., 1993; Wong & Woolsey, 1989).

Data Collection and Analysis

The best times to regularly monitor and increase Mary's rate of social interaction is during the last 10 minutes of lunch, leisure therapy, afternoon break, and dinner. During these periods, staff assigned to the client's area will place hash marks on Mary's data sheet to record the frequency of the following *unprompted responses*:

1. Making eye contact.
2. Acknowledging a staff member or a fellow client's statements (by saying, "Oh really" or "Yes" or repeating back part of what the other person said).
3. Asking a question related to what the other person just said.

Treatment Procedures

Baseline

Mary's primary therapist will make her aware of the three conversational skills targeted for training. Mary will also be asked to use these skills during the monitoring

COMMUNITY LIVING PROGRAM
In Melbourne

RESIDENT: CARLA R.
CASE MANAGER: FRANCIE GOODE
DATE: SEPTEMBER 10, 1995

DOA: 06/5/93
LEVEL: VI
ID#: R-188

TIME	SUNDAY	MONDAY	TUESDAY	WEDNESDAY	THURSDAY	FRIDAY	SATURDAY
6:00		Wake up	Wake up	Wake up	Wake up	Wake up	
						Grooming	
7:00		Grooming	Grooming	Grooming	Grooming	BREAKFAST	Wake up
		BREAKFAST	BREAKFAST	BREAKFAST	BREAKFAST	Toothbrushing	Grooming
		Toothbrushing	Kitchen clean up	Toothbrushing	Toothbrushing		BREAKFAST
8:00	Wake up	Bus ride to Community	Appointment with Cottage	Bus ride to Community	Bus ride to job trial at	Cottage chores	Toothbrushing
	Grooming	Mental Health Program	Supervisor, Ms. Peterson	Mental Health Program	Bayshore Industries		Kitchen clean up
9:00	BREAKFAST	CMHP	Money Management	CMHP	Bayshore Industries	Break	Read morning paper
	Toothbrushing					Shuttle to Human Serv. Dept.	T.V./socialize
10:00	Read morning paper		Menu Planning			Appointment with Social	
	Bedroom cleaning					Worker, Ms. Francie Goode	
11:00	Cottage chores		Cooking			LUNCH	
12:00	LUNCH	LUNCH	LUNCH	LUNCH	LUNCH	Volunteer work at	LUNCH
			Kitchen clean up			St. John's Day Care Cntr	
1:00	Kitchen clean up	CMHP	Appointment with Psycho-	CMHP	Bayshore Industries	St. John's Day Care Cntr	Prepare for Sat. Outing
			gist, Dr. Mann				Community Outing
2:00	Shopping trip, go to		Grocery shopping				
	park, or for a walk						
3:00							
4:00		Bus ride home	Laundry	Bus ride home	Bus ride home	Behavioral Program Meeting	
		Break (reading)		Break (reading)	Break (knitting or reading)	Individual Weekly Review	
5:00	Break /T.V.	Community Meeting	Community Meeting	Community Meeting	Stress Management Group	Community Meeting	
					Community Meeting	Cooking	
6:00	DINNER	DINNER	DINNER	DINNER	DINNER	DINNER	DINNER
				Kitchen clean up			
7:00	Community Meeting	T.V./socialize	Evening Group Activity	Group Community Outing	Break (letter writing)	Kitchen clean up	T.V./socialize
		Exercise Group			Exercise Group		
8:00	Break (knitting)	Break (reading, music)	T.V. or reading		Weekend Activity Planning	T.V./socialize	Break (knitting)
	T.V./socialize						
9:00	Shower	Shower	Shower	Shower	Shower	Shower	Shower
	Bedtime	Bedtime	Bedtime	Bedtime	Bedtime	Bedtime	Bedtime

Figure 7.1 Carla's schedule of weekly activities.

periods mentioned above. Data should be collected as planned. (If Mary begins using the desired skills after these simple instructions, training will be deemed unnecessary and she will merely be encouraged to interact appropriately more often.)

Training Procedures

Mary will first be taught eye contact, then acknowledgments, and finally conversational questions. The staff member at Mary's table will verbally prompt her to employ and demonstrate the skill ("Mary, when someone tells you something, you can show you are listening by saying, 'Oh really' or 'Yes' "). Discreetly reinforce Mary with praise ("You used an acknowledgment—that's good!") and tokens for using the skill with a staff member or any peers who are present.

After Mary has used the trained skill during *three** consecutive sessions, begin training on the next skill in the list. To maintain training gains, make reinforcement contingent on performance of the current target skill *and* all previously trained skills. Tell Mary what new skill you will be teaching her, and that, to earn reinforcement, she must utilize the new skill *and* all skills she has already been taught. After Mary uses all three skills during *six* consecutive sessions, begin thinning tangible reinforcement by omitting token rewards every third session. If Mary's performance remains stable, continue to gradually thin the tangible reinforcement by thirds until Mary is responding appropriately for natural social consequences.

PROGRAM TO IMPROVE GROOMING AND HYGIENE—BRIAN P.

Background

Staff report that Brian's dress is sloppy and at times looks dirty and smells bad. The treatment team intends to collect 3 days' baseline data on Brian's self-care behavior, and, if the data confirm staff impressions, to initiate a structured grooming and hygiene program (Nelson & Cone, 1979; Wong, Flanagan, Kuehnel, Liberman, Hunnicutt, & Adams-Badgett, 1988a).

Data Collection

At 8:00 A.M. every weekday morning (when all of the clients have completed their morning grooming routine), rate Brian using the Grooming-Skills Checklist (see Table 7.5). Check each item that is completed correctly and that is self-initiated (performed without staff prompts). If Brian is self-initiating an average of less than 70% of these grooming skills during baseline sessions, he should be taken through the following training sequence:

Treatment Procedures

Rationale

Brian's primary therapist will meet with him to explain why the grooming program is being initiated and how it will benefit him (i.e., people will like him more, he will be able to

---

*The criteria of three and six consecutive sessions were selected as reasonable cutoff points to either begin training on the next skill or to thin reinforcement. If Mary's performance regresses following a change in criterion, the treatment procedure will revert back to the previous criterion level.

Client _____ Date _____

Staff member _____ Time _____

Task	Performed correctly?	Self-initiated?
1. Hands and fingernails are clean. Hands, fingernails, and wrists free of dirt, grime, food, etc.		
2. Face is clean. Face and neck have no dirt or foreign material on them (e.g., dandruff, food, shaving cream).		
3. Face is shaved. Face is smooth and without facial hair except for beard or mustache.		
4. Hair is clean. Hair is free of excessive dandruff, oil, dirt, and foreign particles (e.g., grass, lint, food).		
5. Hair is combed. Hair is out of eyes and flows in same direction on each side, back, and top of head.		
6. Teeth are clean. Teeth are free of food particles or excessive film. (Engage client in casual conversation to observe this self-care item.)		
7. Clothes are clean. Clothes are free of excessive dandruff, lint, dirt, food, and other foreign material.		
8. Clothes are of proper size and length. Pants and shirt should not be too long, short, or baggy.		
9. Clothes are properly buttoned, fastened, zipped, and tied. Buttons are in the right button holes; shirt cuffs are buttoned or rolled up evenly; zippers on pants are all the way up; shoes with laces are tied correctly; and belts are buckled.		
10. Clothes are of proper amount. Amount of clothing worn is appropriate for temperature and weather conditions.		
11. Clothes worn properly, shirt tucked, collar straight. Pants hanging on waist (not too high or low on body); shirt tucked in pants or left completely out; collar turned out.		

keep his job at the warehouse). In the first few grooming sessions, Brian will be reminded of these reasons for his program.

Training Procedures

At the start of training, the staff member assigned to work with Brian in the morning will escort him to the bathroom and guide him through the complete grooming sequence. Using the grooming-skills checklist, the staff member will describe the first step in the sequence, demonstrate that grooming skill, then have Brian perform the task. As Brian performs the task, the staff member should cue him on how to get better results or do the task more efficiently (e.g., "The razor will work better if you shave against the grain" or "Try wetting your comb between strokes and your hair will stay in place"). After Brian has completed the task, the staff member will describe, model, and coach Brian through the next task and repeat this process until the entire sequence is completed. Brian will receive verbal encouragement for completing individual tasks and 25 points for successfully completing the whole grooming sequence.

After the second or third training session using this format, staff should begin fading prompts so that Brian will perform the grooming sequence on his own.

1. Bring Brian to the bathroom area and allow him to begin the first grooming step by himself.
2. If he initiates the task within 10 seconds, praise him for remembering how to start grooming.
3. If he does not, ask him, "What do you do first?"
4. If Brian does not begin performing the first step correctly within 10 seconds, describe and, if necessary, model the step and then have Brian complete the task.
5. Allow Brian 10 seconds to perform the next step in the sequence.
6. If he initiates the next task within 10 seconds, praise him for remembering what to do.
7. If he does not, ask him, "What do you do next?"
8. If Brian does not begin performing the next step correctly within 10 seconds, describe and, if needed, model the step and then have Brian complete the task.
9. Repeat steps 5 through 8 and continue through the remainder of the grooming sequence.

PROGRAM FOR PREVOCATIONAL TRAINING—RALPH C.

Background

Ralph's major behavior problems (e.g., disruptive outbursts, noncompliance) have declined significantly over the past 3 months. His self-care has also improved to the point that he is grooming independently and keeping his room presentable. Over the past month, he has received the maximum number of available points for grooming and room cleanup, in addition to earning bonus points for various chores around the facility (Ayllon & Azrin, 1968; Paul & Lentz, 1977). After reviewing this information and talking with Ralph, it appears that he is ready for a more demanding work assignment.

Treatment Procedures

Rehabilitation staff have arranged for Ralph to receive prevocational training as a food services aide in the facility kitchen. He will be responsible for clearing and wiping tables, sweeping the floor, restocking snack trays, and occasionally serving drinks and hot-food items. Ralph will start working at 10:00 to 11:00 A.M. and at 1:00 to 3:00 P.M., Monday through Friday, earning $2.50 per hour. (When Ralph has learned his job well enough that he requires minimal supervision, his salary will be increased to minimum wage.) Based on Ralph's ability to handle the work and the amount of business at the kitchen, these hours may be extended or shortened.

Besides frequently reviewing the quality of his work (i.e., completeness, speed), the food services supervisor and rehabilitation staff will help Ralph with four behaviors related to job performance:

1. *Getting to work on time.* To be considered on time, Ralph must arrive 5 minutes before the hour he is scheduled to start work. To assist Ralph in being punctual, a

clock will be placed in his bedroom and he will purchase a digital watch that can be programmed to ring daily at 9:45 A.M. and 12:45 P.M. During his first few weeks on the job, staff will remind Ralph to check the clock and, if necessary, help him set his watch.

2. *Talking to self.* This behavior is defined as any nondirected vocalizations that can be heard by another person who is standing at least 5 feet from Ralph. Ralph often mumbles and talks to himself, and his psychologist has been teaching Ralph alternative responses to displace these inappropriate behaviors. Because there is usually a radio in the kitchen playing music, Ralph has been prompted to hum and sing along with the tune being broadcast.

3. *Accepting directions and feedback.* This is defined as listening to instructions and corrective remarks without becoming annoyed or angry. Using social skills training procedures, Ralph's psychologist is also teaching him to repeat back instructions that are given to him (e.g., "So you want me to throw away the soup and the sauce, but not the other food, Okay") and to report problems that arise on the job (e.g., "I couldn't get any more chips because they were out of stock").

4. *Requesting information and feedback.* Ralph also needs to become more comfortable asking for information on how to do his job better, especially the first few times he performs a task. His psychologist is having him practice soliciting specific feedback (e.g., "Where would you like me to store these cases?" or "Does the grill look clean to you?").

WEEKEND COMMUNITY ACTIVITY PLAN—ALVIN C.

(Addressing skill areas of Transportation Planning, Using Public Transportation, Meal Planning and Preparation, Money Management, and Leisure Planning)

Background

In recent months, Alvin has planned and successfully completed short trips to the museum, shopping mall, and his relatives' homes. This weekend he is proposing a longer and more costly trip to the Shrimp Festival in Cocoa Beach. The outing will allow him to apply many of the independent living skills that he has been learning in his community reintegration classes.

Independent Living Skills

Money Management

For this event, Alvin has set aside $20, which will be spent on food, drinks, bus fare, and possibly, a small souvenir. Rehabilitation staff have suggested that he stretch his day's allowance by bringing a bag lunch. This will leave him more money to purchase a sumptuous seafood dinner in the evening.

Meal Planning and Preparation

Alvin will make a simple breakfast of cold cereal or a donut, and for reasons described earlier, take a lunch with him. He will pack a sandwich (ham, lettuce, and mayonnaise, or peanut butter and jelly), chips, and a soda. The client will eat during the bus ride or at the park hosting the festival.

Transportation Planning and Using Public Buses

Alvin has never ridden the bus to this park before, so with assistance from staff he has worked out his route on a city map and his timetable based around the bus schedule. He will need to make two transfers, and he has rehearsed with rehabilitation staff how he will sit near the front of the bus and ask the driver to alert him as his stop approaches. The entire activity, including travel time, will occupy the hours from 10:00 A.M. to 8:30 P.M.

Leisure-Activity Planning

Alvin intends to spend his time at the festival browsing through the arts-and-crafts booths, eating, and listening to live band music. Alcoholic beverages will be available at the festival and this could present a problem. However, Alvin says that he does not feel a strong temptation to drink at the event, and he would probably not do so unless encouraged by peers. There is a good likelihood that he will see one of his old friends at the gathering; however, this person is currently a member of Alcoholics Anonymous and probably will be a positive influence.

CONCLUSIONS

In this chapter we have examined two sets of biobehavioral interventions for disorders of schizophrenia. The first, represented by excerpts from two modules of the UCLA Program for Training Social and Independent Living Skills, consists of highly prescribed, professionally designed and validated protocols for teaching functional and self-management skills. Because these modules were expressly developed for the purpose of dissemination, they come in the form of standardized instructional curricula and training materials (e.g., videocassette tapes, training manuals).

The second set of interventions focused on skills training through individualized behavioral programs that restructured antecedent and consequent stimuli in the client's living environment. These programs resemble the hospital contingency-management systems from which they were derived, with a couple of important differences. First, the present programs focus on preparing clients to successfully perform normal activities in the community. This leads to instruction in more varied and advanced skills, and to greater consideration of clients' preferences when establishing treatment goals. Second, the programs attempt to deal with undesirable behavior using proactive (problem prevention) and nonrestrictive interventions. This difference reflects the lessened feasibility of restrictive interventions in open settings as well as the current trend in behavioral technology toward reducing the motivation for inappropriate behavior by providing the client with alternate responses that produce the same reinforcers as the inappropriate behavior (Iwata, Vollmer, Zarcone, & Rodgers, 1993; Mace & Roberts, 1993). The drawback to this second set of interventions is that despite their apparent simplicity, their construction requires an understanding of how to apply behavioral interventions with chronic psychiatric patients. Of course, no set of interventions is ideal for all purposes or situations. Clinicians must decide which sets of interventions best suit their needs.

Ayllon, T., & Azrin, N. H. (1965). The measurement and reinforcement of behavior of psychotics. *Journal of the Experimental Analysis of Behavior, 8*, 357–383.

Ayllon, T., & Azrin, N. (1968). *The token economy: A motivational system for therapy and rehabilitation.* Englewood Cliffs, NJ: Prentice-Hall.

Backer, T. E., Liberman, R. P., & Kuehnel, T. G. (1986). Dissemination and adoption of innovative psychosocial interventions. *Journal of Consulting and Clinical Psychology, 54*, 111–118.

Bellack, A. S., Morrison, R. L., Wixted, J. T., & Mueser, K. T. (1990). An analysis of social competence in schizophrenia. *British Journal of Psychiatry, 56*, 809–818.

Bowen, L. (1988). *Assessment and effect of attentional deficits in schizophrenics.* Unpublished doctoral dissertation, California School of Professional Psychology, Los Angeles.

Chadwick, P. D. J., & Lowe, C. F. (1990). Measurement and modification of delusional beliefs. *Journal of Consulting and Clinical Psychology, 58*, 225–232.

Chadwick, P. D., & Lowe, C. F. (1994). A cognitive approach to measuring and modifying delusions. *Behaviour Research and Therapy, 32*, 355–367.

Chadwick, P. D. J., Lowe, C. F., Horne, P. J., & Higson, P. J. (1994). Modifying delusions: The role of empirical testing. *Behavior Therapy, 25*, 35–49.

Corrigan, P. W., Liberman, R. P., & Wong, S. E. (1993). Recreational therapy and behavior management on inpatient units: Is recreational therapy therapeutic? *Journal of Nervous and Mental Disease, 181*, 644–646.

Corrigan, P. W., Schade, M. L., & Liberman, R. P. (1992). Social skills training. In R. P. Liberman (Ed.), *Handbook of psychiatric rehabilitation.* New York: Macmillan.

Corrigan, P. W., & Storzbach, D. (1992) *Cognitive remediation in schizophrenia.* Unpublished manuscript available from first author at Department of Psychiatry, University of Chicago.

Donahoe, C. P., Carter, M. J., Bloem, W. D., Hirsch, G. L., Laasi, N., & Wallace, C. J. (1990). Assessment of interpersonal problem-solving skills. *Psychiatry, 53*, 329–339.

Eckman, T. A. (1992). *Training schizophrenics in social problem solving.* Unpublished manuscript.

Graziano, A. M., & Katz, J. N. (1982). Training paraprofessionals. In A. S. Bellack, M. Hersen, & A. E. Kazdin, (Eds.), *International handbook of behavior modification and therapy.* New York: Plenum.

Iwata, B. A., Vollmer, T. R., Zarcone, J. R., & Rodgers, T. A. (1993). Treatment classification and selection based on behavioral function. In R. Van Houten & S. Axelrod (Eds.), *Behavior analysis and treatment* (pp. 101–125). New York: Plenum Press.

Kiesler, C. A., & Sibulkin, A. E. (1987). *Mental hospitalization: Myths and facts about a national crisis.* Newbury Park, CA: Sage.

Liberman, R. P. (Ed.). (1992). *Handbook of psychiatric rehabilitation.* New York: Macmillan.

Liberman, R. P., & Green, M. F. (1992). Whither cognitive behavior therapy for schizophrenia. *Schizophrenia Bulletin, 18*, 27–35.

Liberman, R. P., Lillie, F. J., Falloon, I. R. H., Harpin, R. E., Hutchinson, W., & Stoute, B. (1984). Social skills training with relapsing schizophrenics: An experimental analysis. *Behavior Modification, 8*, 155–179.

Liberman, R. P., Massel, H. K., Mosk, M. D., & Wong, S. E. (1985). Social skills training for chronic mental patients. *Hospital and Community Psychiatry, 36*, 396–403.

Liberman, R. P., Nuechterlein, K. H., & Wallace, C. J. (1982). Social skills training and the nature of schizophrenia. In J. P. Curran & P. Monti (Eds.), *Social skills training: A practical handbook for assessment and treatment.* New York: Guilford.

Liberman, R. P., Wallace, C. J., Blackwell, G., Eckman, T. A., Vaccaro, J. V., & Kuehnel, T. G. (1993). Innovations in skills training for the seriously mentally ill: The UCLA Social & Independent Living Skills Modules. *Innovations and Research, 2*, 43–60.

Liberman, R. P., Wallace, C., Teigen, J., & Davis, J. (1974). Interventions with psychotic behaviors. In K. S. Calhoun, H. E. Adams, & K. M. Mitchell (Eds.), *Innovative treatment methods in psychopathology* (pp. 323–412). New York: Wiley.

Lowe, C. F., & Chadwick, P. D. J. (1990). Verbal control of delusions. *Behavior Therapy, 21*, 461–479.

Mace, F. C., & Roberts, M. L. (1993). Factors affecting selection of behavioral interventions. In J. Reichle & D. P. Wacker (Eds.), *Communicative alternatives to challenging behavior: Integrating functional assessment and intervention strategies* (pp. 113–133). Baltimore: Brooks.

Massel, H. K., Corrigan, P. W., Liberman, R. P., & Milan, M. A. (1991). Conversation skills training of thought disordered schizophrenic patients through attention focusing. *Psychiatry Research, 38*, 51–61.

Morrison, R. L., & Bellack, A. S. (1984). Social skills training. In A. S. Bellack (Ed.), *Schizophrenia: Treatment, management and rehabilitation*. Orlando, FL: Grune and Stratton.

Moss, G. R., & Liberman, R. P. (1975). Empiricism in psychotherapy: Behavioural specification and measurement. *British Journal of Psychiatry, 126*, 73–80.

Nelson, G. L., & Cone, J. D. (1979). Multiple-baseline analysis of a token economy for psychiatric inpatients. *Journal of Applied Behavior Analysis, 12*, 255–271.

Patterson, R. L., & Teigen, J. R. (1973). Conditioning and post-hospital generalization of nondelusional responses in a chronic psychotic patient. *Journal of Applied Behavior Analysis, 6*, 65–70.

Paul, G. L., & Lentz, R. J. (1977). *Psychosocial treatment of chronic mental patients*. Cambridge, MA: Harvard University Press.

Psychiatric Rehabilitation Consultants. (1995). *Social and independent living skills: Symptom management module*. Camarillo, CA: Author.

Psychiatric Rehabilitation Consultants. (1995). *Social and independent living skills: Medication-management module*. Camarillo, CA: Author.

Sullivan, G., Marder, S. R., Liberman, R. P., Donahoe, C. P., & Mintz, J. (1990). Social skills and relapse history in outpatient schizophrenics. *Psychiatry, 53*, 340–345.

Wallace, C. J., Boone, S. E., Donahoe, C. P., & Foy, D. W. (1985). The chronically mentally ill: Independent living skills training. In D. Barlow (Ed.), *Clinical handbook of psychological disorders*. New York: Guilford Press.

Wincze, J. P., Leitenberg, H., & Agras, W. S. (1972). The effects of token reinforcement and feedback on the delusional verbal behavior of chronic paranoid schizophrenics. *Journal of Applied Behavior Analysis, 5*, 247–262.

Wong, S. E., Flanagan, S. G., Kuehnel, T. G., Liberman, R. P., Hunnicutt, R., & Adams-Badgett, J. (1988a). Training chronic mental patients to independently practice personal grooming skills. *Hospital and Community Psychiatry, 39*, 874–879.

Wong, S. E., Martinez-Diaz, J. A., Massel, H. K., Edelstein, B. A., Wiegand, W., Bowen, L., & Liberman, R. P. (1993). Conversational skills training with schizophrenic inpatients: A study of generalization across settings and conversants. *Behavior Therapy, 24*, 285–304.

Wong, S. E., Massel, H. K., Mosk, M. D., & Liberman, R. P. (1986). Behavioral approaches to the treatment of schizophrenia. In G. D. Burrows, T. R. Norman, and G. Rubinstein (Eds.), *Handbook of studies on schizophrenia, Part 2: Management and research* (pp. 77–99). Amsterdam, The Netherlands: Elsevier.

Wong, S. E., Terranova, M. D., Bowen, L., Zarate, R. Massel, H. K., & Liberman, R. P. (1987) Providing independent recreational activities to reduce sterotypic vocalizations in chronic schizophrenics. *Journal of Applied Behavior Analysis, 20*, 77–81.

Wong, S. E., & Woolsey, J. E. (1989). Re-establishing conversational skills in overtly psychotic, chronic schizophrenic patients: Discrete trials training on the psychiatric ward. *Behavior Modification, 13*, 415–430.

Wong, S. E., Woolsey, J. E., Innocent, A. J., & Liberman, R. P. (1988b). Behavioral treatment of violent psychiatric patients. *Psychiatric Clinics of North America, 11*, 569–580.

Wong, S. E., Wright, J., Terranova, M. D., Bowen, L., & Zarate, R. (1988c). Effects of structured ward activities on appropriate and psychotic behavior of chronic psychiatric patients. *Behavioral Residential Treatment, 3*, 41–50.

8

Community Reinforcement Training with Concerned Others

Robert J. Meyers, Thomas P. Dominguez,
and Jane Ellen Smith

INTRODUCTION

It is widely acknowledged that problems related to alcohol misuse can seriously affect the lives of family members, friends, and close associates of the drinker (Collins, Leonard, & Searles, 1990; Orford & Harwin, 1982; Paolino & McCrady, 1977). Very often those individuals closest to the drinker are the first to feel the negative effects of problematic drinking. In the past, self-help programs advised individuals who were concerned about someone else's drinking to disengage or "detach" from the problems of the user and to concentrate on taking care of themselves. In recent years counseling approaches have been developed that include procedures for training concerned others (COs) in more active strategies for dealing with someone else's drinking. Furthermore, they help COs address areas of their own lives, such that they are better able to recognize and cope with the problems and stresses associated with being close to a problem drinker.

Initiation of Treatment through the Concerned Others

Aggregate data on the number of clients entering alcohol treatment at the urging of COs are generally lacking (Institute of Medicine, 1990). However, instances of COs contacting treatment facilities for advice or help regarding the drinking of others are widely known and commonly encountered. Also, problem drinkers already engaged in treatment

---

Robert J. Meyers • University of New Mexico, Center on Alcoholism, Substance Abuse, and Addictions, Albuquerque, New Mexico 87106.   **Thomas P. Dominguez and Jane Ellen Smith** • Department of Psychology, University of New Mexico, Albuquerque, New Mexico 87131.

Sourcebook of Psychological Treatment Manuals for Adult Disorders, edited by Vincent B. Van Hasselt and Michel Hersen. Plenum Press, New York, 1996.

often report that the decision to seek help was prompted by the direct influence of COs, or COs acting in concert with courts, employee assistance programs, or informal social networks. Surveys by Room (1987) and Hingson, Mangione, Meyers, and Scotch (1982) support the notion that pressure from family and friends about drinking is a common experience among clients currently in treatment for alcohol abuse. What seems clear from these reports is that, in many cases, COs can come to serve as important facilitators in helping problem drinkers and drug users to initiate treatment (cf. Thomas & Santa, 1982).

The general success rates of COs in actively promoting treatment for loved ones can only be estimated from a few published clinical trials. These reports are for specific procedures carried out by relatively small numbers of screened COs, who were actively directed by well-trained clinicians. Under these conditions, success rates in persuading unmotivated problem drinkers to enter treatment ranged from 86% for a cognitive–behavioral procedure (Sisson & Azrin, 1986) to 24% for a programmed social-network intervention (Liepman, Nirenberg, & Begin, 1989).

Characteristics of Concerned Others in Clinical Samples

The question of whether COs could or should be instrumental in efforts to obtain treatment for the problem drinker has been debated for years. Initial beliefs were that COs could only be detrimental to the process, because their own personality deficits were contributing in some way to the alcohol problem in the first place. But early attempts by researchers to document unique patterns of personality disturbance among spouses of alcoholics yielded few positive findings (reviewed in Paolino & McCrady, 1977). In summary, Paolino and McCrady concluded that spouses of alcoholics do not appear to be distinguishable by any particular personality type, nor do spouses of alcoholics tend to exhibit elevated rates of psychopathology compared to control spouses when matched for age, income, and level of education. These authors further criticized the conclusions of some of the researchers in this area for their pathologizing of the family-role adaptations undertaken by some of the wives of alcoholics. In particular, these reviewers were critical of the dependency–dominance studies that tended to view wife-dominant marriages as evidence of aberrant mental states or pathological coping strategies on the part of the wives. For Paolino and McCrady, such conclusions were taken as evidence of a prevailing social reaction by traditional-minded researchers against women who adopted nontraditional roles and duties.

Several recent studies have continued to explore CO characteristics, but primarily out of interest in the type and range of stress being experienced by them. Data from intake profiles of treatment-seeking COs of unmotivated problem drinkers generally indicate moderate levels of self-reported CO distress. Thomas and Ager (1993), for example, reported levels of CO distress that were elevated compared to normals, yet lower than levels for patients receiving general outpatient psychotherapy. On measures of marital adjustment, the same CO sample reported levels of marital distress that were greater than normal couples, less than divorced couples, and comparable to couples in marital counseling.

For a sample of 26 COs presenting for treatment, Dominguez, Miller, and Meyers (1995) detected increased levels of depressed mood and physical symptoms, and decreased levels of self-confidence, compared to a referent sample of community controls. The findings were based on indices and norms from the Health and Daily Living Schedule (Moos, Cronkite, Billings, & Finney, 1987). Interestingly, levels of CO distress on these measures did not reach levels reported by a referent sample of clients entering treatment for major or minor depression.

Today it is more widely believed that reports of psychosocial distress from COs seeking help because of a loved one's drinking should not be taken as evidence of a debilitating underlying syndrome. The condition of being close to a problem drinker or drug user can pose a wide array of stressors for the CO. For example, Velleman et al. (1993) found in his sample of 50 families that relatives of drug abusers commonly reported experiences of physical violence at the hands of the drug abuser (50%), along with verbal aggression (44%), unpredictable behavior (42%), stealing from family members (42%), and embarrassing behavior in front of others (38%). Dominguez et al. (1995) noted that of 26 COs presenting for treatment, 38% reported an alcohol-related arrest for the drinker within the prior 12 months. Descriptions of COs as they present for treatment suggest that these are individuals experiencing moderate to severe situational stress. However, it is important to note that this information generally is obtained from samples acknowledging the need for treatment and specifically recruited to participate in clinical trials. Therefore, generalizations should not be made to other populations of COs who may be coping adequately with their particular situations, or who otherwise may not present for treatment. Furthermore, the findings still do not suggest that COs experiencing stress will somehow compromise attempts to obtain treatment for a drinker, or that COs will be poor treatment collaborators.

The Outcomes of Concerned Other Treatment Approaches

Important theoretical guidelines for conceptualizing and conducting CO treatment were proposed by Thomas and Santa (1982) and by Szapocznik, Kurtines, Foote, Perez-Vidal, and Hervis (1983). Both research teams proposed that change in the behavior of unmotivated problem drinkers or drug users could be achieved by working with and through COs. Thomas and Santa further proposed that outcomes for this type of treatment be assessed by monitoring change in the functioning of the problem drinker (the identified patient, or IP), the CO, and the IP–CO relationship system.

In two companion studies, Szapocznik et al. (1983, 1986) developed and evaluated procedures based on strategic family therapy that was delivered to only one person in the family. In these studies, the IPs were drug-abusing adolescents from Cuban-American families. After initially agreeing to participate in either treatment condition, 37 families meeting entry criteria were randomly assigned to receive strategic therapy delivered either to the entire family (conjoint family therapy) or primarily to one person in the family (one-person family therapy). In most cases the one person was the identified patient. Results showed the two treatment approaches to be similarly effective in reducing IP symptomatology and improving family functioning. The Szapocznik team's conceptualization of one-person family therapy differed significantly from what Thomas and Santa (1982) have termed "unilateral family therapy." In the latter approach, interventions are more clearly designed for cases of an unmotivated, treatment-resistant IP. Nevertheless, Szapocznik et al. provided important theoretical and empirical support for family interventions carried out through one person.

In a clinical trial of unilateral family therapy, Thomas, Santa, Bronson, & Oyserman (1987) assigned 15 COs to receive either immediate or delayed unilateral family therapy. Ten additional COs and their problem-drinking partners were followed as a nonrandom, no-treatment control group. Selected comparisons were made between COs receiving immediate versus delayed treatment, and between COs receiving versus COs not receiving treatment. Usable outcome data were available for 13 of the 15 COs receiving treatment and for 6 out of the 10 not receiving treatment. Improvement was defined as a reduction in drinking greater than the reported average of 53%, or entry into treatment, or both. Results showed that 62% of drinkers whose COs received treatment were classified as "improved," whereas none of 6 drinkers whose COs did not receive treatment were improved.

In a test of a more traditional form of CO counseling, Dittrich and Trapold (1984) conducted a comparative trial of Alanon-focused group therapy versus a delayed-treatment control for wives of alcoholics ($N = 23$). At the conclusion of 8 weeks of treatment, significant improvements were found for treated wives on measures of anxiety, depression, self-concept, and enabling behavior. By the 12-month follow-up, 48% of IPs had entered treatment. Unfortunately, no data were reported on the impact of the intervention on IP drinking.

Liepman et al. (1989) reported a quasi-experimental evaluation of a widely used but relatively unexamined CO counseling procedure (Johnson, 1986). The authors trained 24 "social networks," composed of several relatives and friends of each IP, to conduct confrontational interventions with the IPs. Nonequivalent comparison groups were formed by those networks that carried out the confrontations ($n = 7$) versus those that did not ($n = 17$). Confronted alcoholics were more likely to enter a detox or treatment program (86%) than were nonconfronted alcoholics (17%). The overall success rate in promoting treatment for the drinkers was 24% when the entire treated sample was taken into account. No significant differences were found between confronted and nonconfronted groups for gender of the alcoholic, number of persons in the social network, or number of prior treatments sought by the networks or the alcoholics. However, the alcoholics in the confronted group were significantly younger ($M = 38.4$) than those in the nonconfronted group ($M = 50.7$). No outcomes were reported for the functioning of individuals in the social networks or for the social networks as a whole.

In a small-sample study, Sisson and Azrin (1986) found Community Reinforcement Training (CRT) for COs to be superior to a regimen of traditional, Alanon-focused counseling in facilitating IP entry into treatment and in reducing IP drinking. In the skills-based Community Reinforcement Training condition, 6 of 7 COs were successful in promoting treatment entry for their alcohol-abusing partners, whereas in the traditional group ($n = 5$) none was successful. In addition, the drinkers had succeeded in reducing their alcohol intake by over 50% by the time they entered treatment. No data were reported for outcomes for the COs or for the IP–CO relationships.

Dominguez et al. (1995) reported results from a group presentation of Community Reinforcement Training (CRT). In this study, 26 COs of problem drinkers were randomly assigned to receive up to seven sessions of either CRT or an Alanon-facilitation approach. At the time of the 6-month follow-up, both groups showed improvements in CO functioning, with the CRT group evidencing more rapid relief of physical symptoms and depressed mood. In terms of overall family functioning, the CRT group reported better outcomes on a measure of family growth called the Family Environment Scale (Moos & Moos, 1986). This indicated a more positive family environment for social, cultural, and recreational activities; independence and self-sufficiency; and achievement orientation. All three cases of the drinker entering treatment were from the CRT condition, whereas in the Alanon-facilitation approach, none entered treatment. Although the latter finding was not statistically significant, it mirrored the general pattern of outcome reported by Sisson and Azrin (1986).

In summary, evidence is mounting in support of treatment approaches that view COs as effective agents for promoting change in the IP and in the larger family system. Although it is clear that COs often present with symptoms indicative of severe distress, it is also becoming apparent that procedures exist for stabilizing these clients and for training them in more productive ways of dealing with the drinking of a loved one.

As noted, CRT is a comprehensive set of procedures for working with the COs of problem drinkers. The basic principle and procedures of CRT were adapted from a larger set of procedures for working with problem drinkers known as the Community Reinforcement Approach (CRA; Meyers & Smith, 1995). Since its introduction in the early 1970s, CRA has been evaluated positively in a number of well-designed studies involving alcohol abusing populations (Azrin, 1976; Hunt & Azrin, 1973; Azrin, Sisson, Meyers, & Godley, 1982). The following sections provide detailed information on the application of these procedures when working with COs.

SESSION 1: INDUCTION AND BASIC INFORMATION

Treatment Philosophy

As noted, Community Reinforcement Training for Concerned Others is an outgrowth of the Community Reinforcement Approach (CRA) for problem drinkers. From its inception, CRA has viewed problem drinkers' COs as crucial collaborators in the treatment of alcohol problems. Within this approach, COs have been included successfully as disulfiram monitors, partners in marital counseling, active agents in resocialization and reinforcement programs, peer advisors, and relapse or problem detectors.

The CRT approach is built upon the belief that family members or friends willing to initiate professional involvement on behalf of a problem drinker are sincere in their desire to help the individual. It does not assume that the COs somehow are responsible for the drinking problem of the loved one, or that the family members prefer the drinking. So, although COs often have adopted some rather ineffective strategies in their efforts to deal with drinking, nevertheless, these strategies are viewed as evidence of caring for the drinker. Not surprisingly, then, the family members or friends typically are open to the idea of modifying their interaction style with the problem drinker. And since a CO tends to be the most influential individual in the drinker's life, that CO is in an excellent position to effect a change in the drinker's behavior.

Treatment Goals

Prior to seeing a client for the first session, it is important to have a full understanding of all that CRT is designed to accomplish. Furthermore, it is useful to remind yourself of these objectives periodically throughout treatment. The goals of CRT are as follows:

1. *Promoting Sobriety.* CRT teaches interested family members and friends behavioral skills and responses aimed at discouraging a loved one's harmful drinking. These include response incompatibility, response cost, positive reinforcement, and others.

2. *Reducing the Risk of Family Violence.* CRT teaches family members to recognize the potential for violence in the family and to take precautions to reduce the risk of harm to themselves and others. This is an important aspect of the training, because family members are being asked to make significant changes in the ways they typically have responded to the drinker.

3. *Minimizing Distress for Family Members.* CRT attempts to reduce other types of stress that are experienced by the COs and to introduce meaningful "rewards" into their lives. The latter is accomplished in much the same manner in which sobriety is reinforced

by the CRA program for the drinker. Namely, the importance of reinforcers is explained by the therapist, and suggestions for rewards are generated in the session. A subset of these is sampled by the CO during the week, and the most enjoyable, viable ones are incorporated into the CO's daily life.

4. *Preparing the Concerned Family Members to Suggest Treatment.* COs often can have a tremendous influence on a drinker's decision to reduce drinking or to enter treatment. Drinkers contemplating treatment frequently look to COs for support and reassurance during what can be a very lonely and confusing time in their lives. Simply hearing from a significant individual that treatment is available may be enough to tip the balance for someone who is reeling from the effects of alcohol and indecision. However, in many cases it takes weeks of preparation and training before the CO feels confident and ready to confront the drinker about the need to seek professional help.

5. *Encouraging Treatment for the Drinker.* Behavioral techniques also are used to motivate the CO's loved one to obtain formal treatment for his or her harmful drinking. The procedures are practiced during role plays, and feedback is supplied.

6. *Preparing the CO to Support the Drinker during His or Her Treatment.* CRT emphasizes the importance of the CO being a positive, supportive influence in the therapy process once the drinker decides to enter treatment. The CO is coached in this role in advance and is supplied with information regarding what will take place in therapy with the drinker.

Reviewing Assessment Information

If you did not conduct your own assessment, review all assessment information thoroughly before beginning the initial therapy session. This information provides you with key ingredients for the therapy process, such as details regarding potential positive reinforcers and incentives to motivate your client. For instance, imagine that the assessment material states that a client is very concerned about the constant bickering with her husband when he is drinking. She fears it might cause emotional harm to the children, because they witness it regularly. This information can be used to encourage the client to examine and alter her role in the bickering. Motivation can be enhanced by highlighting how the whole family will benefit in this situation if therapy is successful.

The assessment report should also contain specific facts about the partner's drinking problem. Clarify key pieces of this information with the client to assure accuracy. For example, the severity of the excessive drinking and the nature of previous treatment attempts should be covered. Explore the client's degree of participation in any prior therapy programs.

Treatment Strategies in the Initial Sessions

The first session is used to set an optimistic tone and establish positive expectations. The client should be instilled with the hope that he or she will be a winner regardless of the outcome. The CO will learn how to deal with his or her own life in a more effective manner, as well as learn ways to help the drinker recognize his or her own situation for what it is.

Early treatment sessions also are designed to build trust and to help clients feel comfortable with you. In many cases COs seeking treatment are skeptical, for they have exhausted all known assistance and are making one last effort to help the drinker. Sensitivity and caution should be major components of the early CRT process. Initial strategies are as follows:

1. Let the client express his or her frustration with the partner's drinking and with past unsuccessful attempts to change it.
2. Have the client describe some of the problems created by the drinking.
3. Build rapport by empathizing with the client's pain.
4. Share general information from your previous therapy experience that shows you understand the client's dilemma.
5. Explore the treatment strategies that have been tried in the past.
6. Advise your client that there are three directions their relationship can take as a result of counseling: (a) The problem may get worse; (b) the problem may stay the same; (c) an effective intervention may create positive change.

COs often experience great emotional pain and distress as a result of the problem drinking, as well as profound economic and social consequences. The first session is a time to allow the client to express feelings in these areas. It is not, however, appropriate or useful to devote excessive therapy time to prolonged "complaining." Instead, begin to move the client forward in a positive way by explaining how he or she will come to serve as a role model for positive functioning within the family.

Community Reinforcement Training Description

At this point you are ready to introduce the treatment that you believe will promote positive change. Begin by explaining that CRT teaches people new strategies for dealing with a problem drinker. Then briefly present CRT's four major goals:

1. To help diminish the CO's pain and anguish associated with his or her relationship to the drinker.
2. To help the CO learn new strategies to reduce the drinking behavior of the loved one, and ultimately to coax him or her into treatment.
3. To reduce the possible risk of violence.
4. To help heal the relationship between the CO and the loved one through CRA couples therapy.

Explain to the client that he or she will be taught basic techniques that will help accomplish these goals. Then discuss how CRT already has been shown to be effective in clinical studies.

Place Responsibility Where It Belongs!

Another issue to make clear early in treatment is that the client is not responsible for the partner's drinking problem. Once the drinking problem has developed, however, the client's ineffective ways of dealing with it may sometimes exacerbate such drinking. Discuss the client's understanding of his or her role in the problem, and explore his or her feelings about this. Explain that one of your goals is to help the client learn how to interact with the problem drinker in a way that supports sobriety. Once the client understands and accepts his or her role in the process, you can implement the skills training mentioned earlier. These specific skills allow the client to substitute new behaviors for his or her earlier methods of dealing with the drinker.

In summary, the initial session is a time to convey a sense of hope, understanding, and opportunity. It should also be used to help the client see that there is a clear set of procedures available to promote positive change in the client's current living situation. Finally, by the end of the first session, the client should realize that there are behaviors that not only can improve home life, but may actually influence the drinker's decision to seek treatment as well.

SESSION 2: ESTABLISHING A WORKING RELATIONSHIP

Rationale

In many ways, the second session is a continuation of the first, for it provides a more detailed explanation of CRT and further emphasizes rapport building. The importance of developing a good rapport with COs cannot be stressed enough. Frequently the CO will feel confused, humiliated, and defeated by the long-standing drinking problem of the loved one. It is necessary, therefore, to move rapidly to establish a comfortable working relationship with the CO. Within this relationship, progress can be made toward accomplishing the goals of treatment.

Suggestions for Building Rapport

Although therapists tend to develop their own methods for establishing rapport with clients, there seem to be some commonalities. A set of clinical guidelines for establishing rapport follows:

1. Gain trust by listening to the client and assuring him or her that the problem is one with which you are familiar.
2. Briefly refer to other similar cases to help the client understand that his or her problem is not unusual or strange.
3. Help the CO identify specific problem areas, and offer hope for addressing them effectively.
4. Continually demonstrate understanding and knowledge of the difficult situation, and reflect back the CO's feelings about it.
5. Keep reminding the client that his or her problems will have some type of solution, and even if the solution is less than perfect, the situation will be improved nonetheless.

The treatment process is never easy for the client. Many times, COs feel as if no one truly understands them, or that they have brought the problem upon themselves. So simply being heard and understood by a caring professional often is a significant first step in the therapy process.

Confidentiality

As in most therapeutic procedures, CRT requires an atmosphere of mutual respect, empathy, and trust. A key ingredient in creating such an atmosphere is client confidentiality. The importance of confidentiality in treatment cannot be overstated, and this is especially true when a type of "unilateral" treatment procedure such as CRT is employed. A unilateral intervention involves provision of services to clients who are seeking to influence the behavior of another person. Generally this is without the cooperation, and sometimes without the direct knowledge and consent of the other person. Under these circumstances it is crucial that client and therapist discuss issues concerning the degree of participation, or nonparticipation, by the drinker.

Certainly there will be cases in which a particular client will not want the problem drinker, or other family members, to know of the client's current involvement in treatment. This needs to be respected for a number of reasons, but most importantly for the safety and well-being of the client. For example, if there have been incidents of domestic violence with a couple, you should be concerned that additional incidents may result if the drinker discovers that the spouse has entered treatment. In most cases it will be necessary to have a client provide specific instructions regarding all potential contact with other family members. For instance, you may need to note in the client's chart that he or she is *never* to be called to confirm an appointment, or never to be sent a bill for services to a home address.

Describing the Treatment Fully

As stated earlier, a brief overview of the goals and philosophy of CRT generally is presented in the initial session. This serves to apprise the CO of what to expect in treatment and to alleviate some of his or her anxiety. A full explanation of the program's components is presented in Session Two. The following information is covered and discussed:

1. CRT is designed for those family members and friends who would like to maintain their relationship with the drinker, but who want to encourage their loved one to reduce his or her drinking.
2. It is a skills-based approach in which the nondrinking family member is viewed as a positive and active force for change within the family.
3. Clients involved in CRT are asked to participate actively in written exercises, homework assignments, role plays, and other forms of behavioral training.
4. The decision to use a particular CRT technique remains entirely up to the client. Clients proceed at their own pace.
5. CRT clients make the decision as to whether to inform the drinker about the client's current involvement in treatment, and if so, when to do it.
6. The CRT therapist offers a commitment of support and training over a specified period of time.
7. Job-search information is offered to all CRT clients who desire assistance in organizing a job search, preparing a résumé, and practicing for job interviews.
8. A client's need for independent, enjoyable activities and other rewards is stressed.
9. Special arrangements are made with a cooperating alcohol treatment program that allows for a rapid intake, in the event that the problem drinker agrees to enter treatment.

Entertain questions and address concerns in the course of presenting this information. Discuss with the client how initially much of the work will be conducted with the nondrinker in the family. In most cases he or she will be the only one cooperating with treatment. Explain that under these circumstances, the prospect of change may seem a lonely and unrewarding enterprise; but it need not be! It is your role to provide the support and encouragement necessary to instill positive expectancies for change.

Realistically, there will be cases in which little or no progress is made in influencing the drinker. Clients need to understand and be prepared for this possibility. However, whether the drinker enters treatment is essentially unimportant at this stage. What is notable is the fact that the client now has taken a number of positive steps toward addressing his or her own distressing situation. By contacting the treatment program and walking into the session, the client has cast a vote of confidence; he or she is acknowledging that there is hope and desire for change.

You can strengthen the working alliance greatly by affirming your role in supporting the client's change efforts and in providing the necessary technical instruction. Thus a "teamwork" approach is fostered, with you serving at various times as guide, consultant, cheerleader, and confidant.

Overall, your task in Session Two is to cement the working relationship initiated in Session One. This includes building rapport using the clinical guidelines outlined previously, but flavored with your own therapeutic style. Also, the parameters of confidentiality should be understood by the client by the end of this session. Finally, you should have outlined the treatment process that you and the client will be following. In doing so, you should have stressed that regardless of what the drinker does, the client can continue to make the positive changes in his or her own life that he or she has begun by coming in for therapy.

SESSION 3: MOTIVATION TRAINING FOR THE CONCERNED OTHER

Rationale

As a CRT therapist, you will commonly be dealing with frustrated clients who have tried numerous, unsuccessful methods to get their family member or friend to stop drinking. These COs may have received advice that has not been very helpful, and in a number of cases, even detrimental. Surely, somewhere in the process they have been told that they are overreacting, and that the drinker does not really have a problem. Or it has been pointed out to them that it is *their* problem, and that they simply need to relax and accept it. Clients also may have been informed that they are responsible for their loved one's drinking problem. Despite all of these messages, and in some cases *because* of them, the client seeks treatment. Regardless of the reason, there is some degree of motivation prompting the CO to act. The key is to discover the source of the individual's motivation and to capitalize on it.

Although there are individualized reasons why a CO initially seeks treatment, in actuality there are several fairly common ones. For instance, COs begin psychotherapy because they feel emotionally distraught over their loved one's drinking problem. Other clients want their loved one to stop drinking so that he or she can find work and help with the bills, and sometimes clients want drinkers to curtail their alcohol use for the benefit of the children.

In general, be prepared to identify early the source of the client's current motivation for treatment, so that a solid and workable treatment program can be established without delay. Both assessment information and client comments regarding reasons for seeking treatment are useful in helping you determine each individual's specific motivators. Once you discover the reason why a client wants the loved one to stop drinking, you can rely on this information to motivate client change later in the treatment process.

"Hooking" the Client into Treatment

Although attendance at an initial therapy session is a sign of some level of motivation for treatment, it is well established within the general psychotherapy literature that *many* clients never return for a second session. And despite the fact that an individual actually may have reached his or her third session, it is still important to incorporate some motivational strategies that will "hook" the CO into further treatment.

There are many creative ways to motivate clients. Usually a good place to start is with a description of the benefits that may be produced from treatment. Certainly you will want to place a greater emphasis on those that appear most relevant to a particular client. Although the specifics may differ for each CO, the general advantages of CRT are as follows:

1. It helps increase the self-esteem of the CO.
2. It works to prevent verbal and physical abuse.
3. Often it leads to the reduction or cessation of the use of alcohol by the drinker.
4. In many cases, it leads indirectly to financial stability.
5. Often it motivates the drinker to enter treatment and work on the relationship.
6. It increases the number of enjoyable social activities for the CO, with or without the drinker.
7. It attempts to have the client change his or her behavior back to the way it was before the problems became severe.

If motivation is low because of past unsuccessful treatment attempts, you need to process the reasons why treatment failed, and then invite the client to come to several CRT sessions on a trial basis. A comparable situation with a problem drinker who is reluctant to commit to abstinence is handled by the CRA's Sobriety Sampling procedure (Meyers & Smith, 1995; Miller & Page, 1991). This technique encourages drinkers to "sample" sobriety for a time-limited period. A variation of this technique can be utilized to motivate CO's to "sample" CRT treatment for an agreed amount of time.

The following dialogue illustrates CRT sampling. The therapist (T) has just outlined the advantages of the approach and is now encouraging the client (C) to make a commitment to trying it.

T: I understand why you are skeptical. I know you have been frustrated with counseling in the past. But I believe this program can work for you. Would you be willing to commit to 12 CRT sessions? Twelve weeks is a very short period considering the number of years you've had to put up with his drinking.

C: I'm not sure. I've tried therapy before and it just cost me a lot of money with very little success. I want to believe it will be different this time, but I'm not totally sold on it.

T: Remember Ann, this program has been shown to be effective with people similar to you. But you're smart to be cautious. After all, I can't give you a guarantee. Probably the only way to convince you is to have you try it for a while to see how it works. How about giving it a try, just for a short period? How about agreeing to eight sessions just to sample the process?

C: I guess I could try it for 2 months. I've got nothing to lose!

This example shows the therapist bargaining down to find an acceptable sampling period. If the CO had been unwilling to commit to eight sessions, the therapist would have reduced the number to six, and then four. Most therapists routinely try to get a 12-week commitment first, and all therapists are willing to negotiate down to even just one more session.

Assistance from Family and Friends

Clients frequently are more motivated to continue treatment if there is a supportive individual accompanying them. Because the problem drinker is *not* the likely candidate, ask the client if he or she confides in a close friend or family member about the current situation. If it appears that this person would be a good resource, see if the client would feel comfortable bringing that person to therapy. In the event that the CO is agreeable with the idea, schedule the next session with both individuals. This will serve several purposes in addition to providing a source of support for the CO:

1. It will allow you to determine whether the friends and family view the problem in a similar fashion to the CO.
2. You will be able to enlist the aid of the client's friend in discovering more reinforcers for the client.
3. Practice exercises and role plays during the session and at home will be easier to conduct, because they will be taught to both the client and the friend.
4. The friend may have useful ideas that the client has overlooked. These may include suggestions for a "safe house" in the case of abuse, or nondrinking alternatives for future competing activities.

Benefits to the Concerned Other Once the Drinker Enters Treatment

Certainly one of the biggest motivators for a CO to remain in treatment is getting the drinker to begin treatment as well. During the course of therapy with the client, it is helpful to periodically review the many advantages to be realized once this occurs. For example, in the case in which domestic violence has happened or is a constant threat, the obvious benefit would be to reduce the risk of future harm. Data from a number of studies suggest that a husband's alcohol abuse represents a significant risk factor in physical abuse of his partner (e.g. Kantor & Straus, 1989; Telch & Lindquist, 1984). In this situation, a woman who is successful in persuading her husband to enter alcohol treatment has taken an important step in preventing future harm to herself and to her family.

Other potential benefits should be elicited on an individual basis and related to the importance of obtaining treatment for the drinker. Some examples might include the following:

1. Improvements in family finances due to the drinker spending less money on alcohol, or as a result of a more stable employment situation.
2. Greater sexual satisfaction due to the enhanced physical attractiveness of a sober partner, and in some cases his or her ability to perform better sexually when not inebriated.
3. Less marital conflict due to a more cooperative and effective problem-solving style.
4. Fewer problems with the children due to more effective role modeling and shared parenting responsibilities.
5. Increases in enjoyable family and social activities due to a less alcohol-centered lifestyle.

The CO should be reminded that the first step toward bringing the drinker into treatment is the CO continuing in the CRT program him- or herself.

Exercises

1. *Reviewing the Negative Consequences of Living with a Drinker.* Review with the client his or her answers provided at intake regarding the negative consequences of living with a problem drinker. Encourage the CO to discuss these responses to the extent that it is comfortable. For some clients, this exercise may represent the first look at the "total

impact" of living with an alcohol abuser. The very negative picture that is likely to emerge can be countered by reminding the client that change is possible and that people can and do recover from severe alcohol problems. Also, note that the client is not a mere passive observer in this process. The CO is an active and important individual who is capable of effecting change not only in his or her own life, but also in the lives of others.

2. *Enhancing the View of the Loved One.* Just as it is important to acknowledge the destructive nature of alcohol abuse, so also is it important to remind the client that the problem drinker is a loved and valued family member. To emphasize this point, have the client draw a line down the center of a blank sheet of paper and instruct as follows: On one side of the line, write a list of the positive attributes of the drinker when he or she is sober. On the other side, write the attributes of the drinker when drinking. Alternatively, the client can be asked to describe the drinker before alcohol became a problem in his or her life, and then to contrast this description with the client's current view of the drinker. The intermediate goal here is to enhance the client's view of the loved one by reminding him or her of those more positive attributes. Ask what the client likes (or used to like) about the drinker. What special qualities or gifts does the problem drinker possess? Ultimately, the goal is to increase motivation for the client by helping him or her realize that the potential benefits of therapy are extremely worthwhile.

3. *Establishing Realistic Goals.* Realistic goal establishment is an important part of changing behavior, but in addition to working toward the long-term goal of obtaining treatment for the drinker, it is important to identify more immediate personal goals for the client as well. Reaching short-term goals is an excellent way to increase motivation. As a simple exercise, ask the client to list five major life goals for the next year, and five for the subsequent 5 years. This can be done as a written exercise or as guided imagery. What changes will be necessary in order to achieve these goals? What role will Significant Others play in his or her future? What small steps can be taken *right now* to achieve these goals?

Summary

In summary, you should use each individual client's motivation for seeking therapy to create an appropriate treatment program. Design the specific program to assist the client without overwhelming or discouraging him or her. Utilize the suggestions for "hooking" the client into treatment initially and for helping the client appreciate the benefits for remaining in therapy. Point out that there are advantages not only for the client, but for the drinking loved one as well.

SESSION 4: HANDLING DANGEROUS SITUATIONS

Rationale

A number of reports have described a significant association between alcohol abuse and domestic violence (Coleman & Straus, 1983; Gelles & Cornell, 1990; and Leonard & Jacob, 1988). One line of evidence for the association comes from studies assessing the incidence of partner violence in samples of identified problem drinkers. For example, in a sample of 52 men enrolled in alcoholism treatment programs, Stith, Crossman, and Bischof (1991) found that 59% admitted to using violence in their relationships in the past year. For a sample of 218 male alcoholics entering an inpatient Veterans Administration alcoholism unit, Gondolf and Foster (1991) discovered that over a third of the men (39%) reported assaulting their partners at least once during the previous year. Interestingly, a subsample of 33 wives or partners of these same men reported rates of assault that were almost double that reported by the men. O'Farrell and Choquette (1991) similarly found elevated rates of partner violence in a sample of male problem drinkers.

Although not all family members and friends of problem drinkers are at elevated risk for physical abuse, CRT includes instructions for all clients in techniques aimed at reducing risk of physical harm. Changes in the way that the CO relates to the drinker as a result of CRT may elicit feelings of confusion, frustration, or even rage in the drinker. The CO must be made aware of this potential response and be prepared to deal with it.

Clients who are fearful of making changes in their home situation, or who are being threatened by the drinker, will need to move more slowly through the treatment process. It is essential that they not place themselves at further risk. Before clients carry out any of the behavior shaping and modification procedures with the drinker, they must be able to recognize the potential for danger and know what steps to take to protect themselves.

Assessment of Violence

The goals of the initial assessment of violence are (1) to determine the level of violence that has occurred in the drinker–CO relationship, and the potential for future episodes; (2) to assess the level of contact the CO maintains with family members and friends, and thereby the extent to which these people might be counted upon as sources of support and refuge in dealing with incidents of abuse; and (3) to work with the client in developing an appropriate protection plan based on this information. This may include plans for escaping an abusive situation or initiating legal remedies to halt abuse. Methods for accomplishing each of these three goals are discussed below.

1. *Assessing current levels of violence.* The intake assessment should include a general screening instrument that assesses use of violence to resolve disagreements. The Conflict Tactics Scale (Straus, 1979) is a reasonable choice, for it examines a variety of strategies that couples use to resolve disagreements, including verbal aggression and physical violence. The *Past Year* scale reports periods of recent violence. The *Ever* scale indicates whether episodes of violence have occurred at earlier stages of the relationship. Endorsements of items e–k generally are indicative of mild forms of aggression, l–n signify moderate violence, and o–s represent severe violence.

Comparing lifetime and past-year reports of violence gives some indication of change in the incidence of violence. However, the client should also be asked directly about recent increases in episodes of abuse. After reviewing the instruments completed at intake, proceed by asking if there have been any incidents of violence during the period *since* intake. It is important at this point to allow the CO to report these incidents in his or her own words and at his or her own pace, without attempts to problem solve. Suggested phrasing for eliciting a description of any abusive events and for inquiring about potential future episodes of violence includes the following:

> "I know it is difficult to talk about this, and I appreciate your courage in being able to discuss this with me."

> "Have there been times when your spouse/relative/friend just seemed to 'fly off the handle' and become violent?"

> "Again, I know this is difficult, but I want you to describe for me one of the times when you were abused. Tell me what was happening before the violence started,

what happened during the incident, and what happened afterward. (And how did the violence stop?)"

"We talked about some episodes in the past, now I'd like to ask you if there have been any recent episodes of violence, particularly since the day you first came in and filled out these forms?"

"Are you currently afraid that your spouse/relative/friend might harm you?" (If "yes") "What is it that you are afraid he or she might do?"

"Does your spouse/relative/friend know that you are seeking help because of his or her drinking?" (If "no") "What do you think might happen if he or she found out you were coming here for counseling?"

"Do you have any concerns about the safety of your children (or the safety of others in the family)?"

2. *Assessing current social support.* The intake assessment should include at least one instrument that indicates the CO's current level of social functioning and resources. One frequently used scale is the Health and Daily Living Form (Moos et al., 1987). Items from a tool such as this will alert you to the range and quality of everyday social contacts that the CO maintains, as well as to the number of people the CO can count on in times of trouble.

In the event that the CO reports abuse, you should also ask directly if he or she has discussed these experiences with a friend or family member, or if others are at least aware of the abusive situation. The occurrence of violence often leads to isolation, making responses to the violence more difficult. If the CO appears to be dealing with the violence in isolation, ask if he or she would consider discussing the problem with a friend or relative, or a support group. Provide assistance in setting this up.

3. *Developing a protection plan.* The primary objective in a domestic violence crisis is to provide for the safety and well-being of the victim. This can be accomplished either by helping the individual escape to a safe haven or by assisting in the removal of the batterer from the home by the police or through court intervention. These options are next described.

Use of a Safe House

COs who report that they are in grave danger should be advised to leave the situation immediately. Incidents of abuse that result in hospitalization or other indications of severe injury should be considered as evidence of grave danger. The CO's subjective report of immediate danger also should be taken as sufficient evidence.

Domestic-violence shelters provide temporary refuge for women who are fleeing an abusive situation. In most cases, the call to the safe house should be made immediately upon the determination of grave danger. Arrangements for transportation for the victim and any children involved can be made in consultation with the safe house.

As an alternative, the CO may choose to escape to the home of a trusted friend or relative. In this case, it is useful for you and the CO to discuss plans for enlisting the aid of the friend and arranging transportation.

Police Intervention

COs who choose to return to a potentially violent home should be reminded that police intervention is available by dialing 911. In some areas of the country, police departments now offer specialized services to victims of domestic violence, including transportation to shelters, medical services, and legal advocacy.

Legal Intervention via Temporary Restraining Order

Many states have the means whereby victims of domestic violence may petition the district court for a temporary restraining order. Although laws differ from state to state, some do not require actual harm to have taken place before issuing an order of protection; a threat is sufficient. You should be familiar with the applicable laws in your area.

The victim of domestic violence can apply for a temporary restraining order simply by filling out a petition under oath that describes the nature of the complaint. Forms and instructions for completion are available from the police or the clerk's office in the local courthouse. In most states, the victim does not need an attorney.

Usually within 10 days a hearing is scheduled with both parties present to determine whether a 90-day protective order is needed. As a result of the hearing, the court may order the respondent to refrain from abusing the petitioner or other persons, to stay away from the victim, to leave the house, and to pay temporary child or spousal support. Additional issues typically considered at this stage include constraints on communication, disposition, and maintenance of property during the 90 days, child visitation arrangements, consequences of violating the order, and a recommendation for counseling. During the time the order is in effect, either party may request a review hearing for the purpose of amending the order. At the request of the petitioner, and with good cause, the order usually may be extended at the discretion of the court.

The temporary restraining order is not intended to serve as a permanent solution. Its purpose is to give both parties a 90-day separation period, during which time they are to seek a more permanent resolution to their problem.

Prevention of Domestic Violence

In cases involving only threats of violence or minor incidents of verbal aggression, the focus of counseling shifts to prevention and problem-solving skills. The basic skills can be introduced in a single session, with additional review and training included in subsequent sessions as the need arises. What follows are some general guidelines regarding issues to cover when working with COs who may have experienced mild abuse.

Open Expression of Feelings

It is important that COs who have experienced abuse be allowed to express their emotions openly and honestly in the treatment session. Expressions of anger directed toward the abuser should not be minimized, for it is important to affirm the CO's right to his or her feelings. This is not to suggest that fantasies of violence or revenge should be supported, but rather the CO's rightful anger should be directed toward purposeful acts of self-control, self-empowerment, and independence.

Recognition of the Buildup of Danger

Individuals who have experienced abuse in their relationships or in their families of origin often come to view violence among intimates as a normal occurrence. Moreover, they have difficulty seeing acts of violence as the unfortunate outcome of a progression of events. Instead, the violence is seen as an explosive and unpredictable act. With this in mind, it is often helpful to ask clients to describe the events that typically occur *prior* to an outbreak of abuse, and those that happen directly afterwards. By slowing the process down and "walking" the client through the sequence of events, you can help him or her see that there may be many warning signs that danger is approaching. Show the CO how these warning signs can be used as cues to take action to escape the violence.

Development of Safety Plans

Clients who are not in a crisis situation but who anticipate the possibility of abuse should be advised to develop plans for responding to the threats of violence. For instance, COs should be cognizant of access routes in and out of the house. Also, be sure to warn them against being backed into a corner or taken into remote areas of the home when arguments or high-risk situations are developing. Encourage clients to keep essential personal items (a change of clothing, extra money or checkbook, identification and other important documents) stored at the home of a friend or packed secretly in their own home for easy access should it become necessary to leave rapidly. Escape plans and a checklist should be reviewed with clients and rehearsed periodically in order to develop confidence in their use.

Advocacy and Referral

Additional community resources exist for dealing with abusive situations. You should become familiar with the different types of resources that exist in the local community (i.e., rape-crisis centers, women's cooperatives, victims' advocacy services). This information can be provided to the CO, along with an offer of help in securing any of the services one might require.

Summary

The correlation between alcohol abuse and domestic violence is a factor that cannot be overlooked when conducting CRT. Although domestic violence is not always present in households where there is problem drinking, its occurrence is common enough that the assessment of its potential should be included in your work with the CO. If violence is a risk, you must be sure the CO understands that changing his or her behavior initially may elicit negative responses from the drinker. Given this possibility, you and the client need to develop plans of action that will ensure the CO's safety.

SESSION 5: INTRODUCING THE NOTION OF ALTERNATIVE RESPONSES TO DRINKING

Rationale

Generally the CO is an individual who maintains a great deal of everyday contact with the drinker. The CO is in a unique position to observe and respond to the daily behavior of the drinker across a wide variety of situations. Thus, even small changes in the behavior of the CO can have great effects on the drinker. Consequently, the CO is an ideal person to train to become more aware of the ways in which his or her own behavior might positively or negatively influence the behavior of the drinker.

Assessing Current Responses to Drinking

**Robert J. Meyers
et al.**

Before beginning instruction in how to react to a loved one's drinking, it is advisable to conduct a brief assessment of the client's current pattern of responding. Essentially you are assessing the degree to which the CO is reacting to the drinking in ways that provide positive reinforcement. Due to their contact with self-help groups or popular media accounts, many clients now recognize that caretaking behavior provides the drinker with powerful reinforcing effects and shields him or her from many of the aversive consequences of excessive drinking.

> I used to be one of those women who'd wait up for him and stay up all night, wondering when he'd get home, and in what condition.... Then when he'd get home, I'd try to make sure that he got to bed.... (It) seemed like I was always trying to take care of him, and get him to bed.
>
> 35-year-old spouse

Other forms of caretaking include lending alcoholics money to buy alcohol, drinking with them, picking them up and getting them home when drunk, saving meals for them, cleaning up after them should they vomit or become incontinent, and bailing them out of jail. By no means is this list exhaustive. Responses such as these carry obvious rewarding and reinforcing value. The drinking behavior results in attention, physical contact and care, emotional closeness, and convenience for the drinker. These are the types of responses that will have to be altered if the CO is to be successful in promoting sobriety.

Principles for Managing Behavior

COs typically report that they have tried any number of different approaches in an effort to get the drinker to stop or control the drinking. Unsystematic "home remedies" such as these generally result in little or no improvement for the drinker and much frustration for the CO (See Wiseman, 1980). In this section, the basic principles of a more systematic approach to changing unwanted behaviors are introduced. It begins with an examination of failed attempts to influence the loved one's drinking. What *doesn't* work in getting a drinker to stop or slow down:

- Pouring alcohol down the drain.
- Nagging the drinker to stop.
- Getting drunk to show the drinker "what it's like."
- Yelling and fighting about the drinking.
- Threatening the drinker.
- Emotional pleading, crying.
- Rational pleading, lecturing.
- Acting "crazy" so the drinker can see what it's doing to you.

In theory, punishing a behavior will serve to decrease that behavior. In practice, a number of problems may arise. First, what is the proper amount of punishment to apply during a drinking episode? Punishment that is too mild actually may reinforce a behavior. Punishment that is too severe may trigger the use of alcohol as a coping mechanism, or it may instigate retaliation by the drinker. Second, punishment affords little opportunity to learn "proper" alternative behaviors. If drinking is a punished behavior, what is a rewarded behavior? Reasonable alternatives to drinking are not apparent from any of these examples. Third, a behavior that is first punished and then rewarded becomes extremely resistant to extinction. If yelling and fighting about drinking are later followed by the family members making up, then the drinking and the fighting simply will come to serve as cues for reconciliation. Finally, use of punishment evokes an emotional reaction toward the punisher. In a family setting, the drinker may end up avoiding, fearing, or resenting a CO who relies on punishment.

Are there any strategies that *are* helpful when responding to a loved one's drinking? If you ask a client what *does* work, be prepared to be met with a moment of stunned silence or an "If I knew that I wouldn't be here" response. Nevertheless, often this will be followed by some rather surprising acknowledgments of successful strategies:

> When I'd see my wife start heading for the bottle after dinner I'd ask her, "Would you like to go to a movie with me?" Sometimes she would, and we'd have a great time. If she didn't go, then I'd know I wouldn't want to be around her anyway.
>
> 52-year-old spouse

> Going to church. When we used to go to church regularly he never drank as much. Even now he doesn't drink on days we go to church.
>
> 33-year-old spouse

> When his uncle gave him a job and just sat on him.... Plus on weekends, Jim started motocross racing again and he never drank when he was racing motocross.
>
> 27-year-old friend

> Getting away from her, going to another room ... and sometimes she'd follow me and say some pretty rotten stuff... so I'd have to tell her pretty forcefully, "I just don't care to discuss this with you when you've had this much to drink"... and she'd get away.
>
> 54-year-old spouse

A common theme running through these four statements is that the actions of a CO resulted in some measure of influence over someone else's behavior. The first two statements represent examples of using the principle of *response incompatibility.* On those occasions when the problem drinkers accompanied their spouses to a movie or church, they were engaging in behaviors that interfered with the opportunity to stay home and get drunk. In the first case, the husband also used the principle of *response cost,* in that he removed a positive reinforcer when his wife drank. The reinforcer was the husband's company, since it was known that the wife found it rewarding. The third statement illustrates *positive reinforcement* for sobriety. Positive reinforcers are defined by their capacity to increase the rate of a given behavior. In this situation, the client's sobriety was reinforced through a job. Both the job and the motocross racing could be viewed as examples of response incompatibility as well.

Using Contingency Management at Home

Applying the basic principles of reinforcement in the home setting is one of the core procedures of CRT. Complete descriptions of these principles and specific examples follow. For instance, *contingency management* is the process of influencing rates of behavior by affecting the consequences that follow those behaviors. Positive and negative reinforcement are two methods of contingency management. A *positive reinforcer* is anything that increases the rate of the behavior it follows. COs who provide pleasant company, small favors, and positive attention *only* when the family member is *sober* are applying positive reinforcers for sobriety. To provide the same pleasantry, favors, and attention when the individual is drinking is to apply positive reinforcement for drinking.

A second method of contingency management is negative reinforcement. Reinforcement of a behavior always results in a greater rate of occurrence of the behavior. In *negative reinforcement,* the behavior of interest is increased by removing something aversive from the situation. Some of the aversive consequences of overdrinking include hangovers, arrests, and even loss of employment. The drinker can learn to eliminate these negative consequences by refraining from drinking. In turn, sobriety is reinforced. The CO's role in this procedure is to make sure that he or she does not soften or remove any of the naturally occurring aversive consequences of excessive alcohol use for the drinker.

Additional related methods of contingency management are extinction, response cost, time-out from positive reinforcement, and response incompatibility. All four procedures result in *decreases* in behavior. In the *extinction* condition, behaviors that previously resulted in reinforcement are no longer reinforced. The result is that the behavior is eliminated over time. In psychiatric hospitals, nursing personnel frequently found that by attending to a patient's "psychotic talk" they were unable to eliminate it. When they were instructed to ignore all psychotic talk and attend only to sensible verbalizations, the psychotic talk diminished. CRT clients are advised to ignore, as much as possible, attempts by intoxicated family members to initiate conversations, arguments, or physical or sexual interactions. This serves to preclude, or at least minimize, possible reinforcement of drunken behavior. The fourth client statement listed earlier serves as an example of this.

In *response cost,* positive reinforcements are withdrawn for emitting a particular behavior. In other words, one is forced to "pay a price" for engaging in the behavior. Response costs are used with problem drinkers when they are required to pay for damages related to drunken behavior. COs can help suppress the drunken behavior by expecting drinkers to pay their own fines, pay for any property damages, make their own apologies and reparations, and otherwise settle accounts for their own behavior.

Time-out from positive reinforcement is a form of response cost in that positive reinforcements are withdrawn. However, time-out is unique since it generally involves removing the individual from the reinforcing situation, thereby eliminating all opportunity for positive reinforcement. In actuality, time-out from positive reinforcement is an ideal rather than an accomplished goal in most applied settings, primarily because a person's entire reward structure rarely is under the immediate control of a single person. But in the event that it is possible and desirable to implement this technique, be certain that the situation from which the person is being removed is indeed a positively reinforcing one and not an aversive one. Removing someone from an unpleasant situation will result in increasing the precise behavior you are trying to eliminate.

The time-out principle plays a prominent role in the CRA treatment of the problem drinker directly. The therapist and the drinker seek to arrange natural reinforcers in such a way that drinking represents a time-out from positive reinforcement. For example, drinking would remove one from satisfying job or family interactions. The more the social environment can be arranged to reflect this condition, the greater are the person's chances of remaining sober.

A final principle related to contingency management is that of *response incompatibility.* In the first of the client's statements listed earlier, a man indicated that when he observed his wife about to begin drinking, he suggested that they go to a movie. Drinking alcohol and watching a movie in a movie theater are, for the most part, incompatible responses. They are behaviors that are difficult to do at the same time, and which interfere with one another when they are attempted simultaneously. Competing responses for drinking behaviors vary tremendously across individuals. For some it may be attendance at church or Alcoholics Anonymous. For others it may mean finding suitable employment, developing friendships with nondrinkers, or developing recreational activities, such as bike-riding, swimming, or tennis (i.e., activities in which you cannot hold a beverage or take a drink while you are engaged in it).

These basic principles form the backbone of any behavior-change program. They can be applied systematically to one's own behavior or someone else's across a wide range of problem areas. Whether the goal is to lose weight, eliminate a child's disruptive behavior in the classroom, help psychiatric patients develop better self-care habits, become more assertive, or influence a loved one's drinking, the principles of learning provide a firm scientific base on which to build a personal program for change.

In training COs how to utilize behavioral principles for decreasing drinking behavior, you should be watchful of their misapplication. Clients sometimes happen upon very useful and creative ways of responding to the drinking, but, for whatever reason, they fail to notice the utility of the response or neglect to employ it in a consistent fashion. Thus, clients may report that they abandoned their efforts to use positive and negative reinforcement, response costs, and so on, because the responses did not produce an immediate and unequivocal halt to the drinking. The solution is to review the principles utilized by the CO during the week, and to incorporate role plays and supply corrective feedback when necessary.

Recognizing Signs of Intoxication

Many of the exercises and procedures suggested in this manual are based on the client's ability to recognize cues to the loved one's drinking. Therefore, the client must become adept at identifying signs of intoxication. For many COs this may seem an obvious task, and they will be quite familiar with the stereotypical drinking behavior of the loved one. For others, it may be quite a revealing exercise when you ask them to identify the typical behaviors associated with their loved one's drinking.

For this exercise, it is better for the client to have his or her own notebook and writing instrument. Have the client write out each question as you ask it, and then instruct them to provide an answer in the space below it. Start with signs of obvious intoxication: What changes does the client notice in the loved one's speech, actions, mood? Are there changes in the drinker's appearance or dress? Are there specific situations or circumstances that are more likely to result in drinking to intoxication (e.g., such as drinking with certain individuals, or drinking in certain bars)?

Next, move to the situation in which the drinker has had only one drink. Review the typical behaviors of the drinker in the same manner as before. Have the client write out these behaviors as a guide to recognizing different levels of intoxication. You might then ask the CO if he or she can describe the cues or triggers that signal the beginning of a bout of drinking. Are there certain mood states? Are there certain days of the week or times of the day? Are there specific events?

Refer back to this exercise when you begin to work with clients in developing new responses to the drinking. If COs plan to provide positive reinforcements for sobriety, they must be reasonably sure that the loved one is, in fact, sober. If they intend to withhold reinforcements when the drinker is intoxicated, can they tell that he or she has been drinking? If they want to suggest a competing activity, can they do so before a drinking bout begins?

Summary

In summary, this session introduces the client to the notion of using alternative approaches to influence the drinker's behavior. Specifically, systematic strategies are suggested that will enable the CO to reinforce the drinker when he or she is engaged in nondrinking, positive behaviors. Alternatively, other strategies are offered that the CO may use to suppress the drinker's less desirable behaviors without direct punishment.

SESSION 6: ARRANGING POSITIVE CONSEQUENCES FOR NOT DRINKING

Rationale

This session is designed to help the CO learn how to appropriately reward his or her partner for *not* drinking. Theoretically, the more rewarding nondrinking behavior becomes, the less drinking will occur. This session focuses on helping the CO first identify and then apply meaningful reinforcers in an effort to promote nondrinking behavior.

A word of caution is in order. Do not be surprised if the CO initially resists the idea of providing rewards to a drinker who has made no commitment to change. Be prepared to support and motivate the CO on this issue. Help the client understand that by rewarding the drinker for nondrinking behavior, such nondrinking behavior should become more and more frequent.

Identifying Current Nondrinking Activities

The first step in training the CO to provide positive reinforcement for his or her family member's nondrinking behavior involves identifying several situations or activities in which the problem drinker does not drink. Next determine whether these situations are enjoyable for the drinker, or whether he or she is actually unhappy during this time because of the absence of alcohol. Be careful not to settle for "artificial" reinforcers, namely, activities that are rewarding for the CO but not necessarily for the drinker. For instance, if the CO identifies an evening of alcohol-free card playing with the family as an example of a reinforcing activity, probe to be certain that the drinker, and not just the CO, truly enjoys this activity. Once you are convinced that several rewarding, nondrinking activities have been identified, speak to the CO about the possibility of increasing the frequency of occurrence of these activities. Explore what the CO's role would be in promoting this. Explain how it is easier and less "risky" to first concentrate on behaviors and rewards that are already in place.

Generating a List of Positive Reinforcers

Typically, a CO is able to generate only a short list of reinforcing nondrinking activities or situations that already are taking place. Consequently it is necessary to assist in generating ideas for new ways to introduce rewards for sober behavior. Support the client's attempt to start this process by explaining that the CO knows his or her partner better than anyone. This knowledge is extremely useful in establishing a list of ways to reward the drinker for abstaining.

Begin the procedure by presenting general guidelines for naming potential rewards. State that the list should contain the following:

1. As many positive reinforcers as possible (e.g., 10–20 items).
2. Several rewards for sobriety that worked in the past.
3. A number of reinforcers that support current nondrinking behaviors that the drinker is presently enjoying.
4. Reinforcers that are obviously rewarding to the drinker.
5. Rewards that are easily fit into the drinker's schedule, and consequently can realistically be used.
6. Reinforcers that are easy for the CO to deliver.
7. Several activities in which concerned friends and family members offer the rewards.
8. Several rewards that are reinforcers for other family members in addition to the drinker.

Once the client understands the guidelines for establishing a list of positive reinforcers, supply several common examples, which may include the following:

1. Preparing the drinker's favorite foods.
2. Talking about topics the drinker enjoys.
3. Giving small, inexpensive gifts.
4. Offering the drinker verbal praise and support.
5. Providing the drinker with his or her favorite sexual activity.

Once a lengthy list of positive reinforcers for abstaining has been established, have the client rank the list from the perspective of what the drinker would perceive as the most desirable reward down to the least desirable reward. Next have the CO rate how comfortable he or she would feel in delivering any given reinforcer. If the number-one reinforcer for the partner is one that the client currently would feel uncomfortable providing, then it should not be considered yet. Check with the CO at a later date about whether he or she would be comfortable supplying that reinforcer. Also be prepared for many CRT clients to be reluctant to introduce *any* new reinforcer until they have spent several weeks in therapy. Some simply need time to process the impending interaction and build confidence before they are ready to take action. Clients should not be pushed to act too quickly.

Somewhere in the course of this process it may be necessary to remind the CO that giving positive rewards for not drinking is simply a show of support. It is not considered enabling or rescuing behavior, because it is introduced when the drinker is *sober*.

Introducing Positive Reinforcers to the Drinker

The client should be encouraged to begin introducing positive reinforcers for nondrinking behavior at home once the following has been accomplished:

1. The client understands the concept and feels comfortable using positive reinforcement.
2. The client has shown proficiency in identifying what would be reinforcing to the drinker.
3. The client has demonstrated during behavioral rehearsal that he or she is capable of delivering the reinforcer appropriately.
4. The CO has successfully practiced using positive reinforcement on a nondrinking family member or friend.
5. Session time has been devoted to considering the possible consequences of the action, and problem-solving exercises have identified solutions when necessary.

6. You have discussed the CO's possible resentment for having to "do all the work" and give rewards when the drinker is the one who has caused so much trouble and pain.
7. The two basic rules for *when* the rewards should be delivered have been reviewed:
   (a) Give positive reinforcers only when the drinker is sober and not hungover.
   (b) Pick an optimal time to use positive reinforcement (i.e., the drinker is both sober and in a good mood, and the CO is in an upbeat and positive mood).

Verbally Linking a Reward with Sober Behavior

As noted earlier, simple communication can be used as a positive reinforcer. Obvious examples include compliments and statements about positive feelings for the drinker. But communication can play another vital role when it creates clear verbal links between the rewards a CO is providing and the nondrinking behavior. In essence, the CO is taught and encouraged to explain the reasons behind his or her actions to the drinker. An example of this type of conversation between a well-trained client (C) and his drinking partner (D) follows:

C: Hi, Connie. I'm glad you're home. I was hoping that if I told you in advance I was going to be cooking dinner on the grill tonight, you'd come straight home after work and not stop off and get a drink with your friends.
D: I wasn't going to stop off and get a drink anyway. I don't drink after work that much.
C: The point is, dear, that I really like you coming home right after work. You're much more fun to be with when you don't drink. So my fixing dinner is a way of showing you how much I want to be with you. I know my grilled steaks are one of your favorites.
D: I do really like it when you grill, but I was coming home anyway, just like I said. Are you saying that you only want to be with me if I don't drink? What's going on around here anyway?
C. I just want you to know that I sometimes can't handle it when you drink, but I love you and really like being around you when you don't drink. And I am willing to do whatever I can to be with you when you're sober. Sometimes I miss the old you; the person I fell in love with.
D: I'm still the same person. I just like to drink a little. Let's forget this stuff now and just enjoy dinner.
C: I just wanted you to know how I feel. Okay, let's eat.

The client told his wife exactly why he made dinner and how he felt about her drinking, yet he did it in a very supportive and nonconfrontational way. He was firm but not angry or accusatory. The drinker was somewhat surprised, but she did not react strongly to his remarks. Ultimately, she ended the discussion about her drinking. The CO was very appropriate, inasmuch as he persisted in making his point, but then stopped pushing when his spouse acted as if she had heard enough. COs should be trained not to force their partner into a confrontation. They should be taught to discuss pertinent issues only up to the point at which it appears that the conversation is on the verge of taking a turn for the worse. If in this last dialogue the wife had become angry after the first statement, then the husband would have tabled the discussion until a later date.

When the drinking partner is aware of the fact that his or her CO is in treatment, the conversation between them about the CO's change in behavior typically is more problematic. Assume, for instance, that the client somewhat unsuccessfully tried new ways to reward the drinker for nondrinking behavior. It would not be unusual for the drinker to become angry and ask questions such as, "Is this the stuff your therapist told you to do?" In many cases the drinker acts sarcastic and belittles the client for going to therapy. The following dialogue is an example of how a CRT therapist and client might process a difficult attempt to reward a partner for sobriety.

> C: Well, I tried to do what we talked about last week, and he was horrible to me. I did just like we practiced. I told him I planned his favorite dinner and invited his parents over to play cards, because I wanted to show him my appreciation for his staying sober. He immediately jumped on me for not consulting him. Then he said it was probably all that damn therapist's idea anyway, and I was doing it to please you, not to please him.
>
> T: This is a common reaction. I would rather have him angry with me than angry with you. I bet you felt hurt and discouraged. How did you handle it?
>
> C: Well, I remembered what we discussed. So, I told him that I love him and want to spend time with him, but it was hard for me to be with him when he was drinking. I told him I could not deal with his drinking and I was trying to do whatever I could to help my life become easier.
>
> T: Great job! You remembered to do all of that? How did he respond to that?
>
> C: He said I sounded like a therapy record, that I was brainwashed and it was all garbage. He said that if I really loved him it wouldn't matter that he drinks.
>
> T: He sounds pretty angry and confused. What happened next?
>
> C: He calmed down and said he didn't mind playing cards, but next time check with him first. He also wanted to know why I really go to therapy, and what we do here.
>
> T: You did an excellent job. I bet it was hard to keep your cool, but you managed. I think, overall, it was a great first attempt to establish positive rewards and competing activities.

You should note that although the drinker in this dialogue was abrasive, it was important for the therapist to reframe some of his statements into a more positive light for the CO. Similarly it is important to reinforce any attempt at a new behavior by a CO. You should focus first on those aspects of the behavior that were effective, and then use the session to role-play and problem-solve the more troublesome segments of the interaction.

Inviting the Drinker to Attend Treatment

It is fairly common for a drinker to start asking questions about *why* a CO has changed some of his or her behaviors, particularly once the client begins to draw a verbal link between rewards and sobriety. As illustrated in the previous dialogue, the drinker who is aware of the CO's involvement in therapy may even start to inquire about the therapy process. Frequently this is an ideal time to invite the curious drinker to attend a session.

The dialogue continues with an example of how to encourage the client to ask the drinker to come in to meet the therapist. The therapist suggests a manner that should be minimally threatening to the drinker.

> T: I think it's a good sign that he is curious about your therapy program. Perhaps we could use his curiosity about our work together as a way to get him into treatment for himself. What do you think?
>
> C: I don't know. He has always said that therapy is a bunch of bull that's only for weak people.
>
> T: That's a pretty common response, especially from people who have never actually tried therapy. As you know from your own experience, therapy actually takes a lot of emotional strength and really hard work.
>
> C: That's for sure!
>
> T: I would like you to continue to tell him that you are working on your problem of how to handle the way you feel when he drinks. Next time he asks about your therapy or puts it down, why don't you tell him that I would like to meet him, that I could use his help even. Let

him know that we do discuss him and that he is welcome to come in and just observe if he doesn't want to participate. Tell him that I am just as curious about him as he is about me. How do you think that would go over?

C: I'm not sure. He does seem inquisitive at times about what we're doing in therapy. I could try it. I'm not afraid to ask him to come, as long as I say it's my therapy and not for him.

T: That's fine. It's a first step. Once he gets familiar with me and the therapy process, it will be easier to begin to focus on his problems. You're doing a great job. Keep it up!

You will need to think of creative ways to entice the drinker to attend a session, while causing a minimal amount of disruption at home. Some drinkers will respond to an invitation simply to hear what you are telling the CO. Or you may have the client tell the problem drinker that you want to ask him or her some questions about the client; that the drinker's input is needed to work on the client's problems. Occasionally, with the client's permission, you can call the drinker and request his or her help in the treatment process. But timing is so critical in these circumstances that you and the client should plan an optimal time to call the drinker. If this cannot be anticipated in advance, you might instruct the client to call you when the time is right. And only the CO, the person who knows the drinker best, knows when the time is right. This implies that you are willing to respond quickly before the peak moment vanishes.

Reinforcement for the Client

Clients need to reward *themselves* for all their hard work, particularly when they have not yet been rewarded through behavior change on the part of the drinker. Certainly they will receive praise from you for their commitment, but many will need more than that to stay motivated. So have them make lists with at least 10 examples of small ways to reward themselves for doing good work. Be prepared to support them in this exercise, since many COs view it as being selfish. Explain that it is part of the program, and even though it may feel uncomfortable, it is in their best interest.

Reinforcers for the client can come in multiple ways. They can be activities done independently of the drinker, or they can be activities with the drinker that double as a reinforcer for both of them. Examples of the first type of reinforcer might include taking a class that has interested the CO for some time, going to see a movie, or having lunch with friends. An example of the latter would be to find a baby-sitter and get away for a romantic weekend with the drinker. Naturally, the drinker may become interested in why the client is changing his or her old behavior. The CO may respond that he or she feels better since beginning to work on personal problems, and therefore wants to reward him- or herself. As illustrated in the previous section, at times this even can be used indirectly to motivate the drinker to enter therapy.

Summary

In summary, this session teaches the CO how to reinforce nondrinking behavior in the drinker through a positive reinforcement process. Not only is the drinker reinforced, but the CO also is rewarded by observing the changes that are brought about by his or her own new behaviors. However, it is important also to assist the CO in setting up more personal rewards. This insures that even in those cases in which change in the drinker is slow or nonexistent, there is still reinforcement for the CO's own change and efforts.

SESSION 7: NEGATIVE CONSEQUENCES FOR DRINKING BEHAVIOR

Rationale

This session teaches COs to extinguish the unwanted drinking behavior of another person through the use of negative consequences and the application of the principles of extinction. It is important to explain that these procedures should be relied on only after use of positive reinforcement has been insufficient to produce the desired behavior change.

Recognizing Subtle Ways the Concerned Other "Supports" Drinking Behavior

An important first step is gently pointing out the ways in which the client may be unintentionally "supporting" his or her partner's drinking behavior. This topic needs to be addressed delicately, because many clients will resist the idea that any of their behaviors actually make drinking an easier choice for their loved one. The following conversation is a typical way for a CRT therapist (T) to help a client (C) see the real impact of his or her behavior, and to encourage the CO to try something new:

T: So why don't you tell me about one of the obvious ways Charlie's drinking makes things more difficult for you. Can you think of something you end up having to do as a result of his drinking?

C: Sure. The first thing that comes to mind is how I end up serving dinner twice each night, once for me and the kids, and then for him when he eventually makes it home from the bar.

T: And why is it that you go ahead and prepare dinner for him on a regular basis like that when he's late because of his drinking?

C: I've always kept dinner in the oven for him. I want to make sure he doesn't get sick. He works hard and needs to eat.

T: But do you see that you're indirectly supporting his drinking habit by helping him get a warm meal? You're taking care of him so he can drink.

C: No I'm not. I'm just getting him some supper. I resent that comment about me supporting his drinking.

T: I'm sorry if I have upset you. I know you really care about him and you're trying to help him *and* you. And it's because you care so much about him that I know you'll want to do what's best for him. So I need to point out that anytime you make it a little easier for him to drink, it's almost like you are supporting it. You see, if he knows that you're going to have his supper ready no matter when he comes home, why should he care when he gets home? He knows his supper will be ready, so he can stay out and drink as long as he feels like it. You are making it easier for him to drink and get his meals, too. Do you like him coming in late at night after drinking? Do you like to reheat his food and go to all that extra effort, just to make it easier for him to drink?

C: I hate his drinking. I just thought that I was doing what was expected of me. I don't want to make it easy for him to drink. I just never looked at suppertime in that way before.

T: I know. It *is* a different way of looking at things. And I know you were doing your best. I'm not trying to make you feel bad. I want to support you and help you get your life the way you want it. Would you be willing to take a look at what happens in your house around suppertime, so we can see if there are ways to influence your husband's behavior?

C: Yes, definitely.

The therapist in this dialogue was unwavering in pointing out the effect of the client's behavior on her partner's drinking. However, it was equally important for the therapist to reinforce the client for showing concern for the drinker. It is this type of concern that can be modified through CRT into more effective responding.

Responding to Unwanted Drinking Behaviors

Once your client realizes that there are probably better ways to respond to the loved one's drinking behavior, it is time to explore the options carefully. The rules that follow allow you to systematically address the unwanted drinking behaviors reported by each client in an individualized manner:

1. Ask the client to discuss examples of unwanted drinking behaviors and their consequences. If necessary, assist with examples from other clients.
2. Instruct the client to list these behaviors on a piece of paper or on a blackboard.
3. Have the client pick one behavior that he or she is comfortable discussing and is prepared to address.
4. Explore the possibility of using positive reinforcement to change the behavior. If it is unfeasible or has not worked in the past when delivered appropriately, discuss the rationale behind using a negative consequence.
5. Select a reasonable, timely, negative consequence for the drinking behavior, and explore its impact on the drinker. Then discuss the possible positive gains for the CO as a result.
6. Role-play how the negative consequences for the drinking behavior will be delivered. Be sure to practice the conversation the CO eventually will have with the drinker, in which the client will explain the negative consequences plan. There are guidelines for all verbal interchanges: Be brief, specific, and state requests or intentions in a positive way (e.g., what you would like as opposed to what you would not like). Furthermore, include the reason for your behavior change.

In the dialogue that continues, assume the therapist (T) has explained each of the steps just outlined and will now practice the relevant steps with the CO (C).

T: Let's try out these steps I've just gone over. We don't need to pick a behavior because we already have one that you're interested in examining, right?

C: Yes … Charlie coming home late for dinner every night.

T: Okay. So we've already finished the first three steps. Pretty easy so far. Now Step 4 says to check and see if some type of positive reinforcement would work here. What do you think about telling your husband on the nights he *does* make it home on time that you love it when he's home in time to have dinner with the family?

C: But I can't remember the last time he's made it home on time. Besides, he tends to ignore me unless I'm yelling at him.

T: So, positive reinforcement is not a good option here. That means we should set up some negative consequences for his behavior. What do you think about keeping to your schedule and feeding the family just once, at six o'clock? If he wasn't home yet, you would just put the supper away the way you normally would if he had come home on time and eaten. Remember, you would be doing this so that he would eventually change his behavior and get home in time for dinner. And getting home by six would automatically mean he'd be drinking less. How does that sound? What do you think?

C: I don't know. I've never done that before.

T: Are you ready to give it a try?

C: Yes. I suppose I could try it and see what happens.

T: Great. Now according to Step 5 we're supposed to discuss fully all the negative consequences for your husband if you went ahead and refused to prepare a second dinner. What would be the negative consequences for him of not having dinner waiting?

C: Well he might get upset. Or he may leave and go get dinner someplace else. That's the only thing I can think of him doing. He may just get the supper out and heat it up himself.

T: So he'd end up having to feed himself in some way. That would definitely be a good start, because you would be making him responsible for his own actions. Let *him* pay the consequences of staying out late drinking. Can you see how he would then have to reevaluate whether it was worth it or not to stay out late? If he wants a warm supper he needs to be home on time.

C: I see what you mean. I just didn't know that my actions affected his drinking one way or the other. But I see what you mean now.

T: Good. Now remember that Step 5 also says to look at some of the possible benefits of this action for you.

C: Well he likes to eat; I know that much. It might work, and that would make me real happy. He just might come home more often to eat if he knew he wouldn't get a good meal otherwise. That way the kids would see him more, too.

T: Good. So are you willing to talk to your husband in advance, letting him know you intend to have supper at six, and that you will not wait around for him to show up?

C: Yes. I'm not too worried about talking to him about it. I know just when to approach him. But I'm not so sure of exactly what to say.

T: Well we can practice that right here. That's Step 6 anyway! What would you like to say to him? You know him better than I do. Go ahead and think out loud and I'll try to help you be brief, specific, and positive sounding.

C: I'd like to tell him that I hate his drinking, and I want him home for supper on time so I don't have to go to all that extra work when he gets home late.

T: That's a good start. You stated briefly what you wanted and why. You might want to be even more specific though and say you want him home by six o'clock. Also, I bet you can make it sound a little more positive. In other words, instead of talking about how much you hate his drinking, tell him how much you love it when he eats dinner with you and the kids.

C: Oh, I see what you mean.

T: It's also good to give the reasons *why* you are making these requests and changes. You might tell him that you love him but you don't like his drinking. And you are not going to support his drinking anymore. You will do anything for him, sober, but you feel by warming up his supper it encourages him to stay out and drink. You're not willing to support that type of activity anymore.

C: That's right. I don't want that kind of thing to go on forever. It's even become more frequent the last year or so.

T: So it's definitely time to take action. There. That takes care of Step 6. We're done in here, unless you have any questions. Now don't forget to stick to your guns once you've started the process. If you say you're going to do something and you back down, it makes him feel even more powerful. He knows then that he can manipulate you. He knows you're making idle threats.

Several of the drinking behaviors on a client's list should be processed in this same manner. The goal is for the client to first become more comfortable acknowledging his or her role in the partner's drinking, while at the same time realizing that one cannot be responsible for the behavior of the drinker. Then a decision must be made regarding whether to try to do anything to change the behavior. If the client is interested, the feasibility of using positive reinforcement for relevant nondrinking behaviors should be explored. If negative consequences appear warranted, the steps listed under "Responding to Unwanted Drinking Behaviors" (p. 284) should be followed carefully.

Difficult Cases for Applying Negative Consequences

There are different types of negative consequences that can be introduced in response to an individual's drinking behavior. These include clients' refraining from bailing their partners out of jail, and refusing to call the employer with excuses about an illness preventing the drinker from reporting to work. These strategies are aimed at decreasing the drinking behavior. Withdrawal of support such as this also shows the drinker that the client is serious about changing his or her ways of coping. If the drinker becomes ill and vomits, the client is instructed to let the drinker handle the problem alone. Of course, common sense always prevails. If the drinker is in a life-and-death or otherwise precarious situation, the client is instructed to act accordingly.

The following is a second example of justifications clients give for doing things for their inebriated partner, and the therapist's attempt to show them that it is not productive in the long run. This conversation is more difficult than the earlier dialogue, because in this situation the consequences of drinking are more immediate and severe, and they affect other family members more directly.

> **C:** Well, she usually comes home after drinking and gets really sick. She vomits and makes a total mess of the bathroom. I always clean it up so our son doesn't see what's happened. I do it for him more than for her.
>
> **T:** You do it for your son? So he doesn't know that she has a drinking problem?
>
> **C:** Well, he's seen her drunk, and he is even afraid of her sometimes when she's drinking hard.
>
> **T:** So let me ask the question again. You clean up the bathroom for your son? It sounds to me like he knows what's going on. How is cleaning up the bathroom protecting him? It is still supporting her drinking. You are making it easier for her to drink and get sick. *You* are paying the negative consequences for her drinking. Remember, we want her to correct her drinking problems on her own, to make her responsible.
>
> **C:** You don't want me to leave the bathroom a mess all night long, do you? It would stink even worse in the morning.
>
> **T:** Who's responsible for the mess? Don't you teach your son to clean up his toys when he's done playing with them? Don't you want to teach him to be responsible for his behavior? Why do you treat her different? Shouldn't she clean up after she plays?
>
> **C:** I think it's a bit different. I'm not sure I can deal with the mess. It stinks.
>
> **T:** The idea is to make her so uncomfortable cleaning up her own mess that she changes her drinking behavior, isn't it? It sounds like your main concern is with the smell. What could you do to resolve that part of the problem?
>
> **C:** I guess I could close the bathroom door, and open the window. Then first thing in the morning I could take our son and leave until she cleans it up. I could go visit a friend or her brother.
>
> **T:** Are you comfortable with that plan? It sounds like a very good idea.
>
> **C:** Well, it's really the only thing I haven't tried yet. I've pleaded with her, talked with her calmly and logically about it, and discussed what it's doing to our son. Nothing's worked, so I think I need to go with it.
>
> **T:** Good. Now let's go over all the negative consequences of this behavior that she may experience, and the positive benefits to you. Then we'll role-play how you're going to explain this change to her.

It is not difficult to see the reason for the client's reluctance in this situation. However, even in unpleasant situations you must insist that the client cease whatever behavior is blocking the drinker from experiencing the negative consequences of his or her drinking.

It cannot be stressed enough that part of the training in how to apply negative consequences also entails anticipating the drinker's reaction to a given consequence. The objective is to troubleshoot each consequence before it is tried, and to plan for extreme reactions from the drinker regardless. Many times it is a good idea to have clients write out and then review the negative consequence they will introduce, the anticipated reactions from the drinker, and the CO's planned response. This may help them clarify exactly what they would like to have happen, while at the same time being prepared for "the worst."

In anticipation of an extremely negative reaction from the drinker, a CO may plan to temporarily leave his or her partner. Such a plan typically should be discussed with the drinker beforehand. Depending on the circumstances, a trial separation period may be in order. This extended "time-out" may take place at a friend's or family member's house. Regardless, the decision to leave a partner must be the client's, but it should be supported by you. If the client chooses this method, he or she must be ready to deal with the drinker's reaction to this negative consequence as well.

A written plan describing the circumstances that will convince the CO to move back home should be developed. The plan should be specific, brief, and stated in a positive manner. It should describe the behaviors desired, as opposed to the behaviors that the CO does not want to see. The plan should be a strong, idealistic one, because some room for negotiation is important. At the same time, the plan must take into consideration the possibility that the drinker will not comply. This negotiation should occur in your office, but if for some reason it gets settled between the couple outside of a session, you should review it with the couple as soon as possible.

Summary

In summary, when suggesting modifications in a client's approach to the drinker's behavior, it is preferable to encourage the use of positive reinforcement for nondrinking behavior. However, that tactic is not always possible or effective. This chapter has offered procedures to be used when the implementation of negative consequences for drinking behavior appears to be the only option remaining for the client.

SESSION 8: INDEPENDENCE: RECREATIONAL AND OCCUPATIONAL LIFE CHANGES

Rationale

Upon entering treatment, COs frequently report a great deal of disruption in various family members' activities as a result of the loved one's excessive alcohol use. The nondrinking individuals simply stop doing many of the fun things they used to enjoy. Clients often report that they no longer invite over friends or relatives. Some COs cease socializing publicly with the drinker in order to avoid high-probability drinking situations. Unfortunately, many clients do not replace these activities with other forms of recreation and consequently become increasingly isolated. In essence, they experience an overabundance of negative events and a relative lack of positive events; a sure prescription for frustration and depression.

In an effort to change this situation, COs must work to increase their *own* opportunities for rewards. The first half of this session focuses on helping the CO learn to develop a more satisfying social and recreational life. Regardless of the current status of the drinker, the client learns to explore new interests, activities, and friendships. The second half of the session concentrates on a different type of independence: new employment opportunities for the CO. Specialized training in how to find a new job is provided. The inherent rewards for the client are discussed.

Developing Independent Activities

One of the most useful pieces of advice to give COs is that they should work to develop hobbies, activities, and interests that are independent of the drinker. This allows for greater control over their own quest for satisfaction in life and makes it less likely that the drinker will disrupt the process. There are two important components for encouraging the establishment of independent social or recreational activities:

1. *Identifying possible social or recreational activities.* Start with a brainstorming session. Help the client develop a list of activities that he or she might enjoy. What are some activities that the client has always wanted to do? If there are events in which the CO regularly participates, he or she might be willing to try a slight variation of these. Examples include joining a jazz dance class instead of the regular country/western dance class; attending a live play instead of a movie; volunteering with friends to work a few hours at a hospital or nursing home, instead of simply socializing.

As an assignment, ask the client to generate 10–15 potentially enjoyable activities. These can be added to a resource manual of fun, nondrinking recreational events in the community. The manual can be available to all of your CRT clients.

2. *Response priming.* The next step is to convince the client to try at least one new activity, and then to "prime" the response so that it actually occurs. If the client appears interested, immediately assist in the planning. Obtain the specifics as to the time and place of the activity, costs involved, and transportation or childcare arrangements. Potential obstacles to attending the activity should be addressed as well. You also can assist in priming new activities by becoming familiar with community resources. A client is more likely to try a new activity if given a specific recommendation, including the name of a contact person(s). If possible, make the actual arrangements for the activity by telephone during the session. This increases the chances that the CO will attend the event.

In the next session, the client should report on the results. The critical questions to address include: Did the CO attend the event? If not, why? If so, did the CO enjoy it? Does he or she plan to continue the activity? (Why or why not?) What can be done to make the event more enjoyable? Is there something else the client might want to try next time instead?

Meeting People and Developing New Friendships

In this section specific suggestions for helping clients meet people and develop a support network are outlined. Several excellent works are available on these subjects, and it is recommended that clients invest in a copy of any of these or a similar book:

Asserting Yourself: A Practical Guide for Positive Change (Bower & Bower, 1976)
Don't Say Yes When You Want to Say No (Fensterheim & Baer, 1975)
Assertiveness Training for Women (Osborn & Harris, 1975)
Shyness: What It Is, What to Do about It (Zimbardo, 1977)

The guidelines that follow are commonly described in these works. More specific exercises can be adapted based on the client's particular needs.

1. *Revive old friendships.* People often find it easier to renew old friendships than to start brand new ones. With this in mind telephone an old acquaintance with whom you have not spoken for some time. Have several conversational topics prepared in advance. Reward yourself for completing a call. If you felt that the initial contact went well, arrange for future calls, or perhaps even coffee or lunch together.

2. *Practice "small talk."* Being sociable is a skill that improves with practice. So take time to say "hello" to people at work, to other parents at your children's school, or to neighbors. Practice striking up conversations with people you do not know. Use lunch breaks to talk to co-workers you may have seen before in your building or work site, but with whom you have never spoken. Initiate brief conversations with others in public places: waiting rooms, ticket lines, sporting events. Talk to people of different age groups. At times these brief, pleasant interactions can even be the beginning of lasting friendships.

3. *Develop basic conversation skills.* There are many different aspects to developing friendships, and one involves carrying on a skilled, lengthy conversation. One component of a skilled conversation is being a good listener. So learn to show interest in what others are saying. Use nonverbal encouragers, such as head nods, a forward lean, direct eye contact, and brief verbal encouragers ("Mm-hmm," "Yes," "Right"). Do not interrupt others or attempt to complete their thoughts or words. Try to identify with the feelings others may be trying to express. You can do this by imagining yourself in their situation and picturing what they might be thinking and feeling. You do not have to agree with what the other person is saying, but try to understand how the other person may be seeing things. If you do not understand what another person is saying to you, ask for clarification. Try summarizing or restating the words of the other person and asking, "Is that correct?" Allow them the opportunity to modify your interpretation, and accept the correction readily.

4. *Develop interests that can be shared with others.* You can enhance your conversations even more by keeping current with either political, cultural, or sports topics. Have in mind some humorous stories, anecdotes, or recent events to share when meeting with a group of old or new friends. Discuss movie or book reviews with others.

Many of these exercises can be practiced in-session and then assigned as homework. In both situations, remember to proceed in small steps and reinforce the client for incremental progress. Also encourage the client to reward his or her own accomplishments. This can be done most easily by the use of coping self-statements: "I handled that pretty well," "It worked," "That was fun," "I'm getting better at this," "I actually got through that," or "It was better than I thought." Examples of other self-reinforcers that the client may select are small gifts, favorite foods or snacks, and time set aside to relax, read, or get a massage.

Job Finding

Sometimes the disruption in a CO's life brought on by a problem drinker is more severe than a mere lack of outside social activities. For many clients, the problem entails surviving on a shrinking paycheck or no paycheck at all. In response, some COs decide that they need to change their own work situation. For some, this means finding a different type of job, whereas for others it implies obtaining outside employment for the first time.

Your clients should understand that finding a job is a full-time job. It requires discipline and organization to maximize opportunities. The process should be addressed systematically using the following basic elements:

1. *Résumé Development.* Developing a good résumé is one of the first and most

critical tasks, because the impression it creates probably will determine whether the CO will be granted an interview. So be sure the client has listed in an organized manner all previous jobs and training. Additionally, have the client include valuable personal traits. Make sure that the résumé and cover letter are professionally typed.

2. *Completion of Job Applications.* Many clients need to be taught how to fill out a job application correctly. Focus them again on emphasizing positive personal attributes, along with good job skills. Help them with difficult questions. For example, many applications ask for employment history. This can be problematic for the CO who may not have worked outside the home for a number of years. In this instance it may be better for the client to list him- or herself as having been "self-employed." Or, the CO could list volunteer work that required the same skills as those requested for the position of interest.

3. *Generation of Job Leads.* One way to begin generating job leads is by asking family and friends if they are aware of any possible employment opportunities. Other ways include inquiring of former employers and co-workers. and using the yellow pages of the phone book. The client also should be required to document job leads in a log. The log would include a place for date, type of work, the company's name, address, and phone number, the contact person's name and a space to jot down details during and after the phone call. At least ten job leads should be recorded before the client makes any phone calls.

4. *Phone Skills Training.* The next step is to rehearse phone calls. Phone skills include introducing oneself in a confident and friendly manner, getting the name of the person who hires, and obtaining necessary information concerning job availability, qualifications, and application procedures.

5. *Interview Skills Training.* Now, role-play the entire interview, including how to handle difficult questions. Once the client is prepared, help in arranging transportation plans. Finally, discuss the realistic possibility of being rejected for employment, since this is common when searching for a job.

6. *Daily Goal Setting.* Each day the client should obtain new leads, make appropriate telephone calls, write necessary letters, and attend interviews. Success is based on making a sufficient number of calls to secure enough interviews.

7. *Reinforcer Review.* Remind the CO about the rewards that often accompany a new job. These may include enhanced self-esteem, new friends, intellectual stimulation, a sense of independence, exciting challenges, and increased income.

Summary

This session has offered processes by which the client can develop social, recreational, or occupational opportunities that are less dependent on the drinker's current status. By focusing more time and energy on their own interests instead of the drinker's exclusively, clients increase the likelihood that they will be involved in positive experiences. These positive events often can help balance the familial disruption so common within the families of drinkers.

SESSION NINE

Rationale

Encouraging the drinker to enter into formal treatment is one of the principal objectives of CRT. The training and exercises designed to improve the CO's coping skills, independence, and communication skills, also serve to prepare the CO for the task of encouraging the drinker to begin treatment. To facilitate this process, COs are trained to recognize periods of high motivation for change in the drinker and to take steps to encourage treatment during those times. But COs also are warned that periods of high motivation may be fleeting, and consequently they should not be surprised if the drinker struggles with rapid shifts in his or her awareness of the problem and commitment to change.

Motivating the Drinker

An essential point to communicate to the CO is that "motivation for treatment" is not an all-or-nothing phenomenon. Why and how people decide to enter treatment for alcohol problems is a complex matter. Prochaska and DiClemente (1986) have proposed a stage model for understanding the processes of change in addictive behaviors. In this model, one is not simply "motivated" or "unmotivated" for change. Instead, one moves through a series of stages, sometimes in a forward direction, sometimes backward, before arriving at the decision to do something about an addiction problem. Thus, progress for the drinker can be an uncertain proposition and there may be a series of starts and stops before there is movement in any clear direction. Even for drinkers who recognize that they have a problem, there may be a great deal of time spent "hanging in the balance" before deciding that there is something they can do about the problem.

Miller (1985, 1987) likewise viewed motivation as a dynamic process, and proposed that motivation for change not be viewed as a personality or trait feature of the alcoholic. A major influential factor is the nature of the interaction between the drinker and the CO. CRT attempts to shape this influential factor in a coordinated effort to increase motivation for change in the drinker.

Community Reinforcement Training prepares COs to assume a positive role in suggesting treatment by first arming them with accurate, up-to-date information concerning "motivation for treatment." Once a client understands the dynamic nature of motivation, he or she will be better able to recognize a period of high motivation in a loved one and then move quickly to suggest treatment. Problem drinkers often are highly motivated after a frightening incident or a crisis directly related to their drinking. These crisis situations thus create a "window of opportunity" during which time the drinker may be more open to the suggestion of treatment. COs who are prepared to recognize these moments and who are ready to offer concrete suggestions are more likely to have a positive impact on the drinker's decision to enter treatment.

Suggesting Treatment to the Drinker

In the course of therapy, COs should be given the opportunity to role-play a situation in which they suggest treatment to the drinker. In these exercises, remind clients to present their suggestions in a clear, calm, and matter-of-fact manner. While this may be relatively easy to accomplish during a practice session, it is understood that the actual situation is likely to be highly emotionally charged. But that is precisely the point of role-plays: To develop the skills and confidence necessary to carry out the task when the time arrives. During the role-play be alert to threatening or accusatory messages on the part of the CO. Help him or her to see how this may draw out a drinker's defenses and undermine the goal of getting the drinker to accept treatment.

It is useful to have clients practice both successful and unsuccessful scenarios; that is, one in which the drinker accepts and one in which the drinker refuses to enter treatment.

COs must be prepared for both outcomes. In a scenario in which the drinker refuses a suggestion of treatment, help the client to see that this is not a personal failure. COs have the right to suggest treatment, and drinkers have the right to refuse it. By suggesting treatment in a firm and caring manner, the CO may be laying the groundwork for future compliance by the drinker. Also, the client does not have to feel as if there is one and only one best moment to suggest treatment, and that if the drinker refuses the moment is lost. There will be other opportunities. It may even be the case that on the next occasion, it is the drinker who proposes that the time for treatment has arrived.

Rapid Intake Procedures

Therapists who work with COs are advised to make prior arrangements to allow for a rapid intake at an appropriate alcohol treatment facility in the event that the drinker decides to accept treatment. This is accomplished most easily if the CO's counseling is being conducted at a facility that also offers comprehensive alcohol treatment services. Typically, drinkers whose COs have received counseling can be admitted on a priority basis. If the therapist is working independently or with a program that does not offer alcohol treatment services, then he or she is advised to develop prior arrangements with several treatment referral sources who may be able to implement the rapid intake procedures.

A *rapid intake system* mandates that the first therapy session should be held within forty-eight hours of the phone call from the CO or drinker. Both are requested to be present at this appointment. If the drinker is unavailable to attend within forty-eight hours, the CO alone should schedule a therapy session for a preview of the material that will be utilized during the first session with the drinker. This session should not take place without already having been rehearsed by the therapist and the CO. In the unlikely case that the drinker wants to attend and the CO is unable, the first therapy session should change only slightly in format from the planned one. In that event, the second session should begin with a summary of the first session.

A rapid intake system implies that the therapist will act as the intake worker, and consequently will administer the intake assessment. This should help the client and therapist develop rapport more quickly. It also provides the therapist with needed information concerning the severity of the problem. The intake and the normal first session should be combined, so that by the end of the first day of treatment the client is motivated, evaluated, and even started on disulfiram in many cases.

One advantage of a rapid fire system is that the client only has time to focus on treatment. He or she should leave knowing that the system works and that there is little left to chance. Once the drinker enters treatment, the Community Reinforcement Approach procedures (Azrin, 1976; Azrin et al., 1982; Hunt & Azrin, 1973; Meyers & Smith, 1995) are used for the duration of treatment. CRT and CRA procedures have been developed to work in harmony for the ultimate goal of abstinence.

Complications to Consider

Another issue to explore relatively early in the process is the possibility that the drinker may enter treatment but then drop out prematurely. The CO should be prepared to have to deal with this. In the event that this actually occurs, there are a number of important questions to pose to the CO:

- Exactly what transpired?
- Do you have some idea of what went wrong?
- Is there anything that could have been done differently?
- What can be done now?
- Is there a chance that the drinker will re-enter therapy?
- If so, upon what does this depend?
- Is the drinker simply at a place with his or her drinking that they are not ready to make a commitment to change?
- Is the drinker upset with the therapy process itself?

The client may feel ready to give up, at least temporarily. At this point the client and the therapist need to re-evaluate the client's goals. Determine if the possibility still exists that the drinker will return to treatment. Client involvement is variable according to individual abilities and needs.

Another important issue to discuss early in therapy with the CO is that the drinker may refuse all attempts to motivate him or her into treatment. The therapist would need to review with the client other options for action: (1) Do nothing, and the situation probably will worsen. (2) Get active and change so that one's life is more rewarding. At the same time, continue to try new strategies to motivate the drinker into treatment. (3) Once all attempts to change the situation have failed, leave the relationship.

Even if the client decides to terminate treatment at this time, there still is the possibility that a traumatic event may occur in the life of the drinker that will motivate the drinker to seek treatment in the future. And since an open door policy will have been established with the client, he or she will know that therapy is available whenever it is needed and wanted.

REFERENCES

Azrin, N. H. (1976). Improvements in the community-reinforcement approach to alcoholism. *Behaviour Research and Therapy, 14*, 339–348.

Azrin, N. H., Sisson, R. W., Meyers, R. J., & Godley, M. (1982). Alcoholism treated by disulfiram and community reinforcement therapy. *Journal of Behaviour Therapy and Experimental Psychiatry, 13*, 105–112.

Bower, S. A., & Bower, G. H. (1976). *Asserting yourself: A practical guide for positive change.* Reading, MA: Addison-Wesley.

Coleman, D., & Straus, M. (1983). Alcohol abuse and family violence. In E. Gottheil, K. Druley, T. Skoloda, & H. Waxman (Eds.), *Alcohol, drug abuse, and aggression* (pp. 104–124). Springfield, IL.: Thomas.

Collins, R. L., Leonard, K. E., & Searles, J. S. (1990). *Alcohol and the family: Research and clinical perspectives.* New York: Guilford Press.

Dittrich, J. E., & Trapold, M. A. (1984). A treatment program for the wives of alcoholics: An evaluation. *Bulletin of the Society of Psychologists in Addictive Behaviours, 3*, 91–102.

Dominguez, T. P., Miller, W. R., & Meyers, R. J. (1995). Unilateral intervention with family members of problem drinkers: A comparison of two group therapy approaches. Under review.

Fensterheim, H., & Baer, J. (1975). *Don't say yes when you want to say no.* New York: Dell.

Gelles, R. J., & Cornell, C. P. (1990). *Intimate violence in families* (2nd ed.). Newbury Park, CA: Sage.

Gondolf, E. W., & Foster, R. A. (1991). Wife assault among VA alcohol rehabilitation patients. *Hospital and Community Psychiatry, 42*, 74–79.

Hingson, R., Mangione, T., Meyers, A., & Scotch, N. (1982). Seeking help for drinking problems: A study in the Boston metropolitan area. *Journal of Studies on Alcohol, 43*, 271–288.

Hunt, G. M., & Azrin, N. H. (1973). A community-reinforcement approach to alcoholism. *Behaviour Research and Therapy, 11*, 91–104.

Institute of Medicine. (1990). *Broadening the base of treatment for alcohol problems.* Washington, DC: National Academy Press.

Johnson, V. E. (1986). Intervention: How to help those who don't want help. Minneapolis: Johnson Institute.

Kantor, G. K., & Straus, M. A. (1989). Substance abuse as a precipitant of wife abuse victimizations. *American Journal of Drug and Alcohol Abuse, 15,* 173–189.

Leonard, K. E., & Jacob, T. (1988). Alcohol, alcoholism, and family violence. In V. B. Van Hasselt, R. L. Morrison, A. S. Bellack, & M. Hersen (Eds.), *Handbook of family violence* (pp. 383–406). New York: Plenum Press.

Liepman, M. R., Nirenberg, T. D., & Begin, A. M. (1989). Evaluation of a program designed to help family and significant others to motivate resistant alcoholics into recovery. *American Journal of Drug and Alcohol Abuse, 15,* 209–221.

Meyers, R. J., & Smith, J. E. (1995). *A clinical guide to alcohol treatment: The Community Reinforcement Approach.* New York: Guilford Press.

Miller, W. R. (1985). Motivation for treatment: A review with special emphasis on alcoholism. *Psychological Bulletin, 98,* 84–107.

Miller, W. R. (1987). Motivation and treatment goals. *Drugs and Society, 1,* 133–151.

Miller, W. R., & Page, A. C. (1991). Warm turkey: Other routes to abstinence. *Journal of Substance Abuse Treatment, 8,* 227–232.

Moos, R. H., Cronkite, R. C., Billings, A. G., & Finney, J. W. (1987). *Health and daily living form manual, revised version.* Palo Alto, CA: Stanford University, Social Ecology Laboratory.

Moos, R. H., & Moos, B. S. (1986). *Family environment scale manual* (2nd ed.). Palo Alto, CA: Consulting Psychologist Press.

O'Farrell, T. J., & Choquette, K. (1991). Marital violence in the year before and after spouse-involved alcoholism treatment. *Family Dynamics of Addiction Quarterly, 1,* 32–40.

Orford, J., & Harwin, J. (1982). *Alcohol and the family.* London: Croom Helm.

Osborne, S., & Harris, G. (1975). *Assertiveness training for women.* Springfield, IL: Charles C. Thomas.

Paolino, T. J., & McCrady, B. S. (1977). *The alcoholic marriage: Alternative perspectives.* New York: Grune & Stratton.

Prochaska, J. & DiClemente, C. (1986). Toward a comprehensive model of change. In W. R. Miller & N. Heather (Eds.), *Treating addictive behaviors: Process of change* (pp. 3–27). New York: Plenum.

Room, R. (1987, June). *The U.S. general population's experience with responses to alcohol problems.* Presented at the Alcohol Epidemiology Section of the International Congress on Alcohol and Addictions, Aix-en-Provence, France.

Sisson, R. W., and Azrin, N. H. (1986). Family-member involvement to initiate and promote treatment of problem drinkers. *Journal of Behavior Therapy and Experimental Psychiatry, 17,* 15–21.

Stith, S. M., Crossman, R. K., & Bischof, G. P. (1991). Alcoholism and marital violence: A comparative study of men in alcohol treatment programs and batterer treatment programs. *Alcoholism Treatment Quarterly, 8,* 3–20.

Straus, M. A. (1979). Measuring intrafamily conflict and violence: The Conflict Tactics (CT) Scales. *Journal of Marriage and the Family, 41,* 75–88.

Szapocznik, J., Kurtines, W. M., Foote, F., Perez-Vidal, A., & Hervis, O. (1983). Conjoint versus one-person family therapy: Some evidence for the effectiveness of conducting family therapy through one person. *Journal of Consulting and Clinical Psychology, 51,* 889–899.

Szapocznik, J., Kurtines, W. M., Foote, F., Perez-Vidal, A., & Hervis, O. (1986). Conjoint versus one-person family therapy: Further evidence for the effectiveness of conducting family therapy through one person with drug abusing adolescents. *Journal of Consulting and Clinical Psychology, 54,* 395–397.

Telch, C. F., & Lindquist, C. U. (1984). Violent versus non-violent couples: A comparison of patterns. *Psychotherapy, 21,* 242–248.

Thomas, E. J., & Ager, R. D. (1993, June). *Characteristics of unmotivated alcohol abusers and their spouses.* Presented at the Research Society on Alcoholism Annual Meeting, San Antonio, TX.

Thomas, E. J., & Santa, C. A. (1982). Unilateral family therapy for alcohol abuse: A working conception. *American Journal of Family Therapy, 10,* 49–58.

Thomas, E. J., & Santa, C. A., Bronson, D., & Oyserman, D. (1987). Unilateral family therapy with spouses of alcoholics. *Journals of Social Service Research, 10,* 145–163.

Velleman, R., Bennett, G., Miller, T., Orford, J., Rigby, K., & Tod, A. (1993). The families of problem drug users: A study of 50 close relatives. *Addiction, 88,* 1281–1289.

Wiseman, J. (1980). The "home treatment": The first step in trying to cope with an alcoholic husband. *Family Relations, 29,* 541–549.

Zimbardo, P. G. (1977). *Shyness: What it is, what to do about it.* Reading, MA: Addison-Wesley.

9

Cognitive–Behavioral Treatment of Sex Offenders

William L. Marshall and Anthony Eccles

INTRODUCTION

We have two general locations in which we operate our treatment programs: Canadian federal penitentiaries, and a community-based outpatient clinic. The treatment program we describe here is adapted to suit the special conditions in each of the locations, but essentially it involves the same components and processes. The only inconsistent process concerns the fact that, in some circumstances, we use closed groups (i.e., all clients start and end group treatment at the same time and progress at approximately the same rate) and in others we use open-ended groups (i.e., clients progress at their own rate and when they complete the program, they are individually replaced by another client). The program we describe here is designed specifically for adult male sex offenders and targets those (including nonfamilial and familial offenders) who have sexually offended against either women or children. We conduct mixed groups because we have found that this helps overcome beliefs in particular offenders that their crimes were not as bad as those of some other types of offenders, or that they are not, in fact, sex offenders.

The largest percentage of our clients are child molesters or rapists, with fewer exhibitionists and very few voyeurs. We also treat female offenders and juveniles, for whom we adapt the present program to suit their particular needs. Most of the elements described in this chapter are equally suited to the needs of female and juvenile clients, but some modifications are needed (see Barbaree, Marshall, & Hudson, 1993, for a description of the treatment of juvenile sex offenders). We rarely see enough female offenders at any one time to run groups for them; therefore, they are typically seen individually.

William L. Marshall • Department of Psychology, Queen's University, Kingston Sexual Behaviour Clinic, Kingston, Ontario, Canada K7L 3N6.   **Anthony Eccles** • Forensic Behavioural Services, Eccles, Hodkinson, and Associates, Kingston, Ontario, Canada K7L 1A8.

Sourcebook of Psychological Treatment Manuals for Adult Disorders, edited by Vincent B. Van Hasselt and Michel Hersen. Plenum Press, New York, 1996.

Many of the offenders treated in our prison programs enter a community program when released and some come to our community clinic. However, we receive referrals for our community clinic from many other sources (e.g., Provincial Probation and Parole, child protection agencies, police, lawyers, health-service providers, courts) in addition to Correctional Services of Canada. The overall structure of the programs that come under the auspices of Correctional Services of Canada, involving a three-tier system, has been described elsewhere (Marshall, Eccles, & Barbaree, 1993a). It essentially involves a cascading system in which offenders get extensive and intensive treatment at Tier 1, then prerelease preparation at Tier 2, followed by community treatment upon release at Tier 3. In this chapter, we do not describe this three-tier system (the reader is referred to the original article), but rather the components and processes involved in treatment.

Our programs employ a cognitive–behavioral approach to group therapy with ancillary pharmacological treatment when necessary (approximately 3% to 5% of our patients), and with individualized behavioral treatment (procedures to alter deviant sexual interests) again when necessary. Our groups are typically facilitated by a male and a female therapist and are conducted with groups of 8 to 10 offenders. There is no evidence indicating the optimal size of sex offender treatment groups, but we find it most manageable with this size. Similarly, there is no evidence concerning the value of one or more therapists, nor on therapists' gender; we just find it easier to manage in this way, although we do conduct single-therapist groups when circumstances demand them.

The general approach in our groups is to be supportively challenging when an offender is denying, minimizing, or otherwise appears to be distorting. We attempt to continually enhance participants' self-confidence by (1) encouraging them to distinguish their aberrant behavior from their global view of themselves, (2) being supportive although firm when challenging distortions, and (3) persuading them to believe in the possibility of change. This is meant not only to increase the likelihood they will move in a prosocial direction in their attitudes, beliefs, and behaviors, but it is also predicated on our belief that people who feel good about themselves are unlikely to hurt others.

We divide the targets of our treatment programs into those we consider to be "offense-specific" (i.e., directly functionally related to offending in all offenders) and those we call "offense-related" targets (i.e., those that bear a functional relationship, not always direct, to offending in some but not necessarily all offenders). Offense-specific treatment targets include denial, minimization, victim empathy, distorted attitudes and beliefs, fantasies, and the development of relapse-prevention plans. This description of our treatment targets is provided in the order in which we present these topics to our groups. We believe the order is quite important. For example, it seems evident to us that progress will not be possible until denial is overcome, and empathic feelings for the victims will not be attained until the client has taken full responsibility for his offenses. Similarly, attitudinal distortions may not be fully evident, nor will offenders realize their connection with offending and the corresponding need to change until they have developed some degree of empathy for the victim. Offenders may not be fully committed to changing their fantasies until they can recognize how intimately related they are to their prior attitudes and how such fantasies increase the chances that they will again hurt an innocent person. Finally, of course, attempting to design relapse-prevention plans cannot occur until all the prior treatment components have revealed to the offenders the many factors that put them at risk and, more to the point, that these factors are likely to recur.

Saying all of this implies that components are not independent of each other, but that, rather, they complement each other. Moreover, each component is not a discrete unit; it simply represents the focus of that point in treatment. The same issues, particularly those that are most salient to each individual, are raised repeatedly in different contexts and the interrelationship between all factors is emphasized. In fact, we believe it is poor clinical practice to adhere to a rigid order. When a relevant issue is raised, we attempt to deal with it at that time, because postponing an issue may lead the offender to drop it, or we may miss taking advantage of an emotional opportunity to explore the issue.

"Offense-related" targets include relationship skills, substance abuse, anger management, social and life skills, and communication. Other idiosyncratic problems are also sometimes apparent and need to be addressed. In order to meet many of these goals, we are usually able to refer clients to other programs (either in the prisons or in the community) that are specifically designed to meet these needs. When special needs cannot be met by available resources, we develop strategies ourselves.

THE TREATMENT PROCESS

Entry to the Program

Offenders are initially thoroughly assessed. This assessment process is meant to address the issues requested by the referral source (e.g., treatment needs; risk for reoffending; suitability for release from prison; suitability for particular placement, such as a return to family or job) and to determine the focus of treatment if the client wishes to enter our program and can access it. All clients are given the opportunity to enter treatment whether they are in denial or are suffering from some other disorder or deficit. If the client meets the diagnostic criteria for a psychiatric disorder other than a paraphilia, he will receive prior (only if so severely disrupted as to reduce effective participation in our program) or concurrent therapy in addition to entering our program. Only if the client's intellectual functioning is below an IQ of 70 is he excluded from the group program; he then is involved in individualized treatment carried out in coordination with his referral-source caseworker.

We do not exclude deniers from entry to our program unless they refuse treatment. Many programs will not accept deniers, with some taking denial to indicate a lack of motivation for treatment. We believe it is the therapist's job to motivate clients, particularly when working with sex offenders, since many of the deniers or unmotivated offenders are just those at greatest risk to reoffend. It has to be kept in mind that when sex offenders do reoffend, they do so against innocent women and children whom their abuse typically damages, leaving them with serious long-term problems. In any case, since the incidence of denial and significant minimization is quite high (ranging from 50% to 70% in our different programs over the years; see Barbaree, 1991 and Marshall, 1994), refusal to treat these offenders would result both in few treatment candidates and an artificially inflated apparent effectiveness of the program. The first main targets in our programs, then, are overcoming denial and minimization.

Treatment Components

When clients first enter our treatment group, one of the facilitators indicates that confidentiality must be maintained by group members. They are told that they should discuss issues relevant to the treatment program with one another outside group sessions but that they should be careful not to let anyone else overhear them. They should not discuss issues with anyone outside the group except their family, nor should they disclose to anyone who else is in the group. Participants are told, however, that the group facilitators will have to provide reports (both verbal and written) to the referral source and that this will require them to reveal whatever relevant facts were exposed during treatment. They are cautioned about the legal requirements of the therapists to report to the authorities certain offenses if sufficient details are revealed. All group members sign a "Consent to Participate form" that describes these aspects of confidentiality and when it may be broken.

The group is then told the goals of treatment. The prime goal is, of course, to help the offenders reduce their risk of reoffending. We tell them that we will try to achieve this by identifying the factors (circumstances, behaviors, emotional factors, and attitudes) that previously placed them at risk, and by engaging procedures that will both eliminate old patterns and entrench more prosocial and personally beneficial ways of dealing with these factors. We will also teach them ways to meet their needs in prosocial ways. They are told that our program does not offer a "cure," because they do not have a "disease." Rather, our goal is to increase their control over their aberrant tendencies and to equip them with the skills and attitudes necessary to achieve their goals in prosocial ways. Clients are advised that an important implication of this view is that the termination of formal treatment should not end their efforts at dealing with their problems. Formal treatment is meant to initiate change that they themselves must sustain and enhance after discharge. Indeed, they can expect backward steps (which we refer to as "lapses"); however, these should not be taken as indications of failure, but rather as temporary setbacks from which they can learn. The notions of relapse prevention are explained and repeatedly emphasized throughout treatment.

We advise clients that their offenses resulted from learned, dysfunctional ways of feeling, thinking, and behaving and that they are quite capable of learning more functionally effective ways of dealing with their world and meeting their needs. We frequently remind them that they are not adequately described as sex offenders (or pedophiles, or child molesters, or rapists, etc.), but rather as individuals who are multifaceted, with positive as well as negative behaviors in their history. We discourage their use of these and other denigrating self-descriptors, such as local colloquialisms for sex offenders. Although we insist that they fully accept responsibility for all aspects of their offenses, this should not obscure the fact that they have the potential to overcome these problems. Throughout treatment we take every opportunity to enhance their self-confidence and their belief in the possibility of change.

To "break the ice" we have each client, in turn, tell the group his name and give a brief history of his life, elaborating on his relationships with family friends, and sexual partners. We then quickly move to the more therapeutic aspects of treatment.

Denial and Minimization

Until denial and minimization are overcome, it is difficult, if not impossible, to proceed with other aspects of treatment.

The Nature of Denial and Minimization.   *Denial* involves not simply a refusal to admit having committed an offense, although this is often the initial stumbling block. Some offenders, who admit to the act, nevertheless deny that it was an offense; that is, they claim it was consensual or that it was not really sexual. Others admit they committed a sexual offense but declare they either are not sexual offenders or that they do not have a problem in need of treatment.

Minimization describes either a refusal to accept responsibility for the offense, a denial that they harmed their victim, or limited admission of the extent and nature of their abusive acts (e.g., they may claim that the offenses occurred less often than the victim says, or that they were less forceful and less sexually intrusive than is claimed). Most of the issues of minimization are obvious, but shifting responsibility requires a brief explanation. Many offenders attribute responsibility for their offense to the effects of some type of intoxicant. They claim they would not have committed such dreadful acts had it not been for the influence of alcohol or whatever drug they were using; that is, they suggest that the intoxicant transforms them into a different person having urges foreign to their usual nature, or that it so disinhibits them that they are unable to control urges that they ordinarily can keep in check. Some claim that the intoxicant so seriously interferes with their consciousness that they either did not know what they were doing, or they have subsequently no memory of what they did. In the latter cases, it is common for the men to indicate that they believe they must have offended so they obviously need help, but claim no recall of the incident. Other offenders also claim memory loss but attribute it to either an injury, a disease, or simply the psychological shock of committing such a heinous crime. In all cases of supposed memory loss we attempt to offer a face-saving strategy to facilitate "recall," because we rarely believe their claim of loss of memory. For example, we typically tell these clients that the more often they discuss as many details of the day of the offense as they can recall, or the more often they try to reconstruct the day, the more details they will be able to recall. Of course, we continually remind them of the benefits of a full, accurate recall and of the negative consequences (i.e., discharge from the program and consequent denial of parole, revocation of parole or probation, and loss of various other desired benefits); this often facilitates a surprising recovery of memory.

Others who minimize their responsibility blame the occurrence of the offense on an uncooperative or boring sexual partner. Many, of course, blame the victim, who they suggest was provocative or careless in some way. Child molesters, for example, very often describe their victim as frequently parading about the house scantily clad, or as physically overaffectionate and even deliberately seductive. Some rapists point out that their victim was either alone in a remote place or was hitchhiking; in both cases they see this as the victim's carelessness and they feel this reduces their blame. Over the past decade, more and more offenders are suggesting that they themselves were sexually abused as children and see this as the cause of the offenses.

Treatment of Denial and Minimization. We begin this segment of treatment by having each offender present his disclosure; that is, his account of the offense or offenses. We then ask each other group member to evaluate the disclosure and if they do not accept some or all of it, they are to supportively challenge the man. The group facilitators model supportive challenges and comment on the quality of each challenge made by other clients encouraging them, if necessary, to be less confrontational. Occasionally, it is initially difficult to have all members of the group strike a balance between being so supportive as to ignore defensiveness and being confrontational. Feedback by the facilitators and appropriate modeling usually correct these tendencies.

In order to facilitate these challenges, we are provided with offense accounts from sources independent of the offender. We always have available one or all of the following: a victim statement, a police report, and the court proceedings. We also have a complete offense history for each participant derived from the Canada-wide official police records. We allow each participant to give his own version of the offense and have the others challenge him before we provide the official account. This strategy is meant to reduce the possibility that the offender will simply repeat the official version without authentically accepting it. It does not, of course, completely obviate this possibility, but it does give us some insight into the typical style the man may adopt. This insight allows us to frame our challenges in a way that may maximize effectiveness and also permits us to make judgments (not, of course, guaranteed to be accurate) about the veracity of any subsequent admissions. Within prison settings, in particular, we find that some offenders, realizing their release may be contingent on meeting the goals of treatment, say what they think we want to hear rather than what they really believe. This is sometimes quite obvious; but in some cases, it is difficult to discern. Therefore, our tactic is to have each participant reveal as much about his own views as possible prior to accurate feedback.

Characteristically, when each offender challenges another man, the challenger uses his own experiences as the basis for disputing the other man's claims. This is valuable because it may be the first time the challenger has revealed his own minimizations.

When each offender discloses, he is required to provide extensive details. If he has more than one offense, we typically ask him to describe the first offense and then a sample of the subsequent offenses, particularly the last one. He must give an accurate and detailed account of his thoughts, feelings, and actions immediately prior to, during, and immediately after the offense. He is also required to describe all the physical circumstances in which the offense took place, and to give his understanding of what the victim was doing and feeling at the time.

A critical assumption underlying this process (and, indeed, the whole therapeutic approach of this program) is that people are most likely to take the risk to admit to acts they believe others view as repugnant, if they know they are not going to be rejected and if they are assured that support and help will continue. The more clients are treated with respect, the more self-confidence they will feel, and the more self-confident they are, the more likely they are to have the courage to admit to heinous crimes. Accordingly, the therapist makes explicit the distinction between their offensive behavior, which is described as harmful and unacceptable, and themselves as whole persons. He or she points out that they have many strengths and good features to their personality and makes it clear that it is their sexual offenses that are unacceptable, not them.

Each member of the group is encouraged to make supportive but firm challenges. If any member of the group simply supports rather than questions the offender's stated position, particularly if that position is clearly self-serving, then they are challenged and their motivation is questioned, again in a supportive yet firm manner. An atmosphere is deliberately created that is as relaxed and as informal as possible, while at the same time focusing on the seriousness of the situation. The offender who is disclosing but denying, minimizing, or distorting is told that hiding the truth and avoiding responsibility is expected but not accepted. Open-ended groups make this process easier. For example, because other members of the group have already gone through the process, they can offer insights not only about the difficulty of honestly disclosing but also about the benefits they experienced once they had done so (e.g., a feeling of relief from the stress of continued lying, an opportunity to start from scratch with a clean slate). This, in fact, reveals one of the great advantages an open-ended group has over a closed group. In the latter format, everyone starts together at the same time so that they are all concurrently afraid to disclose, and are consequently afraid to challenge for fear it will be turned on them.

The therapist's task is to help clarify what the offender's disclosure reveals, to assure him that dissimulation is expected but not valuable to him, to make clear to the offender the disadvantages of not being honest and the advantages of telling the truth (e.g., earlier release from prison, a sense of personal relief, a chance to put his life together and overcome his problems), to point to the self-serving nature of the offender's account, and to offer alternative, more realistic views of the offense and of the offender's behavior, thoughts, and feelings during the offense. On the latter issue, it is frequently apparent to the group that the offender has engaged in various manipulations to get access to a victim, to disarm others who might prevent molestation, and to silence the victim. In most cases, these manipulations seem not to be obvious to the offender, or at least he expects his listeners to believe his version of the offenses. Presumably, this is because he has told his story so many times without being challenged that he has come to accept his account as free from any self-serving intentions. One aspect of these manipulations that is particularly evident in many child molesters is their grooming of the victim. This grooming involves behaviors by the offender that are aimed at preparing the victim to participate in the offense, and offenders all too often appear (or present themselves as) oblivious to these manipulations. Rapists also often fail to recognize or acknowledge how they set up a situation to get access to a victim.

Each offender repeats his disclosure, which is followed by further challenges from the group and reconceptualizations by the therapist, until his account of every aspect of his offense(s) is acceptable to the group. Some offenders, of course, admit all facets of their offenses and take full responsibility at their first disclosure; however, most do not, and even those who do initially admit the facts frequently display some distortions. Those who deny or minimize the extent or nature of their offenses, or minimize their responsibility, are the ones who typically need to repeat their disclosure several times. Characteristically, these offenders have told their distorted story many times before they enter treatment, without being appropriately challenged. Indeed, in many cases, family and friends offer them support for their accounts. It is therefore unrealistic to expect anything but initial resistance to challenges. This tendency to resist challenges is all too frequently exacerbated by the fact that their defense lawyer has, perhaps unintentionally, encouraged them to present an exculpatory view of the offense. Sometimes professionals who have evaluated them for the courts have failed to challenge the offender's account, however much they later expressed doubts about it. This encouragement by lawyers and a failure to challenge by professionals are characteristically seen by the offender as confirmation of his claims and this, of course, makes him all the more resistant to challenges. Repeated disclosures followed by supportive challenges are therefore necessary.

Whereas these are the procedures specifically aimed at overcoming denial and minimization, subsequent processes (most particularly the victim-impact component) in the program also facilitate a reduction in minimization and may lead to a full admission in otherwise initially resistant participants. Indeed, we repeatedly return to the more subtle aspects of minimization and distortion throughout the program.

In a recent study (Marshall, 1994) we found that these procedures produced the desired effects. Prior to treatment, 63% of 81 sex offenders (15 rapists, 26 incest offenders, and 40 nonfamilial child molesters) either denied or minimized their offense. With treatment, this was reduced to 13%. Of the 9 sex offenders who continued to minimize after treatment, their scores on a 6-point minimization scale averaged 0.5, whereas the average prior to treatment had been 3.7. So even when we do not completely succeed, we are able to markedly reduce the degree of minimization. The two men who remained in denial were discharged from the program after five sessions due to their recalcitrance.

Homework

Throughout this component, offenders are encouraged to discuss relevant issues with other group members between treatment sessions, keeping in mind the issue of confidentiality. In particular, group members can be very helpful in assisting one another to overcome distortions, denial, and minimization. On occasion, particularly recalcitrant offenders are asked to write out, as homework, the specific features of their offense and the hours and circumstances surrounding it, in order to assist them in recalling details.

One of the most important homework assignments in this component requires each offender to admit complete guilt and responsibility to their family, spouse, partner, or whoever is the most important person in their life, from whom they have withheld the facts. We often assist the offender in doing this by being present when he tells his intimate person.

Victim Harm and Victim Empathy

It is thought necessary by most clinicians who work with sex offenders to have them come to an understanding of the harm that befalls victims of sexual abuse. The belief is that such an understanding will facilitate the development of empathy for potential future victims and that this experience of empathy will inhibit offending. In fact, 94% of sex-offender programs in North America employ empathy training, making it the most commonly employed treatment component (Knopp, Freeman-Longo, & Stevenson, 1992).

No one has yet offered any evidence in support of these ideas, perhaps because they appear to be self-evident truths. There is, in fact, only limited and somewhat confusing evidence indicating that sex offenders are unempathic (Marshall, Hudson, & Jones, 1994b). Except for a single recent study of our own (Marshall et al., 1994b), all of the research to date has assessed a general, nonspecified disposition to be empathic; that is, these studies accepted the assumption that empathy is a trait that is relatively unaffected by the situation or the person to whom empathy might be directed. In our research (Marshall et al., Jones, 1994b; Marshall, Jones, Hudson, & McDonald, 1993b), we have found either no deficits among sex offenders on measures assessing nonspecific empathy, or mild deficits having relatively little clinical meaning. On the other hand, we (Marshall et al., 1994b) have found that child molesters (we have not yet extended our research to rapists) display quite significant deficits in empathy toward children who have been sexually abused and even greater deficits in empathy toward their own victim(s). The targets in treatment for enhancing empathy, then, should not be directed toward people in general, but rather toward both their own victims and the class of people who are potential future victims of the offender (i.e., adult females for rapists, and children for child molesters).

The general body of literature on empathy has often confused the concept, and it is only recently that its multicomponent nature has been recognized. We (Marshall et al., 1994b) have conceptualized empathy as a staged process involving (1) recognition of another person's emotional state; (2) an ability to perceive the world from that person's point of view; (3) an ability to replicate the emotional state of the other person; and (4) a change in behavior toward the other person (i.e., either a cessation of harmful behavior or the offer of sympathy). We (Hudson et al., 1993) have shown that sex offenders are deficient at recognizing emotions in others and that they are particularly unable to recognize anger, disgust, surprise, and fear (just the emotions victims can be expected to show). Thus, in training empathy, we initially teach sex offenders to recognize emotions in the victims of sexual abuse, and we attempt to have them understand the meaning for the victims of these emotional upsets. This latter aspect is what the victim-harm component attempts to accomplish. In order to achieve this goal, we have offenders attempt to take the perspective of their victim and experience distress over the consequences of what they have done. In order to achieve the latter, it is sometimes necessary to train offenders to be emotionally expressive, because many of them appear to have very successfully learned to inhibit their feelings.

Emotional Expression

We ask each offender in turn to describe an emotionally distressing experience they have had other than being arrested. They are instructed to try to relive the experience as they describe it and not to hold back any emotions they feel. Some of them describe being sexually assaulted as children and this usually has a significant impact on the rest of the group as well as the offender himself. Others describe the loss of a loved one, the breakup of a relationship, or the emotional rejection they experienced as children. Typically, this generates a good deal of emotion in both the speaker and the listeners. If the distress of any of the speakers is very intense or prolonged, we arrange counseling so that they can deal with their unresolved emotional problems.

After each description, other participants describe how they felt while listening to the account, and they are encouraged to express their emotions freely. We point out that their expressed feelings are empathic responses.

Victim Harm

In this subcomponent, we have each participant, in turn, indicate what he believes to be the harmful consequences of sexual abuse. We ask participants to distinguish immediate (i.e., during the offense), postabuse, and long-term consequences that might befall victims. As each client describes the consequences he believes may occur, the group facilitator writes them on a flipchart. If a subsequent offender simply says that he agrees with what has been said before, we press him to provide some of his own ideas or at least elaborate on what he understands the consequences to be.

When all participants have given their suggestions, we use the list as an impetus for a general discussion; this is followed by having each offender discuss the extent to which his victim may have experienced any or all of these consequences. We repeatedly emphasize that the offender may not have realized, at the time of the offense, how much the victim was suffering or just what emotions the victim was experiencing. This does not, however, mean that the victims did not suffer and were not upset, but rather that either they did not show their feelings, or that the offender was so preoccupied with what he was doing that he was not aware of the victim's distress.

Next, we have each participant describe the offense from the victim's perspective. Offenders typically find this hard to do and often need prompting to begin. Also, they characteristically present a self-serving account and are challenged on this by other group members who, again, reveal much of their own distorted thinking to illustrate how well they understand the distortions displayed by the target offender's description. By dealing specifically with each offender in turn and having the other participants challenge him, it forces each offender to consider issues from the victim's perspective in a way, and at a depth, that he typically has not recognized before.

Finally, we have each participant write (between group sessions as a homework assignment) two letters: one supposedly from the victim, and the other as a response to the victim's letter (which, of course, he is instructed *not* to send). The letter, supposedly from the victim, should describe the victim's anger, self-blame, loss of trust, and various other emotional, cognitive, and behavioral problems. This letter is read to the group by one of the facilitators, and each member provides feedback and offers challenges to the account. Prior to the next session, the offender revises the letter according to the feedback, and it is read again with additional feedback. This process is repeated until the letter meets the satisfaction of all group members. Then, the offender writes the second letter in response to the victim. This letter is meant to express an understanding of the concerns and problems the victim said he or she was suffering and should acknowledge the legitimacy of the victim's anger and distress. It also provides the opportunity for the offender to express his full acceptance of responsibility and to indicate that he is doing what he can to ensure that he does not offend in the future. Although offenders are encouraged to apologize to the victim in these letters, they are not to ask for forgiveness, because that is seen as an unfair demand on the victim. Once again, this letter is read to the group and feedback is provided. The letter is revised, reread, and revised repeatedly until it meets the satisfaction of the group.

Victim Empathy

The group facilitator either reads to the group a description written by a victim of his or her abuse and its consequences, or shows them a videotape of an actual victim describing an assault and its consequences. In each case, we select an account that is dramatic, emotionally evocative, and believable. We do not typically use a live victim, as we have had problems on occasion when we have tried this, with either the victim getting unexpectedly distressed, or, more usually, the offenders becoming angry with the victim, no doubt out of defensiveness. When the negative experiences have occurred, it has taken considerable effort and time to overcome the resentment or defensiveness generated in the participants.

After we have read the account or shown the videotape, we ask each client to indicate his response. In particular, we ask them to describe how they felt while listening to or watching the victim. Other group members challenge each offender if they consider he either is not expressing himself honestly, or is not exhibiting appropriate emotions.

We then define empathy for them and ask each member to describe the degree of empathy they now feel for their own victim(s) and for other victims of sexual abuse. Again, all group members challenge each offender's remarks. We remind the group at this point that the style of the group is supportive, and as we point out, most of them have shown by their style of responding and acceptance of each other, a degree of empathy.

Finally, we ask each of them to describe how they would feel if their mother, sister, or daughter or son (depending on their own crime) was sexually assaulted. We ask them to describe this sexual assault and then to reveal how they feel toward the offender and toward the victim. Other offenders appraise their responses and offer feedback about its adequacy. They repeat the exercise if the group is not satisfied.

Homework

In the emotional-recognition subcomponent, as noted, we have offenders write letters from the victim and to the victim. They are encouraged to discuss these with other group members, but are told not to allow someone else to write the letters for them. In the emotional-expression subcomponent, offenders are told to practice expressing even low-intensity emotions by discussing emotional issues with their family, friends, and other offenders. In the victim-empathy section we provide participants for their reading between sessions, brief articles and books (e.g., Guberman & Wolf, 1985; Woods, 1992) written by sexual abuse survivors describing their suffering during and after the abuse. They are told to read these in order to better understand the effects on the victim and in order to facilitate their own emotional responses.

Recently, two studies have demonstrated the value of these types of procedure for enhancing offender empathy. Pithers (1994) has shown that a very similar, although perhaps more extensive treatment component effectively increased the general nonspecific empathic responses of sex offenders. We (Marshall, O'Sullivan, & Fernandez, in press) have shown that our procedures markedly enhanced the empathy child that molesters expressed for their own victims and for the whole class of child victims of sexual abuse.

Inappropriate Attitudes and Beliefs

Nature of These Beliefs

Sex offenders typically hold offense-supportive beliefs (Segal & Stermac, 1990) and these must be changed if we are to reduce their risk to reoffend.

Rapists, for example, accept the truth of many rape myths. They believe that (1) women cannot be raped unless they want to; (2) women secretly harbor fantasies of being raped; (3) if a woman is raped, it is because she put herself at risk or was deliberately sexually provocative; and (4) many women falsely report being raped, to name just a few of these myths. Rapists also accept that violence directed toward women is acceptable and sometimes necessary to keep women from overstepping their proper boundaries. And, finally, rapists affirm beliefs that women are inferior to men, should not hold positions of authority, deliberately humiliate men, and can readily behave in a contemptuous and devious manner toward men.

Accepting that women are radically different from and inferior to men allows rapists to view women as alien figures. And research has shown that when male subjects in laboratory studies view others in this way, they are more apt to behave aggressively toward them (Bandura, 1973; Bandura, Underwood, & Fromson, 1975). Presumably, the same alienation facilitates aggression, including sexual aggression, in the real world. Of course, believing that women who are raped both deserve and desire the attack similarly facilitates sexual assaults. Add to this the belief that it is acceptable to aggress against women, and rape becomes all but inevitable.

Child molesters hold equally offense-facilitating attitudes and beliefs. They typically believe that children (at least some, and particularly their own victims) deliberately engage in behaviors that are meant to invite adult males to have sex with them. If a child does not actively resist an adults' sexual advances, or does not say "no" to their sexual proposals, then child molesters believe this means that the child wants to have sex. Some child molesters consider sex between adults and children to be normal and construe society's response to be inappropriate. Many child molesters claim to be educating children by having sex with them. All of these attitudes and beliefs are clearly self-serving and obviously facilitate offending.

Exhibitionists hold many attitudes similar to those held by rapists. However, many of them also believe that sooner or later one of their victims will either be so impressed with the offenders' genitals, or feel sorry for him, or simply be so sexually aroused at the time he exposes, that she will approach him for consensual sex.

Treatment of These Beliefs

We begin this section of treatment by asking each offender, in turn, his view of the proper roles of women and children, and their associated rights. Each offender's views are appraised by the others, and this typically initiates extensive and sometimes heated discussion. We attempt to encourage challenges while defusing hostility. The discussions generated by this process characteristically become far-ranging and most of the attitudes and beliefs outlined previously find ample and clear expression. We point to the offense-facilitating nature of these beliefs and suggest that, unless they change, the offender will remain at serious risk to reoffend.

Our goal is not necessarily to convert our offenders into militant advocates of feminist views; rather, we aim for the more modest goal of having them move toward a more tolerant, less hostile, view of women. It would be pleasing if they were to become enlightened feminist sympathizers. For most of our offenders, however, that is too monumental a goal and might serve to alienate many of them from the therapeutic process. We do, however, attempt to model egalitarian and respectful male–female relations by the behavior of our two therapists: one male and one female. Of course, all of us have a lot to learn about truly egalitarian relationships and we (the therapists, that is) are continually learning from one another. It is all too easy to be self-righteous and dogmatically certain when dealing with these complex issues, but too heavy a hand and too much self-certainty do not encourage change in either our patients or ourselves.

With the child molesters, who also typically have much to learn about adult male–female relationships, we also attempt to have them recognize the rights and feelings of children. In particular, we want them to understand that a child's view of sexual activities is quite different from that of an adult. Children are invariably curious about sex and may ask questions or attempt to observe naked adults. Yet, this does not mean that they are sexually aroused or interested in doing anything sexual. Similarly, many children innocently adopt poses or disport themselves in a manner that in an adult may be construed as sexually inviting, but is not so in a child. Many children enjoy physical interactions with an adult, which offenders all too often see as indicating a desire to be sexually touched. We attempt to have our offenders appreciate these differences between adults and children and have them come to respect children's right to their innocence. In particular, we point to the relative powerlessness of children and remind the offenders of their own childhood and how powerless they felt. If children are respected, we suggest, they will feel more self-confident, and their greater self-confidence will serve to better protect them from molestations. We try to personalize these issues by having the offenders reflect on how much happier their lives might have been had they been treated respectfully as children. Again, discussions usually provide the basis for each offender to reveal their attitudes about children, which can then be challenged and their self-serving nature identified.

Although the focus of this component is on these offense-supportive attitudes and beliefs, these issues are repeatedly raised throughout the program, and many offenders are slow to change. We keep drawing attention to these attitudes whenever even a glimmer of them surfaces. We repeatedly emphasize our respect for each offender and point out that his attitudes are not something he must accept forever. We frequently note that his attitudes are inconsistent with other more positive features of him and that he would earn everyone's greater respect if he became more tolerant and respectful of women and children.

Homework

The primary homework task in this component is to have offenders write brief essays outlining how a woman or a child might challenge their prejudicial views. They are assisted in this task by reading books or articles (depending on their educational sophistication) that present women's and children's views. These essays are passed around the group for comments and challenges that typically engender further discussion of relevant issues. On this point of the offender's educational sophistication, some of our clients are unable to read or write, so that much of their required homework (in this and other components) can present problems. In these cases, we assign a responsible and insightful fellow offender to assist the man. This assistant offender is carefully instructed not to prompt the client and not to use his (i.e., the assistant's) language, but rather to simply read something to the man or write out verbatim what the offender tells him.

Fantasies

Most cognitive–behavioral treatment programs for sex offenders have a significant component dealing with fantasizing. However, in most of these programs, fantasizing is construed as strictly sexual in nature. These ways of viewing fantasizing and its role in sexual offense derives from the sexual-preference hypothesis (Barbaree & Marshall, 1991). In our view, the importance of deviant sexual preferences in initiating and maintaining deviant sexual behavior has been exaggerated. We (Blader & Marshall, 1989; Eccles, Marshall & Barbaree, 1994; Marshall & Eccles, 1991, 1993) have questioned the empirical bases of the sexual-preference hypothesis and have pointed to data that seem incompatible with claims that deviant sexual desires motivate deviant sexual acts. For example, we (Barbaree & Marshall, 1993) have found that in a large sample of rapists, only 30% showed responses at phallometric evaluations that met the criteria for deviance; 26% of a group of nonoffenders also met the deviance criteria. Among incest offenders, only 28% displayed an attraction to children at phallometric evaluation, while 48% of nonfamilial child molesters responded in a deviant manner (Barbaree & Marshall, 1989). Thus, many child molesters and most rapists do not appear to have deviant sexual preferences, at least as these are assessed by laboratory procedures.

In fact, we (Marshall, 1993a) have challenged the very notion of sexual preferences. As presently formulated, the sexual-preference hypothesis (see Barbaree, 1990, and Barbaree & Marshall, 1991, for detailed analyses of the various forms of this hypothesis) claims that men who engage in deviant sexual acts do so because they prefer these acts (i.e., the particular behaviors or the particular partner, or both) to all other acts. There is a clear suggestion that these preferences remain fixed and unvarying, such that any enactment of other sexual behaviors or of sexual acts with other types of partners is to be explained as either a "cover-up" or as substitute responses. If this is true, then sexual behavior is distinctly unique among appetitive behaviors. Many people repeatedly enjoy chocolate and may, at a taste preference test, consistently choose chocolate over various other foods. No one, however, would take this to mean that these people prefer chocolate above all other foods and that whenever these people eat other foods, it is simply to cover up their passion for chocolate. In fact, food preferences continually shift over time and these shifts are, to a very significant extent, dependent on recent eating history and current availability. Why would we not expect the same to be true of sexual behaviors?

With sexual desire, three factors seem likely to affect its specific expression. First, in a few individuals, a persistent preference may increase the likelihood that they will act in a deviant way; however, they will also quite likely engage in nondeviant sex, and there is no reason to suppose that they will not enjoy these acts. Second, there is reasonably solid evidence that men enjoy novelty in sexual behavior (Symons, 1979) and the sexual molestation of children may, in some cases, simply reflect this search for novelty. Third, opportunity may tempt some men to engage in sexual acts that are otherwise low on their preference hierarchy, and it appears that a variety of transitory states (e.g., emotional distress, intoxication) increases the probability of acting deviantly. If a man acts deviantly in such circumstances, whereas he otherwise typically engages in prosocial sexual practices, can we reasonably infer that this reflects a hidden "real" preference? A more parsimonious explanation might simply account for the behavior in terms of circumstantial factors.

Sexual-preferences hypotheses treat sexual preferences as arranged on a fixed hierarchy; thus, these accounts are "trait" theories and, as such, remain untouched by the "situational-specificity" controversy that refocused research and theorizing in the field of personality (Epstein & O'Brien, 1985; Mischel, 1984). It is equally reasonable to hypothesize that sexual assault has as much (if not more) to do with nonsexual motives than it has to do with sexual preferences. Dominance and control over the victim are features that all sexual assaults share in common, just as they do sexual elements. Yet, while many theorists mention these motivational factors, very few treatment programs attempt to measure or explicitly attempt to change them. As described in the previous section, these and associated attitudes and beliefs are targets in our program. We believe that deviant sexual acts are multidetermined. They satisfy many needs and the number and rank order of needs satisfied may vary across offenders, and within each offender they may vary over occasions. The specific sexual acts involved in offending may also satisfy various desires, and sexual desire (deviant or nonspecific) may not necessarily be the strongest. For example, forcing a woman to have sex may make the assailant feel powerful and satisfy his desire to humiliate or degrade her. Having sex with a child may satisfy a man's desire for control over others and over his own sexual activity. Furthermore, it may reduce any performance-based threats to the man's self-concept.

Our view of the motivational nature of sexual offenses and the factors that maintain such behaviors, is, nevertheless, such that we believe thoughts and associated feelings about deviant acts are frequently entertained by offenders. These thoughts and feelings appear certain to occur for a period prior to an actual offense, although the duration of this period of prior fantasizing may vary considerably. We also believe that such thoughts will typically occur at least intermittently at times when opportunities to offend are not present. And they will, at least for some individuals, be repeatedly or occasionally associated with masturbation. On many of the occasions when these fantasies occur independent of masturbation, the associated arousal may not be sexual. This arousal may have more to do with general excitement induced by the possibilities suggested in the fantasy for satisfying power, aggression, dominance, control, humiliation, and perhaps other nonsexual motives. Whatever the nature of this induced arousal, it will be satisfying and may serve in a nonsexual conditioning process that enhances the attractiveness of the deviant thoughts and acts. On this point, it is important to note that we would expect the probability of thoughts that produce feelings of power and control, and so on, to increase when the person is in any negative emotional state (e.g., induced by stress, argument, disappointment) because the excitement produced by such fantasizing would not only attenuate negative feelings, but would also make a powerless man feel in control. This, we believe, is why such fantasy-induced feeling states increase the likelihood of actual offending.

Accordingly, we believe that all sexual offenders will have, or have had, at least occasional thoughts about deviant acts that have come to be associated with feelings of satisfaction. These feelings of satisfaction are, however, not necessarily sexual in nature. Whether these thoughts and their associated feelings reflect sexual motivation is, to a large extent, irrelevant. Treatment must attempt to reduce the probability of these thoughts and/or their ability to produce satisfaction. Because we believe that all sex offenders entertain these thoughts and find them satisfying, we contend that all sex offenders should receive treatment aimed at reducing these thoughts. Of course, changing pro-offense attitudes and beliefs, as described in the previous section, is one aspect of a comprehensive attempt to deal with the need offenders have to engage in deviant fantasizing. So also are our attempts to enhance self-confidence and to provide offenders with the skills necessary to meet their needs in prosocial ways. In this section, we deal specifically with methods to reduce the frequency and attractiveness of the deviant thoughts themselves.

Covert Sensitization

Most programs carry out covert sensitization with sex offenders on an individual rather than a group basis. Indeed, most procedures that attempt to modify sexual preferences are presented and monitored individually. The rationale for this is unclear, as it seems an unnecessary waste of resources. Also, there is no evidence or compelling reason to think that these procedures will be more efficacious if conducted on an individual basis. In any case, we are persuaded that these procedures (in so far as they are effective) are just as effective when training in their use is done in groups. In fact, we believe group processes can enhance their clinical utility.

Our method of employing covert sensitization may be somewhat different from that used by other therapists, but essentially the process and the goal are the same: to have clients repeatedly associate imagined unpleasant consequences with thoughts about engaging in deviant acts in order to reduce the attractiveness, and thereby the frequency, of these thoughts.

The group facilitator describes covert sensitization and its rationale to the group. Each participant is then instructed to produce, in his own time between group sessions, at least three detailed deviant fantasies, one of which must describe an actual offense. These written scripts are refined with the group's assistance until they reflect a response sequence that involves several steps and identifies the feelings, thoughts, and actions of the man. For example, a predatory child molester might produce the following offense scenario:

- *Step 1:* I am sitting at home feeling bored, so I think I will go downtown to check out the local video arcade.
- *Step 2:* I leave the house in order to drive my motorcycle downtown to the arcade.
- *Step 3:* I find a parking spot and go into the arcade.
- *Step 4:* I enter the arcade and check out all the kids until I see one who looks approachable.
- *Step 5:* I begin a conversation with the kid and offer him money to play the games.
- *Step 6:* After spending some time and money on the kid, I ask him if he would like to go for a ride on my motorcycle.
- *Step 7:* We go for a ride and I take him to a deserted area on the pretense that he can steer the bike when we get there.

- *Step 8:* We stop at the deserted spot to talk some more, and I shift the conversation to sex.
- *Step 9:* Once the conversation becomes sexual, I make a pass at him.

Each of these scripts is written on one side of a pocket-sized card that the offender can carry with him.

We then have offenders describe all of the unpleasant consequences they can imagine occurring within each script. Many of the consequences they describe are catastrophic and probably rarely happen; nevertheless, they are often imagined by the offender, although typically postoffense. Once again, these consequences are discussed and refined. When a satisfactory list of several consequences has been produced, appropriate ones (three or four of them) are written on the back of the cards that have on the front of them the offense fantasies or sequences. These cards are to be carried by the offender at all times.

Offenders are instructed to read each card at least three times each day and, at one of the steps, turn the card over and read each consequence at least three times. They are told to begin by reading most of the sequences through to the end before turning over the card to read the consequences. With daily practice, they are to move the consequence reading further back in the sequence. By the third week, they should be reading consequences on most occasions immediately after the first or second steps. In addition, participants are told that should they have a spontaneous fantasy, they are to immediately take out their cards and read the consequences only. Under all conditions, when the offenders complete their catastrophizing thoughts, they are told to imagine some positive sequence, such as turning away from the deviant pursuits and executing a prosocial alternative-response sequence.

Prior to treatment, the catastrophizing that offenders engage in most commonly occurs shortly after an offense has taken place. Although this has a short-lived impact on reducing the risk to reoffend, these concerns gradually fade; with the absence of actual consequences, confidence builds and the probability of reoffending increases. The main aim of covert sensitization is to keep the idea of these unpleasant consequences at the forefront of the offender's thoughts and, most particularly, to have the catastrophic cognitions occur contingent on contemplating the early steps (e.g., feeling bored and thinking about going to the video arcade) in the offense or fantasy sequence so that they will abort the sequence.

Monitoring the use of these procedures presents a problem, because we have to rely on the offender's self-report. However, we attempt to have someone in their everyday environment continually remind them to maintain practice. For incarcerated offenders, one or more of the other participants can fill this role very effectively, whereas for community clients, it has to be a friend or family member.

The supporting evidence for covert sensitization applied to sex offenders is not at all strong and is quite limited. Nevertheless, there are at least theoretical reasons for supposing it will work and it certainly enjoys popularity among clinicians. Until such time as research demonstrates (if it ever does) that these procedures have no impact, we will continue to use them.

Masturbatory Reconditioning

Again, unlike most other programs, we present these procedures within a group setting and have the offenders report their use and progress to the group. One of us (WLM) always uses these procedures in groups, whereas the other (AE) prefers to apply them on an individual basis. Either way, the instructions and monitoring are the same.

Masturbatory reconditioning has two components: (1) a procedure for enhancing interests in appropriate sexual activities, and (2) a method for reducing deviant interests. The first component has sometimes been called "orgasmic reconditioning." In our review of the literature (Laws & Marshall, 1991) we found little evidence to support any of these enhancement procedures. However, the strategy that seemed to offer the most promise was "directed masturbation."

In direct masturbation, the client is instructed to masturbate to orgasm while imagining appropriate sexual behaviors with a consenting appropriate partner. Assistance is offered in generating a set of appropriate fantasies, but we discourage the use of pornography (soft- or hard-core) to facilitate this process. Rather, we encourage the man to think of women (or men, if that is his gender preference) with whom he has had a sexual relationship, or with whom he is currently involved, or with at least a potential partner. He is told that should he have trouble initially generating arousal to these images, he may use a deviant fantasy to get started. However, immediately upon attaining full arousal he should switch to an appropriate fantasy. If he loses arousal during masturbation to the appropriate fantasy, he may switch to deviant thoughts until rearoused and then switch back to the appropriate fantasy. It is hoped that repeatedly associating appropriate fantasies with the excitement of self-induced sexual arousal will eventually enhance the attractiveness of these fantasies. It is not, in our view, the association of these fantasies with orgasm that is important, as has been claimed (e.g., Marquis, 1970), but rather their association with ongoing arousal. Orgasm is a state that is too extreme (i.e., very high arousal) for associative conditioning to occur that will transfer easily to other less extreme arousal states (e.g., those occurring when initiating a sexual response). In any case, most of our clients report that as far as they can recall, their thought processes are suspended during orgasm.

The second part of our masturbatory reconditioning procedures is adapted from our original descriptions of "satiation therapy" (Marshall, 1979; Marshall & Lippens, 1977). The patient is told that after ejaculating, he is to stop masturbating and immediately commence verbalizing (subvocally if necessary) every variation he can think of on his deviant theme. Once men have ejaculated, they enter what Masters and Johnson (1966) call "the relative refractory period." This period typically lasts from 20 minutes to well over 1 hour in most men, and it is a time when they are relatively unresponsive to sexual stimuli. Indeed for most men, sexual stimuli have little or no provocative power during their refractory period. Thus, we attempt to associate deviant fantasies with this unresponsive state. The patient is told to continue verbalizing deviant fantasies during this refractory period for 10 or more minutes but never more than 20 minutes.

In our original accounts of this procedure, we had subjects fantasize deviant themes from the beinning of their masturbatory sequence and continue masturbating and fantasizing for up to 1 hour even if they ejaculated once or several times. Not only was it difficult to get clients to cooperate with this, it did not seem either wise or necessary, upon reflection, to have them associate masturbation-induced arousal with deviant fantasies. We now combine procedures so that arousal and orgasm are associated with appropriate fantasies, while postorgasm, nonstimulation, and low levels of sexual potential are associated with deviant thoughts. Of course, if satiation is effective, it may not be simply the result of associating low arousal with the deviant fantasies. Rather, it is possible that simply rehearsing the fantasies over and over again extinguishes their attractiveness.

Research examining the effectiveness of "satiation therapy" is limited but consistently supportive (Laws & Marshall, 1991). However, in one of our recent studies (Johnston, Hudson, & Marshall, 1992), employing the combination of directed masturbation and satiation as described earlier, we found not only highly significant reductions in deviant arousal, but also significant (although not quite so startling) reductions in appropriate arousal. Deriving deviant indices from the data in the Johnston et al. study, we found dramatic changes in the pedophile indices (i.e., arousal to children divided by arousal to adults) from pre- to posttreatment. It appears that the combined procedure is effective. However, we obviously need to obtain additional data and possibly refine the procedure so that reductions in appropriate arousal are not evident.

Other Approaches

We do not use electric aversive therapy and have not done so for many years. It not only generates bad publicity, but it also causes serious ethical problems (especially when working with incarcerated offenders). Also, it can counteract the development of trust in clients, and there is also very little evidence supporting its value (Quinsey & Marshall, 1983). Furthermore, Rice, Quinsey, and Harris (1991) demonstrated that electrical aversion is ineffective in producing long-term reductions in offending.

In those cases in which, after using the aforementioned procedures, the man displays clear deviant preferences at phallometric evaluation, or complains that he continues to be plagued by deviant thoughts and impulses over which he feels he has little control, we adopt one of the following courses of action: (1) pharmacological treatment by our psychiatrist, (2) olfactory aversion in the laboratory, or (3) self-administered ammonia aversion.

The pharmacological interventions we use are one of two types. Antiandrogenic or hormonal treatments (i.e., cyproterone acetate or medroxyprogesterone acetate) might be expected to reduce overall arousal and thereby reduce the intensity of urges to a controllable level. This may provide the opportunity for the offender to benefit from the rest of our program and acquire sufficient control so that the medication can be withdrawn. However, there is evidence that in some cases, cyproterone acetate has selective effects by only reducing arousal to deviant activities (Bradford & Pawlak, 1993). We do not like to maintain clients on either of these pharmacological agents for too long a period of time. Therefore, we gradually wean them off the drugs when they appear to be acquiring controls by our other training procedures. The other type of pharmacological intervention we use is to place the client on serotonergic drugs. An accumulating body of evidence in recent years strongly suggests the value of such drugs for bringing unwanted sexual urges under control (Pearson, 1990). And we have recently demonstrated the value of Buspirone with one patient whose deviant urges were very frequent, very strong, and all but irresistible (Pearson, Marshall, Barbaree, & Southmayd, 1992). Again, we do not maintain patients on these medications longer than is necessary. Therefore, as soon as their control is stable, we gradually withdraw the serotonergic agent.

Olfactory aversion refers to the presentation to the client of an offensive odor contingent upon his response to a deviant stimulus. We avoid the use of obnoxious chemical agents, because some of these may be carcinogenic or otherwise harmful to the client. Typically, we use rotted meat enclosed in a glass jar. Initially the patient is instructed to imagine a deviant act, or he listens to, or watches, a deviant act, or he listens to, or watches, a deviant stimulus. When he feels aroused, he raises the jar, lifts the lid, and takes a deep nasal inhalation. It is an extremely rare person who does not find the odor or rotten meat to be aversive. Indeed, we have found that olfactory aversion consistently produces changes in remarkably few trials. The reason we do not use it more routinely is that like electrical aversion, it does not enhance the therapist–client relationship and it can generate bad publicity. Furthermore, it is difficult to administer without the odor spreading throughout the treatment room, if not farther; this makes it somewhat aversive to treatment staff.

The final procedure we employ for these unresponsive men is ammonia aversion. Actually, we use ammonia aversion quite frequently with exhibitionists, whether or not they respond to other procedures. However, we use it more sparingly with child molesters and rapists. The deviant acts of exhibitionists seem more consistently triggered by environmental cues than is the case with most other offenders, and many exhibitionist claim to be plagued by urges every day. In ammonia aversion, the client carries either single vials of ammonia salts that can be split open or small bottles of the salts. In either case, these can easily be carried unobtrusively in the man's pocket. He is told that whenever he feels an urge, he is to take out the bottle or vial, open it, and, holding his nose about one inch from the bottle, he is to take a deep, rapid nasal inhalation. This is meant to both interrupt ongoing thoughts and to punish the deviant thoughts. Once the deviant thoughts are interrupted in this way, the offender is told to turn his attention to some more prosocial, although preferably nonsexual, thoughts. Although our experience with ammonia aversion has been positive, there is little evidence regarding its efficacy with sex offenders.

Homework

Participants are instructed to practice using their covert sensitization scripts, and at each group session we check to see how each person is doing. It is impossible to generate a reliable checking system short of audiotaping practices, which has the disadvantage of making the practice seem somewhat artificial. We very rarely have clients audiotape any type of practice sessions, partly for the reason of artificiality, but also because we would have to have on hand a large number of portable recording machines and many tapes, both of which are beyond our budget. The best we can do is ask the participants to honestly report what they have done. We try to arrange it so that the cost of admitting they did not practice is not so great that they will withhold the truth, while balancing this against the need to have some consequences for persistent failures.

Similarly, we do not employ audiotaped recordings of masturbatory or satiation procedures, as do some clinicians. Once again, we feel that such recordings make the practices artificial and, especially for the sequence up to orgasm, interfere with the necessary processes. Also, the time involved in checking such recordings to ensure appropriate practice is being carried out would severely stretch our staff resources, which could more usefully be directed toward therapy. We ask each participant to report the frequency of his masturbatory reconditioning sessions; we deal with any problems in the implementation of these procedures within the group.

We also have those clients who are using ammonia aversion report on their use of the salts. We remind clients of the need to use them every time they have an urge. The group assists in helping each participant define the occurrence of an urge. Typically, we find that as clients practice inhibiting urges by using the ammonia, they become progressively more sensitive to lower intensity urges. Although this is valuable initially, we want them to learn that they can exercise control over low-intensity urges without the use of the salts.

RELAPSE PREVENTION

The approach to treating sex offenders within the framework of a *relapse-prevention model* grew out of the efforts of those working with alcohol and drug addictions (e.g., Marlatt 1982). Marques and Pithers pioneered the modification and application of the model with sex offenders and published this work in the early 1980s (Pithers, Marques,

Gibat, & Marlatt, 1983). As a result, it has become perhaps the most commonly used approach for the treatment of sex offenders, at least within programs that are primarily cognitive–behavioral in their orientation. Also, adopting a relapse-prevention model did not entail a radical departure from the treatment strategies previously used by cognitive-behavior therapists. For the most part, the relapse-prevention model has provided an approach to the treatment of offenders that is compatible with and incorporated much of the work that these clinicians had been conducting previously. Furthermore, the model created a cohesive framework within which the various elements of therapy could be understood. And it undoubtedly added further impetus to the trend that began in the late 1970s and early 1980s toward an increasing emphasis on the cognitive aspects of sexual offending. The relapse-prevention framework also provided for a pragmatic approach to dealing with the treatment of cognitions using a common model and a language in which the terms are reasonably well defined.

In the following pages, we summarize the relapse-prevention model and its application to the treatment of sex offenders. For a more comprehensive review of relapse prevention, we refer the reader to Laws (1989), who provides an excellent overview of many issues relevant to relapse prevention with this population.

We outline the relapse-prevention model here in the form that we typically employ. In our treatment programs, we typically eschew some of the terminology that has the appearance of being "jargon" (e.g., decision matrix, abstinence-violation effect). We find that this makes the model more accessible to many our clients, particularly those who have not had the benefit of adequate educational opportunities. Nonetheless, we feel that it is important that the integrity of the relapse-prevention model and its language be maintained. Consequently, we will frequently make cross-references during therapy to terms used in the formal model (e.g., "Today we will be discussing the *excuses* that many of you used to facilitate your abusive behavior. At other times, some of you who have been in other treatment programs may have heard these referred to as *cognitive distortions* or *rationalizations*"). We believe that this permits us to provide a more readily comprehensible relapse-prevention program for our clients that maintains the essential elements of the formal model in a manner that protects its academic integrity.

Using the Relapse-Prevention Model

It is essential for an offender to acknowledge that there is some risk he will reoffend. If there really were no future risk, there would be no triggers or high-risk situations that he would need to prepare for, and the whole exercise would be futile. We point out to the group members that although it is alright for them be optimistic about their chances of not reoffending, it is nonetheless sensible for them to understand that they cannot entirely rule it out. After all, many, if not most, offenders who reoffend were convinced after their initial offense that they would never do it again. So although optimism is reasonable and perhaps even desirable, it should not interfere with sensible planning and precautions for the future.

Offense Chains

Perhaps the two most fundamental tenets of the relapse prevention model are that (1) sexual offenses do not occur "out of the blue" or in a vacuum, and (2) offenders are not "out of control." Rather, offenses occur in a context whereby many situations arise and many decisions are made prior to the offense itself. Furthermore, they occur in a sequence or chain, and each situation increases the likelihood that the chain of events and behaviors will eventually culminate in the commission of a sexual assault.

Studies of recidivistic offenders show that their offenses tend to occur at times when things are not going well in their lives and their emotional state is a negative one, such as depression or anger (Pithers, Kashima, Cumming, Beal, & Buell, 1988). Typically, these men encounter stressors (e.g., divorce, job loss) with which they are unable to cope satisfactorily. The consequent negative mood may serve to erode their sense of self-esteem and well-being, which makes them more vulnerable to choosing not to suppress deviant sexual thoughts or urges. The result can be an unfolding series of events (referred to as *lapses*) that may include deviant masturbatory fantasies, "cruising" to seek out a victim, victim selection, planning, and grooming. These lapses, if uninterrupted, will ultimately lead to a sexual assault (i.e., a relapse). Progressing along each "link" is facilitated by thoughts, attitudes, and perceptions that serve to excuse or justify the subsequent behavior.

Figure 9.1 outlines the general sequence through which most offenders will proceed in committing an offense, and this is presented to offenders in our groups. Not all offenders will necessarily advance through all stages, nor will they necessarily progress in this order. Nonetheless, the sequence represents a good starting point for understanding the process of offending and reoffending. It must be strongly emphasized to group members that an offense chain does not imply a *causative* role for the elements that comprise the chain. Therefore, if alcohol abuse, for example, is part of an offender's chain, this does *not* mean that alcohol caused the offense. We emphasize the offender's responsibility for choosing to offend, while at the same time pointing to the importance of factors that increase risk. More accurately, drinking makes an assault more likely for an offender already predisposed to be abusive.

When we have introduced the general notion of an offense chain, and have outlined the pattern that this generally take into group members, they are asked to consider a fictitious case history in an effort to further demonstrate to them how offenses consist of a series of events and poor decisions based on faulty thinking. The following is an example of the kind of case we use to accomplish this:

> Derek has been in jail for sexually assaulting a woman but has been out for 2 years now. He has participated in a treatment program and completed his parole and probation without any problems. He also attended Alcoholics Anonymous (AA) for a while, although he has not bothered to go for over 6 months now. Derek is not concerned about this. He is extremely confident that he will not reoffend because he thinks to himself that he sure doesn't want to go through the experience of court and imprisonment again. That part of this life is over now, so he has decided to shut it out completely and get on with his life. Derek thinks that his only problem right now is his boss at the construction site where he works, who he feels has been giving him a really hard time recently. Derek has been late for work a lot lately, and there have been complaints about the quality of his work. For a while now, life at home has not been great either. He and his wife Nancy have not been getting along too well, and so Derek meets his friends at the bar more often now just to get away from the house. He knows that in the past his therapists have urged him not to drink, but he feels that he needs to so that he can relax a little. That makes it difficult to get up in the morning. However, Derek tells himself that he works hard and so it's no big deal if he is a little late for work. He figures that he more than makes up for it later in the day and feels that he knows himself best and will know when his drinking is affecting his work.
>
> One day, Derek is at work installing some tiles on the kitchen wall of a house that is being built. He is preoccupied over an argument he had with his wife that morning. She

William L. Marshall
and Anthony Eccles

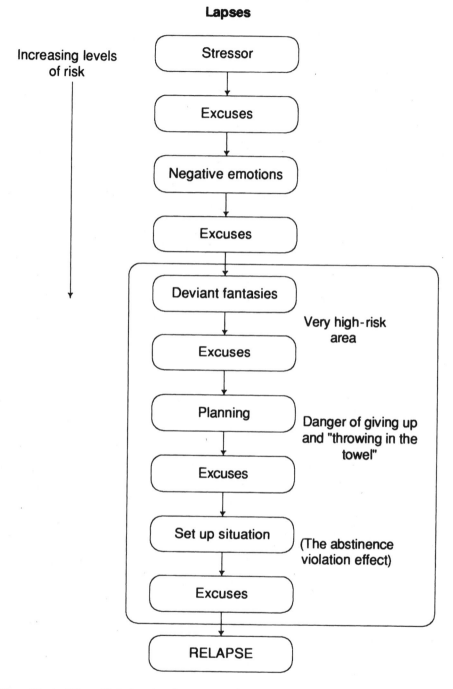

Figure 9.1. An Offense Chain lists the relevant events (i.e., lapses) that precede an offense. Shown here is a simplified generic description of the features of an offense chain for many offenders.

told him that they were running into debt and that he would have to cut down on his drinking. He got angry because, as far as he was concerned, this was how he relaxed. What was the use of working his butt off, he had shouted, it he couldn't even enjoy a drink every now and again with the money he had earned. He still felt a great deal of anger over what he felt were his wife's unreasonable demands. His anger was fueled as he went over and over the argument in his head. Just then his boss came by and started complaining about the job he was doing. Derek could see that it was not very good, but he was sure not going to give his boss the satisfaction of admitting it. He thought that his boss was just giving him a hard time and looking for any excuse to get on his case. Derek felt as if he was going to explode. He told his boss to get lost and to shove his job "where the sun doesn't shine." As he stormed off the site, his pulse and his thoughts were racing. He kept telling himself how unfair it was that no one would give him a break. He jumped into his car and drove around looking for a bar. He found himself outside a strip-bar that he had not been in since before his offense. He felt a flicker of excitement as he thought about going inside. "Screw it," he said, as he parked his car and went into the bar. He told himself that Nancy would never know and that he needed a real distraction right now.

When he got inside the bar, he ordered a drink and started to watch the strippers. They made him feel horny, and he liked the feeling. "Too bad Nancy doesn't look like these babes," he thought to himself. He and the other guys at the bar traded comments and jokes about the strippers for several hours. It was some time before Derek decided that he had better go home. He got into his car and steadied himself as he grabbed the wheel. He thought he would be okay to drive if he took it easy. As he drove home he noticed a lone woman walking along the street. He looked about and couldn't see anyone else around anywhere. He told himself that he would see if she wanted to party with him. He pulled over and grabbed a map out of the glove compartment as an excuse to talk to her. He got out of the car and looked lost as he walked over to inquire about directions. He felt a rush of excitement as she stood beside him and pointed to the next street over. Before he knew it, she smiled and was about to leave. He felt frustrated and angry that she was walking away, so he reached around and covered her mouth with one hand while opening the car door with the other. He managed to shove her inside, where he threatened to kill her if she didn't shut up. He then drove her out of town and raped her.

Derek was arrested a short while later. He admitted raping the woman but expressed astonishment that he had reoffended. It had not been planned, he said, and he had not meant to hurt her. It was impulsive, he pleaded. He was standing beside her and it just suddenly happened. Of course, he was certain that now he had finally learned his lesson and that noting like this could ever happen again.

Despite Derek's opinions to the contrary, there is clearly a buildup to the offense over a period of time. Group members are asked about the sequence of events that led to the offense, and they are encouraged to see a chain of poor decisions and behaviors that are linked together and eventually result in the assault.

When group members understand that offenses are not acts isolated from the rest of their lives and behavior, they are asked to examine the links in the chain more closely. Specifically, we want them to understand how their behavior is dependent on their thoughts and feelings. Some offenders who are somewhat limited intellectually find this exercise to be beyond their abilities, and so we typically simplify it for them. Thus, we expect them to produce a reasonable chain that may not have a behavioral and cognitive element at each link. Most offenders, however, do not have any difficulty with the exercise, which is usually introduced in a manner similar to the following:

Whenever we do something, it is a decision we make based on our thoughts and feelings. For example, when we decide to wear a heavy sweater, it might be based upon feeling cold and our thoughts about the forecast for that day. It is important to understand how this happens, particularly when the decisions we make are to hurt or abuse others. Each group member must try to learn what his thoughts and feelings were prior to his offense, because very often these are different for different people, even though the end behavior is the same. So two guys, for example, let's call them Joe and Ted, might each abuse his 13-year-old stepdaughter, but each will make the decision in a very different way. For example, Joe might be convinced that he is responding to a pass his stepdaughter made at him, whereas Ted might be telling himself that he will get away with it if he scares the hell out of his stepdaughter so that she won't report it. For example, the first sections of Derek's offense chain might look something like this:

1. *Thought*: "I don't need to worry about reoffending any more. It's time to put all that behind me, forget about it, and get on with my life. I know I'm not going to reoffend. Why can't people just believe me?"
   Feeling: Optimistic about himself. Pissed off with others.
   Behavior: Stops attending AA and becomes careless about problems.

2. *Thought*: I wish Nancy would get off my back. Can't she see I'm doing my best? She's such a bitch.
   Feeling: Pressured. Stressed.
   Behavior: Argues with his wife.

3. *Thought*: "I need to relax. The guys will be down at the bar. I'll just have a quick one with them."
   Feeling: Relief.
   Behavior: Goes to the bar. Gets drunk.

4. *Thought*: "Man, I feel awful. Take it easy. I'll be a bit late for work, but I'll make up for it."
   Feeling: Sick. Short-tempered and irritable.
   Behavior: Shows up late for work, again.

5. *Thought*: "I can't take this shit any more. This damn supervisor is always on my back."
   Feeling: Angry.
   Behavior: Quits his job.

6. *Thought*: "I can't believe I just did that, but the bastard gave me no choice. I've got to get out of here."
   Feeling: Angry. Scared.
   Behavior: Walks off the construction site.

7. *Thought*: "Nobody gives me break. Boy, am I ever wound up. I really need a drink."
   Feeling: Angry. Scared. Confused.
   Behavior: Looks for a bar.

8. *Thought*: "Hey, a strip-bar. Gee, I probably shouldn't … Ah, screw it! It would really help me unwind. Besides, Nancy need never know."
   Feeling: Excitement. Anticipation. Relief.
   Behavior: Goes into strip-bar.

Group members are provided with this example, although they are told that it only partly completes the offense chain. They are then asked as a group to complete the rest of the chain. This serves as practice for developing their own offense chains, which they will do prior to the next meeting. Going through this example serves to emphasize to group members just how offenses are preceded by many relevant thoughts and behaviors and serve as a model for developing their own offense chains. Tying the thoughts and feelings to each of the behaviors helps to emphasize how an offender is continually making active choices as he puts himself into increasingly risky situations. Each group member is encouraged to produce a minimum of nine stages. When each member has produced his offense chain, it is presented to the group by the group leader, and all group members are required to appraise it. Feedback from the group guides the offender to modify his offense chain, and then it is again presented, with further feedback and modifications as necessary. This process is repeated until the offense chain is deemed satisfactory.

Warning Signs

Once group members have developed a reasonable offense chain, this is used as the basis for proceeding to the next section, which is the development of *warning signs*. As an individual's coping mechanisms fail and he proceeds along an offense chain, his mood, judgment, and behavior deteriorate, and this is reflected in the offense chain that he develops. It is helpful if offenders have a clear set of specific indicators in mind that can serve as signals to them that their level of risk might be increasing. Ideally, each individual has an idea of what sorts of things to look for both *internally* (i.e., cognitively, and therefore only observable to themselves) and *externally* (i.e., behaviorally, and therefore observable to others). There are a number of advantages to this, which will be outlined later.

It is not unusual for men, in general, and perhaps sex offenders, in particular, to have a difficult time identifying, labeling, and expressing a wide range of emotions. Although anger is probably an exception to men's difficulty in reading their own emotional states, there are other moods with which offenders may have difficulty, and this is important if these moods put them at risk. For example, many offenders may feel depressed but may not label their mood in this way. For these men, it is helpful if they have an idea of what concrete, behavioral indicators would suggest that they were depressed. For example, an offender might more readily recognize external warning signs, such as difficulty sleeping, loss of appetite, and a general lack of concern over his health and hygiene. These signs can serve as cues to him that he is probably in a low mood state that he must cope with effectively if he is to maintain his risk at a minimal level. With many risky moods states, of which depression is one, it is certainly an advantage to arrest their development early, because an offender's judgment and resolve will likely diminish as the mood worsens.

An additional advantage of specifically developing a set of external warning signs is that these are particularly useful to others assisting the individual in his relapse-prevention efforts. We will return to this a little later on, but suffice it to say here that in many cases, others might see warning signs before an offender himself might be aware of them. Of course, certain behaviors will only serve as warning signs if others are primed to see them for what they are. Thus, the warning signs developed by each offender become an important part of the information that he shares with those involved in his overall supervision.

In addition to getting group members to identify both external and internal warning signs, they are asked to break them down further according to the risk level with which they are associated. Thus, although "failing to meet financial responsibilities" might be a warning sign that indicates a mood and frame of mind that elevates an offender's risk, in all likelihood this will signify a lower level of risk than would, say, "collecting flyers that contain pictures of kids modeling underwear." Thus, group members are required to identify warning signs at each of three risk levels: *Moderate Risk*, *High Risk*, and *Very High Risk*. We do not have a low-risk category, because we assume that when an offender is no longer completely abstinent and has lapsed into his offense chain, he can no longer be seen as a low risk.

It is worth emphasizing what on the one hand seems obvious but is frequently overlooked, and that is the dynamic nature of an individual's risk. Courts and parole boards that seek assessments on offenders frequently want some indication of the risk that a given offender poses. There is often an implicit notion here that this risk is a fixed and static feature of the offender. In actuality, a perpetrator's risk level is something that can change over time depending on the decisions he makes and his circumstances. Clearly, there are some offenders who are a very high risks and who are not particularly interested in changing; there are other offenders who can be categorized as generally stabilized at a low-level risk to reoffend. However, the principles of the relapse-prevention model are that an individual's risk level rises incrementally as he makes decisions that advance him along his offense chain. On the other hand, of course, his risk diminishes as he makes decision that abort his movement along the chain.

Each group member is asked to try to identify three external and three internal warning signs at each of the three risk levels. Group members are asked to examine their offense chains in an effort to establish these warning signs. Those offenders who have developed reasonable offense chains will have little difficulty translating these into a series of behavioral and cognitive indicators. To assist them in this, they are given some examples such as those illustrated in Figure 9.2.

As in all the other processes in our program, when an offender has outlined an initial set of warning signs and their estimated risk level, it is presented to the group for evaluation, feedback, and subsequent revision. Once group members have identified their offense chains and the warning signs that these chains may be active, they are in a position to examine more closely how it is that their individual chains advance. It is at this point that we turn the group's attention to the excuses and rationalizations that they have used in the past to engage in high-risk behaviors.

Excuses and Challenges

Whenever a person does something he knows he should not do, he will typically make excuses to make it seem like a more reasonable thing to do. For example, someone who burgles a home might convince himself that "I would not have to do it if this society was not so unfair. The rich get richer while the poor folks like me get screwed and get poorer. Besides, this stuff will all be covered by insurance anyway." To fully appreciate this point, group members must remember that when someone engages in a high-risk behavior or an actual offense, they are making a *decision* to do so. Whenever someone makes a decision, there are a number of factors that determine what the outcome of this decision will be. These have to do with the individual's thoughts and attitudes concerning the act that is being considered, the likely outcomes of the various options the person feels are available at the time, and what that person thinks of others involved in or affected by the act.

It is probably helpful if it can be demonstrated how the process outlined earlier holds

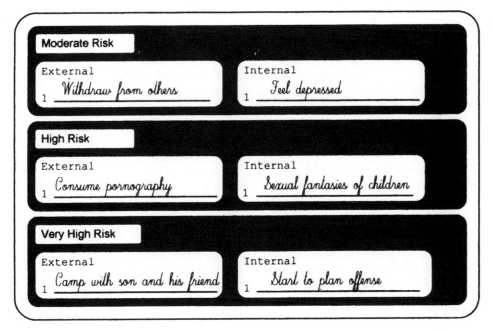

Figure 9.2. In developing a list of warning signs, an offender should be able to identify both external, behavioral events in addition to internal, cognitive events. The list should also reflect different levels of risk. The figure shows this structure with one example; however, group members are asked to generate at least three in each of the six categories.

true for behavior in general and not just for criminal acts. For example, if someone is trying to quit smoking, he might break this attempt on occasion by making excuses that have the effect of giving him permission to do so. The following will be familiar to many smokers who have tried to give up the habit: "Well, it would not hurt to have just one. I won't inhale too much, and besides that, I can't be expected to give them up completely right away. What is important is that I cut down, and I have surely done that." When group members have been able to identify this process in their everyday lives, it becomes easier to see how they use it to maintain their offense-related behaviors.

When offenders use excuses to facilitate their behavior, these rationalizations often seem extraordinary, even to those who have been working with sexual abusers for a long time. In fact, it is not surprising that these distortions are frequently peculiar. After all, if someone allows himself to commit an extreme act such as sexually abusing a child, then any rationalizations that serve to excuse this must necessarily be extreme themselves. Sometimes offenders in group will recognize the absurdity of their thoughts at the time of the offense, whereas others will remain convinced, for example, that "The relationship that I had with my stepdaughter was special. It was not abuse—she was just extremely mature for 13. People just do not understand. Besides, if she wanted me to stop, she would have said so. She only ratted on me in the end when she thought her mother would find out." When working with offenders who are still thinking in these terms, it becomes patently clear why it is so crucial to have offenders accept unqualified responsibility for their abusive behavior at the start of treatment. The more than an offender fails to do so, the greater the extent to which his subsequent efforts in treatment will be compromised.

Clearly, offenders must first be able to identify thinking errors before they can become adept at challenging them. In developing their offense chains, group members are asked to identify the thoughts that accompanied each behavior. This should provide a useful basis for compiling a list of excuses that they have used in the past. It is important that they compile a list that includes the justifications for the preoffense risk behaviors that are components of the offense chain and not just the offense itself. All of these need to be avoided and offenders must prepare for this accordingly.

Each of the thinking errors that is identified must be challenged appropriate if offenders are going to cope effectively with them in the future. Once group members recognize that excuses facilitate proabusive behaviors, they must generate effective and realistic counterarguments, as illustrated in Figure 9.3.

When group members have understood this rationale they are given instructions similar to the following:

> Use the *Thoughts* from your Offense Chain as a guide to help you to identify nine *Thinking Errors* that you have used to "talk yourself into" doing things related to your offenses, as well as the offenses themselves. Find an appropriate challenge to each of these thinking errors that you identify. Your changes of avoiding a reoffense in the future are much greater if you can identify these self-deceptions for what they are and challenge them vigorously. Going through this exercise will make it harder to use the same excuses again, because they are likely to seem rather phony. You should regard this exercise as rehearsal or practice for a strategy you may need to use in the future.

Table of Decision Consequences

Traditionally known as a *Decision Matrix* in the formal model, we prefer a term that is less intimidating to most group members. Quite frankly, our commitment to this component has perhaps not always been what it should be, and we have omitted it from several groups when time was limited. More recently, we have reinstated it as a core part of the program on the basis of some recent research by Marques and her colleagues (Marques, Nelson, West, & Day, 1994), indicating that the quality of an offender's work on this exercise is related to

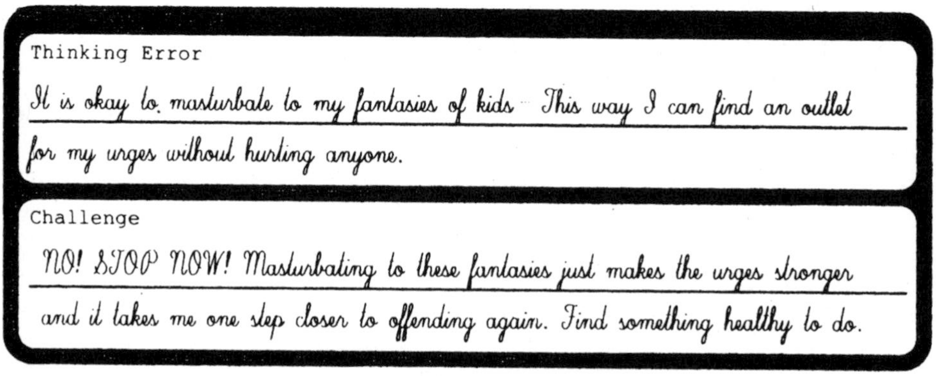

Thinking Error

It is okay to masturbate to my fantasies of kids This way I can find an outlet for my urges without hurting anyone.

Challenge

NO! STOP NOW! Masturbating to these fantasies just makes the urges stronger and it takes me one step closer to offending again. Find something healthy to do.

Figure 9.3. This example shows how an offender might justify an offense-related behavior, in this case masturbation to deviant fantasies. Also illustrated is an example of a challenge for countering this.

his probability of recidivism. It is relatively straightforward, although many group members have difficulty with it initially.

In essence, this portion of the program requires group members to think about the consequences of the various response options they have when considering whether to reoffend. Again, we stress to the group that when perpetrators reoffend, it is because they make a choice to do so. It is worthwhile to have them go through the process of imagining that they are contemplating a decision: Either have sexual contact with a child, or refrain from doing so and remain offense-free. There are a wide range of consequences for themselves and others based on the decision they will make. Some of these will be short-term (e.g., excitement) and some will be *long-term* (e.g., lack of self-respect) consequences. Each of these outcomes can also be classified as *positive* or *negative*. In the cases of the two earlier examples, "excitement" would be positive and the "lack of self-respect" would be negative. Some group members are reluctant to list the positive consequences of offending. Clearly, however, there have to be consequences for the offenders or else they would not choose to do it. Nonetheless, some categories can be difficult to complete (e.g., positive, long-term consequences of a decision to reoffend). However, this serves, in part, to illustrate that the appropriate decision an individual should make (i.e., to remain offense-free) is clearly dictated by the consequences.

In Figure 9.4 we provide the table that group members are given, with one example in each category. We would caution against giving group members more than this in the way of examples, because many will simply repeat what they have seen or heard in this regard. We do not give them opportunities to redo this exercise, because their initial production is probably of the most value from an assessment perspective. However, those who produce poor tables are expected to attend to the work of others and at least express improvements to their own in group sessions.

Support Network

Avoiding a reoffense is the responsibility of each individual offender, and it will depend on his commitment and resolve to remain abstinent. Each man can, however, increase his chances of succeeding if he has a support network of family, friends, and professional services available to him. In most cases, these people should be informed of his offense history and be aware of his relapse-prevention efforts. Group members are asked to list those who are able to play a role in this regard. The list should contain the names of people to whom the perpetrator can realistically be expected to be able to talk to in the event that he is having difficulty coping. Each group member is also expected to seek out and to list the telephone number of a crisis line in his locality.

Some years ago, we had a client who wrote to us saying that he had reoffended despite recognizing for some time prior to his reoffense that he was using deviant fantasies while being aware of the implications of this. He said that he had thought about calling our clinic but did not do so because he did not want to let us down. Apparently, he felt that by having to call he would have failed both us and perhaps himself. We now tell our clients about this letter and stress that if a group member were to call us in the future, then we would see that action as a *success* and not a failure. The occasional return of deviant thoughts and other difficulties is to be expected, and so simply having this happen is not a failure. It is a failure only when these issues are not addressed properly. By getting in touch with a therapist in such a situation, the client is showing a far better way of dealing with the problem than he did in the past. This is very definitely a success. By stressing this aspect, we hope to

Choose to remain OFFENSE-FREE

	Short-Term Consequences	Long-Term Consequences
+	No longer scared	Self-Confidence
−	Sexually frustrated	No child centered lifestyle

Choose to REOFFEND

	Short-Term Consequences	Long-Term Consequences
+	Excitement	Fulfill fantasies
−	Terrify & hurt another child	Lose family

Figure 9.4. A table of decision consequences lists the short- and long-term outcomes, both positive and negative, of the decision to remain offense-free and to reoffend.

increase the chances that group members will use their support network when they really need to.

Relapse-Prevention Plan

Having established an offense chain and the thinking errors and warning signs that are associated with it, offenders are in a position to develop a relapse-prevention plan. The plan describes what they will do in order to avoid or cope better with all the elements in their offense chain that might put them at some risk.

The coping strategies that are developed must be concrete and specific, and each element of the offense chain should be addressed. Early precursors are typically events that precipitate negative mood states, and they can be quite varied. The requirements for dealing with these can sometimes be quite challenging. For example, if an offender is prone to bouts of depression when he is working night-shift, and there is reason to believe that his probability of offending is higher at these times, then he may need to change jobs. In today's economic climate, this is not done lightly or easily. Other kinds of treatment program may be required (e.g., marital counseling, drug and alcohol-abuse treatment) if there are ancillary problems that put the offenders at risk. It is worth stressing to group members again at this point that this does not imply a *causative* role for these problems. In other words, marital problems, for example, might "put fuel on the fire," so to speak, by increasing the risk that an offender with abusive tendencies will act on them. This is very different from compelling him to abuse someone. In fact, he exercises a conscious choice if he does this.

Strategies will also be required to deal with later elements in the offense chain. As such, group members will have to know how to deal with urges and what to do in high-risk situations. We point out that it is not too late to escape from a situation until they have actually touched a child, exposed themselves, or otherwise abused someone. Therefore, even if they find themselves sitting beside a child and about to put their hand between the child's legs, for example, it is still possible for them to come to their senses, get up, and escape the situation.

It is important to instill in group members the view that no matter how desperate things seem to them, no matter how much they feel that they are out of control, it is possible to extricate themselves from the situation right up until the last second before they initiate the assault. The reason this is so important is that many offenders who find themselves at this point can give up or throw in the towel. This phenomenon is often referred to as the *abstinence-violation* effect in the formal relapse-prevention model. This sounds highly technical. However, group members usually grasp the principle fairly quickly, if not the term itself. We caution offenders that the day might come when they lapse and masturbate to deviant fantasies, for example. We want them to be prepared for what might follow, which is a profound sense of dejection and discouragement, and the feeling that their treatment has been a failure and that they have lost all that they worked so hard to achieve. Some might believe that this is further evidence of the fact that they are unable to control themselves. If they are prepared for this happening, it may still be difficult to deal with, but recognizing it for what it is reduces much of its power. Group members are urged never to "throw in the towel" but to fight strongly to keep front and center in their minds that they have a choice, and to constantly remind themselves that they have a plan in place to deal with the situation and to keep a realistic focus on the consequences of offending. Above all, they must tell someone about the struggle they are having at this point so that they can enlist support and assistance in getting over this hurdle.

It is also crucial that group members understand that although occasional lapses are expected and in some cases perhaps inevitable, the further along an offense chain a perpetrator is, the less likely it will be that he will regroup and intervene to cope effectively with the situation. Thus, an offender who lapses into loneliness is in a better position to effectively come to grips with the situation than is an offender who has lapsed to the point where he is drunkenly wandering into his stepdaughter's bedroom at two o'clock in the morning. Furthermore, offenders should avoid using the expectation of lapses to give themselves "permission" to engage in offense-related activities. We have heard several offenders justify their lapses, such as pornography use, by shrugging their shoulders and saying something like: "Well, I cannot be expected to be perfect. Like you said, lapses are probably going to happen, so its not worth getting too worried about them. It's better than offending, isn't it?" Lapses have to be vigorously avoided and then taken seriously when they occur. Group members have to use lapses as learning experiences in which they try to ascertain what went wrong and how they can add to their relapse-prevention efforts to ensure that it does not happen again.

It is worthwhile to consider another potential pitfall for offenders. In our experience, some offenders are inclined to convince themselves that they should deliberately expose themselves to high-risk situations in order to "test" themselves to find out if they can handle it. No doubt, this is simply another example of a rationalization for engaging in these behaviors. However, it occurs sufficiently often that it should be strongly emphasized in group that under absolutely no circumstances should an offender ever test himself by exposing himself to any risk factors.

Generating Potential Lapses/High-Risk Situations.   As a starting point, group members are asked to compile a list of *Lapses*. These are the high-risk situations that increase the probability of their reoffending. The elements of their offense chain will figure prominently here. Usually, either a single behavior, thought, or feeling is selected from each state, or sometimes more if the choice is not considered redundant. Group members are also asked to generate other situations that may not have played a role in their offenses to date, but which may threaten their future commitment to an offense-free lifestyle. For example, many offenders have put their marriages in jeopardy. Although some relationships will have already ended, many offenders have marriages that remain intact but are unstable and face an uncertain future. The end of a relationship is typically a high-risk stressor for many offenders, even though they may not have faced that before. Consequently, it may make sense for them to work in a focused manner toward strengthening the relationship and to have contingency plans in place in the event that these efforts are unsuccessful. Relapse fantasies, which require offenders to imagine scenes of failure and to describe them as vividly as they can, are useful ways to elicit information pertaining to idiosyncratic risk factors (Sandberg & Marlatt, 1989).

Occasionally group members have difficulty generating a list of potential lapses. This arises from their reluctance to specify a series of risk factors, many of which they currently feel competent to handle. Itemizing risk factors in this fashion concerns some offenders who feel that to do so may alarm others who will interpret the list to mean that the offender is a "time bomb," primed and ready to offend whenever any of a plethora of situations arise. Group members anticipating an appearance before a parole board are most likely to feel this. They can be reassured by stressing that these situations do not in any way imply offense certainty. They simply reflect the reality that sex offenders, like all of us, will face problematic situations in the future. The failure to anticipate these, so that appropriate actions can be planned, can have serious consequences for offenders and any future victims. What therapists and others, such as the parole board, want to see from perpetrators are realistic plans for how they will deal with difficulties that will undoubtedly arise. Far more concern will be induced by an offender who says that there are no high-risk situations to consider and prepare for because he "just knows" that he will not reoffend.

Generating Avoidance Strategies.   It is always better to avoid lapses than to have to cope with them. Thus, group members are encouraged to provide strategies that they will use to prevent these high-risk situations from arising. In doing this, it is essential that they be as specific as possible. For example, if "loneliness" is a part of an offender's offense chain, he might consider ways of countering this in the future; however, it would not be good enough to simply put down "make more friends" as an avoidance strategy. Instead, he should indicate *exactly* how he is going to achieve this. Thus, he might list the specific activities, hobbies, or clubs he will join (e.g., "Go to the socials at the County Hall on Friday and Sunday evenings") to minimize the possibility of feeling lonely.

Generating Coping Strategies.   Having established potential lapses and ways of avoiding them, offenders are required to delineate how they will cope with, or escape from, these situations in the event that their avoidance strategies have not been implemented or have otherwise failed. They are asked to prepare both an internal coping strategy that is based on straightening out their faulty thinking, in addition to a behavior that they can engage in to remedy the situation. Again, specificity of the action planned is the key here, as is the incorporation of a support network. Figure 9.5 outlines how this might be applied to

Lapse : _Stop attending Alcoholics Anonymous; Become careless in avoiding risk situations and complacent about future risk._

Avoidance Strategy : _Form strong links with sponsor John. Inform him about my offense and the need to abstain from alcohol use. Arrange for John to call me if I miss any meetings and get him to remind me of why it is important to keep attending._

Coping Strategy (Thought) : _"Hey, wake up and smell the the coffee! They warned us in group about getting careless and this could be happening to me now. I want to lead a normal life but I can not trust my own judgement on this one. Maybe I could make it on my own without going to A.A., but that sure is a gamble. I must do all I can to stay out of trouble and if that means attending A.A. then so be it. I must stay focussed, stay clean and STAY SOBER!"._

Coping Strategy (Behavior) : _Call John to pick me up and take me to the next A.A. meeting (in case I change my mind); Read my material from the group to remind me what this is all about; Go over my relapse prevention plan; Go to the Drop-In Centre for a talk with the counsellor there._

Figure 9.5. A relapse prevention plan identifies a series of lapses that constitute high-risk situations for that offender, who will then develop a plan designed to avoid these lapses and to cope effectively with them in the event that they occur.

the first step in the offense chain that was outlined, in part, earlier. The final elements of the relapse-prevention plan should delineate what group members can do to cope with deviant fantasies. We remind them of the procedures they used in the earlier "deviant fantasy" component. They are told that occasional deviant thoughts are almost certain to occur after they leave formal treatment, but they are not to take these as signs of failure. They must view them in the context of their history since entering treatment. If, for example, prior to treatment they were having deviant fantasies several times each day, then a single deviant thought some weeks after treatment should be viewed as an indication of very positive changes. However, it should also provide the opportunity for determining the factors that led to deviant thinking so that these can be identified and avoided in the future. In fact, we advise patients that their list of risk factors should be under consistent revision as they encounter previously unanticipated problems.

Implementation and Follow-up. Once group members have designed a relapse-prevention plan, they must then begin to implement it. Thus, the specific strategies identified by the client must now be enacted. For example, if a client identified adult education courses as part of his relapse-prevention plan, he would be required to seek out course schedules and register accordingly. This allows for an assessment of the client's willingness to do more than just talk about what he needs to do. Furthermore, it permits adjustments in the relapse-prevention effort as the practical limitations of implementing the plan become evident.

It is important for those involved in the supervision of a sex offender to be familiar with his relapse-prevention plan. This provides the supervisor with more resources than might otherwise be available and allows for a more coordinated and extended level of supervision. Most of the incarcerated clients will be released under parole or probation conditions that require supervision, and most of the supervising officers have some training in relapse-prevention concepts and procedures. For those offenders who are being treated in the community, we require each group member to identify at least one community-support person who will come to the clinic for training. This person must be in regular contact with the client, and he or she must believe the client to be guilty of the offense(s) for which he was convicted. They are briefed on the offender's offense history (to ensure they have been completely informed) and his relapse-prevention plan. Both general and specific warning signs are discussed both in regard to behaviors the client might exhibit if his risk level is increasing, and (where relevant) behaviors that a child might exhibit if they are being sexually abused by the offender. For his part, the client is encouraged to speak to his designated support person(s) in the event that he experiences problems. The support people themselves are asked to raise issues of concern with the client. Furthermore, they sign an agreement whereby they will call us if their concern becomes considerable or if they are unable to resolve issues with the offender. We warn the group members that it may well be that their initial reaction upon learning that a support person has called us will be to become angry and feel betrayed. We counsel them against this, reminding them that they have agreed and encouraged this person to do so, and to remember that their support person is acting in the offender's own best interest when they do call.

In addition to their parole/probation supervisor and community-support person, we require that offenders share their relapse-prevention plans with any other therapists with whom they may become involved, but only if such treatment concerns their offending behavior. For most of the men released from prison, the parole board will require continued treatment in an approved community program. In those cases, the treatment providers are directly sent the offender's relapse-prevention plans by the institutional program. We also, however, encourage the offenders themselves to disclose to these therapists their offense chain, their warning signs, and their relapse-prevention plan. We believe that this encourages the client to take responsibility for his future. After their first three or four meetings, we arrange for the supervising agent to complete a follow-up record on which they rate the offender's understanding of his relapse-prevention plan and their impression of how well he is implementing it. This procedure is repeated at various intervals determined by the offender's progress. These sheets also inquire about the presence of a number of general risk factors. We find that probation and parole officers are an excellent resource in this regard, because they obtain a considerable amount of information from a number of sources.

We endeavor to follow up our clients on a 3-month, 6-month, and subsequently on a yearly basis. At these times, we request an update from the supervisors on the follow-up sheets. These reports are usually supplemented by frequent telephone contacts. During the follow-up period, this communication is essential, because the therapist is unlikely to remain fully informed of the day-to-day activities of each group member.

If they remain committed to their relapse-prevention plans and if therapists and the others in their supervision networks remain informed and coordinated, these offenders will be maximally prepared to reduce their probability of reoffending.

TREATMENT EFFECTIVENESS

We have already noted the value of some of the components of our program in producing the expected changes. Now we will briefly address the overall effectiveness of treatment. There are various indices that might be used to assess efficacy, but the most pertinent are those that attest to reductions in recidivism. In Canada, the Royal Canadian Mounted Police maintain computer records of every person who has ever been charged or convicted of any criminal offense. We have access to these records and count as a failure every discharged patient who has been charged, whether or not a conviction was secured. We are also fortunate to have, at least for our community program, access to the unofficial records on accusations held by the police and the local child-protection agencies.

In the evaluation of our community clinic program (Marshall & Barbaree, 1988), we found reductions in recidivism rates for the treated clients that were significantly lower than those for matched groups of untreated offenders. Table 9.1 shows the recidivism rates for our outpatient community clinic and our early program in Kingston Penitentiary. The untreated offenders are subdivided into volunteers (i.e., those who admitted their offenses but were unable to enter our program, usually because they lived too far away) and intractable deniers (for the deniers, we were only able to obtain data on the nonfamilial child molesters).

As can be seen, each treated subtype had fewer failures than did its corresponding untreated volunteer or denier group. Table 9.1 also indicates the recidivism rates for two groups of exhibitionists (one untreated and one treated group). Again, it is apparent that the treated group was less likely to reoffend. Similarly, an evaluation of an early version of our prison-based program revealed benefits for treatment (Davidson, 1984). More recently we (Marshall & Fernandez, in press) have reported tentative data on our Tier 2 program for which we found one failure out of 87 released offenders, although to date the follow-up period is rather short (slightly more than one year).

Table 9.1. Treatment Outcome

	Recidivism Rates		
	Untreated	Treated	Deniers
Kingston Community Clinic			
Nonfamilial child molesters[a]			
(a) female victims	43 (18)[d]	18 (8)	49 (22)
(b) male victims	43 (19)	13 (5)	51 (24)
Incest (father/daughter)[a]	22 (7)	8 (3)	—
Exhibitionists[b]	57 (24)	24 (12)	—
Kingston Penitentiary			
(Mixed group of rapists and nonfamilial child molesters[c])	35[e]	11	—

[a]Data derived from Marshall and Barbaree (1988).
[b]Data derived from Marshall, Eccles, and Barbaree (1991).
[c]Data derived from Davidson (1984).
[d]Figures are derived from unofficial information with parenthetic figures derived from official police records.
[e]Official data only.

We (Marshall, Jones, Ward, Johnston, & Barbaree, 1991b) have also reviewed the more general outcome literature on similar cognitive–behavioral programs for sex offenders and were satisfied that the evidence was, at the very least, encouraging. Furthermore, we concluded that integrating relapse prevention into the earlier cognitive–behavioral approaches added to their effectiveness (Marshall, Hudson, & Ward, 1992). Subsequent challenges (Quinsey, Harris, Rice, & Lalumiere, 1993; Rice, Harris, & Quinsey, in press) to these conclusions were countered (Marshall, 1993a; Marshall & Pithers, in press), and we believe there is every reason to remain optimistic about the effectiveness of these comprehensive cognitive–behavioral programs. However, we do not seem to be quite so effective with rapists as we are with child molesters, and we (Marshall, 1993b) have suggested ways in which we might improve programs for these problematic offenders.

REFERENCES

Bandura, A. (1973). *Aggression: A social learning analysis.* Englewood Cliffs, NJ: Prentice-Hall.
Bandura, A., Underwood, B., & Fromson, M.E. (1975). Disinhibition of aggression through diffusion of responsibility and dehumanization of victims. *Journal of Research in Personality, 9,* 253–269.
Barbaree, H.E. (1990). Stimulus control of sexual arousal: Its role in sexual assault. In W.L. Marshall, D.R. Laws, & H.E. Barbaree (Eds.), *Handbook of sexual assault: Issues, theories, and treatment of the offender* (pp. 115–142). New York: Plenum Press.
Barbaree, H.E. (1991). Denial and minimization among sex offenders: Assessment and treatment outcome. *Forum on Corrections Research, 3,* 30–33.
Barbaree, H.E., & Marshall, W.W. (1989). Erectile responses amongst heterosexual child molesters, father–daughter incest offenders and matched nonoffenders: Five distinct age preference profiles. *Canadian Journal of Behavioral Science, 21,* 70–82.
Barbaree, H.E., & Marshall, W.L. (1991). The role of male sexual arousal in rape: Six models. *Journal of Consulting and Clinical Psychology, 59,* 621–630.
Barbaree, H.E., & Marshall, W. L. (1993). *An analysis of erectile response profile in rapists.* Unpublished manuscript, Queens University, Kingston, Ontario, Canada.
Barbaree, H.E., Marshall, W.L., & Hudson, S. M. (Eds.). (1993). *The juvenile sex offender.* New York: Guilford Press.

Blader, J.C., & Marshall, W.L. (1989). Is assessment of sexual arousal in rapists worthwhile? A critique of current methods and the development of a response compatibility approach. *Clinical Psychology Review, 9,* 569–587.

Bradford, J.M.W., & Pawlak, A. (1993). Double-blind placebo crossover study of cyproterone acetate in the treatment of sexual deviation—Phase 1. *Archives of Sexual Behavior.*

Davidson, P. (1984, March). *Outcome data for a penitentiary-based treatment program for sex offenders.* Paper presented at the Conference on the Assessment and Treatment of the Sex Offender, Kingston, Ontario.

Eccles, A., Marshall, W.L., & Barbaree, H.E. (1994). Differentiating rapists and nonoffenders using the Rape Index. *Behaviour Research and Therapy.*

Epstein, S., & O'Brien, E. J. (1985). The person–situational debate in historical and current perspective. *Psychological Bulletin, 98,* 513–517.

Guberman, C., & Wolf, M. (Eds.). (1985). *No safe place: Violence against women and children.* Toronto, Canada: Women's Press.

Hudson, S.M., Marshall, W.L., Wales, D., McDonald, E., Bakker, L.W., & McLean, A. (1993). Emotional recognition skills of sex offenders. *Annals of Sex Research, 6,* 199–211.

Johnston, P., Hudson, S.M., & Marshall, W.L. (1992). The effects of masturbatory reconditioning with nonfamilial child molesters. *Behaviour Research and Therapy, 30,* 559–561.

Knopp, F.H., Freeman-Longo, R.E., & Stevenson, W. (1992). *Nationwide survey of juvenile and adult sex-offender treatment programs.* Orwell, VT: Safer Society Press.

Laws, D.R. (1989). *Relapse prevention with sex offenders.* New York: Guilford Press.

Laws, D.R., & Marshall, W.L. (1991). Masturbatory reconditioning: An evaluative review. *Advances in Behaviour Research and Therapy, 13,* 13–25.

Marlatt, G.A. (1982). Relapse prevention: A self-control program for the treatment of addictive behaviors. In R.B. Stuart (Ed.), *Adherence, compliance and generalization in behavioral medicine* (pp. 329–378). New York: Brunner/Mazel.

Marques, J.K., Nelson, C., West, M.A., & Day, D.M. (1994). The relationship between treatment goals and recidivism among child molesters. *Behaviour Research and Therapy.*

Marquis, J.N. (1970). Orgasmic reconditioning: Changing sexual object choice through controlling masturbation fantasies. *Journal of Behavior Therapy and Experimental Psychiatry, 1,* 263–271.

Marshall, W.L. (1979). Satiation therapy: A procedure for reducing deviant sexual arousal. *Journal of Applied Behavior Analysis, 12,* 10–22.

Marshall, W.L. (November, 1993a). *Proper uses of phallometric assessment and aversive counterconditioning in treatment.* Paper presented at the 12th Annual Research and Treatment Conference of the Association for the Treatment of Sexual Abusers, Boston, MA.

Marshall, W.L. (1993b). The treatment of sex offenders: What does the outcome data tell us? A reply to Quinsey et al. *Journal of Interpersonal Violence, 8,* 524–530.

Marshall, W.L. (1993c). A revised approach to the treatment of men who sexually assault adult females. In G.C. Nagayama Hall, R. Hirschman, J.R. Graham, & M.S. Zaragoza (Eds.), *Sexual aggression: Issues in etiology, assessment and treatment* (pp. 143–165). Bristol, PA.

Marshall, W.L. (1994). Treatment effects on denial and minimization in incarcerated sex offenders. *Behaviour Research and Therapy.*

Marshall, W.L., & Barbaree, H.E. (1988). The long-term evaluation of a behavioral program for child molesters. *Behaviour Research and Therapy, 26,* 499–511.

Marshall, W.L., & Barbaree, H.E. (1990). Outcome of comprehensive cognitive–behavioral treatment programs. In W.L. Marshall, D.R. Laws, & H.E. Barbaree (Eds.), *Handbook of sexual assault: Issues, theories, and treatment of the offender* (pp. 363–385). New York: Plenum.

Marshall, W.L., & Eccles, A. (1991). Issues in clinical practice with sex offenders. *Journal of Interpersonal Violence, 6,* 68–93.

Marshall, W.L., & Eccles, A. (1993). Pavlovian conditioning processes in adolescent sex offenders. In H.E. Barbaree, W.L. Marshall, & S. M. Hudson (Eds.), *The juvenile sex offender* (pp. 118–142). New York: Guilford.

Marshall, W.L., Eccles, A., & Barbaree, H.E. (1991a). Treatment of exhibitionists: A focus on sexual deviance versus cognitive and relationship features. *Behaviour Research and Therapy, 29,* 129–135.

Marshall, W.L., Eccles, A., & Barbaree, H.E. (1993a). A three-tiered approach to the rehabilitation of incarcerated sex offenders. *Behavioral Sciences and the Law, 11,* 441–445.

Marshall, W.L., & Fernandez, Y.M. (in press). Cognitive–behavioral treatment of the paraphilias. In V.E. Cabello

& R.M. Turner (Eds.), *International handbook of cognitive/behavioral treatment of psychiatric disorders.* Madrid: Siglo XXI Press.

Marshall, W.L., Fernandez, Y.M., Lightbody, S., & O'Sullivan, C. (1994a). *The assessment of victim specific empathy in child molesters.* Submitted for publication.

Marshall, W.L., Hudson, S.M., & Jones, R. (1994b). Sexual deviance. In P. H. Wilson (Ed.), *Principles and practice of relapse prevention* (pp. 235–254). New York: Guilford Press.

Marshall, W.L., Hudson, S.M., & Ward, T. (1992). Sexual deviance. In P. H. Wilson (Ed.), *Principles and practice of relapse prevention* (pp. 235–254). New York: Guilford Press.

Marshall, W.L., Jones, R., Hudson, S.M., & McDonald, E. (1993b). Generalized empathy in child molesters. *Journal of Child Sexual Abuse, 2,* 61–68.

Marshall, W.L., Jones, R., Ward, T., Johnston, P., & Barbaree, H.E. (1991b). Treatment outcome with sex offenders. *Clinical Psychology Review, 11,* 465–485.

Marshall, W.L., & Lippens, K. (1977). The clinical value of boredom: A procedure for reducing inappropriate sexual interests. *Journal of Nervous and Mental Diseases, 165,* 283–287.

Marshall, W.L., O'Sullivan, C., & Fernandez, Y.M. (in press). The enhancement of victim empathy among incarcerated child molesters. *Legal and Criminological Psychology.*

Marshall, W.L., & Pithers, W.D. (1994). A reconsideration of treatment outcome with sex offenders. *Criminal Justice and Behavior, 21,* 10–27.

Masters, W.H., & Johnson, V.E. (1966). *Human sexual response.* Boston: Little, Brown.

Mischel, W. (1984). Convergences and challenges in the search for consistency. *American Psychologist, 39,* 351–364.

Pearson, H.J. (1990). Paraphilias, impulsive control and serotonin. *Journal of Clinical Psychopharmacology, 10,* 133–134.

Pearson, H.J., Marshall, W.L., Barbaree, H.E., & Southmayd, S. (1992). Treatment of a compulsive paraphiliac with Buspirone. *Annals of Sex Research, 5,* 239–246.

Pithers, W.D. (1994). Process evaluation of a group therapy component designed to enhance sex offenders' empathy for sexual abuse survivors. *Behaviour Research and Therapy, 32,* 565–570.

Pithers, W.D., Kashima, K., Cumming, G.F., Beal, L.S., & Buell, M. (1988). Relapse prevention of sexual aggression. In R. Prentky & V. Quinsey (Eds.), *Human sexual aggression: Current perspectives* (pp. 244–260). New York: New York Academy of Sciences.

Pithers, W.D., Marques, J.K., Gibat, C.C., & Marlatt, G.A. (1983). Relapse prevention with sexual aggressives. In J.G. Greer & I.R. Stuart (Eds.), *The sexual aggressor* (pp. 214–239). New York: Van Nostrand Reinhold.

Quinsey, V.L., Harris, G.T., Rice, M.E., & Laumière, M.L. (1993). Assessing treatment efficacy in outcome studies of sex offenders. *Journal of Interpersonal Violence, 8,* 512–523.

Quinsey, V.L., & Marshall, W.L. (1983). Procedures for reducing inappropriate sexual arousal: An evaluation review. In J.G. Greer & I.R. Stuart (Eds.), *The sexual aggressor: Current perspectives on treatment* (pp. 267–289). New York: Van Nostrand Reinhold.

Rice, M.E., Harris, G.T., & Quinsey, V.L. (1993). Evaluating treatment programs for child molesters. In J. Hudson & I.V. Roberts (Eds.), *Evaluating justice: Canadian policies and programs* (pp. 189–203). Toronto: Thompson.

Rice, M.E., Quinsey, V.L., & Harris, G.T. (1991). Sexual recidivism among child molesters released from a maximum security psychiatric institution. *Journal of Consulting and Clinical Psychology, 59,* 381–386.

Sandberg, G.G., & Marlatt, G.A. (1989). Relapse fantasies. In D.R. Laws (Ed.), *Relapse prevention with sex offenders* (pp. 147–151). New York: Guilford Press.

Segal, Z.V., & Stermac, L.E. (1990). The role of cognition in sexual assault. In W.L. Marshall, D.R. Laws, & H.E. Barbaree (Eds.), *Handbook of sexual assault: Issues, theories, and treatment of the offender* (pp. 161–174). New York: Plenum Press.

Symons, D. (1979). *The evolution of human sexuality.* New York: Oxford University Press.

Woods, G. (Ed.). (1992). *Voices: A collection of writings by survivors of sexual abuse.* Ontario, Canada: Community Mental Health Program of Hastings and Prince Edward Counties.

10

Treatment of Sexual Dysfunctions

Nathaniel McConaghy

DESCRIPTION OF THE DISORDERS

Impairments of sexual functioning, the dysfunctions, are classified in the fourth edition of the *Diagnostic and Statistical Manual of Mental Disorders* (DSM-IV; American Psychiatric Association, 1994) in seven categories. Sexual Desire Disorders include Hypoactive Sexual Desire involving deficient (or absent) sexual fantasies and desire for sexual activity, and Sexual Aversion, involving extreme aversion to and avoidance of all or almost all genital sexual contact with a partner. Sexual Arousal Disorders include Female Sexual Arousal Disorder, an inability to attain or maintain an adequate genital lubrication–swelling response of sexual excitement until completion of the sexual activity, and Male Erectile Disorder, an inability to attain or maintain an adequate erection until completion of the sexual activity. Orgasm Disorders include Female and Male Orgasmic Disorders and Premature Ejaculation. Female Orgasmic Disorder is delay or absence of orgasm following a normal sexual-excitement phase. It is pointed out that women vary widely in the type or intensity of stimulation that triggers orgasm and that the diagnosis should be based on the clinician's judgment that the woman's orgasmic capacity is less than would be reasonable for her age, sexual experience, and the adequacy of sexual stimulation she receives. Presumably, such absence of orgasmic capacity would not be accepted as a disorder in such women as those who reported in many surveys that they enjoyed intercourse very much, although they did not reach orgasm (McConaghy, 1993), provided it did not cause marked distress or interpersonal difficulty (Criterion B).

In a 60% representative sample of British men and women aged 16 to 59, 50% of women disagreed with the statement that sex without orgasm or climax cannot be really satisfying for a woman; less expectedly, 35% of men disagreed with the same statement with regard to orgasm in men (Johnson, Wadsworth, Wellings, Field, & Bradshaw, 1994).

Nathaniel McConaghy • School of Psychiatry, Psychiatric Unit, The Prince of Wales Hospital, Randwick, New South Wales, Australia 2031.

Sourcebook of Psychological Treatment Manuals for Adult Disorders, edited by Vincent B. Van Hasselt and Michel Hersen. Plenum Press, New York, 1996.

Male orgasmic disorder is delay or absence of orgasm following a normal sexual-excitement phase during sexual activity that the clinician, taking into account the person's age, judges to be adequate in focus, intensity, and duration. It is commonly an inability to reach orgasm by ejaculation in the vagina, orgasm being possible with other types of stimulation. Premature ejaculation is ejaculation with minimal sexual stimulation before, upon, or shortly after penetration and before the person wishes it. The clinician must take into account factors that affect duration of the excitement phase, such as age, novelty of the sexual partner or situation, and frequency of sexual activity. The fourth category of dysfunctions, Sexual Pain Disorders, includes Dyspareunia, genital pain in either males or females before, during, or after sexual intercourse; and Vaginismus, involuntary spasm of the musculature of the outer third of the vagina that interferes with sexual intercourse. Vaginismus usually prevents penetration of any object above a certain size into the vagina, including the subject's finger or a tampon. If intercourse is attempted, vaginismus is commonly accompanied by spasm of the adductor muscles of the thighs preventing their separation. Vaginismus does not prevent women from experiencing sexual arousal and orgasm from activities other than coitus. To receive the diagnosis of sexual disorder in the aforementioned four categories, the DSM-IV (APA, 1994) requires that the condition is persistent or recurrent, causes marked distress or interpersonal difficulty, and does not occur exclusively during, or is not better accounted for by another Axis I disorder (such as Major Depressive or Somatization Disorder).

Apart from leaving so many issues to the judgment of the individual clinician, DSM-IV criteria for male erectile disorder may not adequately deal with diagnostic problems evident in the research literature, where the condition is commonly referred to as *impotence*, particularly by urologists. The criteria used for its diagnosis have frequently not been specified in this literature. It is possible that, in some studies, all men who complained of reduced sexual interest and activity and absence of spontaneous erections were diagnosed as impotent; whereas, in other studies, when it was established that some of these men could obtain erections with manual stimulation, they were diagnosed as showing reduced sexual desire rather than an erectile problem. This could account for the inconsistency in research findings in which some studies reported the presence and others the absence of impotence in men with low levels of testosterone. Schiavi, Fisher, White, Beers, and Szechter (1984) diagnosed men who had never been able to achieve intercourse, although they obtained full erections with masturbation and had adequate sexual desire as suffering from primary impotence. It is possible that some clinicians would interpret their condition as not meeting the DSM-IV criteria for Male Erectile Disorder, as these do not state the nature of the sexual activity for which erection is required to be maintained.

Clinicians' judgment concerning the degree of deficiency or absence of sexual fantasies and desire for sexual activity necessary to make the diagnosis of hypoactive or inhibited sexual desire have appeared arbitrary. In one study, women were so diagnosed, although they had engaged in premarital intercourse significantly more often and showed no difference in frequency or duration of intercourse or duration of foreplay compared to those not so diagnosed (Stuart, Hammond, & Pett, 1987). In another investigation, men who received the diagnosis reported a frequency of masturbation 20% higher than that of men reporting a healthy sex life (Nutter & Condron, 1985). In making the diagnosis, it should be established that subjects who report acceptable frequencies of sexual activity are having intercourse out of obligation to their partner rather than out of sexual desire (Wincze & Carey, 1991), and those who report low frequency are not avoiding sexual activity due to dissatisfaction with their sexual relationship rather than reduced desire (Nutter & Condron, 1985).

DSM-IV criteria specify that the four categories of dysfunctions discussed earlier are not due to the direct effect of a substance (e.g., drugs of abuse, or medication) or a general medical condition. When they are, they are classified as Substance-Induced Sexual Dysfunction or Sexual Dysfunction Due to a General Medical Condition. A wide range of medications and drugs of abuse impair sexual desire, arousal, and orgasm. These include antihypertensive agents, diuretics, vasodilators, and psychiatric and anticonvulsant drugs (Segraves & Segraves, 1992). The final category of Sexual Dysfunction Not Otherwise Specified consists of substantially diminished or no subjective erotic feelings despite otherwise normal arousal and orgasm, and sexual dysfunctions that the clinician cannot determine are primary or due to a general medical condition, or substance-induced.

Frank, Anderson, and Rubinstein (1978) investigated the presence in white, well-educated, happily married American couples of what they termed sexual difficulties. These were problems related to the emotional tone of sexual relations, such as the partner choosing an inconvenient time or not using appropriate foreplay. These difficulties, which would appear to reflect the couples' failure to communicate their sexual feelings and needs to each other, correlated more highly with their lack of sexual satisfaction than did the presence of sexual dysfunctions. In the case of the men, the correlations between presence of dysfunctions and lack of sexual satisfaction were not statistically significant. In reporting a similar finding in older men Schiavi, Schreiner-Engel, Mandeli, Schanzer, and Cohen (1990) considered that as older healthy couples continued to engage in satisfying sexual intercourse in the face of significant decrements in erectile function, it may be as important to focus attention on attitudinal factors and coping strategies as on the mechanisms involved in erectile capacity.

In Swedish and British studies (Nettelbladt & Uddenberg, 1979; Reading & Wiest, 1984), again, no association was found between the presence of the dysfunctions of premature ejaculation or erectile difficulties and men's sexual satisfaction. In the Swedish study, the presence of these dysfunctions in the men were also not correlated with the sexual satisfaction of their female partners. Like Schaivi et al. (1990), Nettelbladt & Uddenberg pointed out that the couples' sexual satisfaction was related to their emotional relationship rather than their sexual function. Snyder and Berg (1983) reached the same conclusion from findings in a clinical population: couples presenting with lack of sexual satisfaction to a sexual-dysfunctions clinic. Dysfunctions were common complaints of both the men and women. However, none reported by the women correlated with their sexual dissatisfaction, and only failure to ejaculate during intercourse correlated with that of men. Dissatisfaction correlated strongly in both sexes with the partner's lack of response to sexual requests and the frequency of intercourse being too low.

The importance of relationship factors, rather than sexual dysfunctions in the sexual satisfaction of subjects who seek treatment for dysfunctions, could account for the common finding of outcome studies that despite minimal improvement of the specific dysfunction with which they presented, many subjects reported increased sexual interest and enjoyment following psychological treatment (Adkins & Jehu, 1985; De Amicis, Goldberg, LoPiccolo, Friedman, & Davies, 1985; Hawton, Catalan, Martin, & Fagg, 1986). Hawton et al. pointed out that improvement in couples' general relationship was a frequently reported outcome of therapy for sexual problems and could result from the equally frequently reported improvement in their communication.

Despite the evidence of the importance of sexual difficulties rather than dysfunctions in couples' sexual satisfaction, most subjects seeking treatment for sexual problems tend to report dysfunctions, accounting for the focus on these conditions in the treatment literature.

ASSESSMENT METHODS

The Diagnostic Interview

The major method of data collection for assessment of sexual dysfunctions would appear to remain the unstructured interview. It allows the clinician to frame questions so that they are comprehensible and acceptable to patients, taking into account their education, value system, and personality. If the clinician detects signs of guilt, embarrassment, or reluctance to talk on the part of patients when particular topics are introduced, he or she can respond with encouragement and support and thus elicit crucial information that may not be obtained if adherence to the rigid format of a structured interview or questionnaire is maintained. This flexibility in interviewing is commonly required with patients who are illiterate, schizophrenic, depressed, or brain-damaged. Also, these patients are rarely motivated or able to complete self-rating scales or questionnaires.

Clinicians usually initiate the interview by asking patients why they have sought help and then adopt a nondirective listening approach, asking a minimum of questions, so as to give patients the opportunity to take charge. This allows the assessment of such aspects of patients' personalities as their confidence, verbal ability, assertiveness, and dominance. At the same time, much of the information necessary to establish the nature of their presenting complaints is obtained. The additional necessary information is gathered subsequently when the clinician becomes more directive in questioning. This information usually includes: any past history of similar problems; other illnesses; previous treatment; childhood and adolescent relationships with parents and siblings; social and sexual relationships and practices, including unwanted sexual experiences and history of contraceptive use where appropriate, educational and work history, and current domestic, social, sexual, and occupational situations, including the nature and extent of recreational interests and activities. Use of recreational drugs, (including alcohol and tobacco) as well as any medications needs to be determined.

Investigation of certain sexual experiences appears to pose special problems. Wyatt and Peters (1986) considered that multiple probing questions needed to be asked about specific types of abusive sexual behaviors by interviewers given special training in ideologically correct attitudes in order to identify women who had been sexually abused in childhood. Studies using this methodology found much higher prevalence rates than did investigations not using them. At the same time, it is necessary to avoid possibly influencing the patient by suggestion to develop false memories of coercion. Damages have been awarded against therapists on the basis that they implanted false memories of child sexual abuse in patients (Arndt, 1994).

Identification of the presence of significant personality disorders or relationship problems in patients seeking treatment for sexual dysfunctions is of major importance clinically. These factors markedly influence patients' ability to provide accurate information, their motivation to change their behaviors, and/or the nature of the relationship they attempt to establish with the clinician. If this relationship is handled inappropriately, lack of compliance with, or major disruption of, the treatment plan can result. Consequently, the patient is not helped or indeed may be harmed, and the clinician may also suffer considerable distress. Personality features most important to detect are those indicative of psychopathy, borderline personality, and dependency.

Psychopathy, more prevalent in male than female patients, is suggested by the patient's confidence, lack of ethical concern or empathy for possible negative effects of his behavior on others, history of adolescent truancy, abuse of drugs, other delinquent behaviors, and subsequent record of occupational and relationship instability. Patients with psychopathic traits are likely to favorably distort their accounts of their behavior and to comply poorly with treatment, frequently missing appointments.

Borderline personality disorder, more likely to be shown by women, may also be associated with a history of adolescent drug abuse. Subjects with the disorder commonly were involved in abusive sexual relationships in childhood and adolescence that may have resulted in pregnancy. Suicide attempts or self-mutilations are frequently repeated, consistent with these subjects' low self-esteem. Their initial presentation may induce the inexperienced therapist to become overinvolved and lose objectivity in response to their account of overwhelmingly tragic life events, accompanied by intense gratitude, possibly tinged with sexual seductiveness at the therapist's concern.

Dependent personality disorder results in failure to cope with inevitable life stresses, either due to the subjects being unable to tolerate the normal levels of anxiety and depression the stresses produce, or by their responding with above-average levels of these emotions. The diagnosis will be indicated in the interview by the subjects' lack of confidence and evident anxiety or depression, and supported by their history of poor school performance, occupational instability, and limitation of social relations to the few people on whom they are dependent.

When it is suspected that patients have a significant personality disorder, it is imperative that attempts be made to corroborate their history by interviewing relatives and contacts. Psychopathic and borderline patients may try to prevent this, saying, for example, that they dislike their relatives too much to allow any contact. If it is considered sufficiently important, it may be necessary to make treatment conditional on their granting permission for such interviews.

Assessment of the presenting patient and partner's relationship appears to be commonly made intuitively from observation of the couple's interaction in the interview, interpreted in the light of both partners' account of their present and previous relationships. In addition to verbal expressions indicative of affection or hostility, or indeed both, the couple's body language, including supportive touching, usually gives the interviewer insight into the nature of the their relationship. Hence, even if the presenting person states that he or she and not the partner has the sexual problem, it is important to emphasize that it is of great value to interview the partner, initially alone and then with the patient.

The accuracy of the information obtained in an unstructured clinical interview depends on the ability of the clinician to correctly assess to what extent the patient's self-report can be accepted without modification, and to what extent it should be regarded as distorted and in need of further confirmation. The assessment of the patient's personality is of value in this regard. The attention-seeking are likely to exaggerate and the psychopathic to lie concerning their symptoms; the depressed or those with high ethical standards commonly associated with obsessional features, may present themselves in a somewhat negative light.

In response to the evidence of low levels of reliability (49% to 63%) for specific psychiatric diagnoses reached by different clinicians using unstructured interviews (Matarazzo, 1983), researchers have developed operational diagnostic criteria aimed at defining every operation or decision that is made to reach the diagnosis. To accomplish this aim, these criteria ideally need to be applied to information standardized by being elicited from the patient via structured interview. And it is now common practice that psychiatric research publications report that the diagnoses of patients with schizophrenia or affective psychoses were made using both standardized diagnostic criteria and interviews. This does not appear to be the case in sexuality research. In none of the studies published from 1989 to 1993 in the *Archives of Sexual Behavior*, a major academic, sexuality-research journal, were structured interviews used to reach diagnoses, and only a minority of those reporting sexual dysfunctions made reference to the use of the definitions that aimed at being operational, provided by the *Diagnostic and Statistical Manual of Mental Disorders*, Third Edition (DSM-III; APA, 1980) or Third Edition, Revised (DSM-III-R; APA, 1987), the precursors of the DSM-IV. Walling, Andersen, and Johnson (1990), in a review of studies of hormonal replacement therapy, pointed out that although the most common sexual dysfunction noted was dyspareunia, a DSM-III-R definition was never cited.

Although the reliability of diagnoses reached by different clinicians using the same structured interview is high, that obtained when they use different structured interviews appears of the same order as the reliability of the unstructured interviews criticized by researchers (McConaghy, 1993). The superior reliability obtained by different clinicians using the same structured interview is of no immediate value to the individual clinician in the diagnosis or treatment of patients. This could explain why sex therapists have so far not been prepared to abandon the advantages of the unstructured interview, which makes it a more cost-effective procedure than the structured interview, as it provides more relevant information in less time, being tailored to most appropriately assess the individual patient.

However, the superior reliability of operational diagnosis has the long-term advantage to the clinician of establishing that the information provided by research studies concerning patients given a particular diagnosis is relevant to the patients that he or she diagnoses as having that condition. The difficulty in this respect of interpreting the literature concerning patients diagnosed as having erectile or sexual desire disorder has been pointed out. Unlike the utilization of structured interviews, use of accepted diagnostic criteria for sexual dysfunctions and difficulties would not seem to entail loss of efficiency on the part of the clinician. Therefore, it is unfortunate that no attempts are being made to develop sufficiently rigorous criteria, and, in particular, that DSM-IV definitions of the sexual dysfunctions have left so many issues to the clinician's judgment, inevitably ensuring this will differ between clinicians. Until such criteria are developed, it would seem advisable that research follow the practice adopted in some studies in the issues of the *Archives of Sexual Behavior* examined, of supplying the diagnostic criteria employed. Kelly, Strassberg, and Kircher (1990) stated that anorgasmia was diagnosed as present in women if they reported that orgasm resulted from 5% or less of all sexual activities with their partners and absent if it resulted from 70% or more of such activities. Strassberg, Mahoney, Schaugaard, and Hale (1990) diagnosed subjects as having premature ejaculation who estimated ejaculation latencies of 2 minutes or less on at least 50% of intercourse occasions and, in addition, perceived lack of control over the onset of orgasm.

Termination of the diagnostic interview requires careful planning and adequate time must be allowed for this. Patients should not leave feeling they have been asked a lot of questions or been allowed to talk freely but have been given no answers. It is my practice at this stage to present the patient with either a treatment plan or an explanation as to why further information or laboratory investigations are required before this can be done. Wincze and Carey (1991) recommend three interviews and use of structured assessments before a decision about treatment is made. When a treatment plan is proposed, the clinician should ensure that patients are fully aware of what it entails, including its likely cost, and why it, rather than alternatives, has been selected. Any reservations patients have concerning the plan should be dealt with fully, so that following its discussion they commit themselves either to accepting the plan, or to making a decision concerning this within the next week, possibly in consultation with the person who referred them.

Rating Scale and Questionnaire Investigations

Wincze and Carey (1991) pointed out that although patient-completed questionnaires provided extensive information at little cost, they have not been widely used. They attributed this to the possibility that their employment appeared time-consuming and inconvenient in a busy practice. Furthermore, they may have limited clinical utility due to many questionnaires having been developed for specific purposes in research studies. Conte (1983), in his review of self-report scales for rating sexual function, found that most provide no measures of important aspects of sexual function, such as the frequency of sexual behaviors or subjects' satisfaction with their current sexual functioning. Wincze and Carey (1991) recommended some scales that they apparently use regularly, but emphasized that they should never be used blindly or without a careful interview.

Just as researchers appear to have shown somewhat greater tolerance with regard to the level of reliability and lack of evidence of validity of structured clinical and behavioral assessments compared to unstructured interview assessments (McConaghy, 1993, 1994), they have displayed similar tolerance of rating scales. Conte (1983) found many of these rating sexual function had test–retest reliabilities in the range of $r = 0.5$. Apart from this evidence of reliability in the range of that of different clinicians' unstructured diagnoses, he underscored the need for studies to establish their validity. Little evidence of validity was also provided in a review of 51 objectively scored, mainly self-rated assessments of sexual function and marital interactions (Schiavi, Derogatis, Kuriansky, O'Connor, & Sharpe, 1979). When referred to, it was usually described as adequate or, as demonstrated by the test's ability to discriminate two groups of subjects, a criterion that can be achieved by tests that misclassify a number of individuals in the groups. Studies identifying lack of validity due to the use of rating scales have been reported in more detail elsewhere (McConaghy, 1993, 1994).

Clearly, in investigations of particular sexual behaviors, the use of questionnaires completed by the patient or the interviewer is of value in ensuring that relevant information is obtained from all subjects. However, when the emphasis is on patient treatment, it is necessary to be aware that the use of structured procedures beyond the diagnostic interview can reduce patient compliance with treatment. Reading (1983) randomly allocated paid male volunteers to report details of their sexual behavior either by interview after 1 and 3 months; by interview after 1, 2, and 3 months; or by the latter procedure plus diary cards completed daily and returned every 3 days. Thirty-four percent allocated to the last form of assessment discontinued it, as compared to 14% with the first, and 16% with the second. Another three subjects dropped out from the diary card assessment prior to first month, believing it was causing them difficulty maintaining their sexual potency.

Observational Assessment

As discussed earlier, observation of patients' and partners' nonverbal behaviors is of major importance in interview assessment. Observations of sexual behaviors are currently rarely reported, although their use either directly or by videotape was briefly popular in the more explorative climate of the 1970s (LoPiccolo, 1990). LoPiccolo argued against their employment on the basis that observed behaviors of patients with sexual dysfunctions would not be similar to their private behaviors, that they would be unacceptable to the majority of couples, and that they allowed the exploitation of patients by the therapist. These issues were certainly relevant to the "sexological exam" described by LoPiccolo, in which sex therapists stimulated the breasts and genitals of the opposite sex partner to assess and demonstrate physiological responsiveness. Nevertheless, with appropriate ethical safeguards, videotaped observational assessment of couples' sexual interactions would seem likely to provide information of value in couples who have difficulty in providing this information accurately. Following preliminary sessions to allow them to adjust to the procedure, their observed behavior should be sufficiently related to their private behavior, as is the case with observed nonsexual behaviors (e.g., phobias) and with the laboratory assessment of physiological evidence of sexual arousal, both of which remain widely used. It is likely that taboos concerning sexuality remain the major obstacle to observational assessment. This assessment, of course, plays a major role in surrogate sex therapy. Observation of erections occurring during sleep or produced by masturbation remains recommended (Karacan, 1978; Wasserman, Pollak, Spielman, & Weitzman, 1980). Davidson, Kwan, and Greenleaf (1982) doubted that the erections of hypogonadal men could lack rigidity, questioning the beliefs of Karacan and other workers that full penile-circumference increases may be present without sufficient rigidity for penetration. Consistent with my patients' reports, Slag et al. (1983) found that nearly one-half of the impotent men they investigated stated that they developed erections both in relation to sexual stimulation and spontaneously, but that the erections were of inadequate turgidity for coitus.

Physical Examination and Laboratory Assessments

Erectile disorder, hypoactive sexual desire, and sexual pain disorders are the sexual dysfunctions for which possible organic causes are sought by physical examination and laboratory assessments. Such investigation is indicated in all men with hypoactive sexual desire and in those whose erectile disorder is not situational. *Situational erectile disorder* is that occurring with some but not other partners, or with all partners but not in private masturbation, where no pressure to produce an erection is experienced. Physical examination is indicated to exclude such physical conditions as Peyronie's disease and hypogonadism. Blood and urine screening is employed to exclude diabetes, hyperprolactinemia, raised levels of the pituitary hormone prolactin (HPRL), and thyroid dysfunction.

The study that appeared most influential in reversing the earlier belief that erectile disorder was almost invariably psychogenically determined found that of 105 men diagnosed as impotent, 34 showed reduced serum testosterone levels (3.5 ng/ml or below; Spark, White, & Connolly, 1980). Of the men, 7 of the 34 as well as 1 with a normal level of testosterone showed HPRL, and 2 showed above-normal levels of testosterone and thyroid hormone. Therapy to normalize the hormonal levels restored potency in 33 of the 37 men. The impact of the finding was greatly enhanced by the addition of case histories of some of these men who had been treated with psychotherapy for many years, without investigation of symptoms or signs they showed suggestive of hormonal abnormalities, including a history of pituitary tumor; small, soft testes; loss of body hair; and lack of beard growth. The subjects were referrals to a medical department: Sixteen of the 37 with hormonal abnormalities had pituitary tumors; 2 had other cerebral tumors; and 12 were noted to have small or soft testes. No other study of men with erectile disorders has reported such a high incidence of these problems, suggesting the sample was not representative. Also, the attribution of impotence in 34 subjects to reduced testosterone levels, which were near the lower limits of normal, conflicts with the more frequent reports that most subjects with testosterone levels somewhat below the normal range reported reduced sexual interest, activity, and spontaneous erections, but continue to obtain erections adequate for coitus with appropriate physical stimulation (McConaghy, 1993). As discussed earlier, given the lack of operational criteria still current in the diagnosis of erectile disorder, it is possible the subjects given the diagnosis of impotence by Spark et al. (1980) showed this type of response.

In a study by Buvat et al. (1985) of 1053 men consecutively referred for sexual dysfunctions without obvious organic causes (drugs, apparent endocrinopathies, diabetes, neuropathy, and arthritis), although only 10 (1%) of the 850 men diagnosed as impotent showed marked HPRL (above 35 ng/ml), 6 of the 10 showed radiological evidence of a pituitary adenoma. Five of the 10 had testosterone levels within the normal range (3 to 10 ng/ml). Failure to estimate prolactin levels and perhaps diabetes and thyroid dysfunction in men with erectile disorder or hypoactive sexual desire could have significant medicolegal consequences. This renders all the more disturbing the evidence that patients are reluctant to report and medical practitioners reluctant to inquire concerning the presence of sexual dysfunctions. Only 6 of 1,080 men attending a medical outpatient clinic were identified as having erectile disorder prior to a direct enquiry that revealed its presence in 401 men (Slag et al., 1983).

The evidence that the level of testosterone to maintain erectile function is markedly below that necessary to maintain sexual interest (McConaghy, 1993) is consistent with Jones's (1985) observation that testosterone levels in impotent men under the age of 50 years is almost invariably in the normal range unless signs of marked reduction in the level are present. These signs include loss of libido, physical signs of regression of male hair pattern, gynecomastia (increased breast development), or small, soft testes. Also, although Korenman et al. (1990) found reduction of bioavailable testosterone due to secondary hypogonadism to be present in about 40% of men over the age of 50, they found no relation between the reduction and erectile disorder. Nevertheless, testosterone levels are usually routinely investigated in men with nonsituational erectile disorder and hypoactive sexual desire, even though they do not show physical signs of hypogonadism.

Of the more expensive laboratory investigations, the assessment of subjects' nocturnal penile tumescence (NPT) has received the most attention by sex therapists; Wincze and Carey (1991) stated that it has been considered the gold standard of differential diagnosis in men. At the same time, they pointed out that it is well beyond the financial means of most clients and there are much more affordable and perhaps more valid psychophysiological measures. NPT assessment by continuous recording of subjects' penile-circumference responses during sleep was recommended by Karacan (1978) on the basis that if men with erectile disorder showed erections during dream or rapid eye movement (REM) sleep similar to those of normal men, their dysfunction was due to a psychological, not an organic cause. The procedure was originally conducted in a sleep laboratory on three consecutive nights. On the third night, men who showed erections were awakened for them to assess their fullness and to have the rigidity determined by the pressure necessary to produce buckling. Wasserman et al. (1980) pointed out that the assumption that NPT can distinguish psychogenic from organic impotence had not been established by studies in which the two conditions were diagnosed by criteria independent of the NPT measurements. Wasserman et al. directed attention to findings of impaired NPT in normally functioning men produced by psychogenic factors, in men with erectile disorder diagnosed on clinical grounds as psychogenic, and in elderly men who reported having erections adequate for intercourse.

Schiavi (1992) considered the assessment of penile buckling impractical in older subjects because of rapid penile detumescence at the time of testing. Thase, Reynolds, and Jennings (1988) found that 40% of depressed men showed reduction of duration of NPT corrected for diminished sleep time, in the same range as that of men with organic erectile disorder. And Schiavi et al. (1984) reported recovery of potency after psychotherapy in a man with primary erectile disorder who showed no episodes of full penile tumescence over five nights. Impaired NPT was found in men with reduced testosterone levels due to hypogonadism or estrogen administration who showed normal erectile responses to sexual films and fantasy (Kwan, Van Maasdam, & Davidson, 1985), suggesting that different neurophysiological mechanisms may be involved in the production of NPT and erections in sexual situations. In their recent critical evaluation of NPT assessment, Meisler and Carey (1990) considered that a conservative estimate was that it may misdiagnose as many as 20% of subjects examined. Despite, or rather, because of this evidence that such factors as illness and pharmacological agents, in addition to psychological conditions (e.g., anxiety or depression) associated with abnormalities of sleep were likely to disrupt NPT patterns, Schiavi (1992) proposed that NPT over three nights in a sleep laboratory should continue to be used when diagnostic uncertainty persisted. Less costly alternatives should be employed only as screening devices, because they failed to provide information to identify sleep disorders and REM activity and were likely to lead to false diagnostic conclusions. The implication that experienced investigators could intuitively use such data to improve the validity of NPT assessment does not appear to have been tested empirically. NPT evaluation is routine in patients complaining of erectile disorder secondary to compensable accidents or injuries.

Less expensive alternatives to sleep laboratory assessment of NPT involve assessing subjects' NPT in their own homes, using a ring of stamps or a snap gauge around the penis that bursts if tumescence occurs, or the Rigiscan portable monitoring instrument. This device provides a continuous recording of the frequency, duration, and degree of NPT using two strain-gauge loops: One is placed at the base of the penis, and one immediately behind the glans. The loops are periodically tightened, indenting the penis and providing a measure of turgidity. However, Allen, Smolev, Engel, and Brendler (1993) reported that penile buckling force and observer ratings of erectile rigidity correlated well. Yet, both correlated poorly with Rigiscan assessment when base and tip rigidity exceeded 60% of the maximum, when the assessment failed to discriminate buckling forces between 450 and 900 gm; a buckling force of 550 gm was considered adequate for vaginal penetration. They concluded that exclusion of mild abnormalities in erectile function may not be possible using Rigiscan assessment, and when it exceeds 60% of the maximum, buckling force or observer assessment may be necessary to do so.

In reaction to the earlier belief that most cases of erectile disorder were psychogenically determined (LoPiccolo, 1982), it is now widely accepted that most are due to impairment in penile blood flow (Meuleman et al., 1992). The technique most commonly employed to assess such impairment is determination of penile-brachial index (PBI): PBI is the ratio of the blood pressure in the penile arteries, originally measured by Doppler ultrasound probe, and conventionally measured blood-pressure in the brachial artery in the arm. There is consensus that arterial insufficiency is very likely to be the cause of the impotence of subjects with a PBI of less than 0.6. However, a higher ratio does not exclude the possibility, although a PBI of over 0.9 should indicate sufficient perfusion to maintain erection (Gewertz & Zarins, 1985). Metz and Bengtsson (1981) provided data supporting these conclusions from a study of healthy men, and men with peripheral arteriosclerotic disease, half of whom were impotent. More than 90% of those with PBIs of 0.6 or less were impotent, and all of the healthy controls had PBIs above this ratio. The investigators emphasized that PBIs above 0.6 did not exclude vascular disease as a cause of impotence.

Saypol, Peterson, Howards, and Yazel (1983) questioned the reliance of clinicians on NPT and PBI assessment in impotence. They contended that many patients could be evaluated adequately by a psychiatrist and a urologist without these expensive tests. They compared the two forms of evaluation in 33 consecutive patients with impotence and found close agreement between diagnoses of the psychiatrist and urologist reached by clinical examination alone, and diagnoses based on results of the patients' fasting blood sugar and testosterone levels and their PBI and NPT assessments. They suggested that expensive tests should be reserved for patients about whom the psychiatrist and urologist disagree or cannot determine the diagnosis.

The pharmacological erection test is increasingly being used to assess the penile vascular supply. Vasodilating chemicals, papaverine alone or with phentolamine, prostaglandin E1 alone or a mixture of all three is injected into one of the cavernous sinuses of the subject's penis. The development of a rigid well-sustained erection within 10 minutes suggests no major vascular abnormality exists (McMahon, 1994). The development of the erection may be recorded using a Rigiscan; a slow onset suggests the presence of some degree of arterial disease, and rapid detumescence, a venous leak. If the subject does not develop an adequate erection following the injection, they may do so if they also view an erotic video. Lee et al. (1993) add this procedure routinely immediately after injection, believing that it negates the anxiety factor inherent in testing. They reported that 17 of 20 healthy men (mean = 49 years of age) obtained a full erection following 10 micrograms (mcg) of prostaglandin E1, the 3 men who did not reporting finding the video somewhat offensive. Lee et al. advised that the physician should inquire about this possibility before using a video. Meuleman et al. (1992) stressed the inhibiting effect of the test setting, reporting that even with the addition of manual stimulation in private, only 31 of 44 men (mean = 53 years of age) with normal erectile potency demonstrated a full erectile response following intracavernous injections of 12.5 mcg of prostaglandin E1. An additional 9 developed a full erection after leaving the test situation. The subjects did not view an erotic video. In patients who failed to produce a full erectile response with the test, Meuleman et al. recommended prolongation of the observation period with addition of manual and/or visual stimulation. The higher percentage of men developing full erections when visual stimulation was used during the test in the study by Lee et al. routinely suggests this procedure is advisable with patients who accept it.

When the pharmacological erection test indicates the presence of vascular pathology, further examinations are required to determine its nature, generally commencing with color Duplex Doppler ultrasonography to evaluate the cavernosal arteries. When the necessary equipment is available, this investigation is usually carried out as part of the pharmacological erection test. Arterial blood flow is assessed in the phase of highest flow rate in the first 5 minutes after injection, on the basis of peak flow velocity, acceleration time, and dilatation of the cavernous arteries. Venous leakage is assessed when arterial inflow and venous outflow are equal, using the resistance index:

$$\text{(peak flow velocity} - \text{diastolic flow velocity)} / \text{peak flow velocity}$$

as a measure (Meuleman et al., 1992). These investigators found that only acceleration time significantly differentiated 44 men with normal erectile potency and 280 consecutive patients with erectile disorder. When test results are equivocal, venous leakage may be further assessed by infusion of saline into the corpora cavernosa after intracavernous injection of a vasodilating chemical, when it is indicated by failure to maintain an erection; the leakage can be visualized by injection of a contrast agent and serial radiography (Krysiewicz & Mellinger, 1989). If no impairment in the arterial or venous blood flow within the penis is demonstrated, it may need to be sought in the arteries providing this flow, as is likely if the subject has a history of pelvic trauma. As these tests increasingly require more expensive equipment and considerable experience in interpretation, the investigation of vascular causes for impotence is being taken over by urologists with an interest in the treatment of erectile disorder.

Neurogenic impotence is usually recognized from the patient's history and physical examination. Diabetes, pelvic pathology, radical prostatectomy, the absence of the cremasteric or bulbocavernosal reflex, and reduced lower limb reflexes are major indicators. McMahon (1994) found simple screening with a vibratory biothesiometer useful, but not the more complex procedures developed to investigate impairment of nerve transmission, such as the latency of bulbocavernous reflex and the latency and form of cerebral potentials evoked by stimulation of the glans penis and the peroneal nerve (Ertekin, Akyurekli, Gurses, & Turgut, 1985).

Physical and laboratory examination of women with sexual dysfunctions are more rarely carried out. However, as with men, the possibility that illness, medications, or substances are responsible for producing reduced sexual interest or ability to reach orgasm needs to be excluded. Gynecological investigation is indicated when dyspareunia is present. Vaginal lesions, dermatitis, or infections are likely to be associated with pain on penetration, and inflammation or disease of the pelvic organs with pain on deep penile thrusting. The effects of neurological and vascular disease and of medications and drugs of abuse on the sexuality of women are much more poorly documented than their impact on men. Many women taking drugs used in psychiatric treatment, including major and minor tranquilizers, monoamine oxidase inhibitors, and tricyclic antidepressants, report reduced libido or ability to orgasm. A double-blind study of two such drugs, phenelzine and imipramine, found them to produce a high incidence of impairment of sexual function in depressed women patients compared with placebo, although not as high as in men (Harrison, Rabkin, & Ehrhardt, 1986). As with alcoholic men, clinical studies of alcoholic women report high rates of sexual dysfunction (Leiblum & Rosen, 1984). However, a U.S. national survey of 917 women found that the relationship between the dysfunction and intake of alcohol was weak (Klassen & Wilsnack, 1986). Moderate drinking was associated with lower rates of several dysfunctions than lighter or heavier drinking or abstinence. A recent British survey showed that both women and men reported more occasions of sexual activity in the last 4 weeks as their alcohol consumption increased from none to heavy (Johnson et al., 1994). Jensen (1981) found no significant difference in the percentage of insulin-treated diabetic women (27.5%) who reported sexual dysfunctions, compared to age-matched controls (25%) who consecutively attended a general practitioner, although peripheral neuropathy was more prevalent in the dysfunctional as compared to the functional diabetic women. As in men, diseases associated with pain, or that result in debility, anxiety, or depression, will significantly impair women's sexual interest.

Hormone studies are rarely considered necessary in the routine investigation of sexually dysfunctional women in the absence of indications of hormonal imbalance (e.g., excessive hirsutism). As discussed in more detail elsewhere (McConaghy, 1993), the nature and significance of the influence of hormonal factors on the sexual interest and activity of women remains largely unestablished. And psychological variables (particularly the presence and nature of a relationship with a male partner) appear to be the major determinants at least in heterosexual women who comprise the majority of those studied. The significant hormonal fluctuations that occur throughout the menstrual cycle have not been demonstrated to be accompanied by consistent fluctuations in sexual behaviors. The effects of removal of women's ovaries, oophorectomy, were so much less apparent than those of castration that Kinsey, Pomeroy, Martin, and Gebhard (1953) considered them negligible. However, there appears to be general agreement that the menopausal symptoms, including hot flashes and atrophic vaginitis that follow oophorectomy, are accompanied by reduced sexual interest and activity. It remains to be established whether the reduction is due to direct effects of hormones on the central nervous system, or is secondary to the hot flashes and atrophic vaginitis.

Physiological assessment of women's sexual arousal to erotic stimuli has been evaluated in laboratory studies by vaginal, clitoral, or labial blood-flow changes. Arousal has been measured either by the associated temperature changes using a thermistor, or vaginal color changes with a photoplethysmograph. Rosen and Beck (1988) considered photoplethysmograph assessment of vaginal pulse amplitude (VPA) the most widely used measure and the most sensitive in distinguishing the responses of groups of women to erotic as compared to nonerotic stimuli, but its correlation with subjectively assessed arousal was insignificant in the majority of individuals studied. Hatch (1981) concluded that there were no consistent reports of differences in physiologically assessed genital arousal to erotic stimuli of sexually functional and dysfunctional women, or of changes in the arousal of the dysfunctional women following treatment. In regard to the lack of consistency of the reports investigating the arousal to stimuli of sexually functional and dysfunctional women, Palace and Gorzalka (1990, 1992) convincingly demonstrated this could be accounted for by such factors as differences in stimuli and assessment procedures, including the use of VPA rather than vaginal blood volume (VBV), which they considered could be the more sensitive indicator of sexual arousal. In their studies, sexually dysfunctional women showed less VBV response and subjective arousal to erotic films; however, there were few significant correlations between genital and subjective measures of sexual arousal. The VBV of dysfunctional women increased to a level equivalent to those of functional women following false physiological feedback combined with preexposure to an arousal-evoking film, while their subjective sexual arousal was unchanged (Palace, 1986). Palace suggested generalized sympathetic arousal associated with anxiety, laughter, or exercise could facilitate genital sexual arousal. This raises the possibility that VBV could be in part determined by nonsexual stimuli, supported by the finding that the VBV of sexually functional women significantly decreased during exposure to anxiety-eliciting stimuli (Palace & Gorzalka, 1990). However, this finding was not replicated (Palace, 1996). If strategies combining physiological feedback and increasing autonomic arousal prove effective in improving the sexual responses of dysfunctional women, this could provide evidence VBV is validly assessing specifically sexual responses, not more generalized genital hemodynamic responses. It should also lead to more attention being given the physiological assessment of genital arousal of sexually dysfunctional women.

TREATMENT/TRAINING PROCEDURES

During the assessment interview, the clinician is also initiating treatment by establishing a relationship with the patients or couples that will maximize their confidence and trust in the clinician's ability. The degree to which this is done successfully will not only increase the nonspecific effects of the treatment instituted, but also the likelihood that the patient will comply with it. In determining how best to establish the relationship, therapists need to decide how much they will modify the personality they project to be more in conformity with patients' values, including those reflecting their cultural and socioeconomic background. Certainly, therapists must ensure that their vocabulary is comprehensible to and does not threaten or antagonize patients. As indicated by the greater rejection of behavioral sex therapy shown by men with erectile disorder referred from a urology department compared to those who self-referred to a sexual dysfunction clinic (Segraves, Schoenberg, Zarins, Camic, & Knopf, 1981), it is important to be sensitive to the fact that many less psychologically aware men believe their erectile disorders are organically determined. Although the presence of significant psychological factors may be evident, it is important not to emphasize this until these patients' trust has been established. Reported attrition rates from treatment for sexual dysfunctions and deviations vary remarkably (McConaghy, 1993). And it would seem likely that this, in part, reflects the varying abilities of clinicians to establish appropriate relationships with their patients.

In the treatment of psychogenic factors contributing to sexual dysfunctions, if it has been decided during assessment that they mainly result from the subjects' personalities or their relationship with their partners, the treatment of these conditions will take priority. However, the majority of patients presenting with sexual dysfunctions are suitable for treatment aimed directly at that problem. The concept advanced by Wolpe (1958) that the major psychological factor responsible for sex dysfunctions was anxiety about sexual activity, provides the basis for the direct therapy of these conditions employed by most clinicians, whether or not it is labeled cognitive-behavioral. Winzce and Carey (1991) considered the focus on anxiety in causing sexual dysfunctions could be misleading, because several studies had shown that anxiety can facilitate rather than inhibit arousal. However, Hale and Strassberg (1990) pointed out that the anxiety was produced by injections of epinephrine; exposure to anxiety-provoking material, such as films of fatal car accidents; or threat of electric shock. Fear of sexual activity itself was not examined.

Hale and Strassberg (1990) investigated the effects of two forms of anxiety on sexual arousal of 54 non-sexually dysfunctional men aged 21 to 45 years. One was produced by threat of a painful but not harmful electric shock, the other by threat of sexual inadequacy created by showing subjects bogus, unusually low tracings of their penile responses during a baseline assessment and informing them that low tracings were associated with increased risk of developing sexual problems. The subjects' sexual arousal was assessed by their penile circumference responses to videos of sexual activity by heterosexual couples. Both forms of anxiety reduced subjects' sexual arousal. Hale and Strassberg suggested that their finding that threat of shock reduced sexual arousal, in contrast to its failure to do so in an earlier study of 12 college students, could have been due to the older age and larger size of their sample. It could also have been due to the fact that the 12 students were exposed to a sample of the electric shock prior to assessing the effect of the threat of its administration. The experience of sampling it may have reduced the threat. Hale and Strassberg concluded that their study provided empirical support for the concept that anxiety about sexual performance was a factor in erectile disorder in men. They commented that if the sexually functional men in their study were sufficiently concerned by the possibility that their sexual performance was subnormal, the effect of such cognitions could be expected to be much greater in men with reasons for concern, such as an episode of erectile failure following heavy alcohol intake. If replicated, Hale and Strassberg's findings provide evidence that anxiety need not be directly associated with sexual activity to impair performance in men.

Cognitive Correction

Following the model introduced by Wolpe (1958), the therapist investigates the patient's attitude toward sexual activity. If it is not one of acceptance, experiences are sought that could explain this. These could include sexual abuse, coercion, or assault, the response to which may require specific treatment (McConaghy, 1993). Childhood observations of sexual activities that have led the subject to believe they are harmful, or feelings that they are evil, are corrected by discussion of the illogical nature of the beliefs, when appropriate. Patients' religious values must be treated with sensitivity, and attempts must be made to work within these values, determining what sexual behaviors they consider acceptable. Concerns about past failures of sexual performance are explored with reassurance about the normality of occasional failures, especially when subjects are tired, stressed, or affected by drugs.

Education will be needed if subjects are unaware of the basic facts of sexual anatomy and activity. My experience has led me to the conclusion, also reached by Marshall and Barbaree (1990) in their program to enhance the enjoyment of heterosexual activities of sex offenders, that extensive detailing of the anatomical or physiological aspects of sexual functioning is unnecessary. They considered that it could result in attention being focused on the objective and physical aspects of sex rather than crucially important interpersonal features. However, older women may require information regarding such possible effects of menopause as atrophic vaginitis and lack of vaginal lubrication resulting in discomfort or pain during intercourse, and the role of hormone replacement and use of lubricants in its therapy; older men may be unaware of the normality of the increasing inability with age to obtain adequate erections without manual stimulation. When this inability develops, a number of men whose female partners do not touch their penises in sexual activities cease approaching the partners for coitus, without giving them any explanation; they are unwilling to request such stimulation and often feeling shame at their inability to be aroused without it.

Desensitization of Anxiety

Wolpe (1958) postulated that the regular evocation of anxiety in relation to thoughts or experiences of sexual activity would result in its being conditioned to such thoughts or experiences. The conditioned component would persist following cognitive correction and require desensitization for its extinction. This could be accomplished by the procedure he developed: systematic desensitization in imagination. In its original form, patient and therapist constructed a hierarchy of situations ranging from the one that provoked minimal anxiety to the one that elicited maximal anxiety. The patient was then trained in deep-muscle relaxation over several sessions. Next, while relaxed, the patient was instructed to visualize hierarchical items of anxiety-provoking situations (beginning with the least anxiety-provoking) and to signal to the therapist when anxiety was no longer experienced by raising the index finger. The state of relaxation was considered to reciprocally inhibit the low level of anxiety produced by this item, and the patient would usually signal within about 30 seconds that no anxiety was experienced while visualizing it. When this item no longer produced anxiety, it was expected that the anxiety produced by the next item would be reduced by generalization. The patient could, therefore, visualize it next with minimal anxiety, which again soon dissipated. The patient thus proceeded to work through the hierarchy, finally being able to visualize the last item without anxiety. Also, as subjects experienced minimal anxiety to the visualized situations in imagination, they were given homework assignments (when possible) in which they were encouraged to enter and remain in the equivalent *in vivo* situations.

Most patients with dysfunctions report feeling anxious about sexual activity, even if only about their inability to meet their own or what they imagine to be their partner's expectation of performance. However, some patients, particularly those with hypoactive sexual desire report that they do not experience any feelings (including anxiety) in sexual situations. To treat these subjects, it is assumed that they have repressed awareness of such anxiety. They are treated by exposure to a hierarchy of sexual situations in which they visualize feeling aroused, from the initiation of sexual activity by stroking, cuddling, and kissing to reaching orgasm in coitus.

For men with erectile disorder, Wolpe (1958) appeared to consider desensitization *in vivo* to be more effective. He instructed them to cuddle naked with their partners, but not to attempt penetration even if they obtained adequate erections, until he gave them permission to do so. Under these conditions, they no longer experienced anxiety about their ability to attain and maintain an erection adequate for coitus. And any anxiety conditioned to past experiences was gradually inhibited by the continued exposure to this nonthreatening sexual situation. Once it was no longer blocked by anxiety, their sexual arousal began to result in adequate erections.

The direct therapies of sexual dysfunctions introduced by Wolpe were initially largely ignored by clinicians and researchers treating and investigating these conditions in the United States; most maintained a psychoanalytic approach. This approach centered on the interpretation of the relationship between the therapist and patient to make patients aware of presumed repressed sexual feelings toward their parents, experienced in the first 5 years of their lives. Views of the therapists using this approach were eclipsed when the enthusiastic media reception given the publication in 1970 by Masters and Johnson's *Human Sexual Inadequacy* ensured that it gained wide public recognition. The book reported excellent results from therapy aimed directly at reducing anxiety concerning sexual activity. The resulting demand for such therapy led to its being provided by a large number of minimally qualified or untrained persons (LoPiccolo, 1978), but also stimulated mainstream therapists to apply it.

Modified Masters and Johnson Approach: Communication

The program developed by Masters and Johnson required patients and their partners to be seen individually by a therapist of the same sex as well as jointly by both therapists. The majority of subjects treated came to St. Louis from other parts of the United States to receive the treatment that was carried out in daily sessions for 2 or 3 weeks. In addition, couples were given nightly homework assignments.

Most therapists do not follow the format of the Masters and Johnson approach precisely, because few people seeking help are able or prepared to give up 2 or 3 weeks for treatment or to make time for hourly homework assignments every night. Also, many sex therapists, finding their results satisfactory when they work as individuals, continue to do so rather than increase the cost of therapy by involving a cotherapist of the opposite sex. With the modified approach, couples are seen weekly or less frequently. In the initial interviews, they are provided with appropriate information, and any faulty cognitions are corrected. They are then given instructions concerning their homework activities. Specifically, they are requested to set aside two or more periods of about an hour's duration weekly when they can be relaxed and undisturbed. This often takes considerable negotiation concerning how interruptions from children, household, and external work demands are to be managed. The couple's performance of homework activities are monitored in the following treatment session. For many patients, the appropriate activities are those used by Masters and Johnson, which elaborated Wolpe's injunction not to attempt intercourse, in two phases.

The couple is instructed that, in homework sessions, one is to be passive and the other active for half the period, and then they are to change roles. In the initial phase, the active partner is to sensuously stimulate the passive partner by massaging, stroking, or kissing how and where he or she is told by the passive partner, except that their genitals, and in the case of female subjects, their breasts, are not to be touched. They are informed that the purpose is to enjoy the sensuous experience as such; they are not to expect to become sexually aroused as this is unlikely to occur initially due to the presence of conditioning of their past negative experiences. This procedure, termed "sensate focusing" by Masters and Johnson, enables the couple to have a physical relationship with confidence that coitus will not take place and without pressure to meet some standard of sexual performance. Conditioned anxieties from past experiences of unpleasant or painful coitus, or of failures to meet standards, can thus start to be extinguished. From the information they provide while in the passive role, they also learn to communicate verbally about what they enjoy in foreplay activities. From their experiences in the active role, they learn how to carry out the activities their partners enjoy.

When given the rationale for the initial phase at the beginning of therapy, some couples say they have been regularly cuddling together and stimulating each others' genitals manually and orally without anxiety and not proceeding to coitus, due to the presence of erectile dysfunction or vaginismus. If the therapist feels that the couple is not experiencing anxiety in this situation, it may be appropriate to omit the initial phase of sensate focusing and to include genital stimulation from the start of homework activities. However, if the couple could benefit from dissociating the sensuous from the sexual aspects of physical contact in order to reduce the emphasis on the sexual aspects, or to increase the range of their nongenital foreplay activities, they should be encouraged to adopt the limitation of the initial phase.

When monitoring of subjects' responses in the initial phase reveals that they are comfortable and relaxed, communicating effectively, and enjoying the sensuous stimulation from their partner, they are instructed to proceed to the second phase. In this phase, stimulation of the genitals and breasts of the partner when he or she is in the passive role is added, but intercourse is still countermanded. If they feel it is appropriate, and it will not involve subjecting either partner to any pressure, one or both can reach orgasm by manual or oral stimulation at the end of the session. Men and women who are unable to ejaculate or to reach orgasm in physical relations are instructed to attempt to do so during the session. They are told that it may take an hour or more of masturbatory stimulation for them to reach orgasm initially and that they will need to experiment to find the type of stimulation that most arouses them. Some women find direct stimulation of the clitoris unpleasant and need to be stimulated near it. Some men may require very vigorous stimulation. Some subjects, more commonly women, do not wish to stimulate their genitals themselves, and it may be sufficient that their partner does so. Others prefer to masturbate on their own in separate sessions. Occasionally, women who cannot touch their own or their partner's genitals in this phase benefit from the addition of individual sessions of desensitization to these activities in imagination. If anorgasmic men or women do not respond to prolonged stimulation when with their partners or alone, they are encouraged to use an electric vibrator. LoPiccolo (1990) recommended the use of "orgasm triggers" to aid women who report being unable to reach orgasm, although they become highly aroused. Orgasm triggers are behaviors that occur involuntarily during orgasm, which if performed voluntarily can initiate orgasm. For example, LoPiccolo suggested holding one's breath, bearing down with the pelvic muscles, pointing the toes and tensing the leg and thigh muscles, throwing the head back, and thrusting the pelvis.

The partners of women with vaginismus are instructed in the second phase of homework to begin digital dilation of her vagina when she is sexually aroused, initially using one finger. Provided she remains relaxed, two and then three fingers are inserted. Some women feel less anxious if they initiate vaginal dilatation with their own fingers, or if graded vaginal dilators are employed at first. If subjects with hypoactive sexual desire continue to report lack of sexual arousal in the second phase, it is suggested they add the use of erotic videos, books, and sexual fantasy. Some people with hypoactive desire seem to have reduced ability to enjoy any sensuous experiences. They are encouraged to incorporate appropriate ones into their recreational life, which frequently requires expansion, as understandably they have previously allocated little time to it. Suggested experiences could include physical activities, walking, sunbathing, swimming, and use of spa baths. Some examples of emotional activities are listening to music at home and at concerts, and attending the theater and art galleries.

Partners of men with premature ejaculation are instructed in the second phase to sit between their legs facing them, and to masturbate them. The men are told to monitor their arousal and when they feel they are about to ejaculate, to tell their partners, who then cease stimulation until told the sensation has disappeared. They then recommence masturbation. Subsidence of erection may occur temporarily. As the subject becomes able to prolong erection prior to ejaculation, his anxiety that he will ejaculate prematurely diminishes. This "stop–start" procedure was recommended for premature ejaculation by Semans in 1956, but it appeared to have attracted little attention. Semans believed that ejaculation occurs more rapidly when the penis is wet and advised that once the subject was responding adequately, a lubricant be used with subsequent masturbation. When the subject showed maintenance of erection with this stimulation, Semans considered the moist surface of the vagina would no longer produce premature ejaculation. He reported case histories of 8 subjects who showed a successful response. Masters and Johnson (1970) also advised the use of masturbation for premature ejaculation, with the modification that when ejaculation was imminent, the partner, instead of temporarily ceasing stimulation, carried out a "penile squeeze." This was done by the partner placing the first finger on the subject's glans penis, the second fingers just below it, the thumb under it, and firmly but not painfully squeezing the glans. This inhibited ejaculation and usually resulted in some loss of erection. Masturbation was then recommenced as with the stop–start procedure.

When in the second phase of homework activities, subjects report that they are adequately aroused and experiencing no anxiety at the thought of having coitus, they are instructed to initiate this in a third phase. Whereas the receptive partner in vaginal or anal intercourse presented with negative feelings toward the activity, or the active male presented with premature ejaculation, the couple is told to initiate penetration with the active male lying on his back and the partner squatting or kneeling over him and sitting on his erect penis. This renders it very unlikely that any anxiety concerning being penetrated will be reactivated in the partners, because they are in control. Also, if following intromission, men being treated for premature ejaculation feel they are about to ejaculate, they can inform their partners, who cease stimulation by raising themselves off the penis and, if necessary, use the penile squeeze. LoPiccolo (1990) reported the use of nocturnal penile erections in 3 men with lifelong erectile failure in all situations who had failed to respond to desensitization. Each wife was instructed to remain in another room while her husband went to sleep. After 1 or 2 hours she was to check every 15 minutes until she observed that her husband had an erection. She then gently stroked his penis until he woke to the unique experience of having an erection during sexual activity with his wife. LoPiccolo said this enabled one wife to accomplish vaginal intromission while her husband was awakening and consummate the marriage after 7 years. He did not report the long-term outcome of this procedure.

Learning to Relinquish Control

The significance attributed to anxiety conditioned to past negative sexual experiences in producing sexual dysfunctions may have resulted in less emphasis being placed on the role of learning to relinquish control. This is particularly true with regard to women's inability to become sexually aroused and to reach orgasm. The gradual reduction in the percentage of women who rarely or never reached orgasm in sexual relations from over 50% in adolescence to less than 10% in middle age (McConaghy, 1993) strongly suggests that learning is occurring. It would seem likely that one of the behaviors acquired is relinquishing control (in view of the social pressure on women to initially develop such control). As Mead (1950) pointed out, adolescent girls are expected to restrict the limits of sexual activities, and boys to extend them. Women who consistently experienced orgasm during coitus were more likely to report inability to control their thinking or movements as they approached orgasm (Bridges, Critelli, & Loos, 1985). They also obtained higher scores on a hypnotic susceptibility scale, which was considered to reflect a greater ability to suspend effortful, controlled cognitive processes.

This concept that women need to learn to relinquish control to experience orgasms with coitus is consistent with anecdotal reports in Hunt's (1974) U.S. survey of sexual behavior in the 1970s; women emphasized the role of individual men in helping them to learn to become aroused, stating that these men encouraged them to move their bodies, feel their rhythms, read books on peak experiences and joy, and "blow their minds." The rarer inability of men to reach orgasm and ejaculate in coitus also usually appears attributable to fear of loss of emotional control.

If it is considered that fear of loss of control or embarrassment at behaving emotionally is a factor preventing subjects from reaching orgasm with their partners when they can do so alone, role-playing loss of emotional control and reaching orgasm in the presence of their partners can overcome this problem. If the subjects feel inhibited about doing this in reality, they may first require desensitization to the behavior via imagery. Men with inability to ejaculate into the vagina or rectum may accomplish this if they masturbate with their partner to the point of orgasm and then penetrate. After doing so on one or a few occasions, the inhibition commonly disappears.

Apfelbaum and Apfelbaum (1985) were critical of informing patients that their failure to experience sexual arousal in response to sexual stimulation indicated that they were fearful of being aroused and that they needed to "let go" or accept their sexual feelings. They felt that this approach encouraged the patient to "bypass" valid emotional responses in focusing on their sexual sensations. Bypassing was natural to many subjects and enabled them to experience sexual arousal without difficulty in situations (e.g., a partner with unattractive features) that would inhibit arousal in subjects who could not bypass them. The latter subjects were likely to be trying to be sexually aroused and already felt guilty that they were not responding to their partner's sexual activity. Apfelbaum and Apfelbaum contended that they experienced not pleasure anxiety, the fear of becoming aroused, but response anxiety, the fear of not responding. To encourage them to try to respond further would increase their guilt and put them under pressure to bypass their valid responses that were inhibiting their arousal. Apfelbaum (1988) singled out Kaplan as the most overt of therapists in this respect in encouraging patients to block their valid responses, citing her statement:

> A woman must learn to "shut out" the nuances of her partner's behavior, at least to the extent that it will not inhibit her sexual response; she must learn, in short, to develop a more autonomous pattern of sexual functioning. (p. 92)

A comparison of sexually functional and dysfunctional subjects (Heiman, Gladue, Roberts, & LoPiccolo, 1986) would appear to support Kaplan's approach in treating dysfunctions. Men without dysfunctions were more likely to obtain pleasure from various sexual activities, to use fantasies, including atypical and deviant fantasies, and to attach less importance to emotional closeness, holding, and caring for good sex. Women without dysfunctions were likely to report more pleasure and sexual arousal, but less emotional involvement with the partner in their first experience of coitus. They also indicated more positive feelings to their current partner's genitals and physical appearance. Dysfunctional subjects would appear to have a more romantic and less physical attitude to sexual activity.

Apfelbaum (1988) reported the case of a woman who experienced lack of sexual responsiveness; his interpretation was that her husband was pressuring her into responding sexually. The treatment was reframed so that he became the identified patient. Certainly, therapists should be alert to the possibility that one partner has been encouraged to seek treatment to meet the other partner's needs. This was frequently the case in the 1970s, when the expectation was widespread that all women should reach at least one orgasm by penis–vagina stimulation on all occasions of coitus. During interview of some couples, it would become apparent that the woman enjoyed their current sexual activity and felt no need to reach orgasm more frequently. Her male partner would emphasize how all his previous partners' always reached orgasm with coitus alone, and it would become obvious that he felt the need to prove his ability as a lover in this way. Pointing out the small percentage of women who do reach orgasm in that way with that frequency, and the prevalence of faking orgasm by women, was usually effective in taking the identified patient role from the woman partner. However, such reframing clearly needs to be done with sensitivity to both partners' feelings. Apfelbaum pointed out that a number of male partners were very threatened by having their sexuality questioned. Before deciding on a treatment goal of helping patients learn to be more sexually responsive, it is important to establish that they are not experiencing underlying resentment concerning the need to change. Also, if it is necessary to encourage patients to focus on their own sexual responses, it would also seem important to determine that they do not do so at the expense of their willingness to remain responsive to their partners' needs. Otherwise, it is possible that the patients' sexual dysfunctions might improve at the expense of their sexual satisfaction. This is especially relevant given the evidence discussed earlier that sexual satisfaction is more related to failures to be responsive to partner needs than to the presence of dysfunctions.

LoPiccolo (1992) described a "postmodern" approach to treating erectile failure that was also critical of the standard anxiety desensitization/sexual skills approach to treatment of sexual dysfunctions. He argued that it failed to take into account the systems theory that dysfunction plays a positive role in the homeostasis of the couple's emotional relationship. As an example, he described a wife who is dominated by her husband and who may gain power if he develops erectile failure; she, therefore, could resist carrying out standard behavioral procedures. Instead of implementing the standard approach and encountering resistance, LoPiccolo suggested that the therapist initially analyze the problem from this point of view and deal with it proactively, possibly by use of the concept of secondary gain. In the initial evaluation, when questioning patients about the effects of the sexual problem, the therapist would suggest that some effects could be positive. It may be that the introduction of direct sexual therapy resulted in an excessive focus on subjects' sexual dysfunctions, reducing the attention given to their sexual and general relationship. However, a reaction is occurring and therapists are beginning to respond to the realities Apfelbaum (1988) pointed out:

> The consciousness raising that has been steadily forcing us to recognize disowned realities regarding sexual oppression: sexual exploitation, sexual demands, and the effects of male dominance. The more we recognize legitimate reasons for lack of arousal, the less responsible for it we will feel, and hence the less response anxiety we will experience, with the result that we will be less likely to be locked into experiences of lack of arousal. (p. 103)

Treatment of Subjects without Partners: Modified Systematic Desensitization

The use of desensitization to actual sexual experiences in treating sexual dysfunctions requires that subjects have cooperative partners. Some individuals who seek treatment when they are without partners may be prepared to work through the program with a surrogate therapist. In my experience, unlike women, most men are prepared to do so and some homosexual male patients are prepared to work with each other when this is appropriate. Fortunately, women appear more likely than men to respond successfully when treated without a partner, possibly reflecting the greater performance demands on male sexuality with a partner in that it requires that the man maintain an erection. Women can complete coitus successfully without experiencing any response, and if they wish, they can fake one to the satisfaction of most partners.

Sexual anxieties of subjects without partners can be treated by education, cognitive correction, and systematic desensitization in imagination. When appropriate, use of erotic literature and videos and directed masturbation in homework sessions is added. In advising the use of masturbation, it is, of course, necessary to explore the patient's ethical and religious values concerning this practice.

When I adopted the use of systematic desensitization for the treatment of phobic reactions (including sexual phobias) in the 1960s, like other clinicians, I found the procedure could be significantly modified without reducing its effectiveness. The most cost-effective modification was marked curtailment of the length of relaxation training. As described by Wolpe (1958), patients receiving the therapy were trained over several hours in a progressive muscular relaxation procedure. As I use it, patients lie comfortably on a couch in a darkened room, with their arms by their sides and their eyes closed. They are then asked to clench their fists and concentrate on their feelings of tension. After about 20 seconds, they are asked to relax their fists and concentrate on the sensation of their hands feeling limp and heavy. They are then asked similarly to tense and then relax progressively their arms, legs, stomach, neck, and then their facial muscles, while concentrating on the accompanying feelings of tension or relaxation. They are finally asked to tense further any muscle groups that feel tense and then to relax them; they are to signal by raising the index finger visible to the therapist when they feel relaxed. This procedure is carried out within 5 minutes, with the therapist conveying complete conviction that the patient will be relaxed at its termination. It is extremely rare for patients not to signal that they are relaxed.

When patients signal that they are relaxed, the therapist instructs them to visualize performing the first behavior of the hierarchy of sexual situations about which they are anxious, and to signal when they are doing so and are relaxed. A few seconds after they provide the signal, the therapist instructs them to visualize performing the next behavior in the scenario; they are asked to signal when they are doing so and are relaxed, and so on. The duration of sessions of treatment is about 20 minutes. Outpatients are given sessions once or twice weekly and inpatients, three sessions daily for 5 days. The last hierarchical items are usually presented by about the eighth session. I have found that if by the sixth to the eighth session the patient did not report marked improvement, therapy was not likely to be effective. If significant change was reported, treatment was continued at less frequent intervals for four or five further session. When patients report improvement, they are encouraged to establish a relationship in which they carry out, *in vivo*, behaviors they visualized in imagination without anxiety.

A typical initial hierarchical item for a heterosexual female patient with sexual aversion or hypoactive sexual desire would be as follows: "You are sitting on your living-room couch beside an attractive man you like, and he touches your hand with his"; a final item would be "As you reach a climax you let your feelings take over, letting your body do what it likes, moving and making whatever noises come naturally."

I have obtained good results in the treatment of subjects without partners who present with hypoactive sexual desire, sexual aversion, and anorgasmia, and with men who report inability to reach orgasm in the presence of a partner. Men with erectile disorder and premature ejaculation respond less well.

Men without partners who were impotent in sexual relationships, but not with masturbation, were treated in a group by two male cotherapists (Lobitz & Baker, 1979). Education, cognitive correction of faulty attitudes concerning women's expectations, and systematic desensitization to a hierarchy of sexual situations of increasing intimacy up to coitus were used with homework assignments of masturbating to full erection, letting the erection subside, and repeating the procedure. Subjects also practiced the stop–start and penile-squeeze techniques, because most had anxieties about premature ejaculation. Three female therapists joined the group for one session for the men to role-play self-disclosure of their sexual problem and communicating the suggestion that they did not have coitus in their initial sexual activities.

Treatment of Organic Factors

When medications may be producing sexual dysfunctions, suitable alternatives are sought where possible. Compared to older antihypertensive, drugs, some of the newer medications, such as atenolol, nifedipine, and capropril, have been found to be less likely to impair erectile function in older men (Morrissette, Skinner, Hoffman, Levine, & Davidson, 1993). The use of yohimbine has been reported to be effective in relieving the sexual side effects of clomipramine (Hollander & McCarley, 1992) and fluoxetine (Jacobsen, 1992).

Use of alcohol, tobacco, and other substances is discouraged, and a diet and activities to increase physical fitness are encouraged. Increase in sexual interest and activity was found in men who improved their fitness by an exercise program and reduction of smoking (White, Case, McWhirter, & Mattison, 1990). The prevalence of the most common dysfunction treated organically, erectile disorder, increases with age, being reported in about 1% of men at 30, 2% at 40, 7% at 50, 18% at 60, 27% at 70, 55% at 75, and 76% at 80 years of age (Kinsey, Pomeroy, & Martin, 1948; Weizman & Hart, 1987). The prevalence in men of the same age is markedly lower in healthy than unhealthy older subjects (McConaghy, 1993). In a survey of British men and women up to age 59, in which those over age 50 were underrepresented, there was only a weak relationship between perceived health and the number of occasions of sexual activity in the previous 4 weeks (Johnson et al., 1994). However, 24% of the subjects with identifiable medical illness perceived their health as good or very good. As stated earlier, Korenman et al. (1990) found reduction of bioavailable testosterone due to secondary hypogonadism to be present in about 40% of men over the age of 50, the group most likely to report erectile dysfunction. Hence, a significant percentage of men with erectile disorder will show this reduction. Korenman et al. found no relation between its presence and reduction of bioavailable testosterone. Nevertheless, when testosterone reduction is found in routine investigation of men with nonsituational erectile disorder or hypoactive sexual desire, most therapists will give testosterone administration a trial. Certainly, younger men with testosterone levels markedly below normal associated with reduced sexual interest and spontaneous erections along with physical signs of hypogonadism benefit dramatically from such administration (McConaghy, 1993). The evidence is much less convincing that it helps older men reporting erectile disorder but normal sexual interest, whose testosterone levels are not markedly below normal limits.

The presence of prostatic carcinoma needs to be excluded in older men before beginning a trial of testosterone. Also, they need to be warned that the risk of its development could be increased by testosterone administration. In making this point, Keogh (1993) stated that men should also be informed of the evidence of the effect of androgens on plasma lipids, which could increase severity of coronary artery disease. The occurrence of liver-function impairment and of hepatoma associated with use of methyltestosterone is less common with the more recently introduced forms of testosterone. Keogh found increased aggression could prove a problem when testosterone was administered to correct the low level in boys with retarded puberty. Nevertheless, he considered its administration justified if the condition was causing severe psychological stress. This was despite the further complication that production by testosterone of premature fusion of the epiphyses would deny these boys their full height potential. If investigation of sexual dysfunctions reveals evidence of diabetes, HPRL, thyroid dysfunction, or other physical illnesses, these conditions will require appropriate investigation and treatment. Vascular surgery is occasionally recommended to improve the blood flow in the penile arteries or to correct venous leaks.

If organic causes for erectile disorder cannot be adequately reversed, or if adequate treatment for apparent psychogenic causes has failed, one of three treatment options is currently available, and a fourth, an oral medication, under investigation. Rosen and Ashton (1993) recently reviewed investigations evaluating oral medications, which they referred to as *prosexual drugs*, or aphrodisiacs. These terms would appear to suggest that these drugs increase sexual desire; however, most studies have used them for erectile disorder. Improvement in men given 18 mg daily of yohimbine was reported in 62% with psychogenic (Reid et al., 1987) and in 43% with organic erectile disorder (Morales et al., 1987);

improvement with placebo in the two comparison groups occurred in 16% and 28%, respectively. The difference in improvement rate in subjects with psychogenic but not organic disorder was statistically significant. Savion, Segenreich, Kahan, and Servadio (1987) reported improvement in 67% of men with erectile dysfunction given a combination of yohimbine, thioridazine, and strychnine sulphate. Morales et al. (1987) concluded that due to its ease of administration, safety, and modest effect, yohimbine could be used in patients who do not accept the more invasive methods to be discussed. Rosen and Ashton (1993) cogently stated that no single drug has proven to be clinically safe and reliably effective for human use, but that further research was justified. They also criticized the dearth of studies on prosexual drug effects in women. Some open trials have reported successful treatment of erectile disorder by use of topical applications of yohimbine (Canale, Cilurzo, Giogi, & Menchini Fabris, 1992) or nitroglycerin ointment (Nunez & Anderson, 1993) to the subject's penis.

One of the three physical interventions currently offered patients with erectile disorder is self-injection of a chemical vasodilator into one of the corpora cavernosa of the penis. This is carried out following demonstration that this procedure produced a satisfactory and persistent erection during laboratory investigation. In a brief review of the literature concerning the use of intracavernous injection, Althof et al. (1987) found that prolonged painful erections, or priapism, was reported in 4 to 16% of subjects using it. They considered that this could usually be avoided by gradually increasing the dose of chemicals to the appropriate amount. Penile plaques, nodules, or fibrosis had been found to occur at the injection site, but the published data indicated this was rare. Althof et al. reported on the first 82 patients admitted to their program. The cause of their erectile disorder was considered organic in 43, psychogenic in 11, and mixed in 28 patients. Fifty-two were in stable relationships and their partners participated in the study. Men with psychogenic impotence received the treatment only if they failed to respond to a 6-month trial of individual, marital, or sex therapy. Injections produced satisfactory erections in 50 of the 52 subjects who progressed through the program's trial-dose phase. One-half of the remaining 30 did not pursue the recommendation to enter the program. Althof et al. attributed the dropout of the other half early in the trial-dose phase to the demoralizing effect of the lack of erection following the initial small dose of medication used, and the need to regularly attend the physician's office and attempt coitus to test the result within a half-hour. Periodic bruising occurred at the injection site in 26% and plaque-like nodules were noted in 21%. However, these did not cause penile bending or pain, and did not require treatment termination. One patient developed priapism. The 29 patients who had completed 3 months of self-injections had used them on an average of 4.8 times a month. Seventy percent of the injections produced erections sufficient for coitus. The failures were considered due to improper self-injection technique and the limited shelf-life of the medication. Supplemental teaching sessions were often necessary, and patients were instructed to dispose of the medication after a month. Compared with the pretreatment condition, frequency of intercourse increased, frequency of masturbation decreased, and satisfaction after sexual activity increased. Subjects' partners also reported greater frequency of intercourse, higher levels of arousal during intercourse, and improved satisfaction after sexual activity. Couples were also reported to engage in regular noncoital sexual activity without using the injection and to be less intercourse focused. The 35% attrition rate indicated that intracavernous self-injection is not the treatment of choice for all impotent patients.

Althof et al. (1991) reported an evaluation of the procedure at 1, 3, 6 and 12 months after its application to 42 men, 28 of whom were in committed relationships; twenty-six female partners participated in the study. The improvement in quality of erections with foreplay and intercourse, sexual satisfaction, frequency of intercourse, and coital orgasm reported at one month persisted throughout the investigation, although sexual desire, which increased at 1 month, returned to baseline level. Partners also reported increases in sexual satisfaction, sexual arousal, frequency of coital orgasm, and intercourse that were sustained over the year. Use of the injection declined from 6.2 times monthly at 1 month, to 4.5 times monthly at 1 year. However, Althof et al. stated that some men resented the biweekly limitation on the frequency of injection. Some clinicians, particularly those using prostaglandin E1, allow triweekly or daily use. Increasing number of men attempted sexual activity without self-injection over the year, although their erections were generally not sufficiently firm to accomplish penetration. Sixty percent of men who were referred for or began self-injection either declined or discontinued treatment, a figure comparable to that reported by other researchers (Irwin & Kata, 1994). Althof et al. (1991) expressed surprise at such poor patient acceptance of an efficacious and relatively safe procedure. It was pointed out, however, that some subjects could not afford the cost of approximately $100 per month. Irwin and Kata considered that 34 of the 76 patients who opted not to initiate, or who discontinued the treatment in their study of its use in 110 men, did so because of loss of interest in sexual activity. With regard to the chemical employed, prostaglandin E1 has been reported to produce a better erectile response (Siraj, Bomanji, & Akhtar, 1990) and a much lower rate of prolonged erection (Meuleman et al., 1992) than papaverine. Pain at the injection site or during erection was the most frequent side effect, occurring in 17% of subjects according to a review by Linet and Neff (1994).

An alternative to intracavernous self-injection is use of a vacuum constriction device (VCD). This consists of an acrylic tube that the subject places over his penis and presses against his body to produce an airtight seal. He then evacuates air from the tube using an attached vacuum pump. The resulting erection is maintained by transferring an elastic band from the base of the acrylic tube to the base of the penis, and the tube is then removed. Subjects are instructed not to leave the band on for more than 30 minutes, and it has loops attached to facilitate its removal. Some subjects have difficulty learning to establish the essential airtight seal, complain that the procedure produces pain or numbness in the penis, and find it unacceptable because its use cannot be concealed from the partner. Turner et al. (1991) reported a 12-month follow-up of 45 men who used this approach. Of the men, 6 ceased because the erections produced were of insufficient rigidity, 2 because of relationship difficulties, and 1 recovered. Two-thirds of the 36 men who continued to use the VCD were in steady heterosexual relationships; sixteen were diagnosed as having organic, 8 psychogenic, 11 mixed, and 1 ideopathic erectile disorder. Twenty-one partners participated in the study. Usage rates began at 6.6/month, declined to 4.5/month, and resulted in erection sufficient for intercourse on about 80% of occasions. The most frequent side effects were blocked ejaculation in 40% and discomfort in 33% of patients. In couples who are trying to conceive, blockage of ejaculation can often be remedied by loosening the tension of the ring at the point of ejaculation. Some subjects complained of the 30-minute time limit of use. However, Turner et al. pointed out that the VCD can be used again after the tension ring has been removed for a few minutes, and there are no limits on the frequency of its use. Improvements in quality of erections and sexual satisfaction were the most marked responses reported by patients; subjective sexual desire and frequency of intercourse increased at 1 month but then returned to baseline. Spontaneous erections during foreplay and attempts at intercourse improved significantly, but remained insufficient for adequate penetration. Partners reported improved arousal during intercourse attempts and frequency of orgasm during intercourse, with the strongest effect being increased sexual satisfaction. Single men often felt uncomfortable using the VCD with a new partner, because unlike self-injection, they could not conceal its use. Althof, Turner, Levine, Bodner, and Resnick (1992) reported that partners reported equally good responses to both procedures when assessed at five periods over a year. They felt more at ease in their relationships and characterized sex as more leisurely, relaxed, and assured. Their negative reactions focused on the lack of spontaneity and hesitation about initiating sex.

Turner et al. (1991) indicated that the dropout rate of only 20% over a year's use of the VCD compared very favorably with that following self-injection. However, it is not clear that the comparison was appropriate. Blackard, Borkon, Lima, and Nelson (1993) reported that 45 of 47 men who were recommended use of the VCD for venogenic erectile disorder responded to a mailed questionnaire. Twenty-nine had purchased the VCD and 20 (42%) reported a satisfactory result. Segenreich, Shmuely, Israilov, Raz, and Servadio (1993) tested the VCD on 150 men with erectile dysfunction of organic or psychogenic origin; 113 (75%) achieved an adequate erection. Yet, only 72 (48%) agreed to buy a VCD, and at 3-months to 5½-years follow-up, 65 (43%) were using it regularly and reported satisfying intercourse at least every 2 weeks. If the attrition rates from the total group to whom the VCD was recommended or on whom it was tested are considered equivalent to the rates from the total group of men who participated in self-injection programs, the rates appear compatible.

Men with erectile disorder who do not accept or respond satisfactorily to intracavernous injections, or use of the VCD, may agree to the penile implantation of a prosthesis. This can be a semirigid silastic rod that increases penile rigidity but not its size, or a device that can be inflated by the subject using a pump placed in the scrotum. Steege, Stout, and Carson (1986) concluded that about one-fourth of recipients had significant dissatisfaction with the procedure, complaining of alterations in penile dimensions or in sensations during arousal or ejaculation. There were no significant differences in relation to the type of implant, and 90% of patients would have the procedure again if confronted with the same therapeutic choices. Steege et al. cited a report in which 31 of 60 men who received semirigid implants allowed their female partners to be interviewed. Less than half the women were totally satisfied with the results of the operation. Their complaints included dyspareunia, the partner's hypersexuality, and the decreased size and rigidity of his penis postoperatively. Fifty percent of partners of men who received the operation privately reported total satisfaction, compared to 33% of partners of men who received it at Veterans Administration (VA) hospitals. Sixty percent of partners of those treated privately, and 20% of those treated by the VA had preoperative consultations with the surgeons. It was suggested that this participation by the partner in the decision-making process may have produced the more favorable response. Schover (1989) was critical of reports of favorable outcomes following penile implants, arguing that (1) there was considerable potential for distorted recall of presurgical sexual functions; (2) the measures of satisfaction employed in these reports, such as questions about whether the men would undergo surgery now, were usually those most responsive to cognitive dissonance; and (3) clinicians who took part in reported research generally worked in an academic setting and tended to be the most sophisticated (not only in regard to their surgical skills) in comparison to colleagues whose results were not investigated. The last criticism could be directed at outcome studies of most therapies.

Some men with situational erectile disorder who seek a nonpsychological cure and resist cognitive–behavioral therapy accept it when the alternatives of self-injection, VCD, or penile implants are discussed. This is also true of some men in whom organic factors are contributing significantly to their erectile disorder. Rather than attempt one of these procedures, they accept a behavioral approach on the basis that it might enable them and their partners to enjoy sexual activity even if they did not develop full and rigid erections. Improved communication may lead to their attempting, for the first time, to achieve coitus by "penile stuffing," manipulating the semierect penis into the vagina, where it may become more rigid. This procedure is sometimes easier if the man lies in the supine position.

As with sexual dysfunctions in men, those in women may require adjustment of medications, discouragement of high alcohol intake, or use of tobacco or other substances, and encouragement to increase physical fitness. There is disagreement concerning the nature of hormonal therapy required to reverse the psychological, somatic, and vasomotor symptoms, including hot flashes, as well as reduction or loss of sexual interest and responsiveness in women following menopause or oophorectomy. Dennerstein and Burrows (1982) found estrogen administration alone produced significant reversal compared to placebo. Sherwin and colleagues (Sherwin & Gelfand, 1987; Sherwin, Gelfand, & Brender, 1985) concluded that a combination of androgen and estrogen was required. In the studies by Sherwin et al., the positive effects produced by the two hormones were associated with above-normal levels of androgen, resulting in the longer term in mild hirsutism in about one-fifth of the women treated. The increased sexual interest reported may have been secondary to hypertrophy and increased sensitivity of the clitoris produced by the abnormally high androgen levels. Adamopoulos, Kampyli, Georgiacodis, Kapolla, and Abrahamian-Michalakis (1988) pointed out that the generally accepted concept that androgen was a libido hormone in women was based on early uncontrolled reports that female cancer patients experienced no change in sexuality following oophorectomy. However, they experienced a severe decline after adrenalectomy, with its associated loss of the androgens produced by the adrenal glands. The effects of the marked physical and psychological effects of this major surgical procedure would need to be excluded before the decline could be attributed to its hormonal effects (Donovan, 1985). Adamopoulos et al. (1988) compared the sexual activity of 38 women with hirsutism due to high androgen levels and a control group of age-matched, nonhirsute women. Prior to treatment, the hirsute women with partners reported a higher rate of masturbation and a lower rate of coitus compared to controls; the frequencies of the combined activities of the two groups did not differ. After 6 months of chemical reduction of the treated subjects' total and free testosterone levels, combined with estrogen to maintain their menstrual periods, the resultant reduction of their hirsutism was not accompanied by any reduction in their total sexual outlets. However, their frequency of coitus rose and rate of masturbation fell. The major rise in frequency of coitus was between 2 and 6 months following treatment. Consequently, Adamopoulos et al. concluded that this alteration in type of sexual outlet was unlikely to be due to the endocrine changes because these had occurred prior to 2 months. Rather, they attributed it to psychosocial factors, such as improved self-image or attractiveness.

Although some women taking oral contraceptives report reduced libido and ability to orgasm, others state their sexual interest and enjoyment is increased; there appears to be no agreement among researchers as to whether these effects are induced hormonally or psychologically. As discussed earlier, there are markedly conflicting findings concerning the nature and degree of direct influences of hormones on the sexual interest and activity of women as compared with that of men. These data suggest that, in women, their influences are much weaker and that psychological and social factors are more important (Mc-

Conaghy, 1993). The lack of evidence of involvement of sex hormones in the common sexual dysfunctions of premenopausal women is consistent with this conclusion. Similarly, there is no convincing evidence of the value of increasing women's androgen levels in the treatment of hypoactive sexual desire.

Flowcharts in Figures 10.1 and 10.2 summarize the assessment and direct desensitization treatment of women and men with the common sexual dysfunctions.

MAINTENANCE AND GENERALIZATION STRATEGIES

An underlying assumption of cognitive–behavioral approaches in the treatment of sexual dysfunctions is that they will result in the subjects learning strategies that will maintain any improvement and which they will utilize if further problems arise. Improved communication during sexual activity should minimize the difficulties identified by Frank et al. (1978), such as the partner choosing an inconvenient time, or not using appropriate foreplay, which correlated more highly with couples' lack of sexual satisfaction than did sexual dysfunctions. Readiness to relinquish emotional control, once learned, could be expected to be maintained, as should awareness of the importance of avoiding pressure to become sexually aroused. Evidence of post-treatment utilization of strategies has rarely been sought, but was reported by Hawton et al. (1986). They followed 106 (76%) of 140 couples who received modified Masters and Johnson therapy for 1 to 6 years posttreatment. At follow-up, recurrence or continuing difficulty with the presenting problem was reported by 64 (75%) of the 86 couples whose relationships were still intact. This had caused little or no concern for 22 couples, and almost half of those who experienced a major recurrence were able to overcome this to a large extent or entirely. Subjects' answers as to how they coped with further difficulties indicated that discussing them with the partner, practicing the techniques acquired during therapy, accepting that difficulties were likely to recur, and reading a book about sexuality were commonly used and effective coping strategies. By contrast, ignoring the problem, simply ceasing to have sex, and pretending the problem was not happening, were relatively ineffective. Only 11 couples sought further help for the original sexual problem. Nine couples reported that a new sexual problem had occurred since the end of therapy. Relapse at follow-up was most common for premature ejaculation in men and impaired sexual interest in women. A little over half of both the men and women reported they were very or moderately happy with their sexual relationship. Significant improvement in the couples' general relationship was found at termination of therapy and was still present at follow-up. Hawton et al. considered that this may have been due to their improved communications.

In view of the frequency with which recurrence or continuing difficulty of sexual problems were noted by Hawton et al. following termination of therapy, it would seem necessary to discuss the likelihood of these occurrences with patients prior to termination, and to recommend the use of the strategies identified in the study as effective.

PROBLEMS IN IMPLEMENTATION

As discussed earlier, the consistent finding of evaluations of therapy of couples with sexual problems is that improvement in their general relationship, which appears to be brought about at least in part by improvement in communication, is the strongest determi-

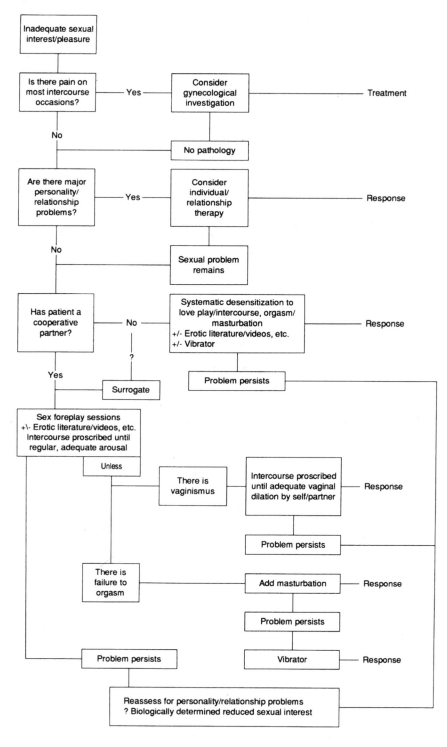

Figure 10.1. Management of sexual dysfunction in women.

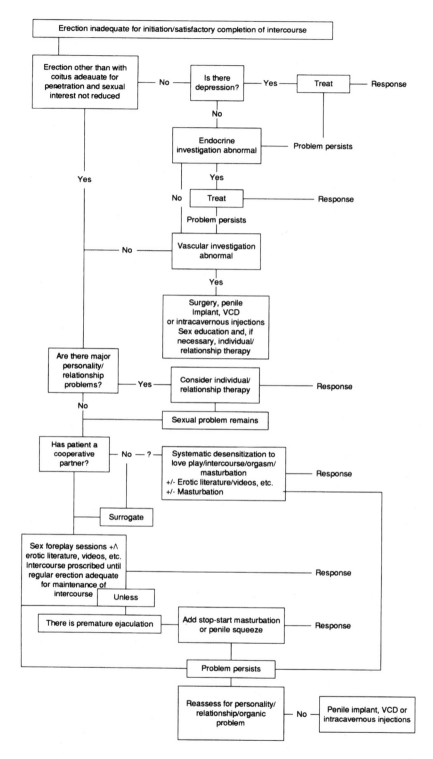

Figure 10.2. Management of common sexual dysfunction in men.

nant of increased sexual satisfaction. Conversely, a hostile relationship with the partner has regularly been found to predict a poor response (Snyder & Berg, 1983; Takefman & Brender, 1984). Therefore, to adequately assess and have the opportunity to maximize improvement in the couple's relationship if only one partner presents for treatment, the therapist must make every effort to interview the other and involve him or her in the treatment program. Inability to achieve this goal is probably the most common problem in implementing treatment. Women are more likely to report that the partner does not wish to be involved; men may be unwilling to involve their partners because they do not want them to know they are seeking treatment, or because they have an additional partner whom they also do not want to involve. Men who feel their masculinity is threatened by their erectile disorder, and who seek a physical solution, are most likely to refuse either to involve their partners or to cooperate with psychological therapy if this is indicated. They are often willing to use intracavernous self-injection or to seek a penile prosthesis, while giving minimal or no information to their partner. At times, they strongly believe that the expected improvement in their sexual ability will transform a relationship that from their account is virtually unsalvageable.

Significant personality problems in one partner or the patient without a partner are other common problems in implementation of therapy. Subjects with borderline personalities, if members of a couple, are likely to sabotage the treatment program, for example, by reporting a variety of reasons for failure to implement homework activities. In those without a partner, after an initial "honeymoon" period when they appear to respond markedly and express excessive gratitude, relapse is usually followed by requests for more time and attention, possibly outside of the therapist's usual working hours. To reduce the likelihood that this second stage will become threatening, inexperienced therapists must avoid initial overinvolvement in response to the patients' flattery. If they decide to accept borderline patients for treatment, therapists should immediately inform them that they will continue to see them for as long as is necessary and define the limits of the amount of time they can provide. In this way, they can ensure that they can maintain the time they give in the initial stage of treatment and will not be forced to reject patients after the "honeymoon period" because they cannot cope with their demands. In view of the disturbingly high frequency with which therapists are reported to become sexually involved with patients, it is important that the therapist is aware that this response, which will totally undermine the aims of therapy, is most likely to be reported by patients with borderline personalities (Gutheil, 1989).

When treating patients with dependent personalities, as with borderline patients, therapists need to guard against the possibility of responding initially with excessive concern and later with rejection. It is necessary to accept that progress is likely to be slow and limited. The partners of patients with dependent personality are typically supportive or controlling in personality and consciously or unconsciously prefer relationships with dependent persons. Therefore, they too may resist the therapist's attempts to change the nature of the patients' dependent relationships, which their sexual dysfunction may be helping to maintain. The therapist must be sufficiently supportive to engage these patients while encouraging the maximum independence of which they are capable. Activities need to be discovered that they are likely to enjoy, but that require some independence. These activities are used to reinforce behavioral changes the therapist is attempting to produce. The partners need to be encouraged to gradually cease reinforcing the patients' illness behaviors and to begin reinforcing their healthy behaviors with encouragement and praise. In patients with vaginismus and dependent personalities, the therapist needs to remain alert to the possibility that fear of the pain of childbirth or of the responsibility of childrearing can be an important factor inhibiting response to treatment.

Psychotic symptoms that have not responded completely to therapy, such as impaired insight or delusional beliefs, often prove major obstacles to the implementation of therapy, as do the hopelessness and negativity of prolonged depression. In their follow-up study, Hawton et al (1986) found a history of psychiatric disorder, particularly in the female partner, to be the major pretreatment predictor of poor outcome at 1- to 5-year follow-ups.

Lack of willingness to consider alternative viewpoints and rigid adherence to beliefs, so that patients are not receptive to cognitive correction, are other significant obstacles to implementation of therapy. This rigidity sometimes results from a degree of intellectual impairment. LoPiccolo (1992) felt that unwillingness by either partner to consider the woman's orgasm reached by manual, oral, or electric vibrator stimulation to provide full sexual satisfaction was a poor prognostic indicator for psychotherapy of erectile failure. Other cognitions that can impede progress include stereotyped views of male and female roles (e.g., husband's belief that it is a wife's duty to respond to her husband's demands for sex in return for his financial contribution to the family), the belief by male and/or female partners that it is unfeminine for a woman to make sexual approaches, or that manual penile or clitoral stimulation by themselves or partners is unacceptable as part of their sexual activities, or the belief that psychological factors are irrelevant to their condition.

CASE ILLUSTRATION

Mr. Peter F. was a 30-year-old male who was referred by a urologist to whom he had presented with a complaint of lack of sexual interest. He was planning to marry in 5 months. The only risk factors reported by the urologist were that he had previously been on steroids and had insulin-dependent diabetes. On examination there were no abnormalities in the genitourinary, vascular, endocrine, or neurological systems. His prolactin, free and bound testosterone, and sex hormone binding globulin were all reported as within normal limits. Mr. F. was a well-built man who currently worked as a bouncer in a nightclub, a position he had held for 3 years. When he began, he was a middleweight boxer weighing 160 lbs. and he said that his slight build did not sufficiently impress clients he asked to leave; therefore, he had to use force on them, which he did not like to do. He took steroids at that time to increase his weight to 185 lbs. However, he related that his loss of sexual interest occurred prior to his taking steroids, and he had not taken any in the preceding 6 months. His diabetes had been detected 10 years ago, but was well controlled by parenteral insulin.

He dated the onset of his problem to 8 years previously, when he was living with a girl to whom he was very attracted. However, he found himself avoiding sexual activity by doing such things as checking the lights to slow up going to bed. He sought counseling, in the course of which he decided "this girl wasn't the one for me" and that he felt intimidated by her. Since then, he had only casual relationships until he met his current girlfriend 3 years ago. He felt that they were both in love and very compatible. They were not living together, but began regular sexual activity soon after the relationship began. He began to notice the same problem of avoiding intercourse 3 or 4 months previously. Asked about the relationship prior to that, he responded that if the problem was there previously, he tried to ignore it. Initially, they were having intercourse once a week or more frequently; then it became weekly, on a Sunday afternoon. He added that it was "very regimented ... no spontaneity." Asked if he had any difficulty getting or maintaining an erection, he said that he did not, but that he had a lot of trouble finishing. With regard to foreplay activities, he said that they were satisfactory, but that "it was up to me to start it," and in relation to oral–genital sex that "she doesn't do it very often." He then repeated, "I'm always worried that I'll not be able to finish … it's on my mind." He added that lately they had not been having sex, only two or three times in the last 3 months, and that he had explained to her how he was feeling. When they last had sex and she had reached a climax, he realized "15 minutes down the line it's not going to finish." Prior to that he said that at times he had faked it, after keeping going and continuing past the time when she would prefer him to stop.

He was continuing to masturbate about once a week, which he said was the frequency of masturbation during periods when he had not been having intercourse. He never had difficulty coming with masturbation; it would take only a couple of minutes. His masturbatory fantasies were usually of coitus and sometimes anal intercourse with girls in magazines. When I said, "Not your girlfriend?" he replied, "No, because I can have sex with her." Asked if he had ever masturbated in her presence, he said "I couldn't … I'd feel ridiculous." They had had anal intercourse a couple of times, and he had come more rapidly; "it was more exciting, as something new … taboo."

He began intercourse at age 17 with a girlfriend of the same age, and the relationship continued for 2 years. They had intercourse several times a week if possible, and it did not decrease in frequency. From the age of 19 to 23 he had brief relationships with fairly frequent intercourse. The relationship then started with the woman with whom he first became aware of a fear of difficulty in reaching a climax. With regard to drug use, he said he had used amphetamines and some LSD in his early 20s, but that this had ceased prior to the relationship. He developed diabetes at the age of 21 or 22, which produced marked sickness with weight loss, constant urination and thirst, and blurring of vision. Since then, he had taken insulin by injection four times daily and consistently monitored his response, adding, "I pride myself to have very good control." He said he had taken a couple of courses of steroids in the last year, but stopped 4 months ago. (Earlier he had related that he had not taken any in the last 6 months.) Initially, he became aggressive on the steroids; however, when he realized this, he was able to control the aggression. He did not drink alcohol regularly or smoke tobacco, and used marihuana about three times a week, but not heavily.

He was the youngest of three siblings and said he had a happy childhood, although he was not close to any family members, saying it was a family that never touched. His mother left the family when he was 17, and he added, "I don't like her." He did not enjoy school— "the idea of having to be there"—and left at age 16 after an average academic performance. He had mixed well at school but was involved in some fighting and truancy. He played soccer initially, but "Mum made us stop—no more team sport till school grades improved." He continued boxing and surfing. After leaving school, he became an apprentice upholsterer, taking 5 years and seven jobs to complete the apprenticeship. He continues to work in this capacity 3 days a week from 8:00 A.M. to 4:30 P.M. He works as a bouncer four nights a week until 3 or 4 A.M. He goes to the gym fairly regularly. Asked if he gets sufficient sleep, he said he sleeps a lot. After he left school, he played bass in a band, but no longer does so. He continued to live with his father until the age of 18, when he moved to the inner city until moving into his grandfather's house at the age of 26, following the latter's death.

Asked about what he enjoys in life, he did not appear to be looking forward to any particular experiences, but said, "Life could be better." Asked in what way, he responded that he could maintain his house better and he did not manage money well; he earned but did not keep it, spending it on day-to-day living, and added "It scares me." Nevertheless, he is purchasing his grandfather's house and he and his girlfriend, who worked as a secretary, were saving money for their wedding in 5 months and were on target for the expenses they had calculated, including those of an overseas honeymoon. He then said spontaneously, "If I wasn't so lazy." When asked if this was related to the diabetes, he said that he has always been lazy; he never has a spare couple of hours to do things, and he prefers to sleep.

My impression was that Mr. F. was significantly self-critical, which could be related to a temporary depressive mood or reflect an aspect of his personality, either possibility being consistent with his failure to report future enjoyable activities. His immediate problem of anxiety concerning retarded ejaculation seemed consistent with this self-critical attitude as reflecting a failure to meet the expectation of his partner. It could also express his dissatisfaction with the regimented nature of their sexual activities. His resentment of school and the variety of jobs he chose were consistent with this dislike of regimentation. My initial treatment plan, therefore, focused on relief of the retarded ejaculation in the context of increasing his ability to enjoy experiences both sexual and nonsexual. I terminated the interview by asking if his fiancé would be prepared to attend the next session with him so that we could discuss the treatment plan jointly. He was confident that she would agree, and he gave permission for me to reveal to her that his retarded climax was evident in their joint sexual activity, but not in masturbation.

Mr. F.'s fiancé, Ms. Jane S., an attractive 26-year-old woman, attended the next interview with him and they both agreed that I could initially interview her alone. She was aware that Mr. F. was slow to reach climax in intercourse, but considered that it was his distress over this being a major problem to her, since the slowness did not significantly affect her enjoyment of their sexual activity. She felt deeply in love with Mr. F., was totally committed to their ensuing marriage, and expressed her willingness to cooperate fully in any treatment to improve their sexual relationship. She had usually reached a climax in coitus, without manual stimulation of the clitoris, following their foreplay activities, which used to take about 20 minutes and rarely involved oral–genital or anal stimulation. Since Mr. F. had told her he was concerned about the difficulty he was experiencing reaching climax, they had only attempted coitus rarely; and on these occasions, foreplay had been briefer and more restricted. Asked if she had any difficulties or distressing experiences in her sexual activities prior to meeting Mr. F., she said she had not. These activities had been limited to three relationships in all of which she was strongly emotionally involved. They had lasted for a year or more, and had terminated nontraumatically when she and the partner considered they were not suitably matched. She had been able to climax with coitus alone soon after starting this activity in the first relationship when she was 20 years of age.

When interviewed together, Mr. F. and Ms. S. showed a warm, supportive relationship, both in their verbal and nonverbal interactions, with no obvious ambivalence. I proceeded to report my assessment that the major problem was Mr. F.'s anxiety about his difficulty in reaching climax in their sexual activity and that this appeared to date back to an earlier relationship. I pointed out that diabetes could be associated with some difficulties in sexual activity, but in relation to his problem, it was unlikely to be even a minor factor, as the problem did not occur when he masturbated. I took the opportunity to point out that although most married men continued to masturbate alone occasionally, Mr. F. appeared to feel some embarrassment about the behavior, and had said to me that he would feel ridiculous if he masturbated during their sexual activity together. I then said, "It is important that we deal with this issue as if you could masturbate during your sexual activity, Peter;

this could give us valuable information about the cause of the problem. In fact, it might be almost essential in the treatment. I'm sure, in any case, it would speed it up. The reason I think this is because the delay only occurs when you are with Jane, so it must be feelings about climaxing with her that are causing it. These feelings could be a concern that the delay is going to occur and this will be unpleasant for Jane, or a sense that you are failing to reach your standard of how sex should be; probably both of these are factors. However, in my experience with other patients who have difficulty coming, a common cause seemed to be that they found it difficult to express strong emotion, particularly emotion which could involve a feeling of surrendering or losing control in front of another person, even someone with whom they were in love and whom they fully trusted. This seems to have been more the case when they grew up in a family which didn't appear to approve of or feel comfortable with showing emotion. I remember you told me, Peter, that yours was a family that never touched and also that you would feel ridiculous masturbating in front of Jane; maybe you have something of the same feeling having a climax in front of her."

Mr. S. said that this was possible, but that he did not think he felt this way when they began sexual activity. Also, he did not then seem to have any difficulty coming, or only a little. I said that perhaps with time, as his feelings for her deepened, his concern about how she felt or the fear of losing control in front of her became stronger. I also took the opportunity his comment offered to introduce the subject of the variety of their sexual activities together, and said, "An additional factor, of course, in the early stages of a relationship is that everything is novel, and most people find novelty exciting. In some ways, this is the most sexually exciting stage and often people have most frequent sexual activity at this time. So it could have been that your sexual excitement when your started having intercourse overcame some of these other feelings. As this novelty excitement subsided, these feelings would have become relatively stronger and so started to produce the delay in your reaching a climax. If this was the case, of course, as the delay became more obvious, you would start to worry about it more, and this would cause it to become greater. Since from my experience, this seems the most likely explanation, I would like to plan the treatment on this basis, if you are prepared to try it. If it doesn't work, the information we get from it should allow us to plan a better one. So initially we will work on reducing your anxiety, Peter, about your delay in reaching a climax, and perhaps try and increase the range of your and Jane's foreplay activities to bring back some element of novelty."

As I intended to use a modified Masters and Johnson approach, I asked them how they could plan their activities to have some periods in the week together that would include an hour when they were not under pressure to do anything else and could devote time to sexual activities. Taking into account their work commitments and their need to maintain their incomes, they felt that they could make two periods available weekly. I then instructed them that initially, to overcome any pressure on Peter to feel he had to climax rapidly, they were not to attempt intercourse. Also, to see if there were foreplay activities one could enjoy of which the other was unaware, they were to concentrate on sensual enjoyment, rather than on sexual arousal. For this purpose, one was to be passive and instruct the other how and where to kiss or massage him or her for half the period, and then they were to reverse roles. Massage oil might be useful in adding to their enjoyment. To maintain the emphasis on the sensuous rather than the sexual, they were not to touch each other's genitals or Jane's breasts until I saw them again. Although I did not specifically prohibit it, I did not suggest that if at the end of the period either felt strongly sexually aroused and wished to climax they could do so in the other's presence by oral or manual genital stimulation. I thought that some degree of frustration could be helpful in increasing their motivation to achieve orgasm at a later stage.

I then made the additional point that, in my interview with Peter, I had gained the impression that he was limiting his life somewhat to work demands at the expense of enjoyment of other activities and that this could mean that he was operating at a mild level of depression that could be a further factor in reducing his ability to fully enjoy and become aroused in sexual activity. I asked if they could consider this and try to plan their lives so that they increased the number of enjoyable activities they carried out, preferably together. In view of Peter's earlier interest in music, I suggested perhaps going to hear bands might be an enjoyable activity, and asked Jane to suggest activities she felt they would enjoy also. I then asked to see them again in about 3 weeks, to assess their response.

In the following session, they reported that they had only been able to carry out the suggested homework on three occasions, due to occupational and social demands, and tiredness. I have become used to this form of apparent resistance by patients in relation to homework assignments. I stated that I commonly found that couples had such difficulties initially in making time for the treatment activities, but that their progress would be expedited if they could carry them out more frequently. On the positive side, they reported that they enjoyed the activities they had carried out and felt they had expanded their knowledge of how to please each other. They had also taken up the suggestion of going to hear a band. In addition, they had selected videos together that they both enjoyed watching and had decided to plan to eat out together every few weeks. I reinforced these changes by positive comments and then asked them to continue the homework activities, extending them to include genital and breast stimulation. I also gave them permission to reach climax by manual or oral stimulation toward the end of the activities. I added that Peter was likely to feel some anxiety concerning this, and if he did and experienced some difficulty coming when Jane masturbated him, it would be very helpful if after about 5 minutes he took over and masturbated himself. If he did not reach climax within about 5 minutes and felt uncomfortable about continuing, he was to stop; however, he was to continue to make similar attempts when he felt sexually aroused after future homework sessions. I explained that with repeated attempts, and provided that the anxiety about delay was not great, it would diminish with repetition. I then asked to see them after 4 weeks.

On their next visit they reported that they had been able to carry out the sexual activities twice weekly. When they initially had attempted to reach orgasm by manual stimulation, Jane said that she had experienced some difficulty, but had done so by a combination of oral and manual stimulation from Peter. Peter said that, initially, he had ceased attempting to reach climax after about 10 minutes, but had enjoyed Jane's manual and oral stimulation of his penis, had been able to masturbate himself in her presence, and that his anxiety about delay had not been strong. After a few weeks, he started reaching a climax within 10 minutes and felt that his anxiety was continuing to lessen. They were planning and carrying out more enjoyable activities together in their social life. I instructed them to continue their homework activities and asked if they thought they would benefit from watching an erotic video prior to initiating, or during, the activity on some occasions. They expressed some reluctance, stating that they felt it was not necessary and that they were not sure that they would be comfortable doing so. I pointed out that this might reflect a lack of comfort in experiencing and expressing sexual arousal in the other's presence, but that they should certainly follow their own feelings while they were continuing to progress.

When I saw them after 4 weeks, they reported that the improvement they had noted previously was continuing, and Peter was reaching a climax without any feeling of difficulty. They were now confident that they would overcome the problem and were looking forward to their wedding, which was in 6 weeks. I suggested that they now include coitus as part of their sexual activity, but not to attempt to reach orgasm using it, and to return to manual and oral stimulation after a few minutes or if they felt the approach of orgasm. In relation to any subsequent oral stimulation of Peter's penis, Jane said she thought she would have no negative feelings toward the taste of her vaginal secretions, but would use a towel to remove them from Peter's penis if she did.

Three weeks later, they reported that they had carried out these activities and were continuing to feel positive and were enjoying them. They were also enjoying their general life activities more. I then said it was satisfactory for them to proceed to reach orgasm by coitus if they felt this was occurring spontaneously, but not if either partner felt they were making an effort to climax. In the latter case, they were to point this out, cease coitus, and return to manual and oral genital stimulation. When seen 2 weeks later just prior to their wedding, Peter reported he had started to feel pressured to reach orgasm during coitus and had not done so, but Jane had on a few occasions. Following the wedding, they were to have a month-long honeymoon in Bali, so that they would have ample time for nonpressured sexual activities. They were not planning to have a child in the near future, and Jane would continue to use oral contraception. I questioned them as to how they would feel about Peter inserting his penis into Jane's vagina when he was about to ejaculate following manual stimulation. The felt that this would be satisfactory. I suggested they do this on some occasions, as men with delayed ejaculation frequently seemed to have some block about ejaculating in the vagina, and this procedure would help if this was a factor in Peter's case. After their return to Australia, Jane and Peter reported they had successfully carried out this further activity after a few attempts in which Peter had experienced inability to reach orgasm. They realized that his inability was due to anxiety about this new experience. And by agreeing not to attempt it on some occasions, they found that the anxiety diminished until Peter was successful first in ejaculating in Jane's vagina in this way, and then in reaching a climax in coitus without having to withdraw.

I complimented them on their increasing ability to understand the problem and to work out effective remedial strategies. I then said I would like them to take further charge of their sexual interactions, with either being prepared to request them, but also to accept that at times the other would not be sufficiently interested. If Peter felt difficulty in reaching orgasm during coitus, he should let Jane know, and they were to decide whether he would continue until she reached a climax or withdraw beforehand and both could climax with manual and oral stimulation. When I saw them 6 weeks later, Peter said he had experienced concern about reaching orgasm on a few occasions, but not sufficiently to withdraw, and I emphasized that if this continued he should withdraw on some occasions, if only to maintain his ability to feel comfortable about doing so. I also pointed out that it was important that they not begin to feel that their sexual activity was becoming routine or regimented, as this may have been a factor in initiating the problem. If they felt themselves or their partner was showing reduced sexual interest consistently, they should discuss this possibility and means to improve it, such as reading together one of the available books about couple's sexual activity. I repeated these instructions when I saw them 3 months and then 6 months later. On both occasions, they reported that the gains had been maintained and that Peter was not experiencing any delay in reaching a climax.

REFERENCES

Adamopoulos, D. A., Kampyli, S., Georgiacodis, F., Kapolla, N., & Abrahamian-Michalakis, A. (1988). Effects of antiandrogen–estrogen treatment on sexual and endocrine parameters in hirsute women. *Archives of Sexual Behavior, 17,* 421–429.

Adkins, E., & Jehu, D. (1985). Analysis of a treatment program for primary orgastic dysfunction. *Behaviour Research and Therapy, 23,* 119–126.

Allen, R. P., Smolev, J. K., Engel, R. M., & Brendler, C. B. (1993). Comparison of Rigiscan and formal nocturnal penile tumescence testing. *Journal of Urology, 149,* 1265–1268.

Althof, S. E., Turner, L. A., Levine, S. B., Risen, C., Bodner, D., Kursh, E. D., & Resnick, M. (1991). Sexual, psychological, and marital impact of self-injection of papaverine and phentolamine: A long-term prospective study. *Journal of Sex and Marital Therapy, 17,* 101–112.

Althof, S. E., Turner, L. A., Levine, S. B., Kursh, E. D., Bodner, D., & Resnick, M. (1992). Through the eyes of women—the sexual and psychological responses fo women to their partner's treatment with self-injection or external vacuum therapy. *Journal of Urology, 147,* 1024–1027.

Althof, S. E., Turner, L. A., Levine, S. B., Risen, C., Kursh, E. D., Bodner, D., & Resnick, M. (1987). Intracavernosal injection in the treatment of impotence: A prospective study of sexual, psychological, and marital functioning. *Journal of Sex and Marital Therapy, 13,* 155–167.

American Psychiatric Association (1980). *Diagnostic and statistical manual of mental disorders* (3rd ed.). Washington, DC: Author.

American Psychiatric Association (1987). *Diagnostic and statistical manual of mental disorders* (3rd ed., rev.) Washington, DC: Author.

American Psychiatric Association (1994). *Diagnostic and statistical manual of mental disorders* (4th ed.). Washington, DC: Author.

Apfelbaum, B. (1988). An ego-analytic perspective on desire disorders. In S. R. Leiblum & R. C. Rosen (Eds.), *Sexual desire disorders* (pp. 75–106). New York: Guilford Press.

Apfelbaum, B., & Apfelbaum, C. (1985). The ego-analytic approach to sexual apathy. In D. C. Goldberg (Ed.), *Contemporary marriage* (pp. 439–481). Homeward, IL: Dorsey Press.

Arndt, B. (1994, May 28–29). An abuse of trust. *The Weekend Australian,* 23.

Blackard, C. E., Borkon W. D., Lima, J. S., & Nelson J. (1993). Use of vacuum tumescence device for impotence secondary to venous leakage. *Urology, 41,* 225–230.

Bridges, C. F., Critelli, J. W., & Loos, V. E. (1985). Hypnotic susceptibility, inhibitory control, and orgasmic consistency. *Archives of Sexual Behavior, 14,* 373–376.

Buvat, J., Lemaire, A., Buvat-Herbaut, M., Fourlinnie, J. C., Racadot, A., & Fossati, P. (19895). Hyperprolactinemia and sexual function in men. *Hormone Research, 22,* 196–203.

Canale, D., Cilurzo, P., Giorgi, P. M., & Menchinin Favris, G. R. (1992). Transdermal therapy of erectile insufficiency. *Archivio Italiano di Urologia, Nefrologia, Andrologia, 64,* 263–266.

Conte, H. R. (1983). Development and use of self-report techniques for assessing sexual functioning: A review and critique. *Archives of Sexual Behavior, 12,* 555–576.

Davidson, J. M., Kwan, M., & Greenleaf, W. J. (1982). Hormonal replacement and sexuality in men. *Clinics in Endocrinology and Metabolism, 11,* 599–623.

De Amicis, L. A., Goldberg, D. C., LoPiccolo, J., Friedman, J., & Davies, L. (1985). Clinical follow-up of couples treated for sexual dysfunction. *Archives of Sexual Behavior, 14,* 467–489.

Dennerstein, L., & Burrows, G. D. (1982). Hormone replacement therapy and sexuality in women. *Clinics in Endocrinology and Metabolism, 11,* 661–679.

Donovan, B. T. (1985). *Hormones and human behavior.* London: Cambridge University Press.

Ertekin, C., Akyurekli, O., Gurses, A. N., & Turgut, H. (1985). The value of somatosensory-evoked potentials and bulbocavernosus reflex in patients with impotence. *Acta Neurologica Scandinavica, 71,* 48–53.

Frank, E., Anderson, B., & Rubinstein, D. (1978). Frequency of sexual dysfunction in "normal" couples. *New England Journal of Medicine, 299,* 111–115.

Gewertz, B. L., & Zarins, C. K. (1985). Vasculogenic impotence. In R. T. Segraves & H. W. Schoenberg (Eds.), *Diagnosis and treatment of erectile disturbances* (pp. 105–113). New York: Plenum Press.

Gutheil, T. G. (1989). Borderline personality disorder, boundary violations, and patient–therapist sex: Medico-legal pitfalls. *American Journal of Psychiatry, 146,* 597–602.

Hale, V. E., & Strassberg, D. S. (1990). The role of anxiety on sexual arousal. *Archives of Sexual Behavior, 19,* 569–581.

Harrison, W. M., Rabkin, J. G., & Ehrhardt, A. A. (1986). Effects of antidepressant medication on sexual function: A controlled study. *Journal of Clinical Pharmacology, 6,* 144–149.

Hatch, J. P. (1981). Psychophysiological aspects of sexual dysfunction. *Archives of Sexual Behavior, 10,* 49–64.

Hawton, K., Catalan, J., Martin, P., & Fagg, J. (1986). Long-term outcome of sex therapy. *Behaviour Research and Therapy, 24,* 655–675.

Heiman, J. R., Gladue, B. A., Roberts, C. W., & LoPiccolo, J. (1986). Historical and current factors discriminating sexually functional from sexually dysfunctional married couples. *Journal of Marital and Family Therapy, 121,* 163–174.

Hollander, E., & McCarley, A. (1992). Yohimbine treatment of sexual side effects induced by serotonin reuptake blockers. *Journal of Clinical Psychiatry, 53,* 207–209.

Hunt, M. (1974). *Sexual behavior in the 1970s.* New York: Dell.

Irwin, M. B., & Kata, E. J. (1994). High attrition rate with intracavernous injection of prostaglandin E1. *Urology, 43,* 84–87.

Jacobsen, F. M. (1992). Fluoxetine-induced sexual dysfunction and an open trial of yohimbine. *Journal of Clinical Psychiatry, 53,* 119–122.

Jensen, S. B. (1981). Diabetic sexual dysfunction: A comparative study of 160 insulin treated diabetic men and women and an age-matched control group. *Archives of Sexual Behavior, 10,* 493–504.

Johnson, A. M., Wadsworth, J., Wellings, K., Field, J., & Bradshaw, S. (1994). *Sexual attitudes and lifestyles.* Oxford: Blackwell Scientific Publications.

Jones, T. M. (1985). Hormonal considerations in the evaluation and treatment of erectile disorder. In R. T. Segraves & H. W. Schoenberg (Eds.), *Diagnosis and treatment of erectile disturbances* (pp. 115–158). New York: Plenum Press.

Karacan, I. (1978). Advances in the psychophysiological evaluation of male erectile impotence. In J. LoPiccolo & L. LoPiccolo (Eds.), *Handbook of sex therapy* (pp. 137–145). New York: Plenum Press.

Kelly, M. P., Strassberg, D. S., & Kircher, J. R. (1990). Attitudinal and experiential correlates of anorgasmia. *Archives of Sexual Behavior, 19,* 165–177.

Keogh, E. J. (1993). Androgen therapy: A powerful biological tool. *Australian Practitioner, 16,* 43–45.

Kinsey, A. C., Pomeroy, W. B., & Martin, C. E. (1948). *Sexual behavior in the human male.* Philadelphia: Saunders.

Kinsey, A. C., Pomeroy, W. B., Martin, C. E., & Gebhard, P. H. (1953). *Sexual behavior in the human female.* Philadelphia: Saunders.

Klassen, A. D., & Wilsnack, S. C. (1986). Sexual experiences and drinking among women in a U.S. national survey. *Archives of Sexual Behavior, 15,* 363–392.

Korenman, S. G., Morley, J. E., Mooradian, A. D., Davis, S. S., Kaiser, F. E., Silver, A. J., Viosca, S. P., & Garza, D. (1990). Secondary hypogonadism in older men: Its relation to impotence. *Journal of Clinical Endocrinology and Metabolism, 71,* 963–968.

Krysiewicz, S., & Mellinger, B. C. (1989). The role of imaging in the diagnostic evaluation of impotence. *American Journal of Roentgenology, 153,* 1133–1139.

Kwan, M., VanMaasdam, J., & Davidson, J. M. (1985). Effects of estrogen treatment on sexual behavior in male-to-female transsexuals: Experimental and clinical observations. *Archives of Sexual Behavior, 14,* 29–40.

Lee, B., Sikka, S. C., Randrup, E. R., Villemarette, P., Baum, N., Hower, J. F., & Hellstrom, W. J. (1993). Standardization of penile blood flow parameters in normal men using intracavernous prostaglandin E1 and visual sexual stimulation. *Journal of Urology, 149,* 49–52.

Leiblum, S., & Rosen, R. C. (1984). Alcohol and human sexual response. In D. J. Powell (Ed.), *Alcoholism and sexual dysfunction: Issues in clinical management* (pp. 1–16). New York: Haworth Press.

Linet, O. I., & Neff, L. L. (1994). Intracavernous prostaglandin E(1) in erectile dysfunction. *Clinical Investigator, 72,* 139–149.

Lobitz, W. C., & Baker, E. L., Jr. (1979). Group treatment of single males with erectile disorder. *Archives of Sexual Behavior, 8* 127–138.

LoPiccolo, J. (1978). The professionalization of sex therapy: Issues and problems. In J. LoPiccolo & L. LoPiccolo (Eds.), *Handbook of sex therapy* (pp. 511–526). New York: Plenum Press.

LoPiccolo, J. (1982). Book review. *Archives of Sexual Behavior, 11,* 273–279.

LoPiccolo, J. (1990). Sexual dysfunction. In A. S. Bellack, M. Hersen & A. E. Kazdin (Eds.), *International handbook of behavior therapy and modification* (2nd ed., pp. 547–564). New York: Plenum Press.

LoPiccolo, J. (1992). Postmodern therapy for erectile failure. In R. C. Rosen & S. R. Leiblum (Eds.), *Erectile disorders assessment and treatment* (pp. 171–197). New York: Guilford Press.

Marshall, W. L., & Barbaree, H. E. (1990). Outcome of comprehensive cognitive–behavioral treatment programs. In W. L. Marshall, D. R. Laws & H. E. Barbaree (Eds.), *Handbook of sexual assault* (pp. 363–385). New York: Plenum Press.

Masters, W. H., & Johnson. V. E. (1970). *Human sexual inadequacy.* Boston: Little, Brown.

Matarazzo, J. D. (1983). The reliability of psychiatric and psychological diagnosis. *Clinical Psychology Review, 3*, 103–145.

McConaghy, N. (1993). *Sexual behavior: Problems and management*. New York: Plenum Press.

McConaghy, N. (1994). Sexual dysfunctions and deviations. In M. Hersen and S. M. Turner (Eds.), *Diagnostic interviewing*. (2nd ed., pp. 211–239). New York: Plenum Press.

McMahon, C. G. (1994). Management of impotence. Part II: Diagnosis. *General Practitioner. CME Files, 2*, 83–85.

Mead, M. (1950). *Male and female*. London: Gollancz.

Meisler, A. W., & Carey, M. P. (1990). A critical reevaluation of nocturnal penile tumescence monitoring in the diagnosis of erectile disorder. *Journal of Nervous and Mental Disease, 178*, 78–89.

Metz, P., & Bengtsson, J. (1981). Penile blood pressure. *Scandinavian Journal of Urology and Nephrology, 15*, 161–164.

Meuleman, E. J. H., Bemelmans, B. L. H., Doesburg, W. H. van Asten, W. N. J. C., Skotnicki, S. H., & Debruyne F. M. J. (1992). Penile pharmacological duplex ultrasonography: A dose-effect study comparing papaverine, papaverine/phentolamine and prostaglandin E1. *Journal of Urology, 148*, 63–66.

Morales, A., Condra, M., Owen, J. A., Surridge, D. H., Fenemore, J., & Harris, C. (1987). Is yohimbine effective in the treatment of organic impotence? Results of a controlled trial. *Journal of Urology, 137*, 1168–1172.

Morrissette, D. L., Skinner, M. H., Hoffman, B. B., Levine, R. E., & Davidson, J. M. (1993). Effects of antihypertensive drugs atenolol and nifedipine on sexual function in older men: A placebo-controlled, crossover study. *Archives of Sexual Behavior, 22*, 99–109.

Nettelbladt, P., & Uddenberg, N. (1979). Sexual dysfunction and sexual satisfaction in 58 married Swedish men. *Journal of Psychosomatic Research, 23*, 141–147.

Nunez, B. D., & Anderson, D. C. (1993). Nitroglycerin ointment in the treatment of impotence. *Journal of Urology, 150*, 1241–1243.

Nutter, D. E., & Condron, M. K. (1985). Sexual fantasy and activity patterns of males with inhibited sexual desire and males with erectile dysfunction versus normal controls. *Journal of Sex and Marital Therapy, 11*, 91–98.

Palace, E. M. (in press). Modification of dysfunctional patterns of sexual response through automatic arousal and false physiolgoical feedback. *Journal of Consulting and Clinical Psychology*.

Palace, E. M., & Gorzalka, B. B. (1990). The enhancing effects of anxiety on arousal in sexually dysfunctional and functional women. *Journal of Abnormal Psychology, 99*, 403–411.

Palace, E. M., & Gorzalka, B. B. (1992). Differential patterns of arousal in sexually functional and dysfunctional women: Physiological and subjective components of sexual response. *Archives of Sexual Behavior, 21*, 135–159.

Reading, A. E. (1983). A comparison of the accuracy and reactivity of methods of monitoring male sexual behavior. *Journal of Behavioral Assessment, 5*, 11–23.

Reading, A. E., & Wiest, W. M. (1984). An analysis of self-reported sexual behavior in a sample of normal males. *Archives of Sexual Behavior, 13*, 69–83.

Reid, K., Surridge, D. H., Morales, A., Condra, M., Harris C., Owen, J., & Fenemore, J. (1987). Double-blind trial of yohimbine in treatment of psychogenic impotence. *Lancet, 2*, 421–423.

Rosen, R. C., & Ashton, A. K. (1993). Prosexual drugs: Empirical status of the "new aphrodisiacs." *Archives of Sexual Behavior, 22*, 521–543.

Rosen, R. C., & Beck, J. G. (1988). *Patterns of sexual arousal*. New York: Guilford Press.

Savion, M., Segenreich, E., Kahan, E., & Servadio, C. (1987). Pharmacologic, nonhormonal treatment of impotence. Evaluation of associated factors. *Urology, 29*, 510–512.

Saypol, D. C., Peterson, G. A., Howards, S. S., & Yazel, J. J. (1983). Impotence: Are the newer diagnostic methods a necessity. *Journal of Urology, 130*, 260–262.

Schiavi, R. C. (1992). Laboratory methods for evaluating erectile disorder. In R. C Rosen & S. R. Leiblum (Eds.), *Erectile disorders assessment and treatment* (pp. 141–170). New York: Guilford Press.

Schiavi, R. C., Derogatis, L. R., Kuriansky, J., O'Connor, D., & Sharpe, I. (1979). The assessment of sexual function and marital interaction. *Journal of Sex and Marital Therapy, 5*, 169–224.

Schiavi, R. C., Fisher, C., White, D., Beers, P., & Szechter, R. (1984). Pituitary–gonadal function during sleep in men with erectile impotence and normal controls. *Psychosomatic Medicine, 46*, 239–254.

Schiavi, R. C., Schreiner-Engel, P., Mandeli, J., Schanzer, H., & Cohen, E. (1990). Healthy aging and male sexual function. *American Journal of Psychiatry, 147*, 766–771.

Schover, L. R. (1989). Sex therapy for the penile prosthesis recipient. *Urology Clinics of North America, 16*, 91–98.

Segenreich, E., Shmuely, J., Israilov, S., Raz, D., & Servadio, C. (1993). Treatment of erectile dysfunction with vacuum constriction device. *Harefuah, 124*, 326–328.

Segraves, R. T., & Segraves, K. A. (1992). Aging and drug effects on male sexuality. In R. C Rosen & S. R. Leiblum (Eds.), *Erectile disorders assessment and treatment* (pp. 96–138). New York: Guilford Press.

Segraves, R. T., Schoenberg, H., W., Zarins, C. K., Camic, P., & Knopf, J. (1981). Characteristics of erectile disorder as a function of medical care system entry point. *Psychosomatic Medicine, 43,* 227–234.

Semans, J. H. (1956). Premature ejaculation: A new approach. *Southern Medical Journal, 49,* 373–377.

Sherwin, B. B., & Gelfand, M. M. (1987). The role of androgen in the maintenance of sexual functioning in oophorectomised women. *Psychosomatic Medicine, 49,* 397–409.

Sherwin, B. B., Gelfand, M. M., & Brender, W. (1985). Androgen enhances sexual motivation in females: A prospective, crossover study of sex steroid administration in the surgical menopause. *Psychosomatic Medicine, 47,* 339–351.

Siraj, Q. H., Bomanji, J., & Akhtar, M. A. (1990). Quantitation of pharmacologically induced penile erections: The value of radionuclide phallography in the objective evaluation of erectile haemodynamics. *Nuclear Medicine Communications, 11,* 445–458.

Slag, M. F., Morley, J. E., Elson, M. K., Trence, D. L., Nelson, C. J., Nelson, A. E., Kinlaw, W. B., Beyer, H. S., Nuttall, F. Q., & Shafer, R. B. (1983). Impotence in medical clinic outpatients. *Journal of the American Medical Association, 249,* 1736–1740.

Snyder, D. K., & Berg, P. (1983). Determinants of sexual dissatisfaction in sexually distressed couples. *Archives of Sexual Behavior, 12,* 237–246.

Spark, R. F., White, R. A., & Connolly, P. B. (1980). Impotence is not always psychogenic. *Journal of the American Medical Association, 243,* 750–755.

Steege, J. F., Stout, A. L., & Carson, C. C. (1986). Patient satisfaction in Scott and Small–Carrion penile implant recipients: A study of 52 patients. *Archives of Sexual Behavior, 15,* 393–399.

Strassberg, D. S., Mahoney, J. M., Schaugaard, M., & Hale, V. E. (1990). The role of anxiety in premature ejaculation: A psychophysiological model. *Archives of Sexual Behavior, 19,* 251–257.

Stuart, F. M., Hammond, D. C., & Pett, M. A. (1987). Inhibited sexual desire in women. *Archives of Sexual Behavior, 16,* 91–106.

Takefman, J., & Brender, W. (1984). An analysis of the effectiveness of two components in the treatment of erectile dysfunction. *Archives of Sexual Behavior, 13,* 321–340.

Thase, M. E., Reynolds, C. F. III, & Jennings, J. R. (1988). Nocturnal penile tumescence is diminished in depressed men. *Biological Psychiatry, 24,* 33–46.

Turner, L. A., Althof, S. E., Levine, S. B., Bodner, D. R., Kursh, E. D., & Resnick, M. I. (1991). External vacuum devices in the treatment of erectile dysfunction: A one-year study of sexual and psychosocial impact. *Journal of Sex and Marital Therapy, 17,* 81–93.

Walling, M., Andersen, B. L., & Johnson, S. R. (1990). Hormonal replacement therapy for postmenopausal women: A review of sexual outcomes and related gynecologic effects. *Archives of Sexual Behavior, 19,* 119–137.

Wasserman, M. D., Pollak, C. P., Spielman, A. J., & Weitzman, E. D. (1980). Theoretical and technical problems in the measurement of nocturnal penile tumescence for the differential diagnosis of impotence. *Psychosomatic Medicine, 42,* 575–585.

Weizman, R., & Hart, J. (1987). Sexual behavior in healthy married elderly men. *Archives of Sexual Behavior, 16,* 39–44.

Wincze, J. P., & Carey, M. P. (1991). *Sexual dysfunction.* New York: Guilford Press.

White, J. R., Case, D. A., McWhirter, D., & Mattison, A. M. (1990). Enhanced sexual behavior in exercising men. *Archives of Sexual Behavior, 19,* 193–209.

Wolpe, J. (1958). *Psychotherapy by reciprocal inhibition.* Stanford: Stanford University Press.

Wyatt, G. E., & Peters, S. D. (1986). Issues in the definition of child sexual abuse in prevalence research. *Child Abuse and Neglect, 10,* 231–240.

11

A Comprehensive Treatment Manual for the Management of Obesity

Michael A. Friedman and Kelly D. Brownell

INTRODUCTION

Obesity is a serious and prevalent problem (Brownell & Wadden, 1992). A recent study shows that 24% of men and 27% of women are at least 20% above desirable weight (Kuczmarski, 1992). Obesity tends to be especially prevalent among minority and low-socioeconomic-status populations (Ernst & Harlan, 1991; Sobal & Stunkard, 1989). The prevalence of obesity also increases with age, particularly among women (Williamson, Kahn, Remington, & Anda, 1990). Furthermore, when these factors come together, as in the case of African-American women ages 45 to 75 years, the prevalence rate of obesity is as high as 60% (Van Itallie, 1985).

Obesity is associated with a substantial risk to health, including hypertension, diabetes, and cardiovascular disease (Bray, 1986; Pi-Sunyer, 1991). Some studies suggest that risk can begin to increase with as little as 8% overweight (Manson et al., 1990). These effects are mediated in part by body fat distribution. Fat found in the upper body, particularly in the intra-abdominal cavity, carries greater risk than does fat stored in the lower body (Bjornthorp, 1985; Sjostrom, 1992). The health-care costs associated with obesity are approximately $40 billion yearly (Colditz, 1992).

Michael A. Friedman and Kelly D. Brownell • Yale Center for Eating and Weight Disorders, Department of Psychology, Yale University, New Haven, Connecticut 06520-7447.

Sourcebook of Psychological Treatment Manuals for Adult Disorders, edited by Vincent B. Van Hasselt and Michel Hersen. Plenum Press, New York, 1996.

CULTURAL CONTEXT OF OBESITY AND WEIGHT LOSS

Michael A. Friedman and Kelly D. Brownell

Obesity exists within a cultural context in which individuals are expected to be thin, physically fit, and to have bodies contoured in specific ways (Brownell, 1991a, 1991b; Rodin, 1992). Vast numbers of individuals are dieting, buying exercise equipment, and undergoing plastic surgery in an effort to achieve this physical ideal. The current cultural norm fostering an extremely lean aesthetic ideal is supported by a dieting industry valued at more than $30 billion per year, which supplies diet books, programs, videos, foods, pills, and devices to help individuals shape their bodies to this ideal.

The drive for the perfect body is rooted in several assumptions: that the body is infinitely malleable, that an imperfect body reflects an imperfect personality, and that the rewards of looking good are so vast as to justify enormous cost and effort (Brownell, 1991a). We exist within a culture that emphasizes that individuals are personally responsible for the state of their lives, including their health and body shape (Brownell, 1991b; Glassner, 1988). In addition, there is a psychological tendency to blame the victims of medical or physical problems to feel less vulnerable ourselves, the concept being that "People get what they deserve and deserve what they get." (Wortman & Lehman, 1985).

SOCIAL AND PSYCHOLOGICAL SUFFERING OF OBESITY

In a culture that not only condemns their physical appearance, but also blames them for their condition, obese individuals face widespread bias and discrimination (DeJong & Kleck, 1986). Obese individuals are discriminated against in employment (Allon, 1982; Larkin & Pines, 1979), housing (Karris, 1977) and college admissions (Canning & Mayer, 1966). Furthermore, obese individuals tend to be described as "lazy," "stupid," "cheats," and "ugly" (Staffieri, 1967). When considering the stigma associated with being obese, it is logical to assume that obese persons suffer emotionally.

Studies investigating the psychological correlates of obesity, which have generally compared the psychological functioning of obese and nonobese individuals, have produced inconsistent results. Some studies show that obese individuals demonstrate more psychological problems than nonobese individuals; other studies find no differences between these two groups; and still others find that obese individuals demonstrate fewer psychological problems than normal-weight individuals. These inconsistent results have led to several broad conclusions, the most important being that obesity is not associated with general psychological problems (O'Neil & Jarrell, 1992; Striegel-Moore & Rodin, 1986; Stunkard & Wadden, 1992; Wadden & Stunkard, 1985).

These early studies sought to find consistent trends across a population that we now know to be heterogeneous (Brownell & Wadden, 1992). Friedman and Brownell (1995) suggest that these studies represent a first generation of research in the area, and argue for a different approach in which a second and third generation of studies occur. Instead of studying whether obese and nonobese people differ, the search would be for factors that explain why some obese individuals suffer negative psychological consequences whereas others do not. They propose a model that would identify factors likely to place an overweight individual at risk for psychological problems, such as gender, dieting frequency, binge eating, weight cycling, and early age of onset of obesity.

Our understanding of the factors that result in obesity has changed markedly over the past 40 years. Originally, in the 1950s, psychoanalytic theorists believed that obesity was the result of a fundamental personality problem in which obese individuals acted out unconscious conflicts (Stunkard, 1988). Subsequently, behavior therapists in the 1960s argued that overeating could be explained by the principles of conditioning, and therefore concluded that obesity was a learned disorder. However, in the 1970s and 1980s, physiologists demonstrated in laboratory animals that weight was tightly regulated by a complex interaction of neural, hormonal, and metabolic factors that together maintained a body-weight set point (Keesey, 1986). Although these theoretical approaches are divergent in their conception of the etiology of obesity, they all share the common error of attempting to explain onset of obesity with a single cause.

We now know that obesity is a strikingly heterogeneous disorder with respect to etiology, and that a convergence of risk factors may contribute to its onset (Brownell & Wadden, 1992). There is now conclusive evidence indicating that there is a substantial genetic component in the maintenance of body weight (Price, 1987; Stunkard et al., 1986; Stunkard, Harris, Pederson, & McClearn, 1990). In fact, Stunkard et al. (1990) found that genetic factors accounted for 66% to 70% of the variance of the body mass index (BMI). The distribution of body fat in either the upper or lower body has also been shown to be heritable (Bouchard et al., 1990).

Furthermore, factors associated with the onset and maintenance of obesity have also been found to be heritable. Resting metabolic rate (RMR), the energy required to maintain vital bodily functions, including respiration, heart rate, and blood pressure, has been found to be highly heritable (Bouchard et al., 1989). RMR may differ by as much as 1,000 kcal a day in obese women of approximately the same age, weight, and height (Foster et al., 1988). Fat (cell number and size) has also been found to have a genetic component. Mildly obese individuals usually have normal fat cell numbers, but the cells are increased in size and weight (i.e., hypertrophy). Fat cell number apparently increases, however, once the individual doubles a normal fat mass.

High rates of obesity also appear to be partially due to decreased physical activity across the population. Daily energy expenditure has relied on agriculture, then industry, and now information. For example, from 1965 to 1977 alone, daily energy expenditure was thought to have dropped by nearly 200 kcal daily (U.S. Department of Agriculture, 1984). In addition, although the caloric intake of the population has remained the same or even decreased, there has been an increase in the consumption of dietary fat. Specifically, since 1910, the percentage of calories consumed from fat increased from 32% to as high as 43%, calories from carbohydrate declined from 57% to 46%, and calories from protein intake has remained at 11% (National Academy of Sciences, 1989).

Common wisdom holds that obesity results from overeating. This age-old explanation was attacked in the 1970s by approximately 20 studies revealing that obese individuals reported consuming no more calories than their lean counterparts (Garrow, 1974; S. C. Wooley, O. W. Wooley, & Dyrenforth, 1979). Studies using direct observation of food consumption revealed no differences between obese and nonobese subjects (Klesges, Hanson, Eck, Durff, 1988; Leibel & Hirsch, 1984). These studies were limited, however, by reliance on self-report or observation of obese persons in public places. Recent studies using more sophisticated metabolic measures, including doubly labeled water, show increased eating in overweight individuals (Lichtman et al., 1992).

CAN PEOPLE LOSE WEIGHT?

Currently, the prevailing belief among professionals is that people simply cannot lose weight or maintain weight loss over a period of time (Garner & Wooley, 1991). This conclusion is based on studies of university-based and has its roots in a paper by Stunkard published more than 30 years ago (Stunkard & McLaren-Hume, 1959). While the long-term results from contemporary clinical programs have also been disappointing (Wadden, Sternberg, Letizia, Stunkard, & Foster, 1989; Wadden, Stunkard, & Liebschutz, 1988), there are problems with interpreting these results to show that all programs fail (Brownell & Rodin, 1994).

Originally, studies of weight-loss treatments utilized only an 8-week follow-up period, and demonstrated losses of approximately 8 pounds. However, programs in the late 1970s and early 1980s consistently utilized techniques such as self-monitoring, stimulus control, and reinforcement, and produced weight losses of about 11 pounds. It was in this second generation of studies that the call for long-term follow-up became so strong (Stunkard, 1975; Wilson, 1978). In the mid-1980s, the third generation of behavioral programs began to appear. Despite the fact that many researchers were, and still are, using the package of the 1970s and were achieving the same 11-pound losses, other investigations began to show larger weight losses, most between 20 and 30 pounds.

There are several plausible reasons for the larger weight losses seen in recent studies. One is that the programs are better. The programs are longer, and from the 1970s to today, the average weight loss in behavioral programs has increased approximately in proportion to increased duration of treatment. Also, there appears to be a greater use of more highly trained group leaders (Bennett, 1986). Current programs place far greater emphasis on cognitive factors. Reinforcement techniques have been refined (Jeffery, 1987), and in some cases, social support techniques are included (Brownell, 1984). In addition, the importance of exercise is being recognized (Brownell, 1995; Brownell & Stunkard, 1980). Finally, issues such as binge eating and body image have become topics of concern, and specific attention is being focused on relapse (Brownell, Marlatt, Lichtenstein, & Wilson, 1986; Marlatt & Gordon, 1985; Perri, 1995; Perri, Nezu, & Vigener, 1992).

A related issue is that only a very small percentage of those who attempt to lose weight do so in university-based weight-loss programs. In a survey of more than 4,000 employed people in the Midwest, Jeffery, Adlis, and Forster (1991) found that 47% of the men and 75% of the women had dieted, but that only 6% of the men and 31% of the women had ever done so in an organized weight-loss program. In a population survey, Jeffery et al. (1984) reported that 6% of the men and 43% of women who were ever overweight had enrolled in a formal weight-loss program. An unknown percentage of these individuals would have enrolled in university-based clinical programs. It is unclear as to the nature or outcome of these weight-loss attempts in this group of individuals. Furthermore, there is evidence that some people do manage to lose weight and maintain their weight loss. Studies by Jeffery and Wing (1983) and Schacter (1982) have shown that 16% to 21% of men and 15% to 18% of women in selected samples were formerly overweight. These studies call into question the prevailing conclusion that it is next to impossible to lose weight or maintain weight loss.

It is not clear whether there are negative health consequences to dieting and weight loss. Few studies have examined the effects of dieting and weight loss on morbidity and mortality, and the results are inconsistent (Williamson, 1995). Furthermore, existing evidence can be questioned on methodological grounds or is difficult to interpret. Typically, the data come from large epidemiological studies in which some individuals lose weight and some do not, and then the mortality experience is compared. These studies do not take into account potentially important mediating variables, such as body-fat distribution and dieting history. Furthermore, subjects may be gaining or losing weight due to factors that themselves are related to the disease (e.g., starting and stopping smoking). The type of study necessary to address this question directly, a longitudinal study with random assignment to weight-loss and no-weight-loss groups, has not been done, and because of practical considerations, will probably never be done.

Even when ignoring methodological considerations, studies of weight loss and mortality are strikingly inconsistent in their results. Early studies suggested that weight loss was associated with unchanged or reduced mortality, as well as beneficial changes in cardiovascular risk factors (Bjornthorp & Brodoff, 1992; Dublin, 1953; Hammond & Garfinkel, 1969; Hypertension Prevention Trial Research Group, 1990). More recent studies on mortality have produced both positive and negative findings. For example, in a prospective study of 7,275 British men, there was a 10% reduction in cardiovascular mortality in individuals who lost more than 10% of their initial weight; the reduction risk was 50% for obese men (Wannamethee & Shaper, 1990). In a study with Type II diabetics, a 10-kilogram weight loss was estimated to restore 35% of the longevity lost due to diabetes (Lean, Powrie, Anderson, & Garthwaite, 1990). There are more studies, however, reporting increased mortality in individuals who lose weight (Andres, Muller, & Sorkin, 1993; Garrison & Castelli, 1985; Pamuk, Williamson, Serdula, Madans, & Byers, 1993; Wilcosky, Hyde, Anderson, Bangdiwala, & Duncan, 1990).

There has also been much concern that dieting is potentially harmful (Wilson, 1995; Wooley & Garner, 1991). Retrospective reports indicate increased depression in overweight individuals during dieting. However, when studied prospectively, dieting seems to be associated with reduced depression. Dieting may also be causally linked to eating disorders and binge eating (Blundell, 1990; Hsu, 1990; Wilson, 1995). Studies show that in many individuals, dieting precedes development of these problems, but a direct link has not been proven. It is clear, however, that dieting is not a sufficient condition, because so many more individuals have dieted than develop eating disorders (Wilson, 1995).

A related question is whether weight cycling ("yo-yo dieting") is harmful. The initial hypothesis in the study of weight cycling was that dieting would increase food efficiency so that on subsequent diets, weight loss would become progressively more difficult (Brownell, et al., 1986). This has been supported by some studies but not others, and the initial hypothesis is very much in question Brownell & Rodin, 1994b; Reed & Hill, 1993; Wing, 1992). More recent studies examining the health effects of weight fluctuation suggest that increased weight variability is associated with mortality, particularly from cardiovascular disease (Blair, Shaten, Brownell, Collins, & Lissner, 1993; Hamm, Shekelle, & Stamler, 1989; Lissner et al., 1991). Because the study of this issue is relatively new, it is still premature to draw final conclusions (Bouchard, 1991).

Collectively, this evidence indicates that dieting and weight loss do have the potential for harm, but it is unclear that this effect is consistent. Whether the mortality is caused by the weight change, whether disease causes weight loss, or whether both are related to a third factor is not known. Weight loss produces clear effects on risk factors, but the effect on morbidity and mortality is not clear, and even raises the possibility of damaging effects of weight loss. However, for overweight persons, weight loss reduces depression and appears to have other salutary effects. Hence, dieting may be harmful or beneficial depending on the individual and the conditions.

MATCHING INDIVIDUALS TO TREATMENTS

The field has made advances in treating obesity by conducting controlled studies with random assignment, parametric statistics, and a search for treatments that provide an increment in weight loss beyond the prevailing standard. Embedded in this approach is the assumption that the population being tested is homogeneous, so that random assignment is effective in establishing equivalent groups, and that a treatment found superior to another should be embraced while the alternative is discarded. However, several treatments have been proposed, and it is not clear across the obese population that any one treatment is superior (Schwartz & Brownell, 1995).

When considering the inconsistent results of studies examining the outcome and consequences of weight-loss treatment, it is possible to hypothesize that the effect is not consistent across individuals. Brownell and Wadden (1991, 1992) have argued that it is likely that different treatments will be effective for different individuals. "The challenge is no longer to conduct only parametric studies to determine if one approach is superior to another, but to develop criteria to match the needs of individuals" (Brownell & Wadden, 1992, p. 510).

Matching Scheme

Many possible approaches are available for matching individuals to treatment, yet none has been validated by experimental studies. Schwartz and Brownell (1995) have begun to identify factors that may inform treatment-matching decisions, such as degree of obesity, weight-loss history, medical profile, and level of eating and general psychopathology. A scheme proposed by Brownell and Wadden (1992) is shown in Figure 11.1. This is a conceptual approach in which three possible matching processes are integrated into a scheme in which a classification decision is made first, followed by a stepped-care decision, then a matching decision. The classification decision is based on percentage overweight and helps narrow the range of approaches that would be relevant to the individual. For instance, a person who is massively overweight would not likely respond to a self-directed program and might need something more intensive. Conversely, a person who is mildly overweight would not be appropriate for surgery.

The second level is based on a stepped-care approach. After a range of approaches has been established by the classification decision, approaches or programs may be ranked according to cost, intrusiveness, side effects (in the case of medication), risk, and other factors used to make a cost-effective judgment. As with the stepped-care treatment of hypertension, the least expensive and least distressing treatments are the first level of intervention. The third step is a matching decision based on the personal needs of the individual. Issues such as probable response to group versus individual treatments, the need

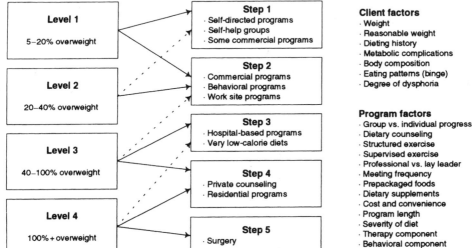

Figure 11.1. A conceptual scheme showing the three-stage process in selecting a treatment for an individual. The first step, the classification decision, divides individuals according to percentage overweight into four levels. This level dictates which of the five steps would be reasonable in the second stage, the stepped-care decision. This indicates that the least intensive, costly, and risky approach will be used from among alternative treatments. The third stage, the matching decisions, is used to make the final selection of a program, and is based on a combination of client and program variables. The dashed lines with arrows between the classification and stepped-care stages show the lowest level of treatment that may be beneficial, but more intensive treatment is usually necessary for people at the specified weight level. Reprinted by permission from Brownell and Wadden (1991).

for supervised exercise, and the degree to which the diet needs to be structured may be considered.

Thus far, very little work has been conducted on matching, so at present, specific matching criteria cannot be specified. In an attempt to determine if a consensus would exist among experts on which treatments would be most appropriate, Schwartz and Brownell (1995) conducted a survey of leaders in the obesity field. There was a diversity of responses obtained in the survey, suggesting that although a matching approach would be essential, there is little research to guide a researcher or clinician in the matching process. However, Schwartz and Brownell (1995) identified an array of factors that may be critical in the matching process (see Table 11.1).

OBESE BINGERS: A NEW CLINICAL SUBTYPE WITHIN THE OBESE POPULATION

One subgroup of obese individuals deserving special consideration when approaching treatment are binge eaters. Stunkard (1959) first described this pattern of obese individuals who ate large amounts of food accompanied by a feeling of loss of control (Stunkard, 1976). Spitzer et al. (1992) argued that this phenomenon represents a distinct disorder, binge-eating disorder (BED). In a national probability sample of U.S. women, the lifetime prevalence of BED across all weight categories was estimated to be 1.6% (Brewerton,

Table 11.1. The Five Most Frequently Cited Indicators for Different Approaches to Weight Control and the Percentage of Experts Endorsing Each Indicator[a]

1. Dieting on one's own (24)	
a. Weight status (mild-moderate)	63%
b. 1st attempt to lose weight (not a weight cycler)	42%
c. No medical complications	38%
d. History of success dieting on own	25%
e. No past or current eating disorders	25%
f. Good social support already in place	25%
2. Twelve-step program (22)	
a. Belief in addiction model; comfort with religious aspect of it	45%
b. Desire social support	41%
c. No medical complications	27%
d. Binge eating disorder	27%
e. Weight status (moderate)	14%
3. Exercise program (24)	
a. Virtually everyone should exercise, regardless of weight status	79%
b. No medical contraindications	63%
c. History of exercise	13%
d. Males	13%
e. Weight status (mild only)	8%
4. Commercial program with group support (23)	
a. Weight status: breakdown as follows:	39%

      indicate   *contraindicate*
      mild 13%   moderate–morbid 17%
      moderate 9%

b. Weight loss history (re: this approach)	35%
Have not tried this approach before 22%	
Past success using this approach 13%	
c. Desire for social support	30%
d. No medical complications	30%
e. Female	17%
5. Commercial program with food provided (24)	
a. Failed with less structured programs and has not tried this one before	33%
b. Weight status: breakdown as follows:	29%

      indicate   *contraindicate*
      mild 4%   mild 4%
      moderate 17%   moderate-morbid 13%

c. No indications/would not recommend to anyone	21%
d. Need/desire for structure	21%
e. Economic resources available	21%
6. University behavioral program (22)	
a. Weight status: breakdown as follows	41%

      indicate   *contraindicate*
      mild 9%   mild 5%
      moderate 32%   morbid 18%

b. History of failure with self-help and lay programs	27%
c. Coexisting psychological diagnosis (Axis I or II)	18%

      indicate   *contraindicate*
      5%   14%

Table 11.1. (*Continued*)

383

**Management of
Obesity**

d. Medical complications	27%
indicate *contraindicate* 9% 18%	
e. Eating disorder diagnosis	9%
7. Very-low-calorie diet (24)	
a. Weight status: moderate–morbid	67%
b. Co-morbid medical condition related to obesity	42%
c. No medical conditions to contraindicate use of VLCD	42%
d. No history of or current Axis I diagnosis	42%

Eating disorder (BED, bulimia, or anorexia) 25%
      substance abuse 4%
      depression 13%	

e. Compliance and willingness to do follow-up work	21%
f. Non-responsive to moderate calorie diets	21%
8. Private counseling (23)	
a. Axis I or II diagnosis	70%
b. Eating disorder diagnosis	22%
c. High SES	17%
d. Previously lost weight and has relapsed	8%
e. Weight status (moderate)	4%
9. Residential program (24)	
a. Weight status	46%

indicate   *contraindicate*
    mild 8%   mild 8%
    moderate 13% morbid 8%
    severe 21%	

b. Economic resources available	46%
c. Time available	29%
d. Want a "jump start" for diet and exercise	25%
e. Nonresponsive to less expensive efforts	25%
10. Medication (23)	
a. Non-responsive to behavioral and other approaches	35%
b. No medical contraindications	30%
c. Weight status (moderate-morbid)	22%
d. Realistic expectations about long-term behavior changes	17%
e. Cannot recommend (due to FDA regulations)	17%
11. Surgery (23)	
a. Weight status (massive-morbid)	74%
b. Medical condition related to obesity	43%
c. Nonresponsive to all conservative approaches	39%
d. No severe Axis I or Axis II diagnoses	35%
e. Compliance and willingness to do follow-up work	26%

[a]From Schwartz and Brownell (1995). Reprinted by permission.
The percentages represent the proportion of the expert sample endorsing a particular indicator for a specific approach to weight control. The numbers in parentheses following the type of program indicate the number of experts who listed matching criteria for that program.

Dansky, O'Neil, & Kilpatrick, 1993). However, rate of binge eating increases with increasing weight (Telch, Agras, & Rossiter, 1988). Prevalence of binge eating in obese persons in the general community is approximately 2% (Bruce & Agras, 1992; Spitzer et al., 1992). Binge eating is particularly common in obese persons seeking treatment, with 25% to 50% having this problem (Marcus, Wing, & Lamparski, 1985; Spitzer et al., 1992).

Comparisons of obese binge eaters versus obese persons who are not binge eaters began only recently, but data thus far suggest key differences. Binge eating in obese persons appears to be associated with poor response to treatment (Keefe, Wyshogrod, Weinberger, & Agras, 1984; Marcus, Wing, & Hopkins, 1988). Bingers tend to eat more than nonbingers and choose a greater percentage of calories from fat (Yanovski et al., 1992). Obese binge eaters presenting for weight-loss treatment have higher levels of psychopathology, particularly affective disorders, than do non-binge eating obese persons also seeking treatment (see Yanovski, 1993, for a review). However, studies have found no differences between BED and non-BED subjects on metabolic variables, such as blood glucose, blood lipids, and resting metabolic rate, after controlling for BMI and age (O'Neil et al., 1992). In addition, studies of body image among binge eaters have produced mixed results (Cash, 1991; Davis, Williamson, Goreczny, & Bennett, 1989).

It is our clinical impression that some binge eaters may require treatment for their disordered eating prior to or during a weight-loss program. However, no studies have tested this assumption. One fruitful area of research would be to examine progress of obese binge eaters in conventional weight-loss treatment compared to others in a program dealing with binge eating first and weight subsequently.

Several promising treatments for binge eating have been derived from work on bulimia nervosa, namely cognitive–behavioral therapy and interpersonal psychotherapy (Fairburn, Jones, Peveler, Carr, & Solomon, 1991; Wilfley et al., 1993). Cognitive–behavioral approaches target dysfunctional attitudes about weight and shape, and aim to create more structured eating from the chaos of binges. Interpersonal psychotherapy does not deal with the core symptoms of the eating disorder *per se*, but rather focuses on key relationships in the client's life.

Essentially equivalent results have been produced by these two fundamentally different approaches, for both bulimia nervosa (Fairburn et al., 1991) and binge eating in obese persons (Wilfley et al., 1993). This raises several important possibilities. First, eating-disordered symptoms may arise from different causes. Second, binge eating *per se*, among some persons, may be a reflection of other pathology, perhaps as a "secondary symptom." Third, matching individuals to treatments may prove to be part of treating obese binge eaters. Research is now underway to examine matching factors, but criteria for matching are not yet available. One might speculate that individuals with serious relationship disturbances, which would include those with one of the personality disorders, might require interpersonal psychotherapy, whereas the symptom-focused cognitive–behavioral approach might be preferable with others. We underscore the speculative nature of this notion.

AN ARGUMENT FOR COMPASSIONATE TREATMENT

We have previously mentioned that obese individuals are subject to pervasive prejudice and discrimination resulting from their weight and shape (Stunkard & Sobal, 1995). Obese individuals may also suffer psychologically from a legacy of shame and failure associated with past cycles of weight loss and regain. These failed efforts to lose weight and maintain weight loss have occurred in full view of family, friends, employers, and health-care practitioners. There are few other medical or psychological conditions that not only occur in such public view, but also are thought by laypersons to result from personal weakness.

The therapist may also experience negative feelings toward the obese client. Working with obese individuals can be rewarding during the first months of treatment as the client achieves relatively easy weight loss. However, practitioners should be aware that the longer they work with an obese individual, the more they are likely to experience feelings of frustration, and even anger. These feelings may arise in response to a variety of failures on the part of the patient (e.g., failure to lose weight for several weeks; apparent inability to control binge eating, etc.). It is during these points in treatment that the practitioner is particularly vulnerable to feeling critical of and expressing frustration toward obese individuals for "not trying hard enough," or suggesting that the client "must not really want to change" (Rand & MacGregor, 1990). This criticism is more likely to diminish the patient's self-esteem than to elicit desired behavior change. It is particularly at such times that practitioners must be most supportive and help patients to understand their weight-related difficulties and their emotional reactions to them (Wadden & Wingate, 1995).

ASSESSMENT

Obesity is an especially complex disorder because of its multiple etiologies, behavioral correlates, psychosocial effects, and medical consequences. Therefore, a broad, thorough assessment is a necessary first step in formulating a treatment plan for obesity. Detailed information must be collected in order to help the individual select the best treatment. A comprehensive list of assessment factors based on the previously presented matching scheme is presented in Table 11.2.

In order to determine whether, to what extent, and with what urgency an individual should lose weight, the practitioner should first consider the medical risk presented by the client's obesity. Clients should be urged to obtain information about their physical health from a personal physician, and clients who have not had a recent medical examination should be encouraged to do so. A medical assessment can also eventually be utilized to demonstrate physical improvement associated with weight loss (e.g., resting heart rate and body circumferences) and can be a strong source of reinforcement for clients. Other medical complications of obesity, such as high blood pressure and diabetes, can also improve with weight loss and need to be monitored by a physician.

The psychosocial correlates of obesity should be assessed both to highlight the need for treatment and to determine whether the client experiences particular psychological or social distress that warrants special attention. An evaluation of the biomedical factors affecting weight and a thorough weight history can help the professional develop an understanding of the potential physical limitations of weight loss for the client. In addition, an assessment of the client's expectations of the process and outcome of treatment can alert the practitioner to psychological factors (e.g., unrealistic notions of how rapidly weight loss will occur) that may interfere with treatment.

Assessment of current eating patterns allows the practitioner to get a picture of the patient's general eating habits, any patterns of aberrant or unhealthy eating (such as binge eating), and the possible factors that may influence particular eating patterns. The best method of assessing eating patterns is through self-monitoring. A number of formats are available to facilitate this process. A sample self-monitoring form is presented in Sidebar 11–1. Once eating records are obtained and reviewed, the therapist should appraise their nutritional meaning and assess their behavioral messages. Whenever possible, a registered dietitian should be consulted to provide feedback and recommend changes on nutritional issues.

Table 11.2. Factors to Be Included in Initial Assessment[a]

I. Medical severity of the weight problem
   A. Current medical problems associated with obesity
   B. Family history of obesity-related medical problems
   C. Body mass index or percentage overweight
   D. Body composition
   E. Body fat distribution (upper body vs. lower body)

II. Psychosocial sequelae of the weight problem
   A. Discrimination encountered at work and socially
   B. Pressure from others to lose weight
   C. Physical limitations on occupational and recreational activities
   D. Dependence of self-esteem on body weight
   E. Overattribution of problems to weight

III. Biomedical factors affecting weight
   A. Family history of obesity
   B. Medications
   C. Resting metabolic rate (when available)
   D. [For women] Menopausal status and parity
   E. Recent medical exam

IV. Weight history
   A. Age at onset
   B. Lifetime adult high and low weights
   C. Previous weight-loss attempts (methods, initial losses, amount and duration of maintenance)
   D. Precipitants of previous relapses

V. Expectations
   A. Weight goal
   B. Rate of weight loss
   C. Ease of weight loss
   D. Requirements for weight loss
   E. Consequences of weight loss
      1. Reality of desired positive effects
      2. Awareness of possible negative effects

VI. Current eating patterns
   A. Nutritional selections
      1. Daily caloric intake
      2. Macronutrient selection
      3. Balance among food groups
      4. Fiber intake
      5. Sodium intake
   B. Eating topography
      1. Number of daily meals and snacks
      2. Eating rate (meal duration)
   C. Behavioral factors influencing eating
      1. Cues for overeating and unplanned eating (time of day, location, concomitant activities, time since last meal, persons, food-cue salience, etc.)
      2. Perceived reinforcers for overeating
   D. Binge eating
      1. Amount eaten
      2. Frequency
      3. Indicators of loss of control

Table 11.2. (*Continued*)

387

Management of
Obesity

VII. Cognitive factors
    A. Self-efficacy for weight loss, maintenance, and program requirements
    B. Self-evaluative style (dichotomous, all-or-none approach vs. continuous, matter-of-degree approach)
    C. Attributional style for success and failure

VIII. Activity patterns
    A. Current exercise program
        1. Type
        2. Frequency
        3. Intensity
        4. Duration
    B. Previous exercise programs
        1. Type, etc. (as above)
        2. Reasons for discontinuation
    C. Current impediments to exercise
    D. Patient preferences about type of exercise
    E. Leisure activities
    F. Extent of physical activity in daily routine

IX. Social support
    A. Persons who can influence patient's success (spouse, family, friends, coworkers, etc.)
    B. Patient's plans to use social support
    C. Reactions of others to previous weight loss and weight-loss attempts

[a]From Brownell and O'Neil (1993). Reprinted with permission.

Although there are no norms for many cognitive factors related to treatment, these factors are crucial to the process and outcome of treatment. For example, client ratings of self-efficacy of achieving weight-related goals have been found to predict subsequent weight loss (Stotland & Zuroff, 1991). Information obtained both from explicit questioning and attention to how the client relates other data can provide a great deal of information for the therapist. One example of this process may be to ask the client to provide ratings on a 10-point scale of his or her confidence in coping with different diet-related situations and in accomplishing the various behavioral changes that will be required. The clinician may also want to listen for how the client evaluates his or her efforts and whether successes and failures are attributed to self or to external factors.

Therapists should assess the client's activity patterns by obtaining actual accounts of specific behavior. The need for specificity is due to the fact that to different clients, "exercise" may mean anything from 45 minutes of step aerobics to a round of golf while riding in a motorized cart. The client who says, "I usually walk a few times a week," may reveal on more careful questioning that 3 months have passed since the last walk. Therapists should also identify physical and lifestyle impediments to exercise, so that they can be considered in devising a realistic program of exercise. If a capable exercise physiologist (with an appreciation of the difficulty of exercise for obese persons) is available, consultation is advisable.

The available and desired social support of the client may vary across the client's relationships. For example, a client may want encouragement from a close friend while preferring that her husband limit his involvement to watching their son while she takes her walks. The clinician should listen for information concerning the reactions of others to the client's previous weight losses, because this suggests how they will react to the next loss. If

Sidebar 11–1

A Self-Monitoring Form for Recording Food Intake and the Situational Factors Related to Eating

List each food item and describe method of preparation (baked, fried, boiled, broiled, raw).

Food item/ beverage	Quantity	Time of day	Duration of eating	Meal/ Snack	Level of hunger before eating: 0 = none, 3 = extreme hunger	Activity during eating	Location of eating	Social situation (family meal, eating out, meal at work, alone)	Feeling/Mood Before eating	After eating

these reactions have been previously unsupportive, the client should be prepared to modify that aspect of the relationship accordingly. Possible ways that the client can reinforce people for the desired type of support should also be considered.

Not all aspects of the assessment presented will be feasible. For example, biomedical variables, such as body composition or resting metabolic rate, may not be easily assessed by a clinical psychologist in private practice. However, core information about weight history, eating and exercise patterns, and various psychosocial factors can be obtained by traditional self-report and interview methods. More detailed information about specific assessment approaches is available from several sources (Brownell, 1980; Brownell & Wadden, 1991; Wadden, 1985).

GETTING STARTED: READINESS AND MOTIVATION

Stages of Change

When approaching the treatment of an obese individual, it is important to identify how motivated the client is to change attitudes and behaviors. We do not view the client's motivation as dichotomous (i.e., the client as either motivated or not motivated). Rather, we view the motivation associated with treatment as a continuous *process*. Throughout a treatment, an individual passes through different stages of change that are associated with different levels of motivation (Brownell et al., 1986). Several attempts have been made to identify the stages that make up this process of change (Prochaska, DiClemente, & Norcross, 1991).

Prochaska et al. (1991) suggested that the process of change consists of five stages: precontemplation, contemplation, preparation, action, and maintenance and relapse. Each stage is associated with different cognitive and behavioral processes. For example, individuals in the contemplation stage may be more motivated to think about their treatment, and may be ready for processes of change such as consciousness raising and self-reevaluation. However, an individual in the action stage of treatment may be more motivated to engage in more behavioral processes such as counterconditioning, stimulus control, and contingency management. It is critical for the therapist to determine what stage of change the client is in when presenting for treatment, and monitor the client's stage throughout treatment. Conceptualizing the client's stage of change will have implications for interventions that would be most appropriate with the client.

Assessing Readiness

Clients enter treatment with different levels of "readiness" to engage in behaviors associated with treatment. Specifically, whereas all individuals present for treatment to lose weight, the degree to which an individual is committed or motivated to begin a program varies across individuals. The challenge of losing weight and sustaining behavioral changes over the long term can be challenging under any circumstances, but can be particularly daunting for a person who is not highly committed or motivated, or who has significant life circumstances likely to interfere. In order to assess motivation and commitment, Brownell (1994) has developed a Diet Readiness Test, which is a 23-item self-report instrument used to assess the degree to which an individual is prepared and motivated to begin a program (see Figure 3). This readiness assessment is divided into six sections. The respondent can add points for the questions in each section and compare these to the criteria provided as part of the test. The focus of each section is clear from the titles shown in Sidebar 11–2. The Dieting Readiness Test could serve as a means for stimulating discussion of important issues between client and therapist, and as a method for identifying factors that may be problematic.

TREATMENT: THE LEARN APPROACH

What follows are the components of a comprehensive, cognitive--behavioral program for the treatment of obesity (Brownell, 1994). The program integrates information in five key areas: Lifestyle, Exercise, Attitudes, Relationships and Nutrition; hence the acronym LEARN. A detailed manual for the client, along with a leader's guide, are available (information may be obtained by calling 1-800-736-7323).

Several concepts are central to this program. First is that whereas changes in eating and exercise must occur for the individual to lose weight, alterations in lifestyle must occur for eating and exercise changes to be permanent. Second, state-of-the-art information from nutritional and exercise science is necessary to ensure a safe and effective program. Third, cognitive changes are critical in this process, especially for maintenance. Fourth, regular exercise is one of the single most important changes a client can make. Fifth, a key aspect of the treatment, which is a focus from the beginning of the program, is relapse prevention.

Program Structure

The program, and programs of its type, are issued in a self-administered fashion, in groups led by professionals, and in individual treatment. Individual client factors determine which format is most appropriate. Where professionals are involved, group treatment is the default choice, because the social support from fellow group members typically overrides any benefit of the professional attention available in individual treatment.

Treatment is generally offered in groups of 8–12 individuals. Fewer can be a problem if some miss sessions and drop out, whereas more create a lecture atmosphere and discourage group interaction. The literature shows that longer treatments produce greater weight losses. Our experience has been that fewer than 16 weekly sessions is insufficient, whereas more can lead to boredom and adherence problems. Therefore, our schedule of meetings involves 16 weekly meetings after an orientation session, followed by less frequent meetings for the next 12 months (meetings every 2 weeks, then every 3 weeks, etc.)

Each participant is given a detailed manual (Brownell, 1994). This ensures that each person receives necessary information, and relieves the professional from having to be an expert on exercise physiology, nutrition, and psychology. It also permits a group leader more flexibility in covering topics that may be important to the group at a particular time, knowing that the basic information is available in the manual. Finally, many clients use the manual after the formal program has ended.

LIFESTYLE COMPONENT

Rationale

Whereas many programs choose to focus on "dieting" as a means of losing weight, we suggest that the behavioral management of obesity should be an effort to create *lifestyle* change. Treatment should be aimed not at short-term weight loss, but rather the development of long-standing, routine patterns of behavior that will support attainment and maintenance of a lower weight in the face of genetic, interpersonal, and environmental influences to the contrary. This approach makes explicit the necessity of long-term change, moves emphasis from weight loss to weight maintenance, and shifts the client's attention from the unpredictability of weight change to the more controllable target of behavior change. In addition, rather than focusing only on eating and exercise, our approach seeks to systematically support client's efforts to develop new hobbies, interests, friendships, or even job skills as an effective way of introducing behavior patterns that would successfully compete with those that precipitate weight gain.

Intervention

Most clients will have histories of weight-loss attempts that do not embrace this "lifestyle" approach. It can be excellent use of initial session time to explain the lifestyle approach to the client in order to overcome the years of contrary messages from weight-loss ads and the client's own quick attempts at weight loss. The explanation of this approach can also put past weight-loss failures into perspective, and help to spare the client unnecessary guilt and impaired self-esteem.

There are several behavioral components to this approach that will help the client make lifestyle changes. The first, and perhaps most important lifestyle behavior is to keep records of eating behavior and weight change. Keeping records accomplishes several goals. Most important, it increases the client's awareness of behavioral patterns. This allows the client to feel more in control of behaviors that have previously seemed beyond control. When considering that many clients find the process of weight loss daunting, and have previously engaged in periods of binge eating or emotional eating, being able to objectify and confront these episodes can be a relief.

One type of record that should be kept is a food diary (see Figure 11.2). The food diary is used to record amounts and calories of foods. The client may resist this part of the program, because it will initially be hard to record everything he or she eats and to estimate calories. Furthermore, as the task eases, adherence may decline if the individual finds the activity repetitive. It is important for the professional and client to work through these obstacles so that record keeping continues. Research has shown this task to be one of the most, if not the most important part of habit change.

There are several steps that the therapist can take in order to ensure that valid information is obtained through the food diary. First, the clinician must adopt and convey an understanding of the effort required to self-monitor accurately. Also, the therapist should ensure that the client records everything that is eaten, even if the types of food or amounts are embarrassing to the client. This process can be aided by assuring the client that the forms are not a means to being "graded" but rather simply a way of bringing his or her customary eating patterns into the therapist's office. Furthermore, it should be made clear that the therapist will not condemn the client on the basis of these data (or anything else, for that matter). For example, the client should be assured that although complete records are desirable, partial records are usable. Finally, the therapist should review the records with the client in order to clarify them. For example, this would allow the client to indicate any eating episodes considered "binges" and to elaborate on related precipitants of loss of control.

The client should also keep a record of weight change. In order to accomplish this task,

Michael A. Friedman
and Kelly D. Brownell

Sidebar 11–2

The Dieting Readiness Test

Answer the questions below to see how well your attitudes equip you for a weight-loss program. For each question, circle the answer that best describes your attitude. As you complete each of the six sections, add the numbers of your answers and compare them with the scoring guide at the end of each section.

SECTION 1: GOALS AND ATTITUDES

1. Compared to previous attempts, how motivated to lose weight are you this time?

1	2	3	4	5
Not at all motivated	Slightly motivated	Somewhat motivated	Quite motivated	Extremely motivated

2. How certain are you that you will stay committed to a weight loss program for the time it will take you to reach your goal?

1	2	3	4	5
Not at all certain	Slightly certain	Somewhat certain	Quite certain	Extremely certain

3. Consider all outside factors at this time in your life (the stress you're feeling at work, your family obligations, etc.). To what extent can you tolerate the effort required to stick to a diet?

1	2	3	4	5
Cannot tolerate	Can tolerate somewhat	Uncertain	Can tolerate well	Can tolerate easily

4. Think honestly about how much weight you hope to lose and how quickly you hope to lose it. Figuring a weight loss of 1 to 2 pounds per week, how realistic is your expectation?

1	2	3	4	5
Very unrealistic	Somewhat unrealistic	Moderately unrealistic	Somewhat realistic	Very realistic

5. While dieting, do you fantasize about eating a lot of your favorites foods?

1	2	3	4	5
Always	Frequently	Occasionally	Rarely	Never

6. While dieting, do you feel deprived, angry and/or upset?

1	2	3	4	5
Always	Frequently	Occasionally	Rarely	Never

Section 1—Total Score _____

If you scored:

6 to 16: This may not be a good time to start a weight loss program. Inadequate motivation and commitment together with unrealistic goals could block your progress. Think about those things that contribute to this, and consider changing them before undertaking a diet program.

17 to 23: You may be close to being ready to begin a program but should think about ways to boost your preparedness before you begin.

24 to 30: The path is clear with respect to goals and attitudes.

SECTION 2: HUNGER AND EATING CUES

7. When food comes up in conversation or in something you read, do you want to eat even if you are not hungry?

1	2	3	4	5
Never	Rarely	Occasionally	Frequently	Always

8. How often do you eat because of physical hunger?

1	2	3	4	5
Always	Frequently	Occasionally	Rarely	Never

9. Do you have trouble controlling your eating when your favorite foods are around the house?

1	2	3	4	5
Never	Rarely	Occasionally	Frequently	Always

Section 2—Total Score _____

If you scored:

3 to 6: You might occasionally eat more than you would like, but it does not appear to be a result of high responsiveness to environmental cues. Controlling the attitudes that make you eat may be especially helpful.

7 to 9: You may have a moderate tendency to eat just because food is available. Dieting may be easier for you if you try to resist external cues and eat only when you are physically hungry.

10 to 15: Some or most of your eating may be in response to thinking about food or exposing yourself to temptations to eat. Think of ways to minimize your exposure to temptations, so that you eat only in response to physical hunger.

SECTION 3: CONTROL OVER EATING

If the following situations occurred while you were on a diet, would you be likely to eat more or less immediately afterward and for the rest of the day?

10. Although you planned on skipping lunch, a friend talks you into going out for a midday meal.

1	2	3	4	5
Would eat much less	Would eat somewhat less	Would make no difference	Would eat somewhat more	Would eat much more

(continued)

Sidebar 11–2

(Continued)

11. You "break" your diet by eating a fattening, "forbidden" food.

1	2	3	4	5
Would eat much less	Would eat somewhat less	Would make no difference	Would eat somewhat more	Would eat much more

12. You have been following your diet faithfully and decide to test yourself by eating something you consider a treat.

1	2	3	4	5
Would eat much less	Would eat somewhat less	Would make no difference	Would eat somewhat more	Would eat much more

Section 3—Total Score _____

If you scored:

3 to 7: You recover rapidly from mistakes. However, if you frequently alternate between eating out of control and dieting very strictly, you may have a serious eating problem and should get professional help.

8 to 11: You do not seem to let unplanned eating disrupt your program. This is a flexible, balanced approach.

12 to 15: You may be prone to overeat after an event breaks your control or throws you off the track. Your reaction to these problem-causing eating events can be improved.

SECTION 4: BINGE EATING AND PURGING

13. Aside from holiday feasts, have you ever eaten a large amount of food rapidly and felt afterward that this eating incident was excessive and out of control?

2	0
Yes	No

14. If you answered yes to #13 above, how often have you engaged in this behavior during the last year?

1	2	3	4	5	6
Less than once a month	About once a month	A few times a month	About once a week	About three times a week	Daily

15. Have you ever purged (used laxatives, diuretics or induced vomiting) to control your weight?

5	0
Yes	No

16. If you answered yes to #15 above, how often have you engaged in this behavior in the last year?

1	2	3	4	5	6
Less than once a month	About once a month	A few times a month	About once a week	About three times a week	Daily

Section 4—Total Score _____

If you scored:

   0 to 1: It appears that binge eating and purging is not a problem for you.

   2 to 11: Pay attention to these eating patterns. Should they arise more frequently, get professional help.

   12 to 19: You show signs of having a potentially serious eating problem. See a counselor experienced in evaluating eating disorders right away.

SECTION 5: EMOTIONAL EATING

17. Do you eat more than you would like when you have negative feelings such as anxiety, depression, anger or loneliness?

1	2	3	4	5
Never	Rarely	Occasionally	Frequently	Always

18. Do you have trouble controlling your eating when you have positive feelings—do you celebrate feeling good by eating?

1	2	3	4	5
Never	Rarely	Occasionally	Frequently	Always

19. When you have unpleasant interactions with others in your life, or after a difficult day at work, do you eat more than you'd like?

1	2	3	4	5
Never	Rarely	Occasionally	Frequently	Always

Section 5—Total Score _____

If you scored:

   3 to 8: You do not appear to let your emotions affect your eating.

   9 to 11: You sometimes eat in response to emotional highs and lows. Monitor this behavior to learn when and why it occurs and be prepared to find alternate activities.

   12 to 15: Emotional ups and downs can stimulate your eating. Try to deal with the feelings that trigger the eating and find other ways to express them.

SECTION 6: EXERCISE PATTERNS AND ATTITUDES

20. How often do you exercise?

1	2	3	4	5
Never	Rarely	Occasionally	Somewhat	Frequently

(continued)

Michael A. Friedman
and Kelly D. Brownell

Sidebar 11–2

(*Continued*)

21. How confident are you that you can exercise regularly?

1	2	3	4	5
Not at all! confident	Slightly confident	Somewhat confident	Highly confident	Completely confident

22. When you think about exercise, do you develop a positive or negative picture in your mind?

1	2	3	4	5
Completely negative	Somewhat negative	Neutral	Somewhat positive	Completely positive

23. How certain are you that you can work regular exercise into your daily schedule?

1	2	3	4	5
Not at all certain	Slightly certain	Somewhat certain	Quite certain	Extremely certain

Section 6—Total Score _____

If you scored:

4 to 10: You're probably not exercising as regularly as you should. Determine whether your attitudes about exercise are blocking your way, then change what you must and put on those walking shoes.

11 to 16: You need to feel more positive about exercise so you can do it more often. Think of ways to be more active that are fun and fit your lifestyle.

17 to 20: It looks like the path is clear for you to be active. Now think of ways to get motivated.

After scoring yourself in each section of this questionnaire, you should be better able to judge your dieting strengths and weaknesses. Remember that the first step in changing eating behavior is to understand the conditions that influence your eating habits.

Note: Reprinted by permission from Brownell (1994).

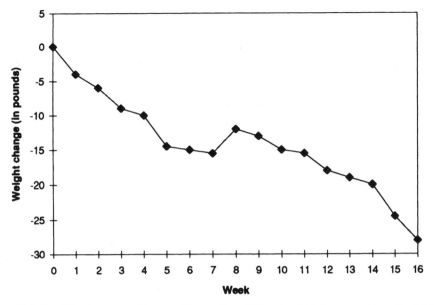

Figure 11.2. A weight change record for recording weekly weight and weight change over time. Reprinted by permission from Brownell (1994).

the client should record the date each week and weight change from the previous week (see Figure 11.2). This chart can serve as a reminder to the client of how he or she is faring in the program. Along with eating and charts, it also shows the client the relationship between behaviors and weight.

EXERCISE COMPONENT

Rationale

Exercise is universally considered a key component to any treatment program. However, there are several hypotheses as to the reason exercise is so effective in helping individuals to lose weight. Exercise can produce both physiological and psychological benefits that may aid in weight loss. Furthermore, the client does not have to become extremely active in order to derive benefit from exercise; these benefits may result from increasing exercise behavior from a very low to a moderate level (Blair et al., 1989; DeBusk, Stenestrand, Sheehan, & Haskell, 1990; Wood, Stefanick, Williams, & Haskell, 1991). Physiological changes resulting from exercise can include increased lean body mass, elevated metabolic rate, or decreased appetite. There is also evidence that exercise may be critical in achieving long-term weight loss (Craighead & Blum, 1989; Foreyt & Goodrick, 1991; Hill et al., 1989; Kayman, Bruvold, & Stern, 1990; Pavlou, Krey, & Steffee, 1989; Sikand, Kondo, Foreyt, Jones, & Gotto, 1988). Most studies of the correlates of long-term treatment outcome show that a regular program of moderate aerobic exercise is a critical factor in weight maintenance.

One hypothesis is that the psychological impact of exercise is the key mechanism that links physical activity to weight control (Brownell, 1995). Exercise can have significant positive psychological effects, even at levels far below those needed to produce a physiological effect (e.g., parking farther from the entrance of a store). One reason may be that even a small amount of activity can be viewed as a tangible symbol of change that can provide the client with a continuous source of motivation and encouragement throughout treatment.

Intervention

Typically, obese individuals are prescribed a regimen of aerobic activity as part of treatment. This approach originated from studies in exercise physiology designed to identify a threshold for activity needed to improve cardiovascular fitness. The resulting belief is that exceeding this threshold is necessary for exercise to have any value. However, attaining this level is often so difficult for many people that exercise is either not attempted or is quickly abandoned.

Although exercise can be valuable in improving cardiovascular fitness, most individuals exercise to lose weight and look better; improving cardiovascular fitness is a lower priority. Therefore, if psychological factors are what connect exercise to weight control, questions should not focus on which types of activity produce the most sustained elevation in heart rate, or are most effective at building lean body mass, but rather should give way to a different question: What exercise will produce the desired psychological effects? As the person defines an effort as exercise, each time he or she exercises is an opportunity for reinforcement and affirmation of lifestyle. The goal, therefore, is to maximize the number of such opportunities and to encourage cognitive changes, such that the individual has a broad definition of exercise and sees any attempt to increase activity as a positive development.

It will often be a considerable challenge for the therapist to help the client initiate and maintain an exercise regimen. The therapist should be aware of the difficulty of exercise for many obese individuals. Excess weight needs to be carried and supported, and medical problems associated with obesity, such as joint or back problems, may limit the types of exercise that are advisable. Furthermore, many clients report stories of jeers and insults that they have received from strangers, and are therefore self-conscious about exercising in public. Finally, many clients have unrealistic expectations about the short-term results of exercise, and may quickly become frustrated and discouraged, as seen in this exchange (from Brownell & O'Neil, 1993) between client (C) and therapist (T):

C: I told you that exercise doesn't work for me. This week proves it. I went out and walked four times this week, and I only lost half a pound. I did better than that the last two weeks, when I didn't walk at all.

T: How did you think the walking would affect your loss?

C: I should have lost at least two more pounds. I was really working up a sweat and breathing hard when I was walking.

T: I know exercise has been a difficult part of this for you, and it would be good to see the results on the scale after you have a good week of exercise. But let's review some of the mathematics of weight loss that we've discussed before. Remember that each pound of body weight contains about 3,500 calories, as a rough estimate. So to lose a pound, you'd need to burn about 3,500 more calories than you take in. Now, how far did you walk?

C: I mapped out a 1-mile route, and did it on 4 days, twice the last time.

T: So you walked 5 miles this week. That's a real achievement. But let's see if maybe you were expecting a little too much to come of it. How many extra calories do you think you burned by walking those 5 miles?

C: I don't know, maybe 1,000 per mile.

T: Actually, a lot less. A really rough estimate is that you burn about 100 extra calories per mile.

C: So I'd have to walk that much for 7 weeks to lose one extra pound? Forget it. I lost that much each day on the Atkins diet and never exercised once.

T: Not so fast. Remember, you said that this time you're trying for long-term success. Let's continue the math for a bit. If you walked the same amount ever week for a year, that would be a little over 7 pounds. That may not seem like much, but I believe you said that you gained about 70 pounds over the last 10 years, that's an average of 7 pounds a year. In the next 10 years, that 500 calorie per week from walking might let you maintain your loss instead of gaining another 70 pounds.

C: But that doesn't help me now.

T: Then we'll need to think of some ways to reward yourself for walking each week, or even each day, to keep you motivated until your walking program gets to be routine and even enjoyable. Even if the walking meant a bigger loss each week, you wouldn't see it because of how your water weight shifts. Let's work on finding some rewards that you control.

One method of dealing with the frustrations associated with exercise (or with other aspects of the weight-loss treatment) is by helping the client to establish behavioral goals and rewards for his or her efforts. The exercise goals that a client sets should be specific and quantifiable, and should require a reasonable effort while still being attainable and realistic. Furthermore, these goals should also be somewhat "forgiving" (i.e., they should not require perfection). Over time, the therapist (T) should help the client (C) to shape the pattern of setting and adhering to these goals that meet these criteria (from Brownell & O'Neil, 1993).

T: It would be helpful for you to focus on one or two goals to really work on this week. Any ideas?

C: I want to work on exercising more.

T: Let's try to get a little more specific about the exercise.

C: Okay, I'm going to walk this week.

T: So the exercise will be walking. How much and how often will you walk?

C: Let's say 5 miles, every day.

T: How much are you walking presently?

C: Well, I haven't been getting out much lately.

T: So it's been a while since you exercised regularly?

C: Yeah, actually I haven't done anything consistently in about 5 or 6 years.

T: Maybe 5 miles is expecting a little too much, too soon. You might injure yourself if you start too quickly.

C: I could say 1 mile a day, but that won't help me lose much weight.

T: You're right, you won't be able to tell when you get on the scale here next week, but we're trying to develop some habits that will make a big difference in your weight over the long haul.

C: Okay, I'll walk a mile every day.

T: If you get tied up at work, or we have bad weather one day, you might not achieve that "every day" goal. How about 4 days? That would be 4 days more than you're doing now, and the success you'd enjoy might help you to reach your next goal.

C: You mean success breeds success? I'll give it a try. I'll walk a mile on 4 days this week.

Whereas most behavioral goals involve behaviors that have short-term costs, they often have only long-term rewards. It is often necessary to help a client develop a reinforcement system to provide short-term rewards for behavior changes until naturally occurring reinforcers take hold. An effective reward should be something that the client finds reinforcing, as well as something that is attainable shortly after the goal is met. In addition, it should be something that the client will forego unless the goal is met. Finally, it should not be food.

Selecting effective rewards can be a difficult task for clients, particularly because many clients have a history of relying on food for reward. In addition, some clients resist the idea of "bribing" themselves in order to engage in health-promoting behaviors. Therapists should encourage clients to not consider tangible items alone. Desirable activities, such as a day at the beach, at the lake, or in the mountains, or attendance at a certain movie or concert might be used as rewards.

THE ATTITUDE COMPONENT

Rationale

Cognitive issues are central to both weight loss and maintenance. A person's goals, expectations, self-imposed rules, and response to eating events affect mood, self-efficacy, and ability to adhere to a program. Clients with weaknesses in this area are extremely vulnerable to lapse and relapse.

As a clinical example, a woman who has lost 20 of the 30 pounds she intends to lose may encounter a high-risk situation, say a restaurant buffet. If she begins eating, and does so with food she considers off-limits, she may feel guilt, shame, and weakening of restraint. This may lead to further eating, and for the sake of discussion, let's say she binges and consumes 4,000 calories. To many, many people, this event would be devastating because this "slip" would be interpreted as a catastrophe, and the likelihood of recovery would be slim.

The real gain in body weight from this episode would amount to little more than a pound, an insignificant gain given that the client had lost 20 pounds and seemed to be making excellent progress. The reaction to the event is the key determinant of future behavior. If the client had learned the necessary cognitive skills, she could place this event in perspective, develop constructive responses, and recover rather than relapse.

There are many cognitive skills taught in modern-day programs (Brownell, 1994). Two examples will be used here—countering dichotomous thinking and establishing reasonable goal weights. *Dichotomous thinking* refers to thoughts that one is either on or off a diet, that a food is legal or illegal, or is either good or bad. This creates an environment in which any deviation from perfection is considered abject failure. Such deviations are inevitable; hence, the need for specific cognitive skills.

One of the most salient attitudes that clients adopt when entering treatment is to orient their program toward achieving a "goal weight." Previously, we have discussed the importance of emphasizing behavioral goals so that changes on the scale are not the only criteria against which clients judge their behavior. However, this concept of "goal weight" is foremost in the minds of most individuals who attempt to lose weight, and clients who fix on this number can become extremely frustrated. One reason is that the criteria used to establish a goal weight can be highly idiosyncratic and may change with time. Many people aspire to a weight they recall from a landmark point in their life. Examples are high school or college graduation, or a wedding. In some cases, individuals have a goal weight based on a health referent, usually "ideal" weights derived from height–weight tables.

Inherent in this concept of goal weight is the notion that the individual can, in fact, reach that weight. This ignores the possibility that the goal weight might be an impossible weight for some individuals. Biological factors such as fat-cell number, resting energy expenditure, or other factors influenced by genetics may impose barriers to weight loss. For others, degree of food restriction and physical activity necessary to lose and maintain the goal weight may be untenable.

Furthermore, goal weight represents an individual's long-range aspirations and could take months or even years to reach. It is our experience that clients may feel that the goal is remote and in some cases unreachable, even when satisfactory progress is occurring. The goal weight can be a significant obstacle rather than a source of motivation and encouragement. This is especially true of people with significant excess weight. It is easy to envision a person who begins a program 60 lb from a goal weight feeling worse about 40 lb yet to be lost than 20 lb already lost, even though the 20-lb loss might have taken 4 months and considerable effort.

Intervention

Training in cognitive skills involves an assessment and functional analysis of an individual's thinking patterns. Once maladaptive patterns are identified, clients can learn to change these thoughts. Table 11.3 presents examples of statements and counterstatements that are typical of this approach. Clients must practice this new thinking repeatedly.

To deal with the problem of inappropriate weight goals, it is possible to abandon the concept of *ideal weight* in favor of "reasonable weight" (Brownell & Rodin, 1990; Brownell & Wadden, 1991, 1992). Reasonable weight would be determined by a number of factors and would represent the weight a person can achieve and maintain by making reasonable changes in lifestyle. This concept runs counter to the stance that elevated weight brings elevated risk, and that all excess weight should be lost. Although that approach is theoretically correct, we feel that it can also be counterproductive. Because the distant goal is likely to discourage people, the goal weight could set the stage for relapse (Brownell

Table 11.3. Maladaptive Thoughts and Counterthoughts[a]

Internal Trap 1—"The diet is the key."
→ *Fat Thought*: The diet and this program are the only reasons I lose weight. When the diet is over, I will have real trouble keeping the weight off.
✓ *Counter*: I am losing weight because of my own efforts. Just because the program ends does not mean my new habits will vanish. The program helps me along, but I get the credit.
Internal Trap 2—"Is this worth the effort?"
→ *Fat Thought*: I have been on my program for weeks and I still have lots of weight to lose. I can't wait till this program ends so I can get back to normal.
✓ *Counter*: Stop this right now! Who said this would be easy? It took a long time to gain the weight, and it will take a long time to lose it. I would like to lose fast and easy, but facts are facts. I don't want to let down now and waste the effort. I can stick with it.
Internal Trap 3—"I have done this before."
→ *Fat Thought*: I have heard this nutrition stuff before, and we covered behavior modification in Weight Watchers. It didn't help me then and will not help me now.
✓ *Counter*: I have never been taught these things in such a concentrated way, and my motivation to learn may be different now. I know deep down this is the only way to get permanent results, so putting down the approach just means I have trouble doing the work. Only I can do it, so I must forge ahead.

[a]From Brownell (1994). Reprinted with permission.

Table 11.4. Questions Used as Clinical Criteria to Help Establish a "Reasonable Weight" for an Individual Client[a]

1. Is there a history of excess weight in your parents or grandparents?
2. What is the lowest weight you have maintained as an adult for at least 1 year?
3. What is the largest size of clothes that you feel comfortable in, at the point you say, "I look pretty good considering where I have been"? At what weight would you wear these clothes?
4. Think of a friend or family member (with your age and body frame) who looks "normal" to you. What does the person weigh?
5. At what weight do you believe you can live with the required changes in eating and/or exercise?

[a]From Brownell and O'Neil (1993). Reprinted with permission.

et al., 1986). In addition, impressive changes in risk factors can occur with relatively small weight losses (Blackburn & Kanders, 1987; Goldstein, 1992). Blood-pressure reduction and improved metabolic control in diabetics are among the changes. Therefore, smaller but better maintained losses may be more beneficial than larger losses followed by relapse (Brownell & Wadden, 1992).

Establishment of reasonable weight must rely on clinical judgment and the intuition of clients. Table 11.4 presents five questions that may be helpful in negotiating a reasonable weight with a client. Research has yet to be done to validate these or any criteria, but we have found them to be helpful in providing the basis for a client to settle on a reasonable weight goal. Clients may be unaccustomed to the concept of *reasonable weight*, so it must be presented with a strong rationale, as illustrated during the following session (from Brownell & O'Neil, 1993) between therapist (T) and client (C):

T: Let's talk about goal weight. What do you think when you hear this?
C: I want to weigh 120 pounds.
T: Why 120 pounds?
C: The nurse at my doctor's office said I should weigh 125 from the tables, but I weighed 120 when I got married and I looked great.
T: Is this the goal you have set before when you joined other programs?
C: Sure. This is what I want to weigh.
T: How long do you figure it will take to get there?
C: Well, I weigh 182 now, so I figure it will take 3 or 4 months.
T: We will talk about this later, because how fast you expect to lose is tied up with how much you expect to lose. For now, let's go back to your weight-loss goal. If 120 is your goal, it is easy to see how you might get discouraged during a program. Can you see how this might happen?
C: Well, I haven't been successful doing this before, so I might feel afraid that I won't make it.
T: True. The fear you feel might be realistic given the circumstances. You want to avoid setting a trap for yourself. What do you think about of setting a goal of 120, when you have not been able to reach 120 before?
C: It might inspire me, but I might also never reach it.
T: Would it make sense to set a different goal—one that you are more likely to reach?
C: How would I do this?
T: This is a good time to talk about a reasonable weight for you. Reasonable weight is the weight you feel you can reach with hard work and persistence. It would be a weight at which you can live with the changes you have made. It is a weight you could maintain.
C: How do I know what weight this would be?

T: Let me ask you several questions. These should help us close in on a reasonable weight. Were your parents or grandparents overweight?

C: My mother was overweight, and so was my grandfather. My grandmother was stocky, but not really heavy.

T: I cannot say for certain, but the history of overweight in your family raises the possibility of an inherited predisposition to gain weight.

C: Does this mean I can't lose weight?

T: No. You may not have such a genetic tendency at all, and even if you do, it should still be possible for you to lose weight. Let's move on to another question and see how the information begins to fit together.

C: Okay.

T: What is the lowest weight you have been able to maintain as an adult for at least 1 year?

C: That's hard to say. I guess I got down to about 140 when I went on the liquid fast.

T: Were you able to stay at 140 for a year or longer?

C: I bounced between 140 and 150 for about a year.

T: The third question. Think about the largest size of clothes you would feel comfortable in— where you would feel you look pretty good. What would you weigh to be able to wear these clothes?

C: Well, I want to say 120, because I'd like to look like I did when I got married.

T: Remember now that we are talking about a reasonable weight.

C: I think I could wear clothes that would make me look much better than I do now at say 140 or 150. When I lost weight with the fast, I looked a lot better and my friends said lots of nice things.

T: Then I will ask the fourth question. Think of a friend or family member, with about the same height and frame as you, who you feel looks "normal." What does that person weigh?

C: My sister-in-law Sally is about my size. She is chunky, but doesn't look real heavy. I'd say she weighs about 135.

T: The final question. At what weight do you think you can live with the changes you would have to make in your eating and exercise? Remember back on diets in the past and think about what you were doing to maintain the lower weights. What did it take, and can you live like that?

C: After the fast, I was eating regular meals. They were small, but I felt good being able to eat normally. I was walking with my friend three times a week or so. I felt great being in better shape.

T: Do you think you could live like this permanently?

C: I guess so. I did it for a year, but then things got crazy at work and my schedule went nuts with the kids.

T: If you could develop some way of handling stress, or perhaps keeping your life on a more even keel, do you think you could live with the eating and exercise habits you were practicing then?

C: I think so.

T: Good. Let's put all this together. You may be susceptible to weight gain because of the family history you described, so getting down to 120 may or may not be possible. You were able to stay between 140 and 150 after the liquid diet program and did so for a year. You think you looked a lot better then. Your sister-in-law looks reasonable to you, and you figure she weighs about 135. Finally, you said you might be able to live with the changes you made after the liquid diet when you were down to 140 to 150. Do these suggest any weight that may be reasonable for you?

C: 140 to 150?

T: This sounds like the right range to me. This 140 might be low, however, because this is at the bottom of the range from 140 to 150. Let's play it safe and pick a weight you think is truly reasonable.

C: I guess 150 sounds about right.

T: How do you think this would work for you?

C: I understand what you are saying, but it will be hard to get the 120 pounds out of my mind.

T: The 120 has been part of your thinking for so long that what you say does not surprise me. If you catch yourself each time you think of the 120 and say something like the following, the 120 will fade and the new weight can take its place. "The 120 sounds good but it may just discourage me. I will be making great progress if I lose to 150, then I can worry about losing more."

Clients can enter treatment with other expectations that are unrealistic or based on faulty assumptions. For example, many clients expect weight loss to be more rapid than is feasible, for the task to be easier than is possible, or for life to improve in a dramatic fashion once weight loss occurs. The rate of weight loss is a common issue when expectation often exceeds reality. The following exchange highlighted one approach to confronting this issue with the client mentioned above (from Brownell & O'Neil, 1993).

T: Before you mentioned that it would take you 3 or 4 months to reach your goal. Would you explain more about where this number comes from?

C: I didn't think about it very much, but this seems like a long time.

T: Let's do some arithmetic and see what we get. How much do you figure you might lose each week?

C: Maybe 3 pounds.

T: That would be a rapid weight loss. You may lose this much in the first week or two, but in a program like ours, where you are making reasonable lifestyle changes, you can count on losing 1 to 2 pounds per week. Just to be on the safe side, let's say 1 pound a week will be your loss. You wanted to lose from 182 to 150, which is a 32-pound loss. How long then, should it take to reach the 150?

C: Let's see. About 32 weeks?

T: Right. This is 8 months, which is double your guess.

C: This is horrible. I can't imagine being on a diet for 8 months.

T: This may be one of the problems that got in your way in the past. It is very common for people to be losing weight at a fine pace, but feel discouraged. The discouragement comes not from lack of progress, but from the way the progress looks when stacked against unrealistic expectations.

C: So what do I do?

T: Many people I work with find it helpful to plot a graph with expected weight loss, so they know what they might expect to weigh at given points in time. Since it is February 1 and you are beginning, you might project a 6-pound loss, to 176 pounds, when your children have their March vacation from school. By tax day, on April 15, you might have lost 10 or 12 pounds, let's say down to 170 pounds. On your birthday in June, you might be down to 160, and by July 4 down to 155. You can work on your own landmark dates and the exact rate of weight loss, but this will give you some idea of how to approach it.

C: This doesn't sound like very exciting weight loss.

T: True, but it is realistic weight loss. What can be different about this time is that you may lose more slowly than you like, but if you make the right changes, you can maintain.

It can sometimes be helpful to have clients write out expectations, how their anticipated performance will compare, and what the emotional response is likely to be. Table 11.5 gives examples of different emotional responses resulting from different goals.

Table 11.5. Producing a Constructive, Positive Emotional Response

Setting Goal	Comparing Performance	Emotional Response
1. Will follow the program as much as possible.	Meet goal on most occasions.	Satisfaction and desire to do better.
2. Will increase level of exercise.	Increase is steady and substantial.	Pride in doing something positive.
3. Will lose most weeks.	Lose weight 10 out of 12 weeks.	Feel good about hard work.

*a*From Brownell (1994). Reprinted by permission.

RELATIONSHIPS

Rationale

Although most clients present for individual weight-loss treatment, weight-loss attempts are rarely private matters that are independent of the client's social network. Rather, body size tends to be a public matter, and changes by the client in dietary and exercise patterns frequently affect the family and close friends. Furthermore, the nature of the client's social support can influence his or her chance of success.

A client's weight may play a critical and complicated role in his or her marriage and other intimate relationships. In such cases, it is often the woman who is the obese partner, and the husband may use the wife's weight as an excuse to withdraw emotionally and avoid sex. In other cases, weight loss by the wife may incite (not always unwarranted) feelings of jealousy and insecurity on the part of the husband, possibly resulting in physical abuse. There are also instances in which the wife's obesity functions as a means of avoiding intimacy with a husband who is no longer desired or loved and, sometimes, as a guard against extramarital affairs. These complicated interpersonal dynamics can often interfere with treatment goals, and must be addressed in treatment in order to achieve long-term weight loss.

The intricacies of these issues are discussed in a book by Stuart and Jacobson (1987) and are illustrated by the dialogue (from Brownell & O'Neil, 1993) that follows between "Nora" (N) and therapist (T). Nora is a 40-year-old, married, small-business owner, mother of two, who had lost 40 lb. She returned to the clinic after an unannounced 3-week absence and a 10-lb weight gain.

T: Looks like you've had a few rough weeks.

N: It's just not fair … (*tears*).

T: What's not fair?

N: When you're a fat woman, you're just fat, not a woman. You're asexual. All of a sudden, men notice you, even though they've known you for years, the bastards. I'm the same person I was 60 pounds ago, but now they're all grins, acting like I'm the best thing they've seen. It's not just "buddies" anymore.

T: Someone came on to you?

N: One of my husband's best friends.

T: Sounds like it made you mad.

N: Yeah, but that's not the problem.

T: What is?

N: I was really tempted. You know, I've been unhappy at home for years, but as long as I was fat, I didn't have to think about it. Now I have to decide, and I'm not sure I can decide to say "no." It scares the hell out of me. It was simpler being fat.

Intervention

It is important for the therapist to alert the client that he or she is not a passive participant in these weight-related interactions, and can influence the amount of support provided by important others. The client should decide how each person can best help with his or her treatment, and how best to solicit that help. At the same time, the client can foster mutuality by asking how to reinforce these people for providing the desired support.

Assertiveness skills are important in this context. To be sure, it is not uncommon for a client who is dissatisfied with others' reactions to reveal on questioning that the preferred type of support has never been communicated to the significant other. Just as most clients have at least one "food pusher" in their lives, food-refusal responses can be rehearsed in therapy sessions so that clients can learn to deal with such individuals. For example, it is often desirable to have clients anticipate events in which they will be encouraged to overeat and notify in advance the relevant people (e.g., hosts) that they are restricting their intake. In addition, compliments about weight loss require assertiveness skills for some clients who feel uncomfortable in such situations. Assertiveness responses are also sometimes needed when requesting modifications to menu items in restaurants.

Difficulties in communicating with a significant other about desirable social support are illustrated in this example of Mary Agnes, a 38-year-old shipyard worker who entered a very low calorie diet (VLCD) program at 220 lb at 5′8″. She had lost 40 pounds. The scenario is between Mary Agnes (M), the therapist (T) and other group members (GM), who are discussing reactions of significant other people to their weight loss (From Brownell & O'Neil, 1993).

M: My husband hasn't said word one about my loss.

T: Are you saying he's ignored all your efforts to lose weight?

M: Yeah, I might as well have skipped the whole thing, as much as he cares.

T: When you lost weight previously, did he react the same way, ignoring it?

M: The last time I lost weight, he drove me crazy by making too much of it every time I lost a few pounds.

T: Did you let him know that?

M: Not in so many words, but he got the message.

T: So up until now he's always made a big deal over your losses?

M: No. Earlier on, he used to act like a cop, always asking me if what I was eating was allowed. After a while, he got the message on that, too.

T: You told him to back off.

M: He figured it out.

T: So he's tried to act like your conscience, and he's tried praising you, but you didn't want either of those. What would you like him to do?

M: What anybody would want their husband to do: show a little understanding.

T: You know what you mean by showing understanding, but it's different for each person. I wonder if the reason he's not saying anything this time might be that he figures whatever he does will be wrong.

M: Do you mean I have to tell him what to do? If I have to draw him a picture, it won't mean anything.

GM: Maybe he wants to help you. Maybe he doesn't. But you won't be able to tell unless you let him know how to help. I used to get furious with my husband because every time I came home from group, he'd ask how much I'd lost. When I finally told him it felt like bringing home a report card, he said he was just trying to show that he wanted me to succeed. Once I told him how to do that, he was great, most of the time.

Learning Communication Skills

Clients generally need more than general advice on social support. They need specific strategies for eliciting support, making specific requests, and reinforcing a partner. Some strategies are provided by Brownell (1994).

Partner Readiness

Others in the client's life may be willing to help, but may be only vaguely aware of how to do so. Increasing their level of readiness can be helpful and can lay the groundwork for specific suggestions by the client to "take hold." One part of our approach is to provide these other people with written material describing how they can best be helpful. Some of the material is in Table 11.6, and was adapted from guidelines developed by Dr. Alberto Cormillot in Argentina.

Dieting Partnership

Some individuals prefer to join a program with another person. Such a partner can provide empathy, support, feedback, and specific advice, and may be enormously valuable. As explained in the following section, weight-loss partnerships are suitable for some individuals and not for others. Where it is a possibility, we have a Partnership Quiz that is helpful in deciding whether a particular person would be a good partner (see Sidebar 11–3).

Once a partnership has been established, the guidelines in Table 11.7 can be helpful in promoting positive interactions.

Solo versus Social Approaches

Engaging others in a weight-loss effort is not the best approach for all people. Some prefer to be private with their efforts, and forcing social support (as in the buddy system) can be counterproductive. We make a distinction between "solo" dieters and use the Solo versus Social Inventory as a guide (Sidebar 11–4). Without providing a scoring key, we have clients complete the inventory to help themselves decide whether a solo or social approach would be best. Future advice is then given on how to best implement each approach (Brownell, 1994; Brownell & Rodin, 1990).

NUTRITION

Rationale

There are certain aspects of an individual's diet that may be related to the onset and maintenance of obesity. Fat intake is one nutritional issue that should be addressed in treatment. Several studies have shown that the lower caloric intake associated with a reduction in dietary-fat intake is not completely compensated for in the individual's diet, thus promoting weight loss (Kendall, Levitsky, Strupp, & Lissner, 1991; Prewitt et al., 1991). Possible explanations for this phenomenon include a general reduction in the

Table 11.6. A List of What Families Should and Should Not Do to Aid a Family Member's Attempt to Lose Weight[a]

Things the Family Should Avoid

→ *Do not hide food from the person losing weight.* He or she will find it and feel resentful.

→ *Do not threaten.* Behavior is best changed with a soft touch, not coercion, so be nice.

→ *Do not avoid social situations because of the person's weight.* This will batter the self-esteem of the family member losing weight and will breed resentment in the family.

→ *Do not expect perfection or 100 percent recovery.* Weight problems are something a person learns to control, not cure. There will be periods of misery, weight gain, and overeating. The individual's achievements should be appreciated and the setbacks ignored.

→ *Do not lecture, criticize, or reprimand.* These rarely help. The person needs to feel better, not worse

→ *Do not play the role of victim or martyr.* Overweight has many causes, both psychological and physiological. It is unfair for the family to blame the overweight family member and to feel victimized. Support and encouragement will do more than guilt and shame.

Things the Family Can Do

✓ *Keep a positive attitude.* This sounds trite, but can be very important. It is not easy to be upbeat and encouraging when a program grinds on for months and months. Extra effort from the family can make life much easier for the person losing weight.

✓ *Talk with others in your situation.* Being in a family where a weight problem exists generates strong feelings in the family members. It can help to talk about these with others who deal with the same issues. Many good ideas can be generated from this process.

✓ *Keep the home and family relaxed.* This will permit the person on a program to pay attention to the task at hand, changing eating and exercise habits.

✓ *Learn to ignore and forgive lapses.* The family can react many ways to mistakes, bouts of weight gain, and binges. The person losing weight feels bad when these occur, so it is best for the family to adopt a hands off policy and to forgive and forget.

✓ *Ask the person losing weight how you can help.* The best way to learn how to help is to ask. Family members are sometimes surprised by what the individual wants.

✓ *Exercise with the person on a program.* This is a wonderful and healthy way to spend time together. If only a daily walk, this provides time to talk and can help the person with the program.

✓ *Develop new interests with the family member losing weight.* There are so many things in life to enjoy, and developing new interests can be good for everybody. Individuals losing weight sometimes feel they are embarking on a new life. New activities can involve the family in this process.

[a]From Bromwell (1994). Reprinted by permission.

individual's fat or the enhanced metabolic activity of the carbohydrate that is likely to replace the fat (Hill et al., 1991).

However, attention only to dietary-fat levels in the diet may be inadvisable. It is still possible to consume a substantial number of excess calories while keeping fat intake at a minimum, especially as more low-fat and fat-free food items are produced, many with caloric content nearly as high as the original versions. In addition, attention to fat or calories only may lead to a diet unbalanced in macronutrients (carbohydrates, protein, fat), vitamins, minerals, and fiber. A sound dietary plan should include foods from all food groups. Recently, the U.S. Department of Agriculture issued revised recommendations for a balanced diet, the "Food Pyramid," which can be used as a guide for food selection.

Intervention

Although it is not always necessary to specify a precise level of caloric intake, a general range, at minimum, should be established based on the client's estimated energy

Sidebar 11–3

Partnership Quiz

	True	False
1. It is easy to talk to my partner about weight.		
	5	1
2. My partner has always been thin and does not understand my weight problem.		
	1	3
3. My partner offers me food when he or she knows I am trying to lose weight.		
	1	5
4. My partner never says critical things about my weight.		
	3	1
5. My partner is always there when I need a friend.		
	4	1
6. When I lose weight and look better, my partner will be jealous.		
	1	3
7. My partner will be genuinely interested in helping me with my weight.		
	6	1
8. I could talk to my partner even if I was doing poorly.		
	5	1

Note: Reprinted with permission from Brownell (1994).

needs, the desired rate of weight loss, the client's ability to restrict intake without precipitating disinhibited binge eating, and the extent to which there will be concurrent medical monitoring. For example, VLCDs are defined as diets providing 800 or fewer calories per day. VLCDs should be restricted to persons who are at least 30% overweight, and must not be used without careful medical screening and monitoring (National Task Force on the Prevention and Treatment of Obesity, 1993). In the absence of monitoring, weight-loss diets should generally provide at least 1,200 calories per day.

Clients should be advised that the reinforcing, rapid weight loss that accompanies highly restrictive, calorically deficient diets is accomplished in part by loss of water and lean body mass. Furthermore, we have observed clinically that dietary adherence is easier if fat intake is limited. Compliance can suffer if fat intake drops to very low levels, so we recommend that fat comprise 20% to 30% of total calories (National Academy of Sciences, 1989).

Therapists should also dismiss the notion that certain foods are "good" or "bad." Declaring certain foods to be taboo can lead to restrictions that cannot be followed for more than a short period of time, setting the stage for lapses that may trigger further dietary deterioration. An alternative approach is to describe foods according to how frequently they are consumed.

Therapists should consider that many obese adults have medical conditions that

Table 11.7. Guidelines for Promoting Positive Interactions around Issues concerning Weight Loss[a]

✓ *Are you both ready for a partnership?* Is your partner ready to listen to requests for help and make the required effort? Is he or she ready to help you during good times and bad? Are you ready to help your partner in return? Some degree of commitment is necessary from both of you.

✓ *Tell your partner how to help.* A common and crucial mistake is to expect your partner to read your mind. If it is your spouse, you may think he or she should know what you want and need. Most people are not good mind readers, so leave nothing to chance. Tell your partner what he or she can do. Do you want to be praised when you do well or scolded when you do poorly? Should the person avoid eating in your presence? Can your partner help by exercising with you?

✓ *Make specific requests.* The more specific your requests, the easier it will be for your partner to comply. If your request is vague and general, like "Be nice," your partner is at a disadvantage. A more specific request is better, such as "Please tell me you love me when I lose weight." Instead of saying, "Don't eat in front of me," say "It helps me when you eat your evening bowl of ice cream in the other room." Replace a general statement like, "Exercise with me" with "Please take a half-hour walk with me each morning."

✓ *State your requests positively.* It is better to ask for something positive than to criticize something negative. Clever changes of words can help. If your partner nags, you can say "It really helps me when you say nice things." If your partner offers you food, you can say "I appreciate the times when you don't offer me food. It is easier to control my eating then." Human nature responds well to the chance to do something positive, so try this approach with your partner.

✓ *Reward your partner.* For your partner to help you, you must help your partner. One-way relationships don't last long. If you are going through this program together, you can work out weight control-related ways of helping. If your partner is not on a program, be forward, and ask what you can do in return. Remember, being a partner can be draining, so you need to acknowledge your partner's help.

[a]From Brownell (1994). Reprinted with permission.

require more specialized dietary prescriptions. Clients with such conditions should be referred to a registered dietitian, who can provide a diet in consultation with the client's physician. For example, diabetes may necessitate greater attention to carbohydrate content and spacing of meals and snacks, and hypercholesterolemia may demand a larger reduction in saturated fat and cholesterol intake.

One technique that can be helpful in limiting the amount of calories consumed is to slow the rate of food consumption. Spiegel, Wadden, and Foster (1991) have shown that weight-loss clients who slow their eating the most lose the most weight. Unfortunately, this same study showed that this slowdown decays over time (i.e., a faster eating rate returns). Clients can be encouraged to slow their eating rate by various means: self-monitoring meal durations, putting down their fork between bites, and building pauses in their meals. This is especially important for clients whose self-monitoring records reveal a pattern of rapid eating. Clients should be reminded that this is one change that does not entail feelings of deprivation and, in fact, may reduce such feelings.

Stimulus-control techniques can be helpful in restricting the client's exposure to eating cues. For example, food in the home should be limited to as few locations as possible and kept out of view. Similarly, clients should do what they can to reduce the prominence and availability of food in the workplace. A single eating location should be chosen and all eating should occur only in that place. This can extinguish associations between other activities or areas of the house and eating, for example, snacking while watching television in the den. Stimulus-control techniques can also be used in helping the client cope with certain high-risk situations. A client who has a long-standing habit of snacking on returning

---

Sidebar 11–4

Social vs. Solo Inventory

	True	False
1. I talk to other people about my weight.	____	____
2. Given a choice, I would rather exercise with others than alone.	____	____
3. I would rather have people compliment me on my weight change than leave me alone.	____	____
4. I feel I could talk to a close friend about my weight and my eating.	____	____
5. I can accept positive comments from others.	____	____
6. In a weight loss program, I would do just fine in a group.	____	____
7. I like others to notice when I am doing well with my weight.	____	____
8. I consider myself more of a sociable person than a loner.	____	____
9. I like to be around other people.	____	____
10. With regard to weight maintenance, I would like to have others support me.	____	____

Note: Reprinted by permission from Brownell and Rodin (1990).

---

home from work may be helped by entering the house through a different door. Declaring the car off limits for eating can, over time, reduce the desire for snacking on trips.

Balancing the Diet: The Food Guide Pyramid

For many years, the tried-and-true method for eating a balanced diet involved food groups, with a recommended number of servings from each group. A widely used alternative, utilized especially by dietitians and physicians working with diabetic patients, was the exchange plan developed jointly by the American Dietetic Association and the American Diabetes Association. Both plans were reasonable ways to encourage healthy eating in the general public.

With new advances in nutritional sciences, a new plan for healthy eating was published in 1992 by the U.S. Department of Agriculture and the U.S. Department of Health and Human Services. Seven general guidelines were issued (Table 11.8). Although these guidelines sound like the advice most Americans have heard repeatedly, they are enormously important to reinforce. These patterns of eating are associated with many of the leading causes of death, and although most people have heard this advice in one form or another, compliance in the general population is low.

Table 11.8. General Nutrition Guidelines Issued in 1992 by the U.S. Department of Agriculture and the U.S. Department of Health and Human Services[a]

1. Eat a variety of foods.
2. Maintain a healthy weight.
3. Choose a diet low in fat, saturated fat, and cholesterol.
4. Choose a diet with plenty of vegetables, fruits, and grain products.
5. Use sugar only in moderation.
6. Use salt in moderation.
7. If you drink alcoholic beverages, do so in moderation.

[a]From U.S. Department of Agriculture (1980). Reprinted with permission.

The new plan for healthy eating was the Food Guide Pyramid (Figure 11.3). The pyramid is similar to the basic-food-group approach, except that fruits and vegetables are in separate groups and a new category has been added for fats, oils, and sweets.

Clients are instructed to use the pyramid in the following way. Foods at the top of the pyramid are to be eaten sparingly. These are foods high in fat or sugar, and tend to be high in calories given their nutritional value (i.e., nutrient density is low). As one proceeds down the pyramid, more servings of food are suggested. As shown in Figure 11.10, specific numbers of servings are recommended in each group. The amounts of specific foods that constitute a serving are discussed elsewhere (Brownell, 1994).

RELAPSE PREVENTION

Rationale

Unfortunately, relapse is a common phenomenon experienced by individuals attempting to lose weight (Brownell et al., 1986). The client's response to relapse may determine the likelihood of success in subsequent attempts to change. It would appear at first glance that relapse has negative emotional effects. Disappointment, frustration, and self-condemnation are apparent in people who relapse, and family and friends are unhappy and sometimes angry. However, learning may occur before or during relapse, so some benefit may exist. One study tracked depression in subjects who lost weight and then regained it (Brownell & Stunkard, 1981). Depression scores dropped as weight declined, but returned halfway to baseline as half of the weight was regained. Although these subjects were not successful maintainers, the net change in mood was still positive.

Relapse can be conceptualized as a process rather than an outcome (Marlatt & Gordon, 1985). Webster's New Collegiate Dictionary gives both definitions. The first is "a recurrence of symptoms of a disease after a period of improvement." This refers to an outcome and implies a dichotomous view, because a person is either ill and has symptoms or is well and does not. The second definition is "the act or instance of backsliding, worsening, or subsiding." This focuses on a process and implies something less serious, perhaps a slip or mistake.

The choice of the process or outcome definition has important implications for conceptualizing, preventing, and treating relapse. We suggest that a lapse may be best described as a process, behavior, or event (Marlatt & Gordon, 1985). A lapse is a single event, or a reemergence of a previous habit, that may or may not lead to the state of relapse.

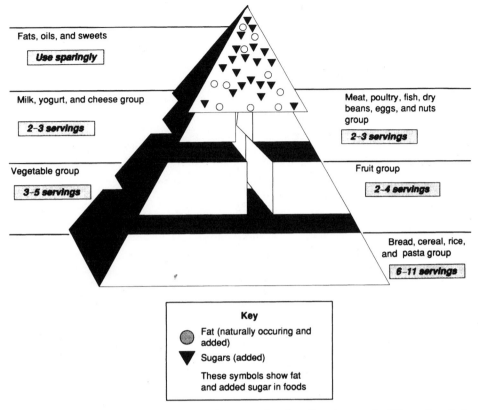

Key

Fat (naturally occuring and added)

Sugars (added)

These symbols show fat and added sugar in foods

Figure 11.3. The Food Guide Pyramid. Foods on the tops, such as fats, oils and sweets should be used sparingly. Foods on the bottom of the pyramid, such as bread, cereal, rice, and pasta, should be used more frequently. Reprinted by permission from Brownell (1994).

When a slip or mistake is defined as a lapse, it implies that corrective action can be taken, not that control is lost completely. The challenge with this approach is defining when one or more lapses becomes a relapse. The individual's response to these lapses determines whether relapse has occurred.

Intervention

When working with the client to implement maintenance strategies to prevent relapse, it is not advisable in treatment to isolate maintenance strategies from weight-loss interventions (Perri, 1995; Perri et al., 1992). This may communicate to the client that implementation of these strategies is optional or postponable. It is preferable to work these techniques throughout the entire span of treatment with an emphasis on long-term change and with institution of cognitive and behavioral methods that will be required to maintain a weight loss over the years. Although it is true that the skills most important for weight loss are often different from those most important for maintenance, they are rarely incompatible; early initiation of maintenance behaviors will allow the client to practice them while under a longer period of supervision by the therapist. There are several strategies that can be useful in achieving maintenance. Some techniques, such as exercise, we have already discussed in detail. Others include extending treatment, providing coping skills, and focusing on certain issues, such as binge eating and body image in clients.

Extend Treatment

Several reviews have shown that length of treatment is positively related to outcome (Bennett, 1986; Brownell & Kramer, 1989; Brownell & Wadden, 1986; Perri, 1995; Perri et al., 1992). Treatment length has increased from an average of 8 weeks in 1974 to 21 weeks from 1987 to 1990. It appears that extending treatment is helpful to approximately 25 weeks, after which weight loss slows substantially. One controlled study, however, found that maintenance was greater in subjects receiving 40 as opposed to 20 weeks in treatment (Perri, Nezu, Patti, & McCann, 1989).

Provide Coping Skills

The use of coping skills has been noted as a central feature in preventing relapse in the addictive disorders (Brownell et al., 1986; Marlatt & Gordon, 1985) and follows logically from relapse prevention and self-efficacy theories (Bandura, 1986; Marlatt & Gordon, 1985). There have been some attempts to use coping skills as the foundation of programs to promote maintenance (Brownell & Rodin, 1990; Perri et al., 1988), but more work is needed to develop skills specific to weight maintenance and to match the skills to the dynamics of the relapse process (Grilo, Shiffman, & Wing, 1989).

A major cause of failure to recover from such lapses is a dichotomous, all-or-none style of evaluating one's success. Clients with this style consider anything less than perfection to be a complete failure. When an inevitable setback occurs, the client overgeneralizes the failure, often attributing this failure to personal flaws rather than to situational factors. Clients who exhibit this evaluative style should be helped to detect implicit all-or-none assumptions in their reactions to lapses during treatment and to rehearse alternative self-statements that embody a continuous, matter-of-degree approach to measuring success.

Anticipating possible problems and developing a set of responses to be used when the problems are encountered can greatly strengthen the client's self-efficacy and the resulting ability to cope with the day-to-day threats encountered during both weight loss and maintenance (Brownell & Jeffery, 1987). The case of "Peter" is a good example. He is a 44-year-old postal supervisor, 5'11" and 205 lb after a loss of 30 lb. Peter (P) slumped dejectedly into his chair after learning that he had gained 1 lb (from Brownell & O'Neil, 1993).

> **P:** I started not to bother coming in today.
> **T:** Why is that?
> **P:** I had a terrible week. I didn't do anything I was supposed to do, and I pigged out at the father–son dinner at my son's school yesterday.
> **T:** Does that mean you didn't meet your exercise goal?
> **P:** I did that, but I didn't do anything else.
> **T:** Like keeping your eating diary?
> **P:** Oh, I did that, it's all here for you to see.
> **T:** So you kept your diary, and you met your exercise goal. What made it such a terrible week besides the father–son dinner?

P: Wasn't that enough? I knew I wouldn't be able to stick to my diet there, I never can, I just don't have any willpower.

T: What do you think gave you trouble?

P: We had an urgent meeting at work at noon, and I didn't get to eat lunch, so I was ready to eat anything when I got to dinner.

T: It's not surprising you overate at the dinner if you missed the lunch. By the way, my mail carrier delivered one of my magazines to the neighbors yesterday.

P: What's that got to do with anything? We handle thousands of pieces of mail each day. What about all of the mail that was delivered correctly? You can't expect people to never make a mistake.

T: Unless we're talking about you and your weight-loss program.

P: (*Pauses*) I guess I get your point. Even though I blow it one day, it doesn't mean that the whole week's a failure.

T: That's right. It might help to remember my magazine the next time you fall a little short of your goals.

Provide Treatment for Body Image Disturbance and Binge Eating

The importance of psychological factors in the management of obesity has been noted for years (Stunkard, 1976), but these factors have been virtually ignored in most programs. There are now signs that the field is recognizing this issue (Brownell & Rodin, 1990; Friedman & Brownell, 1995; Wadden & Bell, 1990). For example, body-image disparagement is common among obese persons (Stunkard, 1976; Wadden & Stunkard, 1985). The body is viewed as an enemy for which there is often hatred and loathing. In addition, some persons overestimate body size even after weight loss. As mentioned earlier, binge eating occurs in a sizable percentage of obese persons who seek treatment and is a negative prognostic sign for weight loss (Marcus et al., 1985, 1988). Early attempts have been made to treat binge eating in obese patients (Marcus et al., 1990).

Stimulated by recognition of the role of body image in psychological health (Cash & Pruzinsky, 1990; Thompson, 1990) and in bulimia (Fairburn & Garner, 1986), researchers have developed programs to improve body image (Butters & Cash, 1987; Rosen, Saltzberg, & Srebnik, 1989). Application of these methods to overweight individuals, taking into account their specific problems with body-size estimation and body image, may be an important development in the field.

The specific interventions necessary during long-term work with the post-weight-loss client will depend on the needs and circumstances of the client, which vary over time. At any given point a client may require assistance with stress management, marital counseling, assertiveness training, body-image remediation, dating skills, exercise compliance, or dealing with commitment and intimate issues. Obviously, one therapist may not be proficient in all these areas. However, the overall role of the therapist in this long-term endeavor may be described rather consistently over time and across clients. According to Perri et al. (1992), the health-care professional's role is to serve as an active problem solver who aids the client in identifying effective strategies to sustain behavioral changes needed for long-term success. To this we add that the role also incorporates the important elements of social support, empathy, and a source of reality testing for client expectations.

The importance of encouraging the client to use the therapist in these ways over an extended period cannot be overemphasized. The idea of a continuous-care approach to obesity is novel to most obese people. Many clients feel the continued reliance on professional help is a sign of weakness. Furthermore, many clients are most reluctant to attend treatment when they most need it: when they are gaining weight. Thus, from the outset, the therapist should use any means available to help the client to accept and act on a long-term model of care (see Table 11.9).

CONCLUSION

Obesity is a complex and heterogeneous disorder with multiple etiologies, medical and psychological effects, and possible options for treatment. When considering the potential negative effects of dieting, as well as the repeated weight cycling associated with dietary failure, it becomes clear that any individual must make a careful, informed decision about whether to attempt to lose weight, and what the appropriate method would be.

There are many approaches other than dieting that are available for the obese person attempting to lose weight. After ruling out unsafe and unsound approaches, there are still many commercial and self-help programs, counseling available from a number of health professionals, and countless plans for losing weight "on your own" that are still available to the individual seeking to lose weight. Professionals can consider these approaches and programs as allies and resources, so that referral to other programs, combining approaches, or using different approaches in sequence can now be part of service delivery for overweight persons.

We suggest several conceptual factors that can increase a person's likelihood of success and should be considered in choosing a treatment approach. The first is a lifestyle-change philosophy in which reasonable changes in eating and exercise are encouraged, and emphasis is on weaving these changes into day-to-day patterns of living. The second

Table 11.9. Suggested Methods for Improving the Maintenance of Weight Loss[a]

1. Consider other treatments for our patients.
2. Develop criteria to match patients to treatments.
3. Develop criteria for screening patients to determine if there would be a better time to diet or a better program to join.
4. Increase initial weight losses.
5. Increase the length of treatment.
6. Be more aggressive about attaining goal weight. Consider the "initial treatment phase" as the period necessary to reach goal weight. "Maintenance" should not be considered until there is a substantial weight loss to maintain.
7. Increase the emphasis on exercise. Structured, supervised exercise programs need to be tested against current programs in which patients are given only verbal or written advice about exercise.
8. Exploit the social environment as a means to improve long-term adherence. More research is necessary to define the factors in the family, work site, community, etc., that can be used to facilitate weight loss.
9. Financial incentives, which have been effective in producing some of the best losses in behavioral studies, need to be extended for use in the long term.
10. Combine behavioral programs with other treatments, such as commercial and self-help programs, aggressive diets, or surgery.
11. Evaluate the cognitive factors that are included in most programs by consensus, but which have not been studied in detail.
12. Possibly extend stimulus control methods into the dieter's daily life by considering different mechanisms for food delivery and for supervised exercise.
13. Study the use and timing of relapse-prevention methods in more detail.

[a]From Brownell & O'Neil (1993). Reprinted with permission.

conceptual factor involves setting reasonable goals and working toward large changes by making small, incremental, and manageable changes. Finally, the third factor is a focus on the maintenance of behavior change. These factors are critical to treating a chronic problem that requires long-term management.

ACKNOWLEDGEMENTS.. Work on this chapter was supported in part by a fellowship from the Jenny Craig Foundation. Some sections of the chapter were adapted from information in a paper by Brownell and Wadden (1992) and a chapter by Brownell and O'Neil (1993). ·

REFERENCES

Allon, N. (1982). The stigma of overweight in everyday life. In B. Wolman (Ed.), *Psychological aspects of obesity: A handbook* (pp. 130–174). New York: Van Nostrand Reinhold.

Andres, R., Muller, D., & Sorkin, J. (1993). *Long-term effects of change in body weight on all-cause mortality. Annals of Internal Medicine, 119*, 737–743.

Bandura, A. (1986). *Social foundations of thought and action: A social cognitive theory.* Englewood Cliffs, NJ: Prentice-Hall.

Bennett, G. A. (1986). Behavior therapy for obesity: A quantitative review of the effects of selected treatment characteristics on outcome. *Behavior Therapy, 17*, 554–562.

Bjornthorp, P. (1985). Regional patterns of fat distribution. *Annals of Internal Medicine, 103*, 994–995.

Bjornthorp, P., & Brodoff, B. (Eds.). (1992). *Obesity.* Philadelphia: Lippincott.

Blackburn, G. L., & Kanders, B. S. (1987). Medical evaluation and treatment of the obese patient with cardiovascular disease. *American Journal of Cardiology, 60*, 55g–58g.

Blair, S. N., Shaten, J., Brownell, K., Collins, G., & Lissner, L. (1993). Body weight change, all-cause mortality, and cause-specific mortality in the multiple-risk-factor intervention trial. *Annals of Internal Medicine, 119*, 749–757.

Blair, S. N., Kohl, H. W., Paffenbarger, R. S., Clark, D. G., Cooper, K. H., & Gibbons, L. W. (1989). Physical fitness and all-cause mortality: A prospective study of healthy men and women. *Journal of the American Medical Association, 262*, 2395–2401.

Blundell, J. E. (1990). How culture undermines the biopsychological system of appetite control. *Appetite, 14*, 113–115.

Bouchard, C. (1991). Is weight fluctuation a risk factor? *New England Journal of Medicine, 324*, 1887–1888.

Bouchard, C., Trembley, A., Despres, J. P., Nadeau, A., Lupien, P., Thériault, G., Dussalt, J., Moorjani, S., Pinault, S., & Fournier, G. (1990). The response to long-term overfeeding in identical twins. *New England Journal of Medicine, 322*, 1477–1482.

Bouchard, C., Tremblay, A., Nadeau, A., Despres, J. P., Theriault, G., Boulay, M. R., Lortie, G., Leblanc, C., & Fournier, G. (1989). Genetic effect in resting and exercise metabolic rates. *Metabolism, 38*, 364–370.

Bray, G. A. (1986). Effects of obesity on health and happiness. In K. D. Brownell & J. P. Foreyt (Eds.), *Handbook of eating disorders: Physiology, psychology and treatment of obesity, anorexia, and bulimia* (pp. 3–44). New York: Basic Books.

Brewerton, T. D., Dansky, B. S., O'Neil, P. M., & Kilpatrick, D. (1993, May). *The prevalence of binge eating disorder in a national sample of women.* Paper presented at the meeting of the American Psychiatric Association, San Francisco, CA.

Brownell, K. D. (1980). Assessment of eating disorders. In D. H. Barlow (Ed.), *Behavioral assessment of adult disorders* (pp. 329–404). New York: Guilford Press.

Brownell, K. D. (1984). Behavioral, psychological, and environmental predictors of obesity and success at weight reduction. *International Journal of Obesity, 8*, 543–550.

Brownell, K. D. (1991a). Personal responsibility and control over our health: When expectation exceeds reality. *Health Psychology, 10*, 303–310.

Brownell, K. D. (1991b). Dieting and the search for the perfect body: Where physiology and culture collide. *Behavior Therapy, 22*, 1–12.

Brownell, K. D. (1994). *The LEARN program for weight control.* Dallas, TX: American Health.

Brownell, K. D. (1995). Exercise in the treatment of obesity. In K. D. Brownell, & C. G. Fairburn (Eds.), *Comprehensive textbook of eating disorders and obesity* (pp. 473–478). New York: Guilford Press.

Brownell, K. D., & Jeffery, R. W. (1987). Improving long-term weight loss: Pushing the limits of treatment. *Behavior Therapy, 18,* 353–374.

Brownell, K. D., & Kramer, F. M. (1989). Behavioral management of obesity. *Medical Clinics of North America, 73,* 185–201.

Brownell, K. D., Marlatt, G. A., Lichtenstein, E., & Wilson, G. T. (1986). Understanding and preventing relapse. *American Psychologist, 41,* 765–782.

Brownell, K. D., & O'Neil, P. M. (1993). *Obesity.* In D. H. Barlow (Ed.), *Clinical handbook of psychological disorders* (pp. 318–361). New York: Guilford Press.

Brownell, K. D., & Rodin, J. (1990). *The weight maintenance survival guide.* Dallas: American Health.

Brownell, K. D., & Rodin, J. (1994a). The dieting maelstrom: Is it possible and advisable to lose weight? *American Psychologist, 49,* 781–791.

Brownell, K. D., & Rodin, J. (1994b). Medical, metabolic, and psychological effects of weight cycling. *Archives of Internal Medicine, 154,* 1325–1330.

Brownell, K. D., & Stunkard, A. J. (1980). Physical activity in the development and control of obesity. In A. J. Stunkard (Ed.), *Obesity* (pp. 300–324). Philadelphia: Saunders.

Brownell, K. D., & Stunkard, A. J. (1981). Couples training, pharmacotherapy, and behavior therapy in the treatment of obesity. *Archives of General Psychiatry, 38,* 1224–1229.

Brownell, K. D., & Wadden, T. A. (1986). Behavior therapy for obesity: Modern approaches and better results. In K. D. Brownell & J. P. Foreyt (Eds.), *The physiology, psychology, and treatment of eating disorders* (pp. 180–187). New York: Basic Books.

Brownell, K. D., & Wadden, T. A. (1991). The heterogeneity of obesity: Fitting treatments to individuals. *Behavior Therapy, 22,* 153–177.

Brownell, K. D., & Wadden, T. A. (1992). Etiology and treatment of obesity: Understanding a serious, prevalent, and refractory disorder. *Journal of Consulting and Clinical Psychology, 60,* 505–517.

Bruce, B., & Agras, W. S. (1992). Binge eating in females: A population-based investigation. *International Journal of Eating Disorders, 12,* 365–374.

Butters, J. W., & Cash, T. F. (1987). Cognitive–behavioral treatment of women's body-image dissatisfaction. *Journal of Consulting and Clinical Psychology, 55,* 889–897.

Canning, H., & Mayer, J. (1966). Obesity—its possible effects on college admissions. *New England Journal of Medicine, 275,* 1172–1174.

Cash, T. F., & Pruzinsky, T. (Eds.). (1990). *Body images: Developments, deviance, and change.* New York: Guilford Press.

Cash, T. F. (1991). Binge-eating and body images among the obese: A further evaluation. *Journal of Social Behavior and Personality, 6,* 367–376.

Colditz, G. A. (1992). Economic costs of severe obesity. *American Journal of Clinical Nutrition, 55*(Suppl. 1), 503s–507s.

Craighead, L. W., & Blum, M. D. (1989). Supervised exercise in behavioral treatment of obesity. *Behavior Therapy, 20,* 49–59.

Davis, C. J., Williamson, D. A., Goreczny, A. J., & Bennett, S. M. (1989). Body image disturbances and bulimia nervosa: An empirical analysis of recent revisions of the DSM-III. *Journal of Psychopathology and Behavioral Assessment, 11,* 61–69.

DeBusk, R. F., Stenestrand, U., Sheehan, M., & Haskell, W. L. (1990). Training effects of long versus short bouts of exercise in healthy subjects. *American Journal of Cardiology, 65,* 1010–1013.

DeJong, W., & Kleck, R. (1986). The social psychological effects of overweight. In C. P. Herman, M. P. Zanna, & E. T. Higgins (Eds.), *Physical appearance, stigma, and social behavior: The Ontario symposium* (Vol. 3, pp. 65–87). Hillsdale, NJ: Erlbaum.

Dublin, L. I. (1953). Relation of obesity to longevity. *New England Journal of Medicine, 248,* 971–974.

Ernst, N. D., & Harlan, W. R. (1991). Obesity and cardiovascular disease in minority populations: Executive summary. Conference highlights, conclusions, and recommendations. *American Journal of Clinical Nutrition, 53,* 1507S–1511S.

Fairburn, C. G., & Garner, D. M. (1986). The diagnosis of bulimia nervosa. *International Journal of Eating Disorders, 5,* 403–419.

Fairburn, C. G., Jones, R., Peveler, R. C., Carr, S. J., Solomon, R. A., (1991). Three psychological treatments for bulimia nervosa. *Archives of General Psychiatry, 48,* 463–469.

Friedman, M. A., & Brownell, K. D. (1995). Psychological correlates of obesity: Moving to the next generation of research. *Psychological Bulletin, 117,* 3–20.

Foreyt, J. P., & Goodrick, G. K. (1991). Factors common to successful therapy for the obese patient. *Medicine and Science in Sports and Exercise, 23,* 292–297.

Foster, G. D., Wadden, T. A., Mullen, J. L., Stunkard, A. J., Wang, J., Feurer, I. D., Pierson, R. N., Yang, M. U., Presta, E., Van Itallie, T. B., Lemberg, P. S., Gold, J. (1988). Resting energy expenditure, body composition, and excess weight in the obese. *Metabolism, 37,* 467–472.

Garner, D. M., & Wooley, S. C. (1991). Confronting the failure of behavioral and dietary treatments for obesity. *Clinical Psychology Review, 11,* 729–780.

Garrison, R. J., & Castelli, W. P. (1985). Weight and thirty-year mortality of men in the Framingham Study. *Annals of Internal Medicine, 103,* 1006–1009.

Garrow, J. S. (1974). *Energy balance and obesity in man.* New York: Elsevier Science.

Glassner, B. (1988). *Bodies: Why we look the way we do and how we feel about it.* New York: Putnam.

Goldstein, D. J. (1992). Beneficial health effects of modest weight loss. *International Journal of Obesity, 6,* 397–416.

Grilo, C. M., Shiffman, S., & Wing, R. R. (1989). Relapse crises and coping among dieters. *Journal of Consulting and Clinical Psychology, 57,* 488–495.

Hamm, P., Shekelle, R. B., & Stamler, J. (1989). Large fluctuations in body weight during young adulthood and twenty-five year risk of coronary heart disease in men. *American Journal of Epidemiology, 129,* 312–318.

Hammond, E. C., & Garfinkel, L. (1969). Coronary heart disease, stroke, and aortic aneurysm. *Archives of Environmental Health, 19,* 167–182.

Hill, J. O., Peters, J. C., Reed, G. W., Schlundt, D. G., Sharp, T., & Greene, H. L. (1991). Nutrient balance in humans: Effect of diet composition. *American Journal of Clinical Nutrition, 54,* 10–17.

Hill, J. O., Schlundt, D. G., Sbrocco, T., Sharp, T., Pope-Cordel, J., Stetsen, B., Kaler, M., & Hime, C. (1989). Evaluation of an alternating-calorie diet with and without exercise in the treatment of obesity. *American Journal of Clinical Nutrition, 50,* 248–254.

Hsu, G. (1990). *Eating disorders.* New York: Guilford Press.

Hypertension Prevention Trial Research Group. (1990). The Hypertension Prevention Trial: Three-year effects of dietary change on blood pressure. *Archives of Internal Medicine, 150,* 153–162.

Jeffery, R. W. (1987). Behavioral treatment of obesity. *Annals of Behavioral Medicine, 9,* 20–24.

Jeffery, R. W., Adlis, S. A., & Forster, J. L. (1991). Prevalence of dieting among working men and women: The Healthy Worker Project. *Health Psychology, 10,* 274–281.

Jeffery, R. W., Folsom, A. R., Luepker, R. V., Jacobs, D. R., Gillum, R. F., Taylor, H. L., & Blackburn, H. (1984). Prevalence of overweight and weight loss behavior in a metropolitan adult population: The Minnesota Heart Survey experience. *American Journal of Public Health, 74,* 349–352.

Jeffery, R. W., & Wing, R. R. (1983). Recidivism and self-cure of smoking and obesity: Data from population studies. *American Psychologist, 38,* 852.

Karris, L. (1977). Prejudice against obese renters. *Journal of Social Psychology, 101,* 159–160.

Kayman, S., Bruvold, W., & Stern, J. S. (1990). Maintenance and relapse after weight loss in women: Behavioral aspects. *American Journal of Clinical Nutrition, 52,* 800–807.

Keefe, P. H., Wyshogrod, D., & Weinberger, E., & Agras, W. S. (1984). Binge eating and outcome of behavioral treatment of obesity: A preliminary report. *Behaviour Research and Therapy, 22,* 319–321.

Keesey, R. E. (1986). A set-point theory of obesity. In K. D. Brownell & J. P. Foreyt (Eds.), *Handbook of eating disorders: Physiology, psychology, and treatment of obesity, anorexia, and bulimia* (pp. 63–87). New York: Basic Books.

Kendall, A., Levitsky, D. A., Strupp, B. J., & Lissner, L. (1991). Weight loss on a low-fat diet: Consequence of the imprecision of the control of food intake in humans. *American Journal of Clinical Nutrition, 53,* 1124–1129.

Klesges, R. C., Hanson, C. L., Eck, L. H., & Durff, A. C. (1988). Accuracy of self-reports of food intake in obese and normal-weight individuals: Effects of parental obesity on reports of children's dietary intake. *American Journal of Clinical Nutrition, 48,* 1252–1256.

Kuczmarski, R. J. (1992). Prevalence of overweight and weight gain in the United States. *American Journal of Clinical Nutrition, 55*(Suppl. 1), 495S–502S.

Larkin, J. E., & Pines, H. A. (1979). No fat persons need apply. *Sociology of Work and Occupations, 6,* 312–327.

Lean, M. E. J., Powrie, J. K., Anderson, A. S., & Garthwaite, P. H. (1990). Obesity, weight loss, and prognosis in Type II diabetes. *Diabetic Medicine, 7,* 228–233.

Leibel, R. L., & Hirsch, J. (1984). Diminished energy requirements in reduced-obese patients. *Metabolism, 33,* 164–170.

Lichtman, S. W., Pisarka, K., Berman, E. R., Pestone, M., Dowling, H., Offenbacher, E., Weisel, H., Heshka, S.,

Matthews, D. E., & Heymsfield, S. B. (1992). Discrepancy between self-reported and actual caloric intake and exercise in obese subjects. *New England Journal of Medicine, 327,* 1893–1898.

Lissner, L., Odell, P. M., D'Agostino, R. B., Stokes, J., Kreger, B. E., Belanger, A. J., & Brownell, K. D. (1991). Variability of body weight and health outcomes in the Framingham population. *New England Journal of Medicine, 324,* 1839–1844.

Manson, J. E., Colditz, G. A., Stampfer, M. J., Willett, W. C., Rosner, B., Monson, R. R., Speizer, F. E., & Hennekens, C. H. (1990). A prospective study of obesity and risk of coronary heart disease in women. *New England Journal of Medicine, 322,* 882–889.

Marcus, M. D., Wing, R. R., Ewing, L., Kern, E., McDermott, M., & Gooding, W. (1990). A double-blind, placebo-controlled trial of fluoxetine plus behavior modification in the treatment of obese binge eaters. *American Journal of Psychiatry, 147,* 876–881.

Marcus, M. D., Wing, R. R., & Hopkins, J. (1988). Obese binge eaters: Affect, cognitions, and response to behavioral weight control. *Journal of Consulting and Clinical Psychology, 56,* 433–439.

Marcus, M. D., Wing, R. R., & Lamparski, D. M. (1985). Binge eating and dietary restraint in obese patients. *Addictive Behaviors, 10,* 163–168.

Marlatt, G. A., & Gordon, J. (Eds.). (1985). *Relapse prevention: Maintenance strategies in addictive behavior change.* New York: Guilford Press.

National Academy of Sciences, National Research Council. (1989). *Diet and Health: Implications for reducing chronic disease risk.* Washington, DC: National Academy Press.

National Task Force on the Prevention and Treatment of Obesity. (1993). Very low-calorie diets. *Journal of the American Medical Association, 270,* 967–974.

O'Neil, P. M., & Jarrell, M. P. (1992). Psychological aspects of obesity and dieting. In T. A. Wadden & T. B. Van Itallie (Eds.), *Treatment of the seriously obese patient* (pp. 252–270). New York: Guilford Press.

O'Neil, P. M., Jarrell, M. P., Hedden, C. E., Cochrane, C., Sexauer, J., & Brewerton, T. D. (1992, August). *Metabolic correlates of binge eating in obesity.* Paper presented at the meeting of the North American Association for the Study of Obesity, Atlanta, GA.

Pamuk, E. R., Williamson, D. F., Serdula, M. K., Madans, J., & Byers, T. E. (1993). Weight loss and subsequent death in a cohort of U.S. adults. *Annals of Internal Medicine, 119,* 744–748.

Pavlou, K. N., Krey, S., & Steffee, W. P. (1989). Exercise as an adjunct to weight loss and maintenance in moderately obese subjects. *American Journal of Clinical Nutrition, 49,* 1115–1123.

Perri, M. G. (1995). Methods for maintaining weight loss. In K. D. Brownell & C. G. Fairburn (Eds.), *Comprehensive textbook of eating disorders and obesity* (pp. 547–551). New York: Guilford Press.

Perri, M. G., McAllister, D. A., Gange, J. J., Jordan, R. C., McAdoo, W. G., & Nezu, A. M. (1988). Effects of four maintenance programs on the long-term management of obesity. *Journal of Consulting and Clinical Psychology, 56,* 529–534.

Perri, M. G., Nezu, A. M., Patti, E. T., & McCann, K. L. (1989). Effect of length of treatment on weight loss. *Journal of Consulting and Clinical Psychology, 57,* 450–452.

Perri, M. G., Nezu, A. M., & Viegener, B. J. (1992). *Improving the long-term management of obesity: Theory, research, and clinical guidelines.* New York: Wiley.

Pi-Sunyer, F. X. (1991). Health implications of obesity. *American Journal of Clinical Nutrition, 53,* 1595S–1603S.

Prewitt, T. E., Schmeisser, D., Bowen, P. E., Aye, P., Dolecek, T. A., Langenberg, P., Cole, T., & Brace, L. (1991). Changes in body weight, body composition, and energy intake in women fed high-and low-fat diets. *American Journal of Clinical Nutrition, 54,* 304–310.

Price, R. A. (1987). Genetics of human obesity. *Annals of Behavioral Medicine, 9,* 9–14.

Prochaska, J. O., DiClemente, C. C., & Norcross, J. C. (1991). In search of how people change: Applications to addictive disorders. *American Psychologist, 47,* 1102–1114.

Rand, C. S., & MacGregor, A. M. (1990). Morbidly obese patients' perceptions of social discrimination before and after surgery for obesity. *Southern Medical Journal, 83,* 1390–1395.

Reed, G. W., & Hill, J. O. (1993). Weight cycling: A review of the animal literature. *Obesity Research, 1,* 392–402.

Rodin, J. (1992). *Body traps.* New York: Morrow.

Rosen, J. C., Saltzberg, E., & Srebnik, D. (1989). Cognitive behavior therapy for negative body image. *Behavior Therapy, 20,* 393–404.

Schachter, S. (1982). Recidivism and self-cure of smoking and obesity. *American Psychologist, 37,* 436–444.

Schwartz, M. B., & Brownell, K. D. (1995). Matching individuals to weight loss treatments: A survey of obesity experts. *Journal of Consulting and Clinical Psychology, 63,* 149–153.

Sikand, G., Kondo, A., Foreyt, J. P., Jones, P. H., & Gotto, A. M. (1988). Two-year follow-up of patients treated with a very-low-calorie diet and exercise training. *Journal of the American Dietetic Association, 88,* 487–488.

Sjostrom, L. (1992). Morbidity and mortality of severely obese subjects. *American Journal of Clinical Nutrition*, 55(Suppl.), 5085–5155.

Sobal J., & Stunkard, A. J. (1989). Socioeconomic status and obesity: A review of the literature. *Psychological Bulletin, 105*, 260–275.

Spiegel, T. A., Wadden, T. A., & Foster, G. D. (1991). Objective measurement of eating rate during behavioral treatment of obesity. *Behavior Therapy, 22*, 61–67.

Spitzer, R. L., Devlin, M. J., Walsh, B. T., Hasin, D., Wing, R., Marcus, M., Stunkard, A. J., Wadden, T., Yanovski, S., Agras W. S., Mitchell, J., & Nonas C. (1992). Binge eating disorder: A multisite field trial of the diagnostic criteria. *International Journal of Eating Disorders, 11*, 191–204.

Staffieri, J. R. (1967). A study of social stereotype of body image in children. *Journal of Personality and Social Psychology, 7*, 101–104.

Stotland, S., & Zuroff, D. C. (1991). Relations between multiple measures of dieting self-efficacy and weight change in a behavioral weight control program. *Behavior Therapy, 22*, 47–59.

Striegel-Moore, R., & Rodin, J. (1986). The influence of psychological variables in obesity. In K. D. Brownell, & J. P. Foreyt (Eds.), *Handbook of eating disorders: Physiology, psychology and treatment of obesity, anorexia and bulimia* (pp. 99–121). New York: Basic Books.

Stuart, R., & Jacobson, B. (1987). *Weight, sex, and marriage: A delicate balance*. New York: Norton.

Stunkard, A. J. (1959). Eating patterns and obesity. *Psychiatric Quarterly, 33*, 284–292.

Stunkard, A. J. (1975). From explanation to action in psychosomatic medicine: The case of obesity. *Psychosomatic Medicine, 37*, 195–236.

Stunkard, A. J. (1976). *The pain of obesity*. Palo Alto, CA: Bull.

Stunkard, A. J. (1988). Some perspectives on human obesity: Its causes. *Bulletin of the New York Academy of Medicine, 64*, 902–923.

Stunkard, A. J., Harris, J. R., Pedersen, N. L., & McClearn, G. E. (1990). A separated twin study of the body mass index. *New England Journal of Medicine, 322*, 1483–1487.

Stunkard, A. J., & McLaren-Hume, M. (1959). The results of treatment of obesity: A review of the literature and report of a series. *Archives of Internal Medicine, 103*, 79–85.

Stunkard, A. J., & Sobal, J. (1995). Psychosocial consequences of obesity. In K. D. Brownell, & C. G. Fairburn (Eds.), *Comprehensive textbook of eating disorders and obesity* (pp. 417–421). New York: Guilford Press.

Stunkard, A. J., Sorenson, T. I. A., Hanis, C., Teasdale, T. W., Chakraborty, R., Schull, W. J., & Schlusinger, F. (1986). An adoption study of human obesity. *New England Journal of Medicine, 314*, 193–198.

Stunkard, A. J., & Wadden, T. A. (1992). Psychological aspects of severe obesity. *American Journal of Clinical Nutrition, 55*, 524S–532S.

Telch, C. F., Agras, W. S., & Rossiter, E. M. (1988). Binge eating increases with increasing adiposity. *International Journal of Eating Disorders, 7*, 115–119.

Thompson, J. K. (1990). *Body image disturbance: Assessment and treatment*. New York: Pergamon.

U.S. Department of Agriculture. (1990). *Nutrition and your health* Publication No. 017-001-00462). Washington, DC: U.S. Government Printing Office.

U.S. Department of Agriculture. (1984). *Nationwide food consumption survey. Nutrient intakes, Individuals in 48 states, year 1977–1978* (Report No. I-2, Consumer Nutrition Division, Human Nutrition Information Service). Hyattsville, MD: U.S. Government Printing Office.

Van Itallie, T. B. (1985). Health implications of overweight and obesity in the United States. *Annals of Internal Medicine, 103*, 983–988.

Wadden, T. A. (1985). Treatment of obesity in adults: A clinical perspective. In P. A. Keller & L. G. Ritt (Eds.), *Innovations in clinical practice: A source book, IV* (pp. 127–152). Sarasota, FL: Professional Resource Exchange.

Wadden, T. A., & Bell, S. T. (1990). Obesity. In A. S. Bellack, M. Hersen, & A. Kazdin (Eds.), *International handbook of behavior modification and therapy* (Vol. 2, pp. 449–473). New York: Plenum Press.

Wadden, T. A., Sternberg, J. A., Letizia, K. A., Stunkard, A. J., & Foster, G. D. (1989). Treatment of obesity by very low calorie diet, behavior therapy, and their combination: A five-year perspective. *International Journal of Obesity, 13*, 39–46.

Wadden, T. A., & Stunkard, A. J. (1985). Social and psychological consequences of obesity. *Annals of Internal Medicine, 103*, 1062–1067.

Wadden, T. A., Stunkard, A. J., & Liebschutz, J. (1988). Three-year follow-up of the treatment of obesity by very low calorie diet, behavior therapy, and their combination. *Journal of Consulting and Clinical Psychology, 56*, 925–928.

Wadden, T. A., & Wingate, B. J. (1995). Compassionate treatment of the obese individual. In K. D. Brownell, &

C. G. Fairburn (Eds.), *Comprehensive textbook of eating disorders and obesity* (pp. 564–571). New York: Guilford Press.

Wannamethee, G., & Shaper, A. G. (1990). Weight change in middle-aged British men: Implications for health. *European Journal of Clinical Nutrition, 44,* 133–142.

Wilcosky, T., Hyde, J., Anderson, J. J. B., Bangdiwala, S., & Duncan, B. (1990). Obesity and mortality in the Lipid Research Clinics Program Follow-Up Study. *Journal of Clinical Epidemiology, 43,* 743–752.

Wilfley, D. E., Agras, W. S., Telch, C. F., Rossiter, E. M., Schneider, J. A., Cole, A. G., Sifford, L., & Raeburn, S. D. (1993). Group cognitive–behavioral therapy and group interpersonal psychotherapy for the nonpurging bulimic: A controlled comparison. *Journal of Consulting and Clinical Psychology, 61,* 296–305.

Williamson, D. F. (1993). Descriptive epidemiology of body weight and weight change in United States adults. *Annals of Internal Medicine, 119,* 646–649.

Williamson, D. F., Kahn, H. S., Remington, P. L., & Anda, R. F. (1990). The 10-year incidence of overweight and major weight gain in U.S. adults. *Archives of Internal Medicine, 150,* 665–672.

Wilson, G. T. (1978). Methodological considerations in treatment outcome research on obesity. *Journal of Consulting and Clinical Psychology, 46,* 687–702.

Wilson, G. T. (1995). The controversy over dieting. In K. D. Brownell & C. G. Fairburn (Eds.), *Comprehensive textbook of eating disorders and obesity* (pp. 87–92). New York: Guilford Press.

Wing, R. R. (1992). Weight cycling in humans: A review of the literature. *Annals of Behavioral Medicine, 14,* 113–119.

Wood, P. D., Stefanick, M. L., Dreon, D. M., Frey-Hewitt, B, Garay, S. C., Williams, P. T., Superke, H. R., Fortmann, S. P., Albers, J. J., Vranizan, K. M., Ellsworth, N. M., Terry, R. B., & Haskell, W. L. (1988). Changes in plasma lipids and lipoproteins in overweight men during weight loss through dieting as compared with exercise. *New England Journal of Medicine, 319,* 1173–1179.

Wood, P. D., Stefanick, M. L., Williams, P. T., & Haskell, W. L. (1991). The effects on plasma lipoproteins in overweight men during weight loss through dieting as compared with exercise. *New England Journal of Medicine, 325,* 461–466.

Wooley, S. C., & Garner, D. M. (1991). Obesity treatment: The high cost of false hope. *Journal of the American Dietetic Association, 91,* 1248–1251.

Wooley, S. C., Wooley, O. W., & Dyrenforth, S. R. (1979). Theoretical, practical and social issues in behavioral treatment of obesity. *Journal of Applied Behavior Analysis, 12,* 3–25.

Wortman, C. B., & Lehman, D. R. (1985). Support attempts that fail. In I. G. Sarason & B. R. Sarason (Eds.), *Social Support: Theory, research, and applications* (pp. 463–490). Boston: Martinus Nijhoff.

Yanovski, S. Z. (1993). Binge eating disorder: Current knowledge and future directions. *Obesity Research, 1,* 306–324.

Yanovski, S. Z., Leet, M., Yanovski, J. A., Flood, M., Gold, P. W., Kissileff, H. R., & Walsh, B. T. (1992). Food selection and intake of obese women with binge eating disorder. *American Journal of Clinical Nutrition, 56,* 975–980.

12

Lifestyle Change

A Program for Long-Term Weight Management

Donald A. Williamson, Catherine M. Champagne,
Lori P. Jackman, and Paula J. Varnado

DESCRIPTION OF OBESITY

Obesity is defined as an excess of adipose (or fat) tissue. Until most recently, *excess weight* was defined in terms of normative tables of weight for a given height, such as the Metropolitan Life Insurance Company (1983) charts or statistics from the National Research Council (1989). This method for defining obesity does not actually measure adiposity, however, and is no longer generally used in research programs on obesity (Bray, 1992b). Methods for estimating body fat range from relatively inexpensive methods, such as measurement of skin-fold thickness, to expensive methods such as magnetic resonance. In recent years, the use of body mass index $(wt/(ht)^2)$ has become a popular method for defining weight status. The body-mass index (BMI) has been found to be highly correlated with other measures of adiposity, except in bodybuilders and other athletes with high muscle mass (Garrow, 1983).

Bray (1992b) has proposed that obesity should be defined in terms of five classes (Class Zero: *Normal*, to Class IV: *Very Obese*) that correspond to the classification system adopted by the American Heart Association. In his classification scheme, a BMI of 25 to 30 defines obesity Class I, which is associated with low risk for cardiovascular and other diseases. Class II is defined by a BMI of 30 to 35, Class III by a BMI of 35 to 40, and Class IV by a BMI greater than 40. The National Center for Health Statistics (Kuczmarski, 1992) shows that about 20% of adults in the United States have a BMI above 30, and that about 1% have a BMI above 40.

Donald A. Williamson, Catherine M. Champagne, Lori P. Jackman, and Paula J. Varnado • Department of Psychology, Louisiana State University, Pennington Biomedical Research Center, Baton Rouge, Louisiana 70803.

Sourcebook of Psychological Treatment Manuals for Adult Disorders, edited by Vincent B. Van Hasselt and Michel Hersen. Plenum Press, New York, 1996.

Morbidity studies of obesity have shown that the incidence of cardiovascular and other diseases increases with increased adiposity, especially for extreme (Class IV) obesity (Sjostrom, 1992). Furthermore, these studies have found that a preponderance of abdominal obesity is highly associated with metabolic disturbances, non-insulin dependent diabetes, hypertension, and hypertriglyceridemia. These findings suggest that regional fat distribution is important for understanding the relationship between obesity and medical risks.

Abdominal obesity in persons with a BMI above 30 defines the group of adults with the greatest health risks. This treatment manual was developed for the implementation of a long-term behavior-therapy program for this type of obese patient. The manual was developed for use in research studies of the long-term administration of drugs for the treatment of obesity (Bray, 1992a), but can also be used in nonpharmacological treatment programs for obesity. The manual is designed to cover a 52-week treatment period, in which the frequency of therapy is faded from once per week in the first 12 weeks to once per month in the last 16 weeks. The treatment program incorporates procedures to modify dietary intake, exercise, eating habits, and emotions and cognitions that interfere with weight management.

ASSESSMENT METHODS

Assessment of obesity should include a thorough medical evaluation, dietary assessment, and a psychological/behavioral assessment. The medical evaluation should include a complete physical, medical history, blood chemistry, and an electrocardiogram. The dietary assessment should evaluate food preference, caloric intake, and macronutrient composition of the diet. Psychological and behavioral assessment procedures are described in more detail in the following sections. We prefer to tailor the psychological assessment protocol to the individual clinical or research project. The procedures described in Appendix A are most commonly used by our staff.

INTRODUCTION TO THE LIFESTYLE-CHANGE PROGRAM

The behavioral program in Table 12.1 is designed for use by a multidisciplinary staff. The staff should include, at a minimum, physicians, nurses, psychologists, and dieticians. Prior to the initiation of treatment, subjects should be scheduled for an individual consultation with a dietician to train the person in the use of a dietary exchange program and to establish the dietary exchange goals for each patient. During this session, the patient should be given a copy of the treatment manual and should be instructed to read the information for Session Week 1. Prior to each session, the subject should read information pertaining to that session. Between sessions, the subject is expected to monitor dietary intake and activity. Over the course of the first five sessions, the patient is introduced to the concepts of meal planning, behavioral contracting, and modification of activity. As shown in the Schedule of Therapy Sessions, the first 12 sessions will meet on a weekly basis. From Week 12 to week 36, sessions are scheduled every other week. From Week 36 through Week 52, sessions are scheduled every 4 weeks. Family members and friends are invited to attend group sessions at Week 6, and are invited to attend group meetings every 4 weeks until Week 36. They are invited to attend the final treatment session at Week 52, as well. We recommend that the

Table 12.1. Schedule of Therapy Sessions

	Family night
Week 1: Orientation	
Week 2: Record keeping, exercise, and behavioral contracting	
Week 3: Dietary exchange program	
Week 4: Exercise goals	
Week 5: Basic principles of lifestyle-behavior change	
Week 6: Family support for behavior change	*
Week 7: Fat and your diet	
Week 8: Modification of exercise habits	
Week 9: Regulation of eating: Hunger, satiety, and taste	
Week 10: Shopping for food	*
Week 11: How has your behavior changed so far?	
Week 12: Increasing physical activity	
Week 14: How can the family help?	*
Week 16: Eating out	
Week 18: Holidays, parties, and special events	*
Week 20: Life history and weight changes	
Week 22: Accidental sabotage of progress	*
Week 24: Evaluation of progress and commitment to the future	
Week 26: Assertion and self-control of eating	*
Week 28: Social problem solving	
Week 30: Community with friends and family	*
Week 32: Mood and eating	
Week 34: Cognitive change strategies	
Week 36: Rational thinking: A family goal	*
Week 40: Relapse prevention: maintenance of weight loss	
Week 44: Relapse prevention: Recognizing risk factors	
Week 48: Relapse prevention: Taking corrective action	
Week 52: Graduation to a new lifestyle	*

patient select one person who can attend all family groups. If they wish to bring others on occasion, this can be accommodated unless the group becomes too large. We recommend starting the group with 12 members and we do not recommend the attendance of children. The program is designed for a closed-group format that remains intact over a 52-week period. The format could be modified to an open-group format with a weekly schedule, however.

Session Week 1: Orientation

Please read this section before attending the first therapy session.

This manual is based on a behavioral approach to the treatment of obesity. A behavioral approach for weight management is designed to modify eating habits, exercise, and other psychological factors that maintain excess weight. Research has shown that behavioral programs are effective for losing weight and maintenance of weight loss. This program is based on extensive research and clinical experience.

A problem-solving approach will be used throughout this program in order to help you identify problem behaviors and situations, and then generate solutions to correct the problems. You will have a very active role in this program. You will be asked to do homework assignments and keep records each week. The assignments are designed to help you become more aware of your eating habits. The specific details of this program will be discussed shortly.

For many of you, this will not be your first time dieting. Therefore, you probably already know that dieting is challenging, but it becomes even more difficult when added to an already hectic lifestyle. One of the most important things to determine before beginning a weight-loss program is your level of commitment and motivation. It will be very important for you to arrange your schedule to allow you to consistently attend treatment sessions. Also, you should ask your family for their support, and ask at least one friend or family member to join you in your efforts to lose weight. That person should be invited to attend therapy sessions once per month throughout the program according to the schedule discussed in the Introduction.

Next, we must discuss the process of active problem solving. As described here, there are six steps in the problem-solving process. When you are having difficulty following the Lifestyle-Change program, remember to use this process to solve your problems.

The Problem-Solving Process

STEP 1—*Define the problem*. Be as specific as possible, using objective, behavioral descriptions of the problem.

STEP 2—*Brainstorm*. Generate as many solutions as possible, regardless of whether they are good or bad solutions. Make sure to write all solutions down; do not eliminate any potential solutions at this stage.

STEP 3—*Conduct a cost–benefit analysis of each solution*. Examine the realistic positive and negative consequence that might be expected if you implemented the solution.

STEP 4—*Choose the most effective solution*. From the solutions you have developed, choose the one with the most positive consequences and least negative consequences.

STEP 5—*Design a plan to implement your solution and then carry it out*. It is often useful to give yourself a time period in which you want this plan of action to be completed.

STEP 6—*Evaluate the effectiveness of your solution*. If it worked, then the process stops here; however, if it was not successful, go back to Step 4 and choose another alternative and try it.

Self-Evaluation of Potential Problem Situations

List the problems that you expect to face while dieting over the next year. These problems may include work problems (busy schedule, fights with your boss), family problems (family prefers high calorie meals, marital distress), cravings, eating when you are emotional, and so on. After you list the problems, also list some potential solutions to each of the problems. Finally, describe potential costs and benefits if you implemented each solution. Please be prepared to discuss your problems and solutions in the first therapy session.

1.

2.

3.

4.

5.

After reviewing the problems that you must solve in order to successfully lose weight, rate your willingness, motivation, and commitment level to a long-term weight-loss program. Be as honest with yourself as possible. Many times, when individuals have trouble losing weight, it is because they have too many other things going on in their lives that take precedence over weight loss.

1	2	3	4	5	6	7	8	9	10
Not ready				Somewhat motivated					Totally committed

If your rating was seven or higher, then you are probably ready to start the Lifestyle-Change program. Be aware that your level of commitment and motivation will change throughout the program. You will have to be your own cheerleader when things get tough. Many people often expect motivation to precede action, but action usually precedes motivation. You may notice that once you begin the Lifestyle-Change program, you may become more motivated.

Causes of Obesity

Obesity is usually defined as being at least 20% above normal weight. Obesity is caused by consuming more energy through eating than is expended. Obesity may be caused by overeating, lack of exercise, genetic predisposition, and thyroid or other medical disorders. Recent research suggests that obesity is probably caused and maintained by a combination of poor eating habits, lack of exercise, and genetic predisposition. Metabolic disorders account for only a small percentage of persons who are overweight.

This Lifestyle-Change program focuses on events that you can control, such as your eating habits, exercise, and attitude. Less emphasis will be placed on methods that produce rapid weight loss. This program is based on an energy-balance model that assumes the following:

1. Weight is maintained if your caloric intake = energy expenditure.
2. Weight gain occurs if caloric intake > energy expenditure.
3. Weight loss occurs if caloric intake < energy expenditure.

Dieting is often unsuccessful, because the short-term, positive consequences of eating (e.g., food tastes good and reduces hunger) are more powerful than the long-term, positive consequences of dieting, such as weight loss and improved health. This program is based on changing long-standing behaviors and attitudes toward food. Lifestyle change means not only changing your habits while dieting, but also incorporating your new habits into your lifestyle.

This program advocates a slow, gradual weight change. Most people can expect to lose 1 to 1.5 pounds per week. Because we encourage lifestyle changes (changes you can live with), we do not recommend that you never eat your favorite foods, but instead learn to eat in moderation when you are hungry.

The Lifestyle-Change program consists of four components: (1) lifestyle or behavioral change, (2) increasing physical activity, (3) nutritional education, and (4) modification of attitudes and emotions that contribute to overeating or underexercising.

One of the major goals of this program is that you become more aware of what, when, where, and why you eat. Awareness is one of the keys to successful weight loss and management. Once you determine your primary problem areas (e.g., times of the day, boredom, depression, parties), then you can develop strategies for coping with each of these problem situations. Awareness of hunger level is also very important. Once you become aware of when you are hungry and full, you will have much more control over your eating.

Assessment of Eating Patterns

My current weight is _____. My goal weight is _____.

- List the things that have been helped you lose weight in the past:

- List the problems that you have had losing weight in the past:

Problem Eating Behaviors (check any that apply):

Eating too fast _____
Taking large portions _____
Not waiting 20 minutes after beginning a meal before having seconds _____
Always cleaning your plate _____
Eating impulsively _____
Eating when you are full or not hungry _____
Excessive snacking _____
Excessive food deprivation _____
Not eating three meals a day _____
Poor meal planning (no low-calorie foods available) at home _____ or at work_____
Meals are not nutritionally balanced _____
Too many sweets (list problem foods) _____
Too many fats (list problem foods) _____

Homework Assignment:

After attending the first session, remember to read Session 2. Next week we will be discussing record keeping, exercise, nutrition, and behavioral contracting. You will be introduced to the monitoring form that you will use every day throughout this program.

Record keeping as related to nutrition involves self-recording of food intake. If done properly, it is possible to get feedback on how well a person follows a diet. Numerous software programs are available to calculate nutrient intake based on how well a person describes and estimates the amount of the food consumed. From a practical standpoint, if a person writes down everything consumed, this leads to a fuller awareness of the total diet and is one way to follow a diet on a long-term basis. Without a doubt, people often have difficulty recording nutrient intake on a consistent basis. Very successful dieters have been known to praise this technique as a sure way to guarantee that weight is managed, cautioning that it takes a high level of commitment.

The Daily Food-Monitoring Form, shown in Sidebar 12–1, is suitable for recording dietary intake and exercise on a daily basis. This form contains areas for planning the food to be eaten and recording the food actually consumed. You should provide a description of the food, the amount consumed, and the number of dietary exchanges for each food.

At the bottom of the Daily Food-Monitoring Form is a section for monitoring exchanges. Each time you consume a particular type of exchange (e.g., meat or vegetable), place an X in one space associated with that food group. By planning your meals in advance and tracking the exchanges as they are consumed, you will be able to control your eating in accordance with the meal plan prescribed by the dietician.

In Session 3, we will discuss how to monitor your eating and dietary intake in some detail. Between the second and third week, you will be instructed simply to monitor your eating. Beginning in Week 3, you will be instructed in the methods of planning meals and using an exchange diet.

The exchange diet, discussed in Session 3, needs to be monitored on a daily basis until you become familiar with the diet and have memorized most of the exchanges.

Importance of Exercise

Exercise is a very important component in the Lifestyle-Change program. Many studies have shown that the combination of dieting and exercise is superior to dieting alone. In addition, exercise has been shown to be one of the best predictors for maintenance of weight loss. Many people do not exercise because of the short-term, negative consequences of exercise, such as the amount of effort required, sweating, being embarrassed because of excess weight, or being out of shape. Although the long-term positive benefits of exercise include improved health and weight loss, many people continue to focus on immediate, negative consequences. Let us examine some of the benefits of exercise:

1. Increases your energy expenditure (burns calories).
2. Numerous health benefits including, decreased heart rate, blood pressure, and cholesterol.
3. Decreases tension and stress.
4. Improves mood.
5. Helps control your appetite.
6. Improves self-esteem and self-image.
7. Research has shown that regular exercise is the best weight-control method for long-term maintenance of weight loss.

The Lifestyle-Change program advocates exercise that can be incorporated into your lifestyle. You do not have to become an Olympic track star or power weight lifter. Instead,

430

Donald A. Williamson
et al.

Sidebar 12–1

Daily Food Monitoring Form

Daily diet plan: Food, description, and amount	Planned exchanges	Actual food consumed: Food, description, and amount	Consumed exchanges
Breakfast		**Breakfast**	
_____	_____	_____	_____
_____	_____	_____	_____
_____	_____	_____	_____
_____	_____	_____	_____
_____	_____	_____	_____
Lunch		**Lunch**	
_____	_____	_____	_____
_____	_____	_____	_____
_____	_____	_____	_____
_____	_____	_____	_____
_____	_____	_____	_____
_____	_____	_____	_____
_____	_____	_____	_____
Dinner		**Dinner**	
_____	_____	_____	_____
_____	_____	_____	_____
_____	_____	_____	_____

we suggest starting an exercise program gradually. For example, walking 15 minutes a day is an excellent goal. However, many of you may have to start with increasing daily physical activity, such as taking the stairs instead of the elevator, or walking around the block.

The Lifestyle-Change program is designed to help you gradually increase your exercise level to achieve a higher level of aerobic fitness. The long-term goal that you will be shooting for is 30 minutes of moderate-intensity physical activity on most days of the week. Each week, you will set realistic, achievable exercise goals for your behavioral contract. A *behavioral contract* is a contract between you and your group and/or therapist. You will set your own goals, and you will also be determining your own rewards. The only restriction is that your reward cannot be food. Other options include a movie, a book, new clothes, or a vacation. You can develop a reward system so that your rewards can add up over time. For example, if you meet your goals all month, then you can go shopping for new clothes. Take a few minutes to determine what kind of rewards would motivate you. You can have daily, weekly, monthly and trimonthly rewards.

The details of this exercise program will be described in a later session. For now, it is important for you to begin walking as many days a week as possible. A good initial goal

Dinner (*cont.*)

_____   _____

_____   _____

_____   _____

_____   _____

_____   _____

Dinner (*cont.*)

_____   _____

_____   _____

_____   _____

_____   _____

_____   _____

Snacks

_____   _____

_____   _____

_____   _____

_____   _____

Snacks

_____   _____

_____   _____

_____   _____

_____   _____

Daily exchanges allowed:	Total planned:	Exchange monitoring 1 2 3 4 5 6 7 8 9 10	Total consumed:
Starch/Bread	_____	_____	– – – – – – – – – –	_____
Meat	_____	_____	– – – – – – – – – –	_____
Vegetable	_____	_____	– – – – – – – – – –	_____
Fruit	_____	_____	– – – – – – – – – –	_____
Milk	_____	_____	– – – – – – – – – –	_____
Fat	_____	_____	– – – – – – – – – –	_____

Exercise Monitoring

Number of METS: Planned: Actual:

                         _____   _____

Type of exercise: _____

if you are not already exercising, is 15 to 30 minutes of walking at least 3 days per week. In Session 4, specific exercise goals will be established. Remember, any type of movement will increase the number of calories that you burn. So Get Moving!!!!

Assessment of Exercise Patterns

List things that have hindered you in starting and staying with an exercise program.

What do you like about exercising or the benefits of exercising?

What physical activities would you enjoy?

Problem Areas (check any that apply):

Insufficient frequency _____
How many days per week _____
Insufficient duration _____
Length of each session _____
Insufficient intensity _____
Sustained heart rate _____
Insufficient unstructured activity _____
Long periods of inactivity _____
Poor or no scheduling of exercise sessions _____
Low priority given to exercise _____
Other _____

Behavior Contracting

The focus of the Lifestyle-Change program is to change eating habits and a sedentary lifestyle that may have developed over many years. A handout that you will use over the course of the Lifestyle-Change program is shown in Sidebar 12–2. This is a behavioral contract to help you *gradually* change your problematic eating behaviors. It would be unrealistic to expect a complete, immediate change to new behaviors. The group leader will explain the contract in more detail during the group meeting. Each week, the group leader will help you identify appropriate behavioral goals for the following week. *It is very important to use the contract for behavioral rather than weight goals.* Remember, weight loss is a variable process; therefore, contracting to lose a certain number of pounds per week may be disappointing.

At the top of the contract are spaces to list your goals for the week and to check off the days that you have met the goals. Another important aspect of the behavioral contract is to reward yourself for your hard work. The section for rewarding behavior change is at the bottom of the contract. Begin thinking about appropriate rewards for yourself. Examples of rewards include giving yourself $5.00 "mad money" each week that you successfully meet the contract. *Never* reward yourself with food. To increase motivation, it is also important to penalize yourself for not fulfilling the contract. Again, using money as an example, you could give $5.00 to a charity (your children) if you do not meet the contract. The group leader will okay your contract during each group meeting.

Homework Assignment

Read Session 3. Next week we will be discussing the exchange program. Remember to do your Food and exercise monitoring each day during the next week.

Session Week 3: Dietary-Exchange Program

The only method of dieting that assures adherence to a prescribed calorie level is the dietary-exchange system. Originally developed for diabetics, the exchange diet is an easy system to follow and can be calculated according to your eating habits. In this diet, foods are categorized into six major food listings: starch/bread, meat, fruit, vegetables, milk, and fat. Table 12.2 illustrates the nutrient levels associated with each food group. The diet

Sidebar 12–2

Handout for Week 2: Contract for Lifestyle-Changes Program

Week(s): _____

Date: _____

Goals: Mon   Tue   Wed   Thu   Fri   Sat   Sun
_____

_____

_____

_____

_____

_____

I understand that if I fulfill my lifestyle-changes contract this week I will reward

myself with _____ . However, if I do not fulfill my contract, then

I agree to _____ .

_____   _____
Group Member's Signature   Therapist's Signature

includes a list termed *free foods* and listings that show how to work *combination foods* into the meal plan.

Each listing contains foods that are sufficiently alike in carbohydrate, protein, fat and calories to be placed in that grouping. The portion sizes in the list differ in many instances, and a great deal of attention must be paid to assure that these variations in portion sizes are accounted for. The advantage of this system is that it is somewhat universal. Many healthy selections of frozen and canned items in the marketplace now contain the number of dietary exchanges per serving on the label, making it easy for you to follow your diet. Some major weight-loss companies devise their diets based on the exchange system and manufacture products that have the exchanges counted for you. The exchange diet is also versatile, because almost any recipe can be analyzed and converted to exchanges by a dietitian. As a result, you may have a favorite food worked into your diet plan either regularly or occasionally, depending on the type of recipe.

A compilation of common foods within each food group and definitions of an exchange for each food are provided in Appendix B.

The exchange list was derived from the American Dietetic Association/American Diabetes Association, Inc. publication entitled *Exchange Lists for Weight Management* published in 1989.

Table 12.2.   Nutrient Levels Associated with Food Group

Exchange List	Carbohydrate (grams)	Protein (grams)	Fat (grams)	Calories
Starch/Bread	15	3	Trace	80
Meat				
Lean	—	7	3	55
Medium-fat	—	7	5	75
High-fat	—	7	8	100
Vegetable	5	2	—	25
Fruit	15	—	—	60
Milk				
Skim	12	8	Trace	90
Lowfat	12	8	5	120
Whole	12	8	8	150
Fat	—	—	5	45

Session Week 4: Exercise

Much has been said about the importance of aerobic activity (raising your heart rate to 60% to 70% of your maximal heart rate). However, lower levels of exercise have also been shown to have many health benefits, including maintenance of weight loss. The Lifestyle-Change program recommends beginning an exercise program gradually. Before you begin any exercise program, make sure that your physician gives you permission to start.

Initially, this exercise program will focus on walking, and as your fitness level improves, you can move on to more vigorous exercise if you want. If you are already involved in a fitness program, continue what you are doing.

Walking has been shown to be an excellent exercise, regardless of speed, because it works all of the major large muscle groups. In addition, walking is something almost anyone can do, and it can be incorporated into most people's lifestyles fairly easily. Walking burns as many calories as running, as long as you go the same distance.

At first any kind of exercise may not feel good. Initially, you may feel sore, bored, or tired. It is really important to start off slowly, at a level that does not hurt, and only go as far as you can. If you push yourself too hard, you will be more likely to be sore and less likely to continue exercising.

Get Your METS (GYM) Fitness Program

The Get Your METS program is a unique exercise program designed to focus on exercise intensity instead of the number of calories burned. This will make it much easier for you to record the amount of exercise that you are doing each week.

Metabolic equivalent terms (METS) will be used to rate your level of intensity. For example, 2 METS = 20 minutes of moderate activity. *Moderate activity* is defined as an activity that uses all of the major muscle groups and is of moderate intensity. As an illustration, a brisk walk using your arms would be classified as a moderate activity. Twenty minutes of brisk walking = 2 METS. Jogging for 20 minutes would be equal to 3 METS, because jogging is a more intense form of exercise. Twenty minutes of racquetball = 4 METS. A slow walk without moving your arms = 1.5 METS.

The Get Your METS program (GYM) is designed to help you gradually increase your activity level. The initial goal of GYM is 10 METS per week. Although this sounds like a considerable amount of exercise, 10 METS are equal to 100 minutes of moderate activity a week. This can be accomplished by doing 20 minutes of moderate walking (2 METS = 20 minutes of moderate walking) 5 days per week, or 20 minutes of jogging 3 or 4 days per week (3 METS = 20 minutes of jogging), or playing racquetball for 20 minutes 2.5 days per week (4 METS = 20 minutes of racquetball).

Guidelines for Exercising

1. *Make exercising fun.* Take a friend, your dog, or listen to music or the radio.

2. *Go at your own pace.* You don't have to set a world record during your first week. The important thing is that you START. Once you put exercise into your routine, you will begin to experience many positive benefits, such as more energy, less tension and stress, and more self-esteem. You will begin feeling better about your body.

What is a good exercise goal? Your exercise goals should depend on your current level of fitness. Make sure your goals are reasonable and flexible. You can always change your goals if they are too high or too low. Remember not to expect perfection. In other words, don't be discouraged if you become sore or if you miss a day, or need to lower your goals. Remember the most important goal is that you start. If you have not been exercising regularly, a good goal is 20 minutes of walking a day. If it is possible, do 20 minutes of *continuous* walking. If this is too much for you at first, start off by walking for 10 minutes two times a day.

Suggestions

1. START TODAY!!!
2. Make sure that you dress appropriately in good shoes and extra clothing if it is cold outside.
3. Try walking in the mall if it is rainy or too cold. Many people go mall-walking as a way to exercise, and for those of you who like to shop, make sure that you finish your walk before you shop.
4. Gradually increase the intensity, duration, and frequency of your exercise. As you feel more comfortable walking 20 minutes, slowly build up to 30, 45, and 60 minutes. If you do not like walking or cannot walk, swimming is a good alternative. Remember not to overdo it. It is very important that you enjoy whatever exercise you choose.
5. At the bottom of the Daily Food-Monitoring Form is a section for recording METS. In addition to recording METS, you should specify your exercise goal for the day. Set a reasonable goal. Missing a day of exercise is not a catastrophe. What is important is that you exercise on a regular basis. In the next session, we will establish your first set of exercise goals.

Homework Assignment

Remember to record your food intake and activity for the next week. In your next therapy session, be prepared to include exercise in your behavioral contract.

Session Week 5: Basic Principles of Lifestyle-Behavior Change

Review: Please answer these questions at the beginning of each session using the rating scale of 0 = Very Poor to 5 = Very Well. Circle the rating that best describes your behavior during the previous week:

1. How well did you accurately record your food moni-   0   1   2   3   4   5
toring?
2. How well did you follow the exchange/calorie guide-   0   1   2   3   4   5
lines?
3. How well did you follow the exercise plan?   0   1   2   3   4   5
4. How well did you complete your behavioral contract?   0   1   2   3   4   5

TOTAL SCORE: _____

If you have been monitoring your eating over the past several weeks, you may have begun to notice several patterns associated with your eating behavior. Do you tend to eat very fast? Do you often eat standing up or on the run? Do you snack at certain times and eat whatever is available? These are only a few of the problematic behaviors that can be associated with eating. In the next session, we will discuss a few techniques designed to help you regain control of your eating, and to help you develop a positive focus for your eating habits. One of the most dangerous things that you can do is to engage in "mindless eating." This form of eating occurs when you are not attending to your eating behavior. Changing these "mindless" eating habits involves the following:

1. Record keeping to identify bad habits, as well as track what you are eating.
2. Learning about the things in your environment that "set you up" to eat.
3. Using the lifestyle-change techniques.

You already have learned about record keeping in an earlier session. Research has shown that there are certain environmental factors that can influence your eating behavior. In Figure 12.1 is a model explaining this process. *Antecedents* are events, thoughts, feelings, and so on, that occur before you eat. Identifying antecedents associated with your eating can help eliminate cues that signal inappropriate eating. Antecedents can include time of day, seeing food, or feeling down. *Behaviors* in this example are eating and other activities associated with eating, such as cooking or shopping. *Consequences* are events, feelings and attitudes that follow eating, and may be positive, negative, or neutral. For example, gaining weight and feeling guilty are negative consequences, whereas feeling satisfied is a positive consequence. Over the course of the treatment program, we will focus on identifying antecedent events that lead to overeating.

To help you focus on your eating and avoid "mindless" eating, there are several basic principles of lifestyle change that you can follow. These principles are summarized here. We will go over these techniques more thoroughly in the next therapy session. Begin thinking about some of these principles to determine which ones you may not engage in and which ones may give you trouble.

1. *Slow Down Eating*. Are you a very fast eater? Do you find that you do not really enjoy your food? There are several reasons to slow down your eating rate. First, you must learn to really enjoy the taste of food. If you enjoy the food more, you are less likely to feel deprived while dieting. Second, it allows you to focus on what you are eating and to make

```
┌─────────────────────────────────────────────────────────────┐
│                 Functional analysis of eating                 │
│                                                               │
│   Antecedents  ———— Behaviors  ———— Consequences              │
│                                                               │
│   Antecedents = Time of day; doughnuts at the office, etc.    │
│   Behavior = Eating, overeating                               │
│   Consequences = Gaining weight                               │
│                                                               │
└─────────────────────────────────────────────────────────────┘
```

Figure 12.1. Handout for Week 5: Functional analysis of eating.

better decisions about your eating behavior. Finally, a more relaxed eating pace will allow you to stop eating when you feel full. There are several techniques that you can use to slow down eating rate. For example, you can put your fork, spoon, sandwich down between bites. Other techniques are to set a timer, pause during meals, or slowly chew your food.

2. *Leave Food on Your Plate/Take Smaller Portions.* This technique is designed to help you rely on the internal cue of being satiated rather than the external cue of a clean plate to determine when you should stop eating. This habit is particularly important when eating in restaurants or at other's homes, when you cannot control portion sizes. Even if you are already eating smaller portions, leaving food on your plate demonstrates that you are paying attention to your eating behavior.

3. *Always Plan Ahead.* Plan your exchanges and food choices before you eat them. Never wait to calculate exchanges at the end of the day. At that point, you may have already eaten too much. In addition, plan your snacks within the diet, so that you decrease your chances of giving in to external cues, such as someone bringing doughnuts to the office. Also, planning your meals cuts down on grabbing whatever you can find. Often, there are not many good food choices when you must eat whatever is available.

4. *Sit Down at the Table to Eat/Only Eat at the Table.* If you eat in a variety of places and situations, you will be more likely to experience hunger in those places and situations. By limiting when and where you eat, you are more likely to experience hunger only at that time in only a few places. How often do you sit down in front of the television to eat? How often do you nibble while cooking, or eat in your car? Again, these behaviors do not allow you to concentrate on how much you are eating or when you are satisfied. Try to make the table your designated place to eat. At work, try to find a nice quiet place, preferably not your desk. How well can you concentrate on eating with all of your work around you and the telephone ringing?

5. *Focus Only on Eating.* Try not to talk on the phone, read the paper, or watch television while eating.

6. *Above All Else, Be Aware!!!* "Mindless" eating adds "unnoticed" calories. These calories add up and make the difference between successful and unsuccessful weight management. For example, have you ever grabbed candy out of a candy dish without

realizing what you were doing? Have you ever tasted so much of what you were cooking that you were not really hungry when it was time to eat? Watch out for these types of behaviors.

7. *Get Back on Track as Soon as Possible*. Remember, it is always better to get back on track as soon as possible, rather than waiting until Monday, next month, and so on. If you overdo it at lunch, get back on track for your evening meal. *Never* skip meals to try to make up for a slip. Skipping meals can lead to problems such as really overeating. Have you ever told yourself that you were going to fast and then gave in? Most of all, do not get down on yourself; instead, realize that every dieter slips on occasion. It is how you handle the slip that determines a successful dieter.

Your goal over the next several weeks will be to begin implementing these changes. Like any other habit, it will require practice. In the next group session (Session 5), we will discuss how you can implement these behavior-change procedures, and you will be instructed in the inclusion of behavior changes into your next behavioral contract. In Week 6, the group will focus on developing family support for your behavioral changes. Remember to invite a family member or friend to attend Session 6.

Handout, Week 5: Summary of Basic Principles of Lifestyle Change

1. *Slow Down Eating.*
   - Put fork down between bites
   - Set a timer.
   - Count the number of times you chew.
2. *Leave Food on Your Plate/Take Smaller Portions.*
3. *Always Plan Ahead.*
   - Never wait to calculate exchanges at the end of the day.
4. *Sit Down at the Table to Eat/Only Eat at the Table.*
5. *Focus Only on Eating.*
6. *Above All Else, Be Aware!!!*
   - Mindless eating adds "unnoticed" calories.
7. *Get Back on Track ASAP.*

Session Week 6: Family Support for Behavior Change

A family member or a friend is invited to this meeting and should read and respond to the questions posed in this manual.

Review: Please answer these questions at the beginning of each session using the rating scale of 0 = Very Poor to 5 = Very Well. Circle the rating that best describes your behavior during the previous week:

1. How well did you accurately record your food monitoring?	0	1	2	3	4	5
2. How well did you follow the exchange/calorie guidelines?	0	1	2	3	4	5
3. How well did you follow the exercise plan?	0	1	2	3	4	5
4. How well did you complete your behavioral contract?	0	1	2	3	4	5

TOTAL SCORE: _____

Now that you have been on the Lifestyle-Change program for 6 weeks, you have probably noticed how important social support (friends or family) is to your progress. We invited your family or significant other for that reason. We want to be able to give them some guidelines as to what to do, what to expect, and how they can help. We will go over the basics today; however, each of you will have to talk with your families about what specifically is important to you. Research has found that social support is very beneficial for weight loss and especially helpful for weight maintenance.

Special Note to Family and Friends

Family and friends can range from helpful to hostile. This program assumes, because you are here tonight, that you want to learn how to be most helpful to your friend or family member who is trying to lose weight. A good idea for anyone who is considering being helpful to the dieter is to read this manual.

Family members can be very helpful by rearranging the home eating environment. The family can also be helpful by reinforcing both a dieter's good food choices and his or her hard work. For example, "Mary, I am really impressed with all the changes you are making" or you can be more specific: "Joan, I am so glad that you are exercising regularly."

Helpful Hints

1. *Help with some of the grocery shopping.* You can actually go to the store for the dieter, go with him or her, or make a list for groceries together.
2. *Eat three meals a day.* This will help the dieter get used to scheduled meal times.
3. *Do not snack in front of the dieter.* Snacking away from the dieter will remove the stimulus for the dieter to eat. Most dieters tend to become hungry when they see or smell food. Out of sight, out of mind.
4. *Do not ask the dieter to serve you snacks or second helpings.* It is important for dieters not to be exposed to food any more than they have to be.
5. *Help with the cooking and the cleaning of dishes.* Often, dieters have trouble snacking or testing the food while it is cooking, and some have trouble with leftovers. (Clearing the dishes off the table can be very beneficial for it removes the opportunity to overeat.)
6. *Help keep high-calorie snack foods out of sight.* Do not leave candy bars or cake on the counter where the dieter can see them (remove the temptation).
7. *Follow many of the same lifestyle changes that the dieter is undergoing.*
   Eat only at the table.
   Eat slowly.
   Do not do any other activities while eating.
8. *Exercise together.* Go for walks together; make exercise an important part of the family routine. The more satisfying the exercise, the more likely the dieter will be to continue exercising.

Special Note to the Weight-Loss Participant

In the next session, you will be asked to discuss with your family or friends how you would like them to help. Please answer the following questions (in writing) in order to prepare for this discussion.

List those things that you would like their help with:

List those things that you do not want them to do:

Make sure that you reinforce your family and friends for helping you. For example, be sure to thank them for eating at the table with you, or removing the dishes from the table.

Note for the Family/Friend

Be a cheerleader, not a watchdog. Do not be critical of the dieter's progress or food choices.

Homework Assignment

Remember to bring a friend or family member to the next session. Remember to monitor your food, activity, and lifestyle changes. Finally, follow your behavioral contract.

Session Week 7: Fat and Your Diet

Review: Please answer these questions at the beginning of each session using the rating scale of 0 = Very Poor to 5 = Very Well. Circle the rating that best describes your behavior during the previous week:

1. How well did you accurately record your food monitoring?   0   1   2   3   4   5
2. How well did you follow the exchange/calorie guidelines?   0   1   2   3   4   5
3. How well did you follow the exercise plan?   0   1   2   3   4   5
4. How well did you complete your behavioral contract?   0   1   2   3   4   5

TOTAL SCORE: _____

Without a doubt, one of the primary culprits in the average American's diet is excess fat. On the average, the percentage of calories from fat is in the range of 37% to 40%. The American Heart Association recommends that this figure should be reduced to include no more than 30% of calories from fat. Many believe that it is even possible to further reduce the percentage of fat calories to 10% to 20%.

Why is dietary fat so important? A high-fat diet appears to be related to many chronic diseases and some types of cancer. Obese people consume more fat in their diets than lean people. Cardiovascular disease is related to obesity and high-fat diets. Although high serum cholesterol is a problem in some of these conditions, dietary intake of cholesterol impacts serum cholesterol to a lesser degree than does the intake of fat and saturated fat in the diet.

In order to control fat intake, one needs to know how to find the sources of fat in the diet. Traditionally, you think of fat as fried foods, fats, oils, spreads, salad dressings, creams, and so on. You must also find invisible fat sources in your diet. This is where knowing how to read the nutrition label comes in handy. The new nutrition label contains information on calories from fat. If this figure is divided by the total calories per serving, then the food can be categorized as to whether it is high or low fat. You should strive for the majority of foods you eat to contain less than or equal to 30% of calories from fat.

Be careful to study the label indicating that the product is low fat. If the product description says 98% fat free, for example, the product contains 2 grams of fat for every 100 grams of product. For example, 1 gram of fat = 9 calories; therefore, 2 grams of fat contain 18 calories (2 gm fat × 9 calories/gm) in the 100 gram portion. If the total calories for 100 grams is 30 calories, and 18 calories are fat calories, then the percentage of calories coming from fat is 60%. This example is a little farfetched, but it should be clear that consuming this particular food on a consistent basis would not be appropriate if you wish to manage your weight.

It is a misconception that food needs to be prepared with fat in order to achieve a better taste. In fact, fats sometime conceal the natural flavor of the food item. As an example, the natural freshness of just-harvested vegetables can be totally destroyed by high amounts of oils used in cooking. Although olive oil is favored by many, too much oil on a vegetable such as green beans results in a slimy and less tasty product.

The key to fat intake is moderation. Keep your fat intake within your daily allotment, as specified in your dietary exchange plan. Cut the fat down even further if you are able to do so. This will help you achieve a much healthier diet. In the next session, we will discuss methods for reducing dietary-fat intake and will incorporate these methods into your behavioral contract.

Homework Assignment

Remember to record food intake and METS. Also, plan your meals in advance and follow your behavioral contract.

Session Week 8: Modification of Exercise Habits

Review: Please answer these questions at the beginning of each session, using the rating scale of 0 = Very Poor to 5 = Very Well. Circle the rating that best describes your behavior during the previous week:

1. How well did you accurately record your food moni-   0   1   2   3   4   5
   toring?
2. How well did you follow the exchange/calorie guide-   0   1   2   3   4   5
   lines?
3. How well did you follow the exercise plan?   0   1   2   3   4   5
4. How well did you complete your behavioral contract?   0   1   2   3   4   5

TOTAL SCORE: _____

During Session 8, we will review your new exercise habits. By now, many of you will have noticed some changes. You may have lost some weight, or maybe your clothes are looser, or you are wearing a smaller size of clothing. We hope that by now you are becoming more aware of your eating patterns when you are full, or whether you are more likely to overeat when you are emotional.

We hope that you have begun to incorporate exercise into your daily schedule (Table 12.3). You should also be noticing how you feel during those days that you exercise. Are you less stressed? Do you have more energy? Are you getting your METS?

It is very important to make exercise a priority; it is just as important as eating healthy

Table 12.3. METS for 20 Minutes of
Activity

Activity		METS
Aerobics	(low-impact)	3
	(high-impact)	4
Bicycling	(slow)	1.5
	(fast)	2
Dancing	(slow)	1
	(fast)	2
Golf	(if you walk)	2
Jogging		3
Running	(9 min/mile)	4
Swimming	(slow)	2
	(fast)	3
Tennis		2
Walking	(without your arms)	1.5
	(with your arms)	2.0

foods. All of the things you have been learning are not only beneficial for weight loss, but they are also beneficial for enjoying life, better health (lower blood pressure, heart rate, and cholesterol), and for being more comfortable as you get older. Our goal for this session is to further incorporate exercise into your lifestyle.

Lifestyle Activities versus Programmed Activities

Lifestyle activities are activities that fit easily into your daily routine, whereas programmed activities are the more traditional types of exercise, such as jogging, aerobics, or sports. The following are examples of lifestyle activities:

1. Parking farther from your destination.
2. Cleaning the house more vigorously.
3. Using the stairs instead of the elevators.
4. Gardening.

Remember, any activity burns calories. The higher the intensity of an activity, the more calories you will burn. However, any activity is better than no activity. You will burn as many calories walking as you will running, as long as you cover the same distance.

Continue your GYM program; gradually increase the duration and the intensity of your exercise. In the next session, we will discuss adding additional lifestyle exercises to your program by incorporating them into your weekly behavioral contract. In the next section, we have provided a more complete description of METS for different types of exercise. Be prepared to discuss changes in your GYM program in the next session.

Any moderate activity should be equal to 2 METS for 20 minutes. If you have been averaging 6 METS a week, try to go up 1 MET per week. Keep increasing your exercise goals.

Homework Assignment

Remember to monitor your food, exercise, and lifestyle changes. In the next session, new exercises will be developed.

Review: Please answer these questions at the beginning of each session using the rating scale of 0 = Very Poor to 5 = Very Well. Circle the rating that best describes your behavior during the previous week:

1. How well did you accurately record your food moni-   0   1   2   3   4   5
   toring?
2. How well did you follow the exchange/calorie guide-   0   1   2   3   4   5
   lines?
3. How well did you follow the exercise plan?   0   1   2   3   4   5
4. How well did you follow you behavioral contract?   0   1   2   3   4   5

TOTAL SCORE: _____

How do you know when you are hungry? How do you know when to stop eating? How often do you eat something because you are craving a certain taste? *Hunger* is a physiological drive. Physiological mechanisms within our bodies signal that we have depleted our store of nutrients. Our bodies need food as fuel, much like a car needs gasoline. However, sometimes people eat when they are not hungry because they are responding to external cues to eat rather than internal cues. *Satiety* occurs when our bodies have received enough fuel. Satiety is regulated by physiological mechanisms, but can also be learned. We can learn the proper amount of food to be eaten for weight management. How often do you eat to the point of being uncomfortably full? This feeling is different from satiety. Satiety means having enough, not too much.

Taste is the perception of sweet, sour, salty, and bitter. Flavor is composed of these four tastes and the aroma of food. Sometimes we eat because we desire or crave a specific food, rather than because we are actually hungry. If you often eat when you are not hungry, eat to the point that you are uncomfortably full, or eat because you crave the taste of a food, you are probably giving in to external cues to eat instead of the internal cue that you have depleted your body of nutrients. The following is a list of techniques to help you rely more on internal cues to regulate your eating. The group leader will discuss these in more detail during the next group meeting. Relying upon internal cues to control eating does not mean depriving yourself. Remember, it is important to eat three meals per day. These techniques are designed to help you cut down on unnecessary eating (e.g., snacking when you are not hungry, or eating dessert even if you are full). Before the group meeting, answer the following questions.

How often do you eat in response to external cues?

Make a list of problem situations to discuss with the group leader to aid in the group discussion.

The following techniques can help you learn to rely upon internal cues for controlling eating.

1. *Avoid eating when bored, angry, etc.* Have a list of other positive activities that you can do in these situations. For example, take a walk, talk to a friend, or use problem-solving.

2. *Distract yourself when you are craving a food*. Find something else to do. Distract yourself for about 20 minutes, so you can decide if you are really hungry. Do not spend that time thinking about food, however. Have you ever thought about a food so much that you became hungry for it?

3. *Keep problem foods out of sight/the house*. Remember the old saying, "Out of sight, out of mind." Try not to loiter around the candy machine at work; you will probably find something that you want if you look long enough. Try to plan your snacks so that they can be calculated into your diet plan. Also, if you plan ahead, you probably will not spend a lot of time rummaging through the pantry. If at all possible, remove yourself from the situation if problem foods are around. For example, if someone brings doughnuts to work, try to have a healthier option around. Do not keep them on your desk, and leave, if you can, while everyone else is eating. Finally, keep good food options on hand.

4. *Follow the Lifestyle-Changes program*. If you are truly hungry, eat a small amount, sit down to eat, and eat slowly.

5. *Wait 5 minutes before getting another helping*. Then ask yourself if you really need a second helping based upon hunger.

6. *Identify problematic situations*. You can identify the antecedents associated with problem eating. Once you have identified the problematic situations, you can use this information to come up with creative solutions for these problem situations, as described in Session 1.

Common problem situations include shopping for food, holidays, parties, and special occasions. In the next group session, we will discuss shopping for food, and in Session 18 we will deal with holidays, parties, and special occasions.

In the next session we will use problem-solving to identify and solve problems that are impeding your progress.

Homework Assignment

Monitor your eating and exercise. Implement solutions to problems and plan your meals in advance.

Session Week 10: Shopping for Food

Review: Please answer these questions at the beginning of each session using the rating scale of 0 = Very Poor to 5 = Very Well. Circle the rating that best describes your behavior during the previous week:

1. How well did you accurately record your food moni-   0 1 2 3 4 5
toring?

2. How well did you follow the exchange/calorie guide-   0 1 2 3 4 5
lines?

3. How well did you follow the exercise plan?   0 1 2 3 4 5

4. How well did you complete your behavioral contract?   0 1 2 3 4 5

TOTAL SCORE: _____

This session is a family session designed to help everyone learn more about shopping. Family members or friends should read this session prior to attending the next session.

Shopping for food is usually either a pleasant experience or an unbearable chore for most people.

Lesson number one when shopping for food is to not shop when you are hungry. There is a tendency to buy additional items that are not needed when you shop while hungry. Planning meals ahead of time will help you to shorten your shopping trip and will allow you to buy only those items you need to stock in your pantry.

Become familiar with the labels on food when you shop. Effective May 1994, labels will have changed to provide consumers with more information. There are few exceptions to the labeling regulations, so it is important to know about the foods you are shopping for.

The ingredients statement on a food product tells you everything that is in the item and lists ingredients from greatest to least content. If the label indicates that something is "fat-free" and there is oil in the ingredient statement, then there still is some fat in the product, even though it may not be enough to make a significant impact if you eat just one serving. However, if you consume more than one serving, then you may indeed add some fat to your diet.

The new food label is intended to clear up confusion about nutrition labeling. The new laws mean that almost all foods will carry the label. Nutrients associated with major health problems will be listed on the label and expressed as a percentage of daily values to show how the food can be worked into one's diet. Descriptors such as "light," "low-fat," and others will be standardized to have the same meaning for all products. Standardized serving sizes will help to make comparisons easier. These and other changes will help to make the consumer more educated about what he or she is eating. An example of the label is provided in Figure 12.2. During this session, we will discuss how to use food labels to improve your shopping habits. In order to facilitate discussion on this topic, we invite you to bring confusing food labels to the next group session.

Session Week 11: How Has Your Behavior Changed?

Review: Please answer these questions at the beginning of each session using the rating scale of 0 = Very Poor to 5 = Very Well. Circle the rating that best describes your behavior during the previous week:

1. How well did you accurately record your food moni-   0 1 2 3 4 5
   toring?
2. How well did you follow the exchange/calorie guide-   0 1 2 3 4 5
   lines?
3. How well did you follow the exercise plan?   0 1 2 3 4 5
4. How well did you complete your behavioral contract?   0 1 2 3 4 5

TOTAL SCORE: _____

Remember, it is much easier to control your behavior and your attitude than to control rate of weight loss. Your behavior has an obvious effect on your rate of weight loss. But how does attitude affect weight loss? Let us say that you overeat at a luncheon at work, and you become very upset with yourself for overeating. Do you think being angry with yourself will help or hinder your weight loss? Becoming angry will most likely hinder weight loss (i.e., you may become upset, tense, or depressed, which may create a "What's the use, I've already blown it" attitude). This attitude may then lead to future overeating.

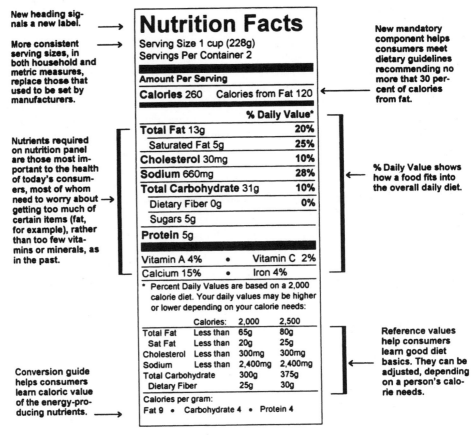

New heading sig-
nals a new label.

More consistent
serving sizes, in
both household and
metric measures,
replace those that
used to be set by
manufacturers.

Nutrients required
on nutrition panel
are those most im-
portant to the health
of today's consum-
ers, most of whom
need to worry about
getting too much of
certain items (fat,
for example), rather
than too few vita-
mins or minerals, as
in the past.

Conversion guide
helps consumers
learn caloric value
of the energy-pro-
ducing nutrients.

New mandatory
component helps
consumers meet
dietary guidelines
recommending no
more that 30 per-
cent of calories
from fat.

% Daily Value shows
how a food fits into
the overall daily diet.

Reference values
help consumers
learn good diet
basics. They can be
adjusted, depending
on a person's calo-
rie needs.

Figure 12.2. Food label.

It is very important to treat yourself kindly (as you would a best friend who is learning to manage weight) when you are changing major habits such as eating and exercise. You did not form these habits in a few weeks; it took a lifetime to form these habits. Consequently, it may take a while to adopt new, healthier habits. So give yourself a break. None of us is perfect, especially at weight management. Just keep practicing the methods of this program.

The next group session will focus on problem solving, evaluation of positive changes, and areas for improvement.

Assessment of Lifestyle Changes

How do you feel about your progress?

List the behaviors you have changed.

List the behaviors you are having problems with.

What was your weight at the start of the program? _____

What is your weight now? _____ What is your goal weight? _____

Rate Your Progress (1% to 100%)

Are you more aware of being hungry and full? _____

How often do you stop eating when you are full? _____

Three meals a day? _____

Leave a bite or more on your plate? _____

Eat slower than you use to? _____

Wait 20 minutes before going for seconds? _____

Treat yourself kindly and get back on track if you overeat? _____

Eat in one designated area (the TABLE)? _____

Focus only on eating? _____

Problem Solving

List the problems that you have encountered during the first 11 weeks of this program, and any problems that you expect to encounter over the next year (review problem-solving section in Session 1). Choose problems that you have not solved and apply this method to these problem areas.

	Problems	Solutions	Costs/Benefits
1.			
2.			
3.			
4.			
5.			

Review of Lifestyle Changes

1. *Slow down eating.* Are you beginning to enjoy and taste your food?
2. *Leave food on your plate.* Are you relying on internal cues, such as hunger and satiety, or is a clean plate your master? One of the major goals of this program is to help you regain control over your eating habits. Leaving one bite of food (one piece of rice, or one bran flake) on your plate shows that you are aware of what you are eating, and we hope you are learning to focus on your hunger level. One piece of rice will not be shipped to starving people living in India.
3. *Always plan your meals ahead.* Planning before eating will help keep you from overeating between meals and during meals.
4. *Only eat at the table.* Are you eating at the table at least 85% of the time? This is one of the most important changes that you can make. It will cut out much of

"mindless" eating and keep the external cues such as the TV from making you want to eat.

5. *Focus only on eating.* Why is this important?
6. *Exercise.* Continue to increase your daily exercise. Burn those calories.
7. *Be kind to yourself.* Everyone falls off the wagon. Just get back on as soon as possible.

Homework Assignment

GET YOUR METS!!! Remember to monitor your food, activity, and lifestyle changes. Remember to reward yourself when you meet your goals.

Session Week 12: Increasing Physical Activity

Review: Please answer these questions at the beginning of each session using the rating scale of 0 = Very Poor to 5 = Very Well. Circle the rating that best describes your behavior during the previous week:

1. How well did you accurately record your food monitoring?	0	1	2	3	4	5
2. How well did you follow the exchange/calorie guidelines?	0	1	2	3	4	5
3. How well did you follow the exercise plan?	0	1	2	3	4	5
4. How well did you complete your behavioral contract?	0	1	2	3	4	5

TOTAL SCORE: _____

Exercising your body is like choosing to drive a Porsche instead of a 1950 Chevy truck. It runs so much smoother and faster, the ride is much more comfortable, and you can do so many more things. It is similar to taking excellent care of your car or house. Exercising is important for weight loss, maintenance, and overall health. We hope that you incorporate exercise not just for this program, but for the rest of your life. It is easier to add exercise to your life if you plan it into your daily schedule. Some people exercise before breakfast, some exercise during their lunch hour, and some exercise after dinner. Take a few minutes and decide the best time of day for you to exercise. Make exercise a habit the same way you are making the lifestyle changes into new habits.

At this point, many of you are getting used to exercising on a more regular basis. Keep increasing your METS, if you are not at 10 METS yet, find a way to get there. Remember to reward yourself whenever you hit your exercise goals.

Suggestions

1. Choose an activity that you will enjoy. Do not start a swimming program if you hate the water. If you have always wanted to learn to dance, take a dance class.
2. Choose an activity that you can do. Do not choose high-impact aerobics if you get winded after 15 minutes of walking; however, you could choose lower impact aerobics.
3. Choose an activity that fits into your schedule.

Remember that any activity is better than no activity. All activities burn calories. The goal of 10 METS a week was chosen, because if you are at this level of exercise, then you are improving your overall fitness level and burning calories. During this session, we will review your progress in the GYM program and discuss the next level of changes in activity that could be made. Be prepared to change your behavioral contract with the goal of increased activity.

Homework Assignment

We will be meeting every 2 weeks for awhile. Remember to bring your family/friends for family night in Session 14. Continue monitoring food intake and exercise.

Session Week 14: How Can the Family Help? (Remember to Invite Family)

Review: Please answer these questions at the beginning of each session using the rating scale of 0 = Very Poor to 5 = Very Well. Circle the rating that best describes your behavior during the previous week:

1. How well did you accurately record your food moni-   0 1 2 3 4 5
   toring?
2. How well did you follow the exchange/calorie guide-   0 1 2 3 4 5
   lines?
3. How well did you follow the exercise plan?   0 1 2 3 4 5
4. How well did you complete your behavioral contract?   0 1 2 3 4 5

TOTAL SCORE: _____

During the first part of this session, we will conduct a family/friend progress check. It is important to talk about how the family/friend is helping or hindering progress toward weight management. How well are you working together? We will break into smaller groups, and each group will discuss what is working and what needs to be changed. It is very important for the family to be able to communicate about these issues. Please be as specific as possible about asking for help from the family/friend. Also remember that the family/friend must be rewarded for being supportive. Be honest and let them know when you do and do not want their assistance.

Helpful Hints and Reminders for Family/Friend

1. *Do not be a watchdog.* Do not hound weight-loss participants by watching everything they eat. Only help in those areas in which they have requested your help.
2. *Be Positive.* Let the weight-loss participant know that you are really proud of them for all the effort they are putting into this program.
3. *Support your family member or friend in making the following lifestyle changes*:
   a. Slow down eating.
   b. Leave food on your plate.
   c. Sit only at the table to eat. If you do not eat on the couch or in the car, the dieter may be less likely to eat there.
4. Focus only on eating. Do not read the paper or watch the news during meals. Use meal times as family time.
5. *Keep your expectations reasonable.* Do not expect a 3-pound weight loss each week. Expect small gradual changes in eating and exercise behavior.

Family support can be very beneficial, especially for weight maintenance. If you can handle changing your eating habits, it will help prevent minor lapses. For example, ask for baked instead of fried chicken—the dieter will be less likely to overeat, and it is a healthier style of cooking.

Homework Assignment

Remember to monitor your food, exercise, and lifestyle changes. Communicate with persons who are trying to support you. Read Session 16.

Session Week 16: Eating Out

Review: Please answer these questions at the beginning of each session using the rating scale of 0 = Very Poor to 5 = Very Well. Circle the rating that best describes your behavior during the previous week:

1. How well did you accurately record your food monitoring?   0   1   2   3   4   5
2. How well did you follow the exchange/calorie guidelines?   0   1   2   3   4   5
3. How well did you follow the exercise plan?   0   1   2   3   4   5
4. How well did you complete your behavioral contract?   0   1   2   3   4   5

TOTAL SCORE: _____

Eating out presents a significant challenge to the dieter. All too often, some of the problems within a diet stem from not knowing which foods one should select in order to follow the dietary-exchange program. Whereas some restaurants offer very healthy menu selections, others do not. The objective in an uncontrolled situation, such as eating in a restaurant, should be to reduce the overall calories and dietary fat that you consume. To achieve this objective, certain habits should become a part of your restaurant visits.

One habit should be always to order salad without salad dressing. Often salads are drowned in high-fat salad dressings that can mask the flavor of the vegetables in the salad. Calories may be significantly reduced by either totally eliminating the dressing or using only a small amount on the tines of a fork before spearing the lettuce greens and other salad components. If a larger amount of dressing is desired, then choose a low-calorie fat-free dressing and carry it with you, or order it, if it is available. There are many good-tasting fat-free dressings on the market today, and we expect more to appear in the future.

Another habit to form when eating out is to order entree items without sauces and gravies. Meat, poultry, and fish should be ordered broiled or grilled. Specify that no fat be added. If the meats are fresh, you will taste their full natural flavor. Even on broiled or grilled items, butter or other fats are added after cooking. Try to prevent this from happening by specifying your desires when first ordering.

Sandwich items should be ordered without mayonnaise and dressings, if possible. If a fat-free alternative is available, specify that it be used. Otherwise, order the dressing on the side, and use as little as possible.

Finally, learn all you can about the items you typically order. The waiter or waitress may tell you about the special of the day and will probably be more than happy to answer questions about other dishes on the menu. Because it is becoming more trendy to inquire about low-fat dishes, a good server will probably be happy to indicate which items on the menu are already low in fat and which can be prepared to cut the fat.

Since restaurant dining for most people is a social occasion, take time to enjoy your meal. Stretch out the time it takes to eat and spend time in conversation with your dining companion. In the next session, we will discuss solving common problems associated with eating out. Prior to this discussion, answer the following questions (in writing).

Do you usually have an idea of what you might order in the restaurant?

Can you actually plan your meal prior to going into the restaurant, because you are familiar with the menu?

Can you anticipate problems (e.g., sauces and gravies that are high in fat) and develop a plan to solve them?

What excuses have you used in the past that have resulted in significant overeating in restaurants? Do your family or eating companions make it difficult to select restaurants with healthy foods on the menu?

Why have you made bad food selections in the past? Are you doomed to repeat this behavior?

Homework Assignment

Be prepared to solve your problems related to eating out. Remember to plan your meals in advance and monitor your behavior.

Session Week 18: Holidays, Parties, and Special Events (Invite family members and friends to this group session)

Review: Please answer these questions at the beginning of each session using the rating scale of 0 = Very Poor to 5 = Very Well. Circle the rating that best describes your behavior during the previous week:

1. How well did you accurately record your food moni- 0 1 2 3 4 5
   toring?
2. How well did you follow the exchange/calorie guide- 0 1 2 3 4 5
   lines?
3. How well did you follow the exercise plan? 0 1 2 3 4 5
4. How well did you complete your behavioral contract? 0 1 2 3 4 5

TOTAL SCORE: _____

Parties, holidays, and special events are particularly hard for persons trying to manage weight. Sometimes you may feel that these occasions are time-off from weight management. However, overeating during these events can lead to guilt or feeling that you have "blown it," which makes relapse much more probable in these supposedly "happy events." Even when you enter one of these situations with the best of intentions, you may still find them difficult. Special events are filled with external cues to eat. There is usually lots of food, and everyone is eating and drinking. The following is a list of techniques to help deal with these situations. The group leader will discuss these in more detail in the next group meeting. Before the group, identify the last party, holiday, or special occasion in which you had a problem with your eating. Try to analyze that situation and determine whether these techniques would have helped. Discuss this situation and any other upcoming events with the group. Remember, alcohol is *NOT* a free food.

Hints for the Family

Try not to pressure the dieter to eat or to abstain from eating. Be encouraging and reinforcing, but do not be a watchdog. Sit down with the dieter to eat. Try to help keep the dieter's mind off food if the dieter is having a problem. Table 12.4 summarizes some helpful hints for successful management of parties and special events.

1. *Eat before you go.* This suggestion is especially useful for parties. Most parties have lots of foods for nibbling. It is very hard to feel full when eating these types of foods. If you eat a small meal before you go (e.g., a salad), it will help to keep you from overeating on chips in an effort to fill up.
2. *Eat only special foods at a party.* Have you ever given in to "family-reunion" eating behavior? That is when you have to try everything, even three different kinds of baked beans, because they are there. Do not feel that you have to eat everything. Stick to the special foods you do not eat every day. Remember, those finger sandwiches and meatballs are the same as what you eat on a routine basis.
3. *Sit down and follow the other lifestyle changes.* Never stand over the food. That makes it more likely that you will eat without paying attention to the amount that you have eaten. Eat smaller amounts, and eat slowly.
4. *Plan ahead.* If you generally know what foods will be served, plan what you are going to eat before you get there. Planning ahead will help reduce temptation and give you the confidence that you can attend a special occasion and still control your eating. Planning ahead also means planning for any dessert you may eat.

Table 12.4 Holidays, Parties, and Special Events: Always Plan Ahead

1. EAT BEFORE YOU GO/NEVER GO HUNGRY.
   —It's hard to fill up on *nibble* foods.
2. EAT ONLY THE SPECIAL FOODS.
   —Don't give in to the urge to try everything.
   —Remember, those cute little sandwiches are the same that you eat for lunch several times a week.
3. SIT DOWN.
   —Never stand over the food. It can lead to mindless eating.
4. FOLLOW THE LIFESTYLE CHANGES.
5. PLAN AHEAD.
6. DO NOT GET DOWN IF YOU OVERDO IT A LITTLE. JUST GET BACK ON TRACK ASAP.

5. *Get back on track.* Remember, do not get down if you overeat at a party. Just get back on track as soon as possible.

Homework Assignment

Be prepared to use problem solving to modify your eating behavior at parties and special occasions. Follow your behavioral contract and exercise program. Plan your meals before eating and be sure to monitor eating and activity.

Session Week 20: Life and Weight History

Review: Please answer these questions at the beginning of each session using the rating scale of 0 = Very Poor to 5 = Very Well. Circle the rating that best describes your behavior during the previous week:

1. How well did you accurately record your food monitoring? 0 1 2 3 4 5
2. How well did you follow the exchange/calorie guidelines? 0 1 2 3 4 5
3. How well did you follow the exercise plan? 0 1 2 3 4 5
4. How well did you complete your behavioral contract? 0 1 2 3 4 5

TOTAL SCORE: _____

This session will focus on weight changes throughout your lifetime. By completing a graph of your weight changes, you may begin to notice patterns in weight gains and losses. Focusing on these patterns may help you become more aware of both the external and internal situations that have contributed to your problems with excess weight. We will also be able to examine other, less obvious behaviors that contributed to your weight gain. For example, many women gain weight during and after pregnancy; however, you may also have reduced your activity during that time period. Examining your weight history may help you determine what to do to take the weight off and keep it off. For example, after losing weight in the past, you may have put the weight back on. What did you do during that time period? Did you go back to your old eating habits? We will examine your weight changes as a method of problem solving for the future—when you are finished with the Lifestyle-Change program.

Weight History Exercise

In preparation for the next group, list 10 weight milestones—the 5 highest and 5 lowest weights that you can remember. For example, you may recall what you weighed when you graduated from high school, got married, got pregnant, dieted, and so on. These weights do not have to be exact, just an estimate.

In the next group session, you are going to construct your own weight history. The group leader will assist you in completing this exercise. In preparation for this group, identify any important events that were associated with significant weight gains or losses, such as marriage, divorce, new jobs, any major stressors, surgery, quitting smoking, hysterectomy, menopause, pregnancy, retirement, or decrease in exercise. Match these events to the 10 weight milestones that you listed. Using this information, we will attempt to uncover potential causes of your current weight problem. The following section will be completed in Session 20.

After completing your weight graph, what patterns between weight change and life events and changes in habits are evident? Did you gain weight gradually or in spurts? What caused you to gain weight after previous weight-loss attempts?

Problem Solving

Looking at your weight history, list the problems that led to weight gains in the past. Then, list potential solutions to these problems. (Remember to go through all the problem solving steps.)

	Problems	Solutions	Costs/Benefits
1.			
2.			
3.			
4.			
5.			

Homework Assignment

Make it a point to discuss what you have learned from this exercise with family and friends. They will be invited to the next group session. Remember to monitor food intake and METS.

Session Week 22: Accidental Sabotage of Progress (Family and friends are invited to this session)

Review: Please answer these questions at the beginning of each session using the rating scale of 0 = Very Poor to 5 = Very Well. Circle the rating that best describes your behavior during the previous week:

1. How well did you accurately record your food moni-   0   1   2   3   4   5
   toring?
2. How well did you follow the exchange/calorie guide-   0   1   2   3   4   5
   lines?
3. How well did you follow the exercise plan?   0   1   2   3   4   5
4. How well did you complete your behavioral contract?   0   1   2   3   4   5

TOTAL SCORE: _____

What is accidental sabotage? Accidental sabotage occurs anytime you give up responsibility for controlling your eating. This form of sabotage often occurs when you are feeling pressured to eat. We have all heard parents say, "I have to keep cookies and ice cream in the house, because my kids like to have dessert after supper," or "My family likes fried food, therefore it is hard for me to eat healthy." This attitude promotes keeping problem foods within reaching distance. Anytime you blame your eating habits on something out of your control (e.g., your family), you are not taking responsibility for what you are doing. Another "excuse" we often hear is that "My friends took me out for lunch, and they ordered dessert, so I felt that I had to have dessert." What is wrong with this type of thinking? If you want to have a small bowl of ice cream for dessert, incorporate it into your meal plan. It is very important to be aware of your food choices. No one else can make you eat. You are the one who says, "I'll have some." If you want a dessert and did not plan to eat it, accept responsibility and compensate at the next meal. It is alright to eat your favorite foods in moderation.

How to Deal with the External Pressure to Eat

Most people know at least one "food pusher," someone who suggests eating, even when you are not hungry. Perhaps a relative expects you to eat everything on your plate and acts hurt if you do not. They may even say, "You really do not like my cooking" or "What about those starving children in India?" Perhaps they made your favorite dessert and expect you to eat a large piece. Friends and family, although they may want the best for you, may at times make dieting very difficult. They may even encourage you to overeat. The way you handle challenges such as these may determine your success at weight loss and maintenance. If you do indulge when you are not hungry, how do you generally feel afterwards? Some of you may feel angry at yourselves and the "food pusher," or some of you may just feel depressed. These feelings are much more likely to lead you to continue overeating. If you do indulge, forgive yourself and get back on track *as soon as possible.*

You may notice that your friends who are not dieting may say, "Go ahead have dessert; it won't hurt you" or they may say, "Why are you dieting, you know that diets never work?" They may not be deliberately trying to sabotage your progress, but on the other hand, they may be jealous that you are losing weight and they are not. It is sometimes hard to watch a friend lose weight, especially if you have not been successful at weight loss. Your family may also give you a hard time about losing weight, or they may continue to eat your favorite foods while watching TV.

What is the best way to handle pressure from friends and relatives? The best solution is to politely say, "No, I am not hungry." After "Aunt Jane" hears "no" a few times, she will be less likely to offer you rich dessert (e.g., cheesecake or chocolate cake). Refusing food from friends and relatives is easier said than done. In the next session, we will practice saying "no" to family and friends. Their job will be to suggest a number of different foods or scenarios, and your job is to practice saying "no." Remember, learning a new habit takes time and practice.

Internal Pressure to Eat (Attitude Traps)

A common problem area for people trying to manage weight is the type of rules they have about dieting. You should pay special attention to any rules that use the words *always*, *must*, or *never*. For example,

- I must always control my sweet cravings.

- I must lose at least 2 pounds a week.
- I must never get depressed, because I tend to eat more when I am depressed.
- I must exercise for 30 minutes every day.
- I will never eat chocolate cake again.

What happens when you eat chocolate cake? Does that mean you have blown it? What are you most likely to do if you break any of your rules? Overeat?

Notice the difference in how you feel if you just modify these statements a little. For example, the following dialogue is very destructive.

Destructive Thinking. "I can't believe that I just had chocolate cake! Why do I bother dieting, I have no willpower, I will never be successful at losing weight." With this style of thinking, you are likely to feel discouraged and frustrated, and you are more likely to give up.

Healthier Thinking. As an alternative, try this style of thinking: "I had a piece of cake. I guess that means that I'll have to eat less at dinner, and do better tomorrow." (*Remember*, skipping meals is not a good idea). With this style of thinking, you provide a solution (eating less at dinner) to solve the problem of eating too much at an earlier time. Table 12.5 provides some further examples of how to modify self-defeating thoughts.

Homework Assignment

List your old rules that contain the words *never* and *always* and make them into more flexible guidelines, as shown in the earlier example. Follow your behavioral contract. Seek support from family and friends. Reward them for helping you. Remember to monitor your food, exercise, and lifestyle changes.

Session Week 24: Evaluation of Progress

Review: Please answer these questions at the beginning of each session using the rating scale of 0 = Very Poor to 5 = Very Well. Circle the rating that best describes your behavior during the previous week:

1. How well did you accurately record your food moni-   0   1   2   3   4   5
toring?
2. How well did you follow the exchange/calorie guide-   0   1   2   3   4   5
lines?
3. How well did you follow the exercise plan?   0   1   2   3   4   5
4. How well did you complete your behavioral contract?   0   1   2   3   4   5

TOTAL SCORE: _____

How do you feel after 24 weeks of the Lifestyle-Change program? We hope you are no longer considering this program a diet, but rather a series of lifestyle changes. Have you met your weekly behavior and exercise goals? I know that you have already realized that losing weight is hard work.

Congratulations, you are half way through the program. In this session, we will discuss the habit changes that have been most helpful for you in your efforts to manage weight. Answer the following questions in preparation for Session 24.

Table 12.5. Modifying Your Dieting Rules (Guidelines)

Old rule	New rule
I must never eat cake.	I will do my best to eat less cake. If I do have a piece, I will compensate for the added calories.
I must exercise every day.	I will do my best to exercise every day. It is okay if I miss a day. I will get back on track *as soon as possible*.

Progress Check

List the positive changes that you have made.

List the areas that you still need to improve.

Rate Your Progress (1–100%)

Are you aware of being hungry and full? _____
How often do you stop eating when you are full? _____
    Three meals a day? _____
Leave a bite or more on your plate? _____
Do you eat more slowly than you did before? _____
Do you wait 5 minutes before going back for second portions? _____
Do you treat yourself kindly and get back on track quickly if you overeat or fail to exercise? _____
Do you eat in one designated area (preferably at the table)? _____
Do you focus only on eating while consuming food? _____
Do you plan snacks in your dietary exchange plan? _____
Do you use stairs instead of elevators? _____
Do you park farther away? _____
Do you engage in regular walking or other activities? _____
Rate your current level of commitment (1 = *None* to 10 = *Total Commitment*). Rating = _____

Describe any other problems that you have encountered.

Homework Assignment

Remember to monitor your food, exercise, and lifestyle changes.

Session Week 26: Assertion and Self-Control of Eating (Family and friends are invited to this group session)

Review: Please answer these questions at the beginning of each session using the rating scale of 0 = Very Poor to 5 = Very Well. Circle the rating that best describes your behavior during the previous week:

1. How well did you accurately record your food monitoring?	0	1	2	3	4	5
2. How well did you follow the exchange/calorie guidelines?	0	1	2	3	4	5
3. How well did you follow the exercise plan?	0	1	2	3	4	5
4. How well did you complete your behavioral contract?	0	1	2	3	4	5

TOTAL SCORE: _____

How assertive are you in response to pressures to eat? One of the most useful skills that you can acquire is assertiveness. This applies not just in relation to pressures to eat, but also in response to your family, friends, and co-workers. *First*, we will define general assertiveness and then discuss how this relates to eating.

What is the difference between passivity, assertiveness, and aggressiveness?

There are three ways to handle a problem situation. As we discuss each of these, decide which sounds most like you.

1. *Passive, nonassertive position.* This type of response violates your own rights by *failing* to express your feelings and thoughts, or expressing your feelings or thoughts in an apologetic, self-effacing manner. By not stating your feelings and thoughts in a direct, honest way, the other person is allowed to take advantage of you. This set of habits is called the "Doormat Syndrome." If you tend to respond in this manner, you may feel anxious, depressed, or angry when you do not express your feelings or do things for others that you do not want to do. You may often end up thinking, "Why didn't I say no?" or "I can't believe I just did that."

2. *Assertive position.* You stand up for your rights, express your thoughts and feelings in a direct, honest, and appropriate way that does not violate another's personal rights. You feel good about being honest and taking care of yourself. The other person respects you for your honesty.

3. *Aggressive position.* You stand up for your own rights, but express your thoughts and feelings in a way that always violates the rights of another. In other words, you take advantage of the other person. To facilitate the discussion in this session, complete the following exercise.

Describe when you behaved in the following manner:

1. Nonassertively:

2. Aggressively:

3. Assertively:

Now, describe how you might behave more assertively in situations 1 and 2 in the next section.

1. *With "food pushers."* If your best friend, Susie, suggests that you go out for triple-layer cheese pizza with everything on it, you can say, "Susie, I would love to get together with you, but I am not hungry" Or "Why don't we go for a walk or go to the movies." Your friends/family will quit suggesting food after you politely refuse to eat unhealthy food a few times.

2. *Internal pressures to eat.* Be assertive with yourself about when, where, and why you are eating. Have you ever "guilted" yourself about eating? For example, you think to yourself, "I really shouldn't have eaten that" or "I really have to have cheesecake or I'll be miserable." If you are going to eat something when you are not hungry, take responsibility for your actions and be honest with yourself. "Even though I am not hungry, I am choosing to have this piece of cake." This honesty allows you to respond appropriately after you eat. "I am doing my best to cut down on sweets. I'll compensate at dinner by eating less."

Homework Assignment

Before the next session, monitor your assertiveness as it relates to eating. Describe at least three situations in which you were or were not assertive.

Describe event	**Describe how you handled it**
1.	
2.	
3.	

Follow your behavioral contract and monitor behavior change. Be prepared to honestly and assertively discuss problems with your family and friends. During this session, we will engage in role playing to help you learn to be more assertive in weight management.

Session Week 28: Social Problem Solving

Review: Please answer these questions at the beginning of each session using the rating scale of 0 = Very Poor to 5 = Very Well. Circle the rating that best describes your behavior during the previous week:

1. How well did you accurately record your food monitoring?   0 1 2 3 4 5
2. How well did you follow the exchange/calorie guidelines?   0 1 2 3 4 5
3. How well did you follow the exercise plan?   0 1 2 3 4 5
4. How well did you complete your behavioral contract?   0 1 2 3 4 5

TOTAL SCORE: _____

Learning how to be more effective at dealing with social problems will help not just with weight management, but also with making major and minor decisions. What types of coping mechanisms do you tend to use if a social problem overwhelms you? Feeling helpless to solve a problem can lead to sadness, anger, and anxiety. These emotions can lead some people to overeat. The problem-solving technique is a form of self-control. Let's review the six steps of problem solving.

STEP 1—*Define the problem*. Be as specific as possible.

STEP 2—*Brainstorm*. Generate as many solutions as possible, regardless of whether they are good or bad solutions. Make sure to write all solutions down. Do not eliminate any at this stage.

STEP 3—*Do a cost–benefit analysis of each solution*.

STEP 4—*Choose the most effective solution*.

STEP 5—*Design a plan to implement your solution and then carry it out*. It is often useful to give yourself a time period in which you want this plan of action to be completed.

STEP 6—*Evaluate the effectiveness of your solution*. If it worked, then the process stops here; however, if it was not successful, go back to Step 4 and choose another alternative.

This problem-solving process is very effective, because sometimes people get so involved and worried about their problem that they can not see more than one solution. This form of "tunnel vision" is especially true when people try to solve social problems that involve potential interpersonal conflict. The following example illustrates how the problem-solving process can be used to solve a common social problem related to eating:

1. *Define the problem*. My spouse suggested that we go to my favorite buffet tonight.
2. *Generate solutions*.
   - Go to the buffet.
   - Tell him that I want to stay home, because I am not sure that I am ready for a buffet.
   - Go with a meal plan.
   - Stay home, pretending that I am sick.
   - Ask for his help in dealing with the buffet.
   Note: There are many other possible solutions.
3. *Cost–benefit analysis*
   a. *Solution*: Go to the buffet.
      Cost: I may overeat.
      Benefit: I can practice my new eating habits.
   b. *Solution*: Stay home, because I do not know if I can handle it.
      Cost: I may miss out on an opportunity to try my new skills.
      Benefit: I will be less likely to overeat.
   c. *Solution*: Go with a meal plan.
      Cost: I may overeat; however, I will be less likely to overeat because I have a plan.
      Benefit: I will get a chance to test myself, and with a plan, I will probably be successful.
   d. *Solution*: Tell him I am sick.
      Cost: I would be lying, and I will feel bad about it later.
      Benefit: Stay home and not overeat.

 e. *Solution*: Ask for his help.
  Cost: I may still overeat, but it's less likely.
  Benefit: I am being assertive and asking for the help I may need. I will probably
   do fine.

 4. *Choose a solution*. Designing a meal plan and asking for help seem to have the most potential benefits with the least costs. You could choose one solution or combine both strategies. Let us suppose you elected to combine both strategies.

 5. *Implement solution*. Next you must develop a meal plan, which is possible because you are very familiar with the foods served in the buffet. Let us assume you planned ahead so that you eat within the allotted dietary exchanges. Now you must talk with your spouse, tell him or her about your problem solving, planned meal, and ask for his or her support.

 6. *Evaluate outcome*. The next step is to carry out this plan of action and see if it results in controlled eating. If it does, then you have more confidence in this strategy. If it does not work, then next time you should try one of your alternative solutions. The key concept: *Do not give up*. Be a persistent and active problem solver.

In the next session, you will be invited to solve one of your problems through group problem solving.

Homework Assignment

Select two problems and use the problem-solving method to determine a solution or course of action that you can follow. If you have trouble solving a problem, bring it up in the next group for group problem solving. Next week, remember to bring your family and friends. Continue monitoring your food, exercise, and lifestyle changes. Follow your behavioral contract.

Session Week 30: Communication with Family and Friends (Family and friends are invited to this group session)

Review: Please answer these questions at the beginning of each session using the rating scale of 0 = Very Poor to 5 = Very Well. Circle the rating that best describes your behavior during the previous week:

1. How well did you accurately record your food monitoring?	0 1 2 3 4 5
2. How well did you follow the exchange/calorie guidelines?	0 1 2 3 4 5
3. How well did you follow the exercise plan?	0 1 2 3 4 5
4. How well did you complete your behavioral contract?	0 1 2 3 4 5

TOTAL SCORE: _____

This session will focus on effective communication skills. People trying to lose weight often report overeating after getting upset with their family and friends. Good communication skills can lessen the likelihood of negative feelings and increase the effectiveness of problem solving.

Good Communication Guidelines

1. Tell others how you want to be helped.
2. Make specific requests.
3. State your requests positively.

The more assertive and honest you are when dealing with friends and family, the better you will feel. Remember to reward your family/friends when they do the things that you ask them to do. One way that many people get their feelings hurt is by engaging in "mind reading." Mind reading usually occurs when you must interpret a person's words or actions that are vague or ambiguous. For example, a friend or family member may say, "Haven't you had enough?" You could interpret this statement as meaning that he or she is suggesting that you are fat and have no willpower, which will likely make you depressed or angry. Another conclusion is that the person is trying to help you. The easiest way to understand what they meant by the comment is to simply ask them and to accept their answer. Many times, you will find that the other person was only trying to help. By effectively listening and communicating, many arguments and negative feelings can be avoided.

Listening Skills

Listening is a very important skill, which many of us believe that we do well. However, many of us listen to our own internal dialogue while appearing to listen to someone else (especially in an argument). If you are concentrating on what to say next, you will not be very effective at hearing and understanding the other person.

Guidelines for Healthy Communication

1. When it is your turn to listen—*only listen*.
2. Paraphrase what you heard to make sure you heard correctly.
3. Do not engage in *mind reading*. Another form of mind reading occurs when we expect the other person to read our minds. "We've been married for over 10 years. My spouse *should* know I'm upset." How is that spouse suppose to know what is wrong unless you tell him or her directly?

Listening Skills Exercise

In the next group session, we will do the following exercise. Be prepared to do the following:

1. Spend 10 minutes listening to your partner.
2. Paraphrase what you heard (ask about any assumptions that you made).
3. Switch positions, and you do the talking.

Homework Assignment

After the next group session, practice the listening skills exercise at least twice the following week with a friend or spouse. If you are serious about changing your communication patterns, continue to work on this skill each week. Remember to plan your meals before you eat. Be assertive with your weight-management program. Be an active problem solver. Follow your behavioral contract.

Review: Please answer these questions at the beginning of each session using the rating scale of 0 = Very Poor to 5 = Very Well. Circle the rating that best describes your behavior during the previous week:

1. How well did you accurately record your food moni-　0　1　2　3　4　5
   toring?
2. How well did you follow the exchange/calorie guide-　0　1　2　3　4　5
   lines?
3. How well did you follow the exercise plan?　　　　　0　1　2　3　4　5
4. How well did you complete your behavioral contract?　0　1　2　3　4　5

TOTAL SCORE: _____

For the next few sessions, we will be discussing how mood and thinking style can affect your eating. Have you noticed that you tend to eat when you are upset? Or, do you eat when you are happy, or to reward yourself? What about eating when you are bored, tired, or sad? Mood, just like time of day or social events, can become a stimulus for eating. Sometimes, people eat to console themselves or to celebrate. Although in the short term food can be positively reinforcing, the long-term consequence may be weight gain because of overeating. Again, it is very important to evaluate if you are eating in response to a physiological drive or in response to other cues, including emotions. This session is designed to help you evaluate mood states and thought processes that may affect your eating. Once these factors have been identified, you can employ problem-solving techniques to situations or mood states that may be affecting your eating. Think back to the last time your mood affected your eating. Using the worksheet in Table 12.6, you can evaluate the events that influence your eating. Be prepared to describe a situation in which mood influenced your eating.

In reflecting on the relationship between mood and eating, do you see a pattern of mood affecting your eating? Sometimes, you must try to change your emotional and behavioral reaction to a problematic situation. Your moods and thoughts are closely related. Most of the time, your moods are strongly influenced by your thinking style. For example, if you are thinking, "I am fat and no good," your mood is probably not going to be very positive. In addition, negative thoughts can set you up for overeating. For example, after eating a cookie, if you think, "Oh boy, I have really blown it!" that may lead to thinking, "Oh well, I might as well eat more." This sequence of thoughts is an example of an internal dialogue. For persons trying to manage weight, irrational internal dialogues revolve around three primary ideas:

1. The impossibility of weight loss (e.g., "I will never meet my goals").
2. Unrealistic goals (e.g., "I have to lose 5 pounds a week").
3. Negative self-image (e.g., "I should not have eaten that chocolate. I am disgusting").

In addition, some internal dialogues can revolve around convincing yourself that it is okay to eat (e.g., "The broken cookies do not count as real calories"). Irrational internal dialogues often stem from *cognitive distortions*. It is important to identify internal dialogues that lead to overeating or negative emotions. Table 12.7 presents a list of common cognitive distortions associated with eating. These examples are presented to aid you in

Table 12.6. Evaluating My Mood and Eating

Donald A. Williamson
et al.

During the next 2-week period, describe two recent episodes that illustrate the influence of positive or negative mood states on your eating habits. For each of these situations, provide information related to mood and hunger:

Describe the first situation: Describe the second situation:

Mood prior to eating: Very Good
                                                          Good
                                                          Neutral
                                                          Bad
                                                          Very Bad

Describe the emotion: (angry, sad, happy, etc.)   _____

Hunger prior to eating: Very Hungry
                                                          Hungry
                                                          Neutral
                                                          Full
                                                          Very Full

Mood after eating: Very Good
                                                          Good
                                                          Neutral
                                                          Bad
                                                          Very Bad

Hunger after eating: Very Hungry
                                                          Hungry
                                                          Neutral
                                                          Full
                                                          Very Full

What were you thinking?

What did you do?

identifying irrational internal dialogues. During the group meeting for Week 32, the group leader will discuss these various cognitive distortions and try to help you identify your mood states that lead to overeating. However, begin evaluating these mood states before the session. Try to determine which of these cognitive distortions pertain to you. During the group meeting, you will be given a homework assignment to help you begin identifying these patterns of thinking. In Session 34, we will focus on changing thoughts about your eating and weight, and deal more appropriately with your moods.

Session Week 34: Thought Monitoring

Review: Please answer these questions at the beginning of each session using the rating scale of 0 = Very Poor to 5 = Very Well. Circle the rating that best describes your behavior during the previous week:

1. How well did you accurately record your food monitoring? 0 1 2 3 4 5
2. How well did you follow the exchange/calorie guidelines? 0 1 2 3 4 5
3. How well did you follow the exercise plan? 0 1 2 3 4 5
4. How well did you follow your behavioral contract? 0 1 2 3 4 5

TOTAL SCORE: _____

Were you successful at identifying internal dialogues associated with eating and weight? If so, how did these thoughts affect you? If they had a negative influence upon eating, the following technique will show you how to modify problematic thoughts.

Sidebar 12–3 is an example of how to modify irrational thinking. Sidebar 12–4 is a blank form to help you systematically work through your problematic thoughts. The group leader will help you go through this process during the next group meeting and assign homework for you to complete before Session 36. The *ultimate* goal is for you to be able to go through this process in your head at the moment it is happening. However, like any other skill, you first have to practice. Going through the process on paper helps you stop the thoughts from repeating themselves, like an internal whirlwind.

On the left side of the handout, write a description of an internal dialogue that you consider bothersome. Now, is there any evidence to contradict the conclusions derived from this thought? If yes, write this contradiction down on the right-hand side under Rational Response. It can be helpful to "switch places" with yourself. What would you tell another group member who repeated this thought to you? What would the group leader say about this reasoning? List all of the rational arguments that you can come up with to contradict the irrational internal dialogue. The following are two examples of this process:

Table 12.7. Common Cognitive Distortions[a]

1. *All-or-nothing thinking*—You see things in black or white. "I have succeeded with my diet because I have lost 5 pounds, but have failed if I have not."

2. *Overgeneralization*—You see a single negative event as a never-ending pattern of defeat. "I went over my exchanges today just like I always do."

3. *Mental filter*—You focus on a single negative detail so that it colors your thinking about everything else.

4. *Disqualifying the positive*—You disqualify positive things because they do not count. For example, focusing on the amount of weight that you have not lost rather than what you have.

5. *Jumping to conclusions*—a. *Mind Reading*—You assume that you can read others minds without checking it out. "My boss doesn't like me because I am overweight"; b. *Fortune-Teller Error*—You predict what will happen in the future. "I will never be able to stick to this diet, so I might as well eat what I want."

6. *Magnification and minimization*—You exaggerate your mistakes or minimize positives. It is also important to not rationalize overeating. For example, "I just ate one cookie, so I won't write it down," or "The broken ones do not count.'"

7. *Should statements*—You use "shoulds" to motivate yourself. "I should have reached my goal weight by now. I should eat this extra helping because my mother cooked it for me."

[a]Adapted from Burns, 1980.

Sidebar 12–3

Handout for Week 34: Example of Rational-Thinking Form

Irrational thought	Rational response
1. I am fat and no good.	1. I may be overweight, but, I am a good person with many good qualities. 2. List those qualities. 3. I am actively trying to lose weight.
2. I blew it again. I will never be able to lose weight.	1. This is just one lapse. I can correct it. 2. I am trying to lose weight. 3. If there is a problem with the program, I can use the problem solving techniques to correct it. 4. It is important for me not to allow this to sabotage my diet.

Session Week 36: Rational Thinking: A Family Goal (Family and friends are invited to this group session)

Review: Please answer these questions at the beginning of each session using the rating scale of 0 = Very Poor to 5 = Very Well. Circle the rating that best describes your behavior during the previous week:

1. How well did you accurately record your food monitoring?   0 1 2 3 4 5
2. How well did you follow the exchange/calorie guidelines?   0 1 2 3 4 5
3. How well did you follow the exercise plan?   0 1 2 3 4 5
4. How well did you follow your behavioral contract?   0 1 2 3 4 5

TOTAL SCORE: _____

One of the most important aspects of a successful weight-loss program is the development of family support. Over the past several weeks, we have been discussing how mood and irrational thinking are associated with eating and weight management. It is also very important for the family members and friends to engage in rational thinking about weight management. Family support can take many forms. The following is a list of goals for the family. The group leader will generate a family discussion during the next group meeting, so encourage your family member of friend to attend.

1. *Keep rational/realistic expectations.* Remember to focus on caloric and behavioral goals rather than weight loss. Weight loss is a gradual, sporadic process. Keep in mind that the person trying to lose weight may have bad days. Try to help, but do not be overbearing.

2. *Be supportive*. Being overly critical or a "watchdog" can lead to resentment and worsen a negative mood. Being a watchdog will not help the dieter. Being a watchdog can lead the dieter to deceptive eating practices, which are a very bad habits to form.

3. *Be involved*. Know what is involved with the program. Help to prepare your own snacks and meals if necessary. Try to engage the dieter in activities that will keep the him or her from overeating.

4. *Encourage the weight-loss participant to communicate*. If there is a problem, see if you can help. Try to talk to the person about the process of controlling eating and increasing exercise.

5. *Try to help the dieter to remain rational*. This includes being reasonable about weight goals, and about the process of reducing caloric intake. Remember that the dieter's ultimate goal is to achieve a healthy status, not to be the same size he or she was at age 18.

After this group meeting, the sessions will be held once per month. For the rest of the lifestyle program, the group will focus on maintenance of weight loss and relapse prevention. If you foresee any problems for the next month, please discuss these with the group leader during the group meeting for Week 36.

Session Week 40: Relapse Prevention: Maintenance of Weight Loss

Review: Please answer these questions at the beginning of each session using the rating scale of 0 = Very Poor to 5 = Very Well. Circle the rating that best describes your behavior during the previous week:

1. How well did you accurately record your food monitoring? 0 1 2 3 4 5
2. How well did you follow the exchange/calorie guidelines? 0 1 2 3 4 5
3. How well did you follow the exercise plan? 0 1 2 3 4 5
4. How well did you follow your behavioral contract? 0 1 2 3 4 5

TOTAL SCORE: _____

Sidebar 12–4

Handout for Week 34: Rational-Thinking Form

Irrational thought   Rational response

In this session, we will begin discussing strategies for the maintenance of weight loss. Maintenance of weight loss is an ongoing process. It can seem overwhelming to think about maintenance of weight loss as a lifetime goal. However, remember that you have already made a number of behavior changes. Many of these new habits are probably well established. In the next few months, we must consolidate behavior changes and learn to stop "backsliding" in its earliest stages. A key to relapse prevention is recognition that you are in danger of returning to old habits. In particular, you must be able to comfortably consume moderate quantities of formerly troublesome foods. Remember, it is unwise to eliminate any food from your diet. It is very important to remember what you have accomplished over the past 40 weeks. Remembering how far you have come can often help prevent your giving in to the temptation of overeating. Finally, continued exercise has been cited by researchers as one of the most important aspects of long-term success with dieting.

For the next several sessions, we will learn about relapse prevention. The format of this program was adapted from research with alcoholism. First, there is a very important distinction between relapse and lapse. *Relapse* is defined as falling back into a former condition. After the completion of a weight-loss program, it is very easy to revert to old habits. However, it was those old habits that caused weight gain in the past. Totally reverting to your old eating habits would be considered a relapse. A *lapse*, however, is somewhat different; it is a slip of much less significance. It is very important to remember that a lapse does not have to lead to a relapse. Try to think of a lapse as a learning experience. You have the opportunity to collect information and formulate a plan of action to help prevent its recurrence. During Weeks 44 and 48, the group will discuss the components of relapse prevention. Analyze any problem situations in order to discuss them in these groups. Very often, irrational thoughts can precipitate relapse. Using the form provided, complete the homework assignment to identify problematic thought patterns.

Cognitive Change / Irrational Internal Dialogues

Over the next week, pay attention to your thoughts. Write down at least three irrational internal dialogues associated with your eating or weight.

These can be instances when you felt guilty, overate, or otherwise became upset with your eating or weight.

1. Situation: _____

   Internal Dialogue: _____

   _____

   _____

2. Situation: _____

   Internal Dialogue: _____

   _____

   _____

3. Situation: _____

   Internal Dialogue: _____

   _____

   _____

Review: Please answer these questions at the beginning of each session using the rating scale of 0 = Very Poor to 5 = Very Well. Circle the rating that best describes your behavior during the previous week:

1. How well did you accurately record your food monitoring? 0 1 2 3 4 5
2. How well did you follow the exchange/calorie guidelines? 0 1 2 3 4 5
3. How well did you follow the exercise plan? 0 1 2 3 4 5
4. How well did you follow your behavioral contract? 0 1 2 3 4 5

TOTAL SCORE: _____

Have you had any problems with eating or exercise over the last month? Have you suffered any lapses? If so, please talk about these during the group session for Week 44. The relapse-prevention section of this program is designed to help you keep a lapse from becoming a relapse. This section can be divided into three parts:

1. Development of social support.
2. Recognizing risk factors.
3. Practice and the utilization of the skills that you have learned (e.g., problem solving, cognitive techniques).

The first part will be described in the group meeting for Week 44. The second and third components will be discussed in Week 48. Another key activity is to set up an objective criterion that signals you are experiencing a lapse. For example, this criterion could be defined as a small but significant weight gain (e.g., 5 pounds) or five consecutive days of not exercising. Be prepared to discuss your criterion for defining a lapse with the group leader during the next group.

The first part of this section is designed to help you evaluate your social support for behavior change. Research has indicated that one of the primary factors involved in long-term weight loss and prevention of relapse is the development of social support. In Table 12.8 is a quiz for you to take during the next group meeting. If you answer "yes" to most of these questions, you may need to engage in problem solving with the group to find higher quality support from friends and family. For example: How can you get your family to serve their own food? How can you refuse second helpings? You have learned problem solving and communication skills. You have the skills, so use them. Your supporters cannot

Table 12.8. Partner Quiz

	True	False
1. I prepare all the meals for my family.	_____	_____
2. I often prepare snacks for my family, even if I am not eating.	_____	_____
3. My pantry contains troublesome foods because my family requested them.	_____	_____
4. I prepare two meals at dinnertime, one for my family and one for myself.	_____	_____
5. My family pushes second helpings on me.	_____	_____
6. My family often makes negative comments about my weight.	_____	_____
7. My family does not think that my losing weight is important	_____	_____

know how to help unless you tell them. If your family has been resistant to change, you will have to take the initiative. During the next group, you will be asked to come up with two examples of what you would like your family to do to help you further. Begin thinking about how to solve these problems, or how to effectively communicate these examples to your family.

Session Week 48: Relapse Prevention—Recognizing Risk Factors and Taking Corrective Action

Review: Please answer these questions at the beginning of each session using the rating scale of 0 = Very Poor to 5 = Very Well. Circle the rating that best describes your behavior during the previous week:

1. How well did you accurately record your food monitoring? 0 1 2 3 4 5
2. How well did you follow the exchange/calorie guidelines? 0 1 2 3 4 5
3. How well did you follow the exercise plan? 0 1 2 3 4 5
4. How well did you follow your behavioral contract? 0 1 2 3 4 5

TOTAL SCORE: _____

In Week 44, we discussed the development of social support. Now we will discuss the second and third components of relapse prevention. The second portion of relapse prevention is recognizing high-risk situations (Perri, 1992). High-risk situations usually can be grouped into three categories:

1. Situations associated with negative emotional states (e.g., depression, frustration).
2. Situations involving interpersonal conflict (e.g., problems at work, or with a spouse).
3. Situations involving social pressure (e.g., parties and holidays).

The worksheet in Sidebar 12–5 asks you to list several high-risk situations that lead to overeating or inactivity. You will be asked to discuss this list during the next group session. After you list high-risk situations, develop at least three techniques you have learned that could be applied to lower your risk for relapse. Planning for the management of lapses is the third component of relapse prevention. If you have a plan of action, you are less likely to become "caught up" in the situation.

The next session (Week 52) will be the last group meeting. If there are *any* problems, please discuss them with the group leader during the last two sessions.

Session Week 52: Graduation to a New Lifestyle

Review: Please answer these questions at the beginning of each session using the rating scale of 0 = Very Poor to 5 = Very Well. Circle the rating that best describes your behavior during the previous week:

1. How well did you accurately record your food monitoring? 0 1 2 3 4 5
2. How well did you follow the exchange/calorie guidelines? 0 1 2 3 4 5

3. How well did you follow the exercise plan?	0	1	2	3	4	5
4. How well did you follow your behavioral contract?	0	1	2	3	4	5

TOTAL SCORE: _____

Congratulations!!! You have completed the Lifestyle-Change program. One of the most important things for you to do now is to maintain your current weight status. Remember, this program is not a time-limited diet. Rather, you have learned how to change your lifestyle. What do you think will happen if you return to your old eating and exercise habits? One of the important things to remember is that there are certain skills you may need to use from time to time. For example, you may not want to continue food monitoring. We suggest that you gradually discontinue this habit. Even if you do okay without it, there may be times when it would be helpful, such as during a lapse. We hope that the specific lifestyle changes have become automatic, and that you will continue to use them. Another technique you can use during minor lapses is behavioral contracting. Remember, a lapse is not a relapse. If you deal with a lapse expediently, you lessen its potential damage to your diet and your self-esteem. The worksheet at the end of this section is designed for you to list all that you have learned and accomplished. You will be asked to complete this list during the final group session. Do not just focus on your weight. Remember all of the lifestyle changes that you have made. Focus on how you have changed your diet and how this has affected your health. If you experience lapses in the future, turn directly to this worksheet. More than likely, you will be reminded of techniques that will prevent a lapse from becoming a relapse.

Sidebar 12–5

Handout for Week 48: Risk Factors Associated with Overeating

1.
   Technique A
   Technique B
   Technique C
2.
   Technique A
   Technique B
   Technique C
3.
   Technique A
   Technique B
   Technique C
4.
   Technique A
   Technique B
   Technique C

> *Sidebar 12–6*
>
> **Handout for Week 52: What I Would Like to Accomplish**
>
>
> Make a list of things that you have not accomplished through the treatment program:
>
> 1.
> 2.
> 3.
> 4.
> 5.
>
> For each of these things, formulate a plan using your problem-solving skills.

A few weeks ago, we discussed the general goals of weight maintenance. In this group session, we will discuss your goals for the immediate future. Do you want to lose more weight? Would you like to increase your exercise? Would you like to loosen your diet regimen? The final handouts in Sidebars 12–6 and 12–7 are designed to help you form a plan of action for these goals. During the group meeting, make a list of the things that you would still like to accomplish. Again, do not just focus on your weight. After you complete the list, use your problem-solving skills to form a plan of action for implementation.

Congratulations again!!!

PROBLEMS OF IMPLEMENTATION

There are many reasons for a diet- or lifestyle-change program to fail. The dieter may not be committed to lifestyle change, or there may be other life problems that compete with compliance. A few common problem areas are as follows:

1. *Unrealistic Goals and Expectations*. If a person's high expectations are not met, this "failure" may cause unintentional sabotage. For example, if you expect to lose 3 to 5 pounds per week, you may be devastated if you have not lost 9 or more pounds in 3 weeks. The person may conclude: "Why bother with this program, I am a failure when it comes to weight loss." He or she may have unrealistic expectations about becoming the same size as when he or she was a high school senior, or that there is no way to ever reach this goal. Unrealistic expectations and goals need to be addressed in the early phases of treatment. Instead of allowing the person to focus on long-term weight goals, we recommend that the therapist emphasize the development of realistic, short-term behavioral goals.

2. *The Impossible Fantasy*. Many dieters feel that once they lose their weight, all areas of their lives will improve dramatically. Their marriage, work, or dating situation will miraculously change. Not only will a woman meet Prince Charming, he will fall madly in love with the "skinny" wonderful woman that she is, and they will live happily ever after.

This type of thinking is very dangerous. If things do not get better, the person may become depressed and sabotage further progress. For example, you cannot make a bad marriage good just by losing weight. The couple may need marital counseling. Many

---

Sidebar 12–7

Handout for Week 52: What I Have Accomplished

1.
2.
3.
4.
5.
6.
7.
8.
9.
10.

---

overweight people blame many of their problems on their weight. Most of the time, weight status is not the cause of these problems.

3. *Negative Social Support.* If participants in the program are experiencing little or no support from their family and friends, it will be much more difficult to be successful. For example, take a woman whose brothers, sisters, and parents are obese and are not trying to lose or manage weight. Every time she sees her family, they may tell her very discouraging things, such as "Why are you dieting? Fatness is in the family genes."

A husband may not want his wife to get thin, because he is jealous and afraid of losing her to another man. In this case, the husband may actively make it very difficult for his wife to follow the Lifestyle-Change program. He may buy her candy to show her how much he loves her, or take her to a very expensive restaurant for her birthday, knowing that it may be for her difficult to control overeating.

4. *Extreme Dietary Restriction.* Some dieters may eat very restrictively. Extreme dietary restriction may cause binge eating or overeating. Careful monitoring of their dietary intake records is very important for the prevention of extreme dieting.

CASE ILLUSTRATION

Brenda was a 41-year-old, white female, who was employed as a school bus driver. Brenda was 5′4″ tall and had gained to 195 pounds by the age of 41 years. She was significantly overweight and very unhappy. Brenda reported that she had not gained her weight gradually. Rather, she described a "stair-step" progression.

Brenda weighed approximately 118 pounds when she married at 18 years of age. She reported that her weight remained relatively stable until she became pregnant 3 years later. According to Brenda, she gained 73 pounds while pregnant. She weighed 191 pounds shortly before her delivery. After her daughter was born, Brenda began dieting in an effort to lose weight. She lost almost 50 pounds utilizing a commercial weight-loss center. After her initial success, she gained approximately 15 pounds over the next several years. Her weight was at 160 pounds when, at 24, she became pregnant again. During this pregnancy, she gained approximately 55 pounds, putting her weight at 215 pounds. Brenda again tried a commercial-diet program, and lost 35 pounds. However, she again regained the weight. Over the last 15 years, she has repeatedly attempted to diet, each time with some success, but always regaining the initial weight and often a little more.

Several patterns were noticed during Brenda's initial assessment. First, she reported that her mother had also experienced weight problems that began after pregnancies. Second, Brenda reported that her job as a school bus driver allowed her to stay at home most of the day. She experienced a great deal of boredom during the day, before her children returned from school. She would often find herself snacking while watching television. In addition, she prepared a snack for her children on their return from school, and she would always eat the snack with the children. She was also responsible for all meal preparation, and related that she would nibble while cooking. Brenda further described a lack of good food choices on hand, because she always bought her family's favorites. Finally, Brenda reported that she did not make an effort to exercise. She stated that, although she had been somewhat active when she was younger, she had never had an exercise routine.

Brenda enrolled in the Lifestyle-Change program at a weight of 195 pounds. She was prescribed fenfluramine and mazindol in an experimental program testing the combination of pharmacotherapy and behavior therapy for long-term weight management. She stated that her goal weight was approximately 130 pounds. Brenda's treatment focused on modification of her problematic eating behaviors and inactivity. Snacking between meals was targeted as a primary habit to be corrected. The group attempted to identify the antecedents for this behavior, which included boredom and eating with her children. Treatment recommendations included purchasing better food choices and putting more responsibility for food preparation in the hands of her family. Efforts were made to increase Brenda's activities during the day and weekends to hinder snacking, as well as to help her to feel better about herself. Additional recommendations included increasing Brenda's exercise and helping her establish a consistent exercise program. It also proved beneficial to help Brenda identify other antecedents for overeating, such as negative mood states.

Initially, Brenda was successful with the treatment program, losing 25 pounds. However, Brenda found it increasingly difficult to comply with treatment after approximately 32 weeks. At that time, Brenda's weight had "plateaued" and she had been unable to lose weight for a few weeks. In addition, she had experienced a small weight gain. Efforts were made to reevaluate her exercise and calorie levels. Her initial diet plan had been targeted at 1,500 calories, and this goal was reduced to 1,250 calories. Brenda also reported that she had resumed some of her old eating habits (e.g., eating in front of the television). Brenda and her therapist reevaluated her behavioral contract and reinforcers for compliance. Also, the dosage of mazindol was increased to help curb her appetite.

Upon completion of the program, Brenda had lost 45 pounds over the 52 weeks. Her goal was to continue the weight-loss program in an attempt to reach her goal weight of approximately 130 pounds. Her goals were reevaluated and the group generated a discussion of realistic expectations, as well as problem solving about ways to achieve her goals.

SUMMARY

The Lifestyle-Change program was designed for long-term weight management of obese persons with significant medical risks. We believe that behavioral programs such as this one can be combined with medical interventions to produce safe and effective weight loss and maintenance. We hope that the development of more comprehensive treatment programs for chronic obesity will result in a significant reduction in the cardiovascular and metabolic disorders associated with this condition.

APPENDIX A: ASSESSMENT MEASURES

1. Interview for Diagnosis of Eating Disorders-IV (IDED-IV)
   I.   *Purpose*: The IDED-IV is a structured interview procedure that screens subjects for the diagnoses of Anorexia Nervosa, Bulimia Nervosa, and Binge Eating Disorder as defined by the fourth revision of the *Diagnostic and Statistical Manual for Mental Disorders* (DSM-IV; American Psychiatric Association, 1994).
   II. *Supplies/Equipment*: The IDED-IV requires photocopying.
   III. *Subject Preparation*: For nonclinical subjects, the interview requires approximately 30 minutes. For clinical subjects, however, the interview may require up to 90 minutes.
   IV. *Personnel Required*: Persons conducting the interview must be trained in psychiatric diagnostic procedures and in the definition of eating disorders as defined by the proposed DSM-IV criteria. They must observe administration of the IDED-IV for three subjects and they must be observed in their administration of the IDED-IV for three subjects before given approval for independent administration of this procedure.
   V.   *Specific Procedures*:
        A. *Interview Procedure*
           The Interview for Diagnosis of Eating Disorders-IV is a structured-interview format for making diagnoses of Anorexia Nervosa, Bulimia Nervosa, or Binge Eating Disorder based on the eating-disorder criteria for DSM-IV. It is administered by a trained professional familiar with the diagnoses of eating disorders, and can be used with either psychiatric populations or with nonpatients.
           The interview protocol has specific questions asked every subject. Rating scales for each of the diagnostic categories are provided. Ratings are made by the interviewer based on the subject's responses during the interview. From this procedure, subjects are diagnosed with a specific eating-disorder diagnosis.
        B. *Reliability and Validity*
           Reliability and validity data for the IDED-IV are currently being analyzed. However, data for the IDED, on which the IDED-IV is based, are available. Recent psychometric studies have supported its reliability and validity. Inter-rater reliability for each of the rating scales was greater than .85.
           Also, diagnostic agreement for Anorexia Nervosa, Bulimia Nervosa, and Compulsive Overeating was 100% (Williamson, Davis, Norris, & Van Buren, 1990).
        C. *Scoring Procedure*
           A total test score is not obtained for the IDED-IV. Rather, the interviewer completes ratings for each of the diagnoses. A total score for each diagnosis is obtained by summing the ratings.
        D. *Copying Procedure*
           The IDED-IV is not copyrighted and can be obtained from Donald A. Williamson, Department of Psychology, Louisiana State University, Baton Rouge, Louisiana 70803.

2. Bulimia Test-Revised (BULIT-R)

I. *Purpose*: The BULIT was initially developed by Smith and Thelen (1984) as a measure of bulimic symptoms. The revised version (Thelen, Farmer, Wonderlich, & Smith, 1991) was developed to follow DSM-III-R criteria for Bulimia Nervosa (American Psychiatric Association, 1987).

II. *Supplies/Equipment*: The BULIT-R can be photocopied. The items of the BULIT-R can be found in an appendix of Thelen, Farmer, Wonderlich, and Smith (1991).

III. *Subject Preparation*: Subjects must be scheduled for administration of the test, which requires approximately 15 minutes.

IV. *Personnel Required*: Persons administering the questionnaire must be instructed as to the purpose of the test. Personnel are not required to be present while the test is completed, however personnel should be available to answer questions for the subject if necessary. Persons scoring the questionnaire must be instructed in the scoring procedure.

V. *Specific Procedures*:

A. *Assessment Procedure*

The BULIT-R is a questionnaire with 36 questions answered using a 5-point rating scale. Thelen et al. (1991) determined that the cutoff of 104 was most accurate in classifying bulimic subjects. Factor analysis determined the presence of five factors as follows: (1) binge eating/loss of control; (2) radical weight loss measures/body image; (3) laxatives/diuretics; (4) vomiting; and (5) exercise.

B. *Reliability and Validity*

Initial reliability and validity data on the BULIT-R were quite good. Test–retest reliability coefficients were reported to be high ($r = .95$). In addition, the BULIT-R correlates highly with the ULIT (.99).

C. *Scoring Procedure*

Each question on the BULIT-R is answered on a scale from 1 (*Agree, Most of the Time, Strongly Agree*, etc.) to 5 (*Never, No, Strongly Disagree*, etc.). Items 6, 11, 19, 20, 27, 29, 31, and 36 are not scored. Items 2, 5, 7, 8, 10, 12, 13, 14, 15, 16, 17, 21, 23, 26, 28, 30, 32, and 35 are reverse scored. On these items, if the test taker endorses 1, the item is scored as 5, 2 as 4, etc. The remaining items are calculated on a 1 to 5 scale. A total score is obtained by adding these values.

D. *Copying Procedure*

The BULIT-R is not copyrighted and can be copied with permission of the author. Copies can be obtained through the Director of Psychological Services.

3. Body-Image Assessment (BIA)

I. *Purpose*: The BIA measures the perception of current and ideal body size in adult women (Williamson, Kelley, Davis, Ruggiero, & Blouin, 1985). Measures of current and ideal body size have been found to significantly predict overall body satisfaction (Williamson, Gleaves, Watkins, & Schlundt, 1993).

II. *Supplies/Equipment*: The BIA requires the use of a testing protocol that includes a set of cards containing female silhouettes. There are nine cards ranging from thin to obese in incremental steps. Each of these 6-inch silhouettes is presented on a separate $5'' \times 8''$ (12.5 cm × 20.5 cm) card. Materials can be obtained by ordering from the Louisiana State University Psychological Services Center.

III. *Subject Preparation*: The BIA can be administered in less than 2 minutes. No special preparation of the subject is required.

IV. *Personnel Required*: Persons administering the BIA must be trained in its administration.

V. *Specific Procedures*:

A. *Testing Procedure*

To administer the Body Image Assessment (BIA), the experimenter randomly places the nine cards in front of the subject on a flat surface and states the following instructions: "Select the card that most accurately depicts your current body size, as you perceive it to be. Please be honest. You must choose only one card and you may not rearrange the cards to directly compare them." After the subject has selected a card, the experimenter records the number from 1 to 9 on the back of that card without it being seen by the subject. This number is the subject's score for current body size (CBS). The cards are then reshuffled and again randomly placed in front of the subject with the following directions given: "Please select the card that most accurately depicts the body size that you would most prefer. Again, be honest and do not rearrange the cards." The experimenter then records the number of the selected card, which is the score for ideal body size (IBS).

B. *Reliability and Validity*

Test–retest reliability of the BIA over relatively short periods is high (CBS: $r = .89$; IBS: $r = .72$; Discrepancy Score: $r = .80$). In addition, there is evidence for concurrent and discriminant validity for this instrument as a measure of body-image disturbances (Williamson, Davis, Bennett, Goreczny, & Gleaves, 1989).

C. *Scoring Procedures for the BIA*

Raw scores for CBS and IBS are interpreted by comparing them to scores of nonclinical subjects of similar height and weight. Norms have been developed for the interpretation of this data and a standard score can be derived from the raw score. A table of norms is attached. A discrepancy score (a measure of body-size dissatisfaction) is derived by subtracting the IBS T score from the CBS T score. A body-image distortion is indicated by an elevation from norms for a particular height–weight group. The amount that the IBS is depressed as compared to norms indicates a preference for thin body size.

D. *Copying the Procedure*

Each of the silhouettes is presented on a separate card. The protocol may be obtained from Donald A. Williamson, Department of Psychology, Louisiana State University, Baton Rouge, Louisiana 70803.

4. Three-Factor Eating Questionnaire (TFEQ)

I. *Purposes*: The TFEQ is a 51-item self-report inventory designed to evaluate dietary restraint as a three-dimensional concept. Stunkard and Messick (1985) found three factors or scales in this questionnaire: (1) dietary restraint, (2) disinhibition, and (3) perceived hunger.

II. *Supplies/Equipment*: The TFEQ is a paper-and-pencil test, and requires only that one have the test available for each subject.

III. *Subject Preparation*: Subjects need approximately 10 minutes to complete the TFEQ.

IV. *Personnel Required*: No special training is necessary to administer the TFEQ. Scoring the TFEQ requires limited training, however.

V. *Specific Procedures*:
  A. *Assessment Procedure*
     The TFEQ is a self-report inventory. The subject responds to the 51 questions without assistance from the evaluator.
  B. *Reliability and Validity*
     The three subscales have been found to have high reliability and validity. The dietary restraint and disinhibition scales have relevance to assessing cases of obesity. The dietary-restraint scale measures the intent to diet and dieting behavior. The disinhibition scale measures episodic overeating. The disinhibition and perceived hunger scales are positively correlated.
  C. *Scoring Procedure for the TFEQ*
     The TFEQ is a two-part measure that consists of items that load on three factors. Factor 1 is the dietary-restraint factor containing 21 questions. Factor 2, disinhibition, is composed of 16 questions assessing the lability in behavior and weight. Factor 3 measures the perception of hunger with 14 items. To score the TFEQ, the number of items that load onto a factor must be determined. Part I of this measure consists of 36 items endorsed as either true or false. Part II includes 14 items endorsed on a scale of 1 to 4, and 1 item with a scale of 0 to 5.

PART I

If the items are endorsed as designated, one point is scored to the corresponding factor.
Factor 1
Items answered as true: 4, 6, 14, 18, 23, 28, 32, 33, and 35.
Items answered as false: 10, 21, and 30.
Factor 2
Items answered as true: 1, 2, 7, 9, 11, 13, 15, 20, 37, and 36.
Items answered as false: 16, 25, and 31.
Factor 3
Items answered as true: 3, 5, 8, 12, 17, 19, 22, 24, 26, 29, and 34.

PART II

All items except for questions 47 and 50 are scored as 1 or 2 equals 0, and 3 or 4 equals 1. Item 47 is reversed, 1 or 2 equals 1, and 3 or 4 equals 0. For question 50, the scale is 0, 1, or 2 equals 0, and 3, 4, or 5 equals 1.
Factor 1
Items: 37, 38, 40, 42, 43, 44, 46, 48, and 50.
Factor 2
Items: 45, 49, and 51.
Factor 3
Items: 39, 41, and 47.
  D. *Copying the TFEQ*
     The TFEQ is not copyrighted and can be photocopied.
5. Eating Attitudes Test (EAT)
  I. *Purpose*: The EAT is a 40-item self-report measure designed to evaluate anorexic attitudes, beliefs, and habits. The primary value of the EAT for assessing obesity is that it has been shown to be a good measure of concern for dieting, body-size

disturbance/dissatisfaction, and overconcern with body size. Recent research related to dietary restraint and bingeing have shown that these "anorexic" characteristics are predictive of bingeing, dietary chaos, and strict dieting. Thus, the EAT
and its subscales are useful for assessing the degree to which a person has extreme
body-size concerns or uses extreme dietary practices to control weight.

II. *Supplies/Equipment*: The EAT is a paper-and-pencil test and requires only that one
have the test available for each subject.

III. *Subject Preparation*: Subjects need approximately 10 minutes to complete the EAT.

IV. *Personnel Required*: No training is necessary to administer the EAT.

V. *Specific Procedures*:

   A. *Assessment Procedure*

   The EAT is self-administered.

   B. *Reliability and Validity*

   Test–retest reliability of the EAT is high ($r = .94$). It has been found to be highly
correlated with other measures of anorexia and bulimia nervosa, and it discriminates anorexics and bulimics from nonclinical groups.

   C. *Scoring Procedure for the EAT*

   The EAT consists of 40 items answered on a 6-point Likert-type scale from 0 to
5. A total score is obtained by adding the answers. For all questions *except* 1, 18,
19, 23, 27, and 39, the following scale is used.

> Always (0) = 3
> Very Often (1) = 2
> Often (2) = 1
> Sometimes (3) = 0
> Rarely (4) = 0
> Never (5) = 0

Items 1, 18, 19, 23, and 39 are reverse scored.
The following scale is used.

> Always (0) = 0
> Very Often (1) = 0
> Often (2) = 0
> Sometimes (3) = 1
> Rarely (4) = 2
> Never (5) = 3

Question 27 is not scored.

   D. *Copying the EAT*

   The EAT is not copyrighted and can be photocopied.

APPENDIX B: EXCHANGE LISTS

The reason for dividing food into six different groups is that foods vary in their carbohydrate, protein, fat, and calorie content. Each exchange list contains foods that are alike.
Each choice contains about the same amount of carbohydrate, protein, fat, and calories.

As you read the exchange lists, you will notice that one choice often is a larger amount
of food than another choice from the same list. Because foods are so different, each food is

measured or weighed so the amount of carbohydrate, protein, fat, and calories is the same in each choice.

If you have a favorite food that is not included in any of these groups, ask your dietician about it. That food can probably be worked into your meal plan, at least now and then.

1—STARCH AND BREAD LIST

Each item in this list contains approximately 15 grams of carbohydrate, 3 grams of protein, a trace of fat, and 80 calories. Whole grain products average about 2 grams of fiber per serving. Some foods are higher in fiber. Those foods that contain 3 or more grams of fiber per serving are identified with the fiber symbol.

You can choose your starch exchanges from any of the items on this list. If you want to eat a starch food that is not on this list, the general rule is that:

½ cup of cereal, grain, or pasta is one serving
1 ounce of a bread product is one serving

Cereals/Grains/Pasta

Bran cereals, concentrated (such as Bran Buds, All Bran)	⅓ cup
Bran cereals, flaked	½ cup
Bulgur (cooked)	½ cup
Cooked cereals	½ cup
Cornmeal (dry)	2½ Tbsp.
Grapenuts	3 Tbsp.
Grits (cooked)	½ cup
Other ready-to-eat unsweetened cereals	¾ cup
Pasta (cooked	½ cup
Puffed cereal	1½ cup
Rice, white or brown (cooked)	⅓ cup
Shredded wheat	½ cup
Wheat germ	3 Tbsp.

Starchy Vegetables

Corn	½ cup
Corn on cob, 6 in. long	1
Lima beans	½ cup
Peas, green (canned or frozen)	½ cup
Plantain	½ cup
Potato, baked (3 oz.)	1 small
Potato, mashed	½ cup
Squash, winter (acorn, butternut)	¾ cup
Yam, sweet potato, plain	⅓ cup

Dried Beans/Peas/Lentils

Beans and peas (cooked) (such as kidney, white, split, blackeye)	⅓ cup
Lentils (cooked)	⅓ cup
Baked beans	¼ cup

Crackers/Snacks

Animal crackers	8
Graham crackers, 2½ in. square	3
Matzoth	¾ oz.
Melba toast	5 slices
Oyster crackers	24
Popcorn (popped, no fat added)	3 cups
Pretzels	¾ oz.
Rye crisp, 2 in. × 3½ in.	4
Saltine-type crackers	6
Whole wheat crackers no fat added (crisp breads, such as Finn, Kavli, Wasa) (¾ oz.)	2–4 slices

Starchy Foods Prepared with Fat

(count as 1 starch/bread serving, plus 1 fat serving)

Biscuit, 2½ in. across	1
Chow mein noodles	½ cup
Corn bread, 2 in. cube (2 oz.)	1
Cracker, round butter type	6
French fried potatoes, 2 in. to 3½ in. long (1.5 oz.)	10

Muffin, plain, small	1	Bread sticks, crisp 4 in. long × ½	2
Pancake, 4 in. across	2	in. (⅔ oz.)	
Stuffing, bread (prepared)	¼ cup	Croutons, low fat	1 cup
Taco shell, 6 in. across	2	English muffin	½ cup
Waffle, 4½ in. square	1	Frankfurter/hamburger bun	½ (1 oz.)
Whole wheat crackers, fat added	4–6	Pita, 6 in. across	½
(such as Triscuits (1 oz.)		Plain roll, small	1 (1 oz.)
		Raisin, unfrosted (1 oz.)	1 slice
		Rye, pumpernickel (1 oz.)	1 slice
Bread		Tortilla, 6 in. across	1
		White (including French, Italian)	1 slice
Bagel (1 oz.)	½	Whole Wheat (1 oz.)	1 slice

2—MEAT LIST

Each serving of meat and substitutes on this list contains about 7 grams of protein. The amount of fat and number of calories varies, depending on what kind of meat or substitute you choose. The list is divided into three parts based on the amount of fat and calories: lean meat, medium-fat meat, and high-fat meat. One ounce (one meat exchange) of these includes:

	Carbohydrate (grams)	Protein (grams)	Fat (grams)	Calories
LEAN	0	7	3	55

You are encouraged to use more lean meat, poultry, and fish in your meal plan. This will help decrease your fat intake, which may help decrease your risk for heart disease. Meat and substitutes do not contribute any fiber to your meal plan. The following is a list of tips on the preparation of meat.

1. Bake, roast, broil, grill, or boil these foods rather than frying them with added fat.
2. Use a nonstick pan spray or a nonstick pan to brown or fry these foods.
3. Trim off visible fat before and after cooking.
4. Do not add flour, bread crumbs, coating mixes, or fat to foods when preparing them.
5. Weigh meat after removing bones and fat, and after cooking. Three ounces of raw, cooked meat is about equal to 4 ounces of raw meat. Some examples of meat portions are:

> 2 ounces meat (2 meat exchanges) =
> 1 small chicken leg or thigh
> ½-cup cottage cheese or tuna
> 3 ounces meat (3 meat exchanges) =
> 1 medium pork chop
> 1 small hamburger
> ½ of a whole chicken breast
> 1 unbreaded fish fillet
> cooked meat about the size of a deck of cards

6. Restaurants usually serve prime cuts of meat, which are high in fat and calories.

Donald A. Williamson et al.

(One exchange is equal to any one of the following items)

Beef:	USDA Good or Choice grades of lean beef, such as round, sirloin, and flank steak; tenderloin; and chipped beef	1 oz.
Pork:	Lean pork, such as fresh ham; canned, cured or boiled ham; Canadian bacon; tenderloin.	1 oz.
Veal:	All cuts are lean except for veal cutlets (ground or cubed); examples of lean veal are chops and roasts.	1 oz.
Poultry:	Chicken, turkey, Cornish hen (without skin)	1 oz.
Fish:	All fresh and frozen fish	1 oz.
	Crabs, lobster, scallops, shrimp, clams (fresh or canned in water)	2 oz.
	Oysters (medium size)	6
	Tuna (canned in water)	1/4 cup
	Herring (uncreamed or smoked)	1 oz.
	Sardines (canned) (medium size)	2
Wild game:	Venison, rabbit, squirrel, pheasant, duck, goose (without skin)	1 oz.
Cheese:	Any cottage cheese	1/4 cup
	Grated parmesan	2 Tbsp.
	Diet cheeses (with less than 55 calories per ounce)	1 oz.
Other:	95% fat-free luncheon meat	1 oz.
	Egg whites	3
	Egg substitutes with less than 55 calories per 1/4 cup	1/4 cup

3—VEGETABLE LIST

Each vegetable serving on this list contains about 5 grams of carbohydrates, 2 grams of protein, and 25 calories. Vegetables contain 2–3 grams of dietary fiber.

Vegetables are a good source of vitamins and minerals. Fresh and frozen vegetables have more vitamins and less added salt. Rinsing canned vegetables will remove much of the salt.

Unless otherwise noted, the serving size for vegetables (one vegetable exchange) is:

½ cup of cooked vegetables or vegetable juice
1 cup of raw vegetables

Artichoke (½ medium)	Eggplant	Rutabaga
Asparagus	Greens (collard, mustard,	Sauerkraut
Beans (green, wax, Italian)	turnip)	Spinach, cooked
Bean sprouts	Kohlrabi	Summer squash (crookneck)
Beets	Leeks	Tomato (one large)
Broccoli	Mushrooms, cooked	Tomato/vegetable juice
Brussels sprouts	Okra	Turnips
Cabbage, cooked	Onions	Water chestnuts
Carrots	Pea pods	Zucchini, cooked
Cauliflower	Peppers (green)	

Starchy vegetables such as corn, peas, and potatoes are found on the Starch/Bread List. For free vegetables, see Free Food List.

4—FRUIT LIST

Each item on this list contains about 15 grams of carbohydrate and 60 calories. Fresh, frozen, and dry fruits have about 2 grams of fiber per serving.

The carbohydrate and calorie content for a fruit serving is based on the usual serving of the most commonly eaten fruits. Use fresh fruits or fruits frozen or canned without sugar added. Whole fruit is more filling than fruit juice and may be a better choice for those who are trying to lose weight. Unless otherwise noted, the serving size for one fruit serving is:

½ cup of fresh fruit or fruit juice
¼ cup of dried fruit

Dried Fruit

Apples	4 rings
Apricots	7 halves
Dates	2½ medium
Figs	1½
Prunes	3 medium
Raisins	2 Tbsp.

Fruit Juice

Apple juice/cider	½ cup
Cranberry juice cocktail	⅓ cup
Grapefruit juice	½ cup
Grape juice	⅓ cup
Orange juice	½ cup
Pineapple juice	½ cup
Prune juice	⅓ cup

Fresh, Frozen, and Unsweetened Canned Fruit

Apple (raw, 2 in. across)	1 apple
Applesauce (unsweetened)	½ cup
Apricots (medium, raw) or	4 apricots
Apricots (canned) or 4 halves	½ cup
Banana (9 in. long)	½ banana
Blackberries (raw)	¾ cup
Blueberries (raw)	¾ cup
Cantaloupe (5 in. across)	⅓ melon
(cubes)	1 cup
Cherries (large, raw)	12 cherries
Cherries (canned)	½ cup
Figs (raw, 2 in. across)	2 figs
Fruit cocktail (canned)	½ cup
Grapefruit (medium)	½ of one
Grapefruit (segments)	¾ cup
Grapes (small)	15 grapes
Honeydew melon (medium)	⅛ melon
(cubes)	1 cup
Mandarin oranges	¾ cup
Mango (small)	½ mango
Nectarine (1½ in. across)	1 whole
Orange (2½ in. across)	1 orange
Papaya	1 cup
Peach (2¾ in. across)	1 peach, or ¾ cup
Peaches (canned)	½ cup, or 2 halves
Pear	½ large, or 1 small
Pears (canned)	½ cup, or 2 halves
Persimmon (medium, native)	2 whole
Pineapple (raw)	¾ cup
Pineapple (canned)	⅓ cup
Plum (raw, 2 in. across)	2 plums
Pomegranate	½ of one
Raspberries (raw)	1 cup

Fresh, Frozen, and Unsweetened Canned Fruit

Kiwi (large)	1 kiwi
Strawberries (raw, whole)	1¼ cup
Tangerine (2½ in. across)	2 whole
Watermelon (cubes)	1¼ cup

Donald A. Williamson et al.

5—MILK LIST

Each serving of milk or milk products on this list contains about 12 grams of carbohydrate and 8 grams of protein. The amount of fat in milk is measured in percent (%) of butterfat. One serving (one milk exchange) includes:

	Carbohydrates (grams)	Protein (grams)	Fat (grams)	Calories
Skim/Very Lowfat	12	8	trace	90

Milk is the body's main source of calcium, the mineral needed for growth and repair of bones. Yogurt is also a good source of calcium. Yogurt and many dry, powdered milk products have different amounts of fat. If you have questions about a particular item, read the label to find out the fat and calorie content.

Milk is good to drink, but it can also be added to cereal and to other foods. Many tasty dishes such as sugar-free pudding are made with milk (see the Combination Foods List). Add life to plain yogurt by adding one of your favorite fruit servings to it.

Skim and Very Lowfat Milk

Skim milk	1 cup
½% milk	1 cup
1% milk	1 cup
Lowfat buttermilk	1 cup
Evaporated skim milk	½ cup
Dry nonfat milk	⅓ cup
Plain nonfat yogurt	8 oz.

6—FAT LIST

Each serving on the fat list contains about 5 grams of fat and 45 calories. The foods on the fat list contain mostly fat, although some items may also contain a small amount of protein. All fats are high in calories and should be carefully measured. Everyone should modify fat intake by eating unsaturated fats instead of saturated fats. The sodium content of these foods varies widely. Check the label for sodium information.

Unsaturated Fats

Avocado	⅛ medium	Other nuts	1 Tbsp.
Margarine	1 tsp.	Seeds, pine nuts, sunflower (without shells)	1 Tbsp.
Margarine, diet	1 Tbsp.	Pumpkin seeds	2 tsp.
Mayonnaise	1 tsp.	Oil (corn, cottonseed, safflower, soybean, sunflower, olive, peanut)	1 tsp.
Mayonnaise, reduced-calorie	1 Tbsp.		
Nuts and Seeds:		Olives	10 small or 5 large
Almonds, dry roasted	6 whole		
Cashews, dry roasted	1 Tbsp.	Salad dressing, mayonnaise-type	2 tsp.
Pecans	2 whole	Salad dressing, mayonnaise-type, reduced-calorie	1 Tbsp.
Peanuts	20 small or 10 large	Salad dressing (all varieties)	1 Tbsp.
Walnuts	2 whole	Salad dressing, reduced-calorie	2 Tbsp.

Saturated Fats

		Coffee whitener, powder	4 tsp.
		Cream (light, coffee, table)	2 Tbsp.
Butter	1 tsp.	Cream, sour	2 Tbsp.
Bacon	1 slice	Cream (heavy, whipping)	1 Tbsp.
Chitterlings	½ oz.	Cream cheese	1 Tbsp.
Coconut, shredded	2 Tbsp.	Salt pork	¼ oz.
Coffee whitener, liquid	2 Tbsp.		

(Two tablespoons of reduced-calorie salad dressing are a free-food.)

FREE FOODS

A free food is any food or drink that contains less than 20 calories per serving. You can eat as much as you want of those items that have no serving size specified. You may eat two or three servings per day of those items that have a specified serving size. Be sure to spread them out through the day.

Drinks

Bouillon or broth without fat
Bouillon, low-sodium
Carbonated drinks, sugar-free
Carbonated water
Club soda
Cocoa powder, unsweetened (Tbsp.)
Coffee/Tea
Drink mixes, sugar-free
Tonic water, sugar-free

Nonstick Pan Spray

Fruit

Cranberries, unsweetened (½ cup)
Rhubarb, unsweetened (½ cup)

Vegetables

(raw, 1 cup)
Cabbage
Celery
Chinese cabbage
Cucumber
Green onion
Hot peppers
Mushrooms
Radishes
Zucchini

Salad Greens

Endive
Escarole
Lettuce
Romaine
Spinach

Condiments

Catsup (1 Tbsp.)
Horseradish
Mustard
Pickles, dill (unsweetened)
Salad dressing, low-calorie (2 Tbsp.)
Taco sauce (1 Tbsp.)
Vinegar

Sweet Substitutes

Candy, hard, sugar-free
Gelatin, sugar-free
Gum, sugar-free
Jam/jelly, sugar-free (2 tsp.)
Pancake syrup, sugar-free (1–2 Tbsp.)
Sugar substitutes (saccharin, aspartame)
Whipped topping (2 Tbsp.)

Seasonings can be very helpful in making food taste better. Be careful of how much sodium you use. Read the label, and choose those seasonings that do not contain sodium or salt.

Basil (fresh)
Celery seeds
Cinnamon
Chili powder
Chives
Curry
Dill
Flavoring extracts (vanilla, almond, walnut,
   peppermint, butter, lemon, etc.)
Garlic
Garlic powder
Herbs
Hot pepper sauce
Lemon

Lemon juice
Lemon pepper
Lime
Mint
Onion powder
Oregano
Paprika
Pepper
Pimento
Spices
Soy sauce
Soy sauce, low sodium ("Lite")
Wine, used in cooking (¼ cup)
Worcestershire sauce

COMBINATION FOODS

Much of the food we eat is mixed together in various combinations. These foods do not fit into only one exchange list. It can be quite hard to tell what is in a certain casserole dish or baked food item. This is a list of average values for some typical combination foods. This list will help you fit these foods into your meal plan. Ask your dietitian for information about any other foods you would like to eat. The *American Diabetes Association/American Dietetic Association Family Cookbooks* and the *American Diabetes Holiday Cookbook* have recipes and further information about many foods, including combination foods. Check your library or local bookstore.

Foods	Amount	Exchanges
Casseroles, homemade	1 cup (8 oz.)	2 starch, 2 medium-fat meat, 1 fat
Cheese pizza, thin crust	¼ of 15 oz. or ¼ of 10″	2 starch, 1 medium-fat meat, 1 fat
Chili with beans (commercial)	1 cup (8 oz.)	2 starch, 2 medium-fat meat, 2 fat
Chow mein (without noodles or rice)	2 cups (16 oz.)	1 starch, 2 vegetable, 2 lean meat
Macaroni and cheese	1 cup (8 oz.)	2 starch, 1 medium-fat meat, 2 fat
Soup:		
Bean	1 cup (8 oz.)	1 starch, 1 vegetable, 1 lean meat
Chunky, all varieties	10¾ oz. can	1 starch, 1 veg., 1 med-fat meat
Cream (made with water)	1 cup (8 oz.)	1 starch, 1 fat
Vegetable or broth	1 cup (8 oz.)	1 starch
Spaghetti and meatballs (canned)	1 cup (8 oz.)	2 starch, 1 medium-fat, 1 fat
Sugar-free pudding (made with skim milk)	½ cup	1 starch
If beans are used as a meat substitute:		
Dried beans, peas, lentils	1 cup (cooked)	2 starch, 1 lean meat

Moderate amounts of some foods can be used in your meal plan, in spite of their sugar or fat content, as long as you can maintain blood-glucose control. The following list includes average exchange values for some of these foods. Because they are concentrated sources of carbohydrate, you will notice that the portion sizes are very small. Check with your dietitian on advice on how often you can eat them.

Foods	Amount	Exchanges
Angel food cake	$\frac{1}{12}$ cake	2 starch
Cake, no icing	$\frac{1}{12}$ cake, or a 3″ square	2 starch, 2 fat
Cookies	2 small (1¾″ across)	1 starch, 1 fat
Frozen fruit yogurt	⅓ cup	1 starch
Gingersnaps	3	1 starch
Granola	¼ cup	1 starch, 1 fat
Granola bars	1 small	1 starch, 1 fat
Ice cream, any flavor	½ cup	1 starch, 2 fat
Ice milk, any flavor	½ cup	1 starch, 1 fat
Sherbet, any flavor	¼ cup	1 starch
Snack chips, all varieties	1 oz.	1 starch, 2 fat
Vanilla wafers	6 small	1 starch, 1 fat

REFERENCES

American Dietetic Association (1989). *Exchange lists for weight management.* Chicago, IL: Author.

American Psychiatric Association (1994). *Diagnostic and statistical manual of mental disorders* (4th ed.). Washington, DC: Author.

Bray, G. A. (1992a). Drug treatment of obesity. *American Journal of Nutrition, 55,* 5385–5455.

Bray, G. A. (1992b). Pathophysiology of obesity. *American Journal of Clinical Nutrition, 55,* 4885–4945.

Burns, D. D. (1980). *Feeling good: The new mood therapy.* New York: Signet.

Garner, D. M., & Garfinkel, P. E. (1979). The Eating Attitudes Test: An index of the symptoms of anorexia nervosa. *Psychological Medicine, 9,* 273–279.

Garrow, J. S. (1983). Indices of adiposity. *Reviews in Clinical Nutrition, 53,* 697–708.

Kuczmarski, R. J. (1992). Prevalence of overweight and weight gain in the United States. *American Journal of Clinical Nutrition, 55,* 4955–5025.

Metropolitan Life Foundation. (1983). 1983 Metropolitan height and weight tables. *Statistical Bulletin, 64,* 2–9.

National Research Council. (1989). Diet and health, implications for reducing chronic disease risk. *National Academy Press.* Washington, DC: Author.

Perri, M. G. (1992). *Improving the long term management of obesity: Theory, research, and clinical guidelines.* New York: Wiley.

Sjostrom, L. V. (1992). Morbidity of severely obese subjects. *American Journal of Clinical Nutrition, 55,* 5085–5155.

Smith, M. C., & Thelen, M. H. (1984). Development and validation of a test for bulimia. *Journal of Consulting and Clinical Psychology, 52,* 863–872.

Stunkard, A. J., & Messick, S. (1985). The three-factor eating questionnaire to measure dietary restraint, disinhibition, and hunger. *Journal of Psychometric Research, 29,* 71–83.

Thelen, M. H., Farmer, J., Wonderlich, S., & Smith, M. (1991). A revision of the bulimia test: The BULIT-R. *Psychological Assessment, 3,* 119–124.

Williamson, D. A., Davis, C. J., Bennett, S. M., Goreczny, A. J., & Gleaves, D. H. (1989). Development of a simple procedure for assessing body image disturbances. *Behavioral Assessment, 11,* 433–466.

Williamson, D. A., Davis, C. J., Norris, L., & Van Buren, D. J. (1990, November). *Development of reliability and validity for a new structured interview for diagnosis of eating disorders.* Paper presented at the annual meeting of the Association for the Advancement of Behavior Therapy, San Francisco, CA.

Williamson, D. A., Gleaves, D. H., Watkins, P. C., & Schlundt, D. G. (1993). Validation of a self-ideal body size discrepancy as a measure of body size dissatisfaction. *Journal of Psychopathology and Behavioral Assessment, 15,* 57–68.

Williamson, D. A., Kelley, M. L., Davis, C. J., Ruggiero, L., & Blouin, D. C. (1985). Psychopathology of eating disorders: A controlled comparison of bulimic, obese, and normal subjects. *Journal of Consulting and Clinical Psychology, 53,* 161–166.

13

Managing Marital Therapy

Helping Partners Change

Robert L. Weiss and W. Kim Halford

> Marriage is one of the most nearly universal of human
> institutions. No other touches so intimately the lives of
> practically every member of the earth's population.
> —LEWIS M. TERMAN, 1938, p. 1

INTRODUCTION

Marriage, the most intimate adult relationship most people experience, is perceived by the majority of adults as their primary source of support and affection (Levinger & Huston, 1990); high quality marriage is a strong predictor of adults' reports of global life happiness (Glenn & Weaver, 1981). Most unmarried adults expect to marry at some point in their lives and for that marriage to be life long (Millward, 1990).

Given the importance people attach to marriage, it is not surprising that marital distress and divorce are perceived as extremely stressful. In fact, after death in the family, marital distress and divorce are rated as the most severe life stressors adults experience (Bloom, Asher, & White, 1978). Marital problems are associated with markedly increased risk for a wide range of psychological problems, including depression, particularly in women (Beach & O'Leary, 1986; Hooley & Teasdale, 1989); alcohol abuse, particularly in men (O'Farrell, 1989; Vanicelli, Gingereich & Ryback, 1983); sexual dysfunction in both sexes (Zimmer, 1983); and increased behavioral problems in the couples' children (Emery, Joyce, & Fincham, 1987; Grych & Fincham, 1990).

Prevalence of marital distress is difficult to estimate. We know that divorce rates vary considerably in Western countries, ranging from 0% in Ireland, where divorce is prohibited, to just over 50% of marriages ending in divorce in the United States (Glick, 1989). The

Robert L. Weiss • Oregon Marital Studies Program, Department of Psychology, University of Oregon, Eugene, Oregon 97403.   **W. Kim Halford** • Department of Psychology, Griffith University, Queensland, Australia.

Sourcebook of Psychological Treatment Manuals for Adult Disorders, edited by Vincent B. Van Hasselt and Michel Hersen. Plenum Press, New York, 1996.

decision about whether to separate or divorce is influenced by multiple factors, including existing legislation about divorce within particular states and countries, financial implications of separation and divorce, personal and cultural expectations about the desirability of separation or divorce, and the person's perception of available alternatives to remaining married. Given all these factors, divorce provides only a very crude index of the prevalence of marital problems. Surveys of representative samples of adults in the United States suggest that, at any given time, approximately 20% of people will report that they have significant marital problems (Beach, Arias, & O'Leary, 1986). Of the majority of adults who report that they do not currently have marital problems, 40% report that they have considered separation or divorce from their current partners, and 38% have already been divorced from a previous partner. All of these figures converge on the point that significant marital distress is a very common problem in most Western countries.

Couples present for marital therapy with a large variety of problems. The most common presenting problems, rank-ordered in their approximate prevalence rates are poor communication, poor conflict management, specific complaints about behavior of the partner, perceived lack of compatibility or common interests with the partner, lack of positive love or affection, and the occurrence of violence within the relationship (Wolcott & Glezer, 1989). With the considerable overlap between individual and couple problems, people present with an individual problem, such as depression or alcohol abuse, but, subsequently, we find significant marital distress as well (Halford & Osgarby, 1993). Adjunctive marital therapy can be a very important component of effective management for a range of individual disorders, including both depression (Jacobson, Dobson, Fruzetti, Schmaling, & Salusky, 1991; O'Leary & Beach, 1990) and alcohol abuse (O'Farrell, 1993), and children's behavior problems (Dadds, Schwartz, & Sanders, 1987).

Violence is one aspect of marital problems that warrants special mention. It is estimated that about one in six of all married couples are violent toward each other in any given year (Straus & Gelles, 1986). Rates of interspousal aggression are considerably higher in maritally distressed couples, with over half of such couples experiencing violence each year (O'Leary & Vivian, 1990). Across all couples, the modal form of spousal aggression is hitting, pushing, or slapping, and women and men seem approximately equally likely to engage in these aggressive acts (Straus & Gelles, 1986; O'Leary et al., 1989). However, men seem more likely to engage in severe violence, and woman are at particular risk for being injured or even killed by their partners (Koop, 1985; Stets & Straus, 1990). Women repeatedly assaulted by their husbands also have a high risk of depression, alcohol abuse, psychosomatic disorders, and are high users of the health-care system (Cascardi, Langhinrichsen, & Vivian, 1992; Jaffee, Wolfe, Wilson, & Zak, 1986; Stets & Straus, 1990). These problems usually seem to postdate onset of violence (Stark & Flitcraft, 1988). To date, there has been no report of an equivalent set of problems for battered husbands, although as Steinmetz and Lucca (1988) noted, there has been little investigation of the impact of wives' violence on their husbands.

Marital violence probably is underdetected in mental health settings where marital therapy is offered. In couples who present with marital problems and have been violent toward each other, less than 3% of males and 12% of females spontaneously report aggression as a problem; in the majority of instances, violence is only detected when each partner is privately and specifically asked about the occurrence of physical aggression (O'Leary & Vivian, 1990). Marital violence also has a major impact on children and is associated with increased behavior problems in the children (Grych & Fincham, 1990) and increased risk of the child entering a violent relationship as an adult (Widom, 1989).

This chapter describes our approach to couples' therapy. This approach is appropriate for couples presenting conjointly, or when an individual presents initially and then the spouse is involved in subsequent therapy sessions. We begin by outlining our model of couple therapy. This is followed by a detailed description of methods of assessment and treatment procedures. Additional topics are presented on maintenance and generalization issues, problems in implementation, together with a case illustration, and a final summary.

A MODEL OF COUPLE THERAPY

Content of Behavioral Couple Therapy

Behavioral couple therapy (BCT) usually is conducted in a conjoint format with a goal of altering interaction between partners (Baucom & Epstein, 1990; Halford, Sanders, & Behrens, 1994; Jacobson & Margolin, 1979). Based on the premise that the exchange of behavior between partners is central to a relationship, BCT began as the application of behavioral contracting to the treatment of marital distress. Couples were trained to identify specific aspects of their partner's behavior that were pleasing and displeasing and, based on such assessments, behavioral contracts were developed to reduce displeasing and increase pleasing behaviors within the relationship (e.g., Azrin, Naster, & Jones, 1973; Stuart, 1969; Weiss, Hops, & Patterson, 1973). Initially, such contracting emphasized tightly structured *"quid pro quo"* agreements, in which spouses were taught to systematically and immediately reward desired behavior from the partner. However, this was replaced with more unilateral "good-faith" contracts in which each partner undertakes to make certain changes for the good of the relationship (e.g., Weiss, Birchler, & Vincent, 1974; Stuart, 1980). Although the details of behavioral contracting have changed, an emphasis on changing relationship behaviors remains an important element of BCT.

The second phase of BCT development saw incorporation of communication and problem-solving skills training. These process skills were conceptualized as providing couples with the means to enhance intimate communication and resolve both their current and future sources of conflict (Jacobson & Margolin, 1979; Weiss, 1978). Typically, the skills targeted for this training were identified by the therapist, based on contrasting the couple's current communication with a model of adaptive marital communication. These models were derived, in large part, by contrasting the communication behaviors of maritally distressed and nondistressed couples in problem-solving interactions held in research laboratories (e.g., Hahlweg et al., 1984; Weiss & Heyman, 1990a, 1990b). This phase in the development of BCT sought to provide couples with process skills intended to maintain therapeutic gains, rather than just addressing immediate presenting concerns.

The next stage in the evolution of the model was represented by cognitive-behavioral couple therapy. BCT had always included recognition of the importance of internal mediators of external experience (Weiss, 1980a, 1984); the more recent developments broadened and placed greater emphasis on cognitive and affective change strategies. Existing behavior-exchange and communication skills training were modified to foster changes in dysfunctional cognitions. For example, the change from bilateral *"quid pro quo"* to "good faith" behavior-change contracts was designed to foster the formation of relationship-enhancing positive attributions for change (e.g., "He made the change to improve the relationship"), rather than negative attributions (e.g., "He changed because the therapist told him to"; Baucom & Epstein, 1990). Additionally, explicit strategies aimed at modification of cognition and affect were incorporated into BCT. For example, self-instructional strategies are used to attempt to modify attributions (Baucom & Lester, 1986) or control anger (Schindler & Vollmer, 1984), Socratic dialogue is used to challenge irrational relationship beliefs (Baucom & Epstein, 1990), emotional expressiveness training is used to enhance intimacy through affect expression (Baucom & Epstein, 1990), and exposure-based procedures are used to reduce intense negative affect (Behrens, Sanders, & Halford, 1990).

BCT also is used when an individual family member has a problem that is the focus of therapy, although this requires some adaption of BCT. For example, when one partner abused alcohol, BCT was modified to incorporate conjoint contracting for Antabuse use (e.g., O'Farrell, 1986). BCT also has been successfully applied with depressed women and their partners; this is particularly useful when there are coexisting marital problems that exacerbate the depression (Beach, Sandeen, & O'Leary, 1990). A brief form of BCT, focused on communication and cooperation between partners about parenting issues, significantly improves the maintenance of behavioral parent training in those families with coexisting marital distress and child-behavior problems (Dadds et al., 1987).

Process of Behavioral Couple Therapy

Those who write about BCT emphasize the need for developing therapeutic alliances with each partner; developing a shared understanding of relationship problems and goals that promote adaptive change, and explicit negotiation with the couple about their roles in therapy (Beach, Sandeen, & O'Leary, 1990; Jacobson & Margolin, 1979; Baucom & Epstein, 1990; Stuart, 1980). In contrast, in some nonbehavioral couple therapy, the therapist determines the goals and process of therapeutic change. In instances of even greater therapist control, an unseen therapy team observes the couple and advises the therapist on what interventions to deliver to the couple. The couple is not informed as to the goals of therapy or provided with a rationale for therapy. Indeed, therapy often is paradoxical (i.e., misinforming clients about the process or goals of therapy). The couple system is viewed as resisting change, and therefore not informing clients about the process of change is seen as desirable. In our view, the ultimate goal of couple therapy is to empower the partners to develop and sustain a mutually satisfying relationship, and we think this necessitates their being active participants in the process of therapy.

Developing a common understanding of relationship problems with couples, one that promotes adaptive change, is often a challenging therapeutic task. Clients do not have a relationship *tabula rasa,* ready to accept the therapist's expert relationship wisdom. The therapist needs to work with the partners to help them develop a constructive, shared view of their relationship problems. BCT therapists conceptualize marital problems largely in terms of the behaviors and communication processes occurring between partners and the internal cognitive and affective reactions of each partner. Each of these factors potentially is changeable within conjoint couple therapy. In contrast, many maritally distressed people attribute their relationship problems to stable, global, negative characteristics of their partner (Fincham & Bradbury, 1990), believe relationship improvement is very difficult or even impossible to attain (Notarius & Vanzetti, 1983), and do not see what they, as individuals, can do to promote change. The challenge to the therapeutic process is how to shape these disparate views into common assumptions and goals, and how to assist each partner in identifying and carrying out changes likely to improve the relationship.

Clinical descriptions of BCT since the mid-1970s have emphasized the crucial role assessment plays in the process of BCT. The therapist seeks both to establish an empathic understanding of each partner's experiences within the relationship, and to promote a shared conceptualization of problems in terms of their relationship interactions. For example, if one partner wanted to spend more time with his or her spouse, but the other wanted to retain current levels of independence, individual partners initially might describe the problem in a partner-blaming manner (e.g., "She is not interested in me, and is too selfish to see my needs"; "He is so insecure, he cannot accept my having interests that don't involve him"). The therapist might describe the problem as "You have never been able to reach a mutually acceptable agreement about the balance of independent and shared time." The rationale for this relationship focus is that it circumvents blame of the partner for marital difficulties and promotes a relationship view more conducive to promoting constructive change.

To achieve an acceptable relationship focus in BCT, the therapist initially assesses key presenting problems from the perspective of each partner. During the assessment process, the therapist uses a variety of strategies to prompt attention to a relationship (or dyadic) focus, by strategic questioning (e.g., "How do you two resolve conflict? What happens between you when you discuss problems? As a couple how do you ensure you have quality time together?"). Reframing summaries, as in the previous example, foster a dyadic focus. On completion of assessment, structured feedback and discussion of assessment results are used as means to define mutually acceptable goals in a relationship focus, and to negotiate the content of therapy (e.g., Baucom & Epstein, 1990; Beach et al., 1990).

After developing a shared-relationship focus, the next step in couple therapy is to have each partner define what he or she can do to change the problematic interactions. This emphasis on self-change, (also known as *self-regulation*), focuses therapy on that which each client has the most direct control over: namely his or her own behavior (Halford et al., 1994). This is not to say changes in the partner are unimportant, but rather that the most productive method to achieve change is for each partner to focus on his or her own opportunities to change.

A self-regulation focus in therapy can be particularly important when partners address seemingly irreconcilable perceptions of what should happen in their relationship. In the traditional BCT approach, differences between partners were assessed in terms of current levels of communication and problem-solving skills in resolving their differences; couples were helped to define what behavior changes should be instituted to resolve their differences. However, it is clear that even in maritally happy couples there are some things that most people would admit dissatisfy them about their partner. One important element of successful long-term relationships, as Christensen, Jacobson, and Babcock (1995) point out, is acceptance of the human failings of one's spouse. To that end, we emphasize having partners monitor their own cognitive and affective responses to their spouse's behaviors. Standard cognitive procedures can be used to help the individual to alter his or her usual reactions to displeasing behaviors. In other words, a self-regulation focus incorporates the option that one solution for dissatisfaction with some aspects of one's partner's behavior is to alter one's own response to that behavior, and to stop unproductive attempts to change the partner. Thus, the self-regulation focus does not attempt to replace a relationship focus, but rather suggests that in order to respond to the variety of problems that a couple presents, it is important to focus partners on what they individually can do to improve their relationship. The process of therapy focuses on moving clients from a powerless, partner-blaming perspective to a consensually agreed relationship focus, and emphasizes initiating self-directed change.

In many instances, partners presenting for couple therapy may be actively considering separation. If either partner has made a clear decision to separate, the therapeutic task may be to mediate the process of negotiating a separation. More often, in couple therapy, one or both partners may be ambivalent about the relationship, so that the goals of therapy initially are difficult to establish. In such instances, the strategic use of assessment can be used to clarify dissatisfactions and to identify those goals necessary to make the relationship satisfactory. In so doing, clients often clarify their own goals for the relationship.

In summary, our approach to behavioral couple therapy makes the interaction between the partners the locus of change. The approach incorporates a combination of behavioral change, communication and problem-solving change, conflict management, and cognitive and affective change (e. g., Halford, Sanders, & Behrens, 1993: Christensen et al., 1995). The process of therapy helps each partner activate self-directed personal changes that will reduce dissatisfaction with the relationship and enhance both current and future relationship satisfaction.

ASSESSMENT

Initial Interview(s)

Assessment of a couple's relationship begins with the very first interview. Assessment provides two kinds of information: content and process. *Content* information refers to the reported concerns of the partners, such as the specific content of conflicts or their current thinking and actions about separation. Content information is what the partners are able to report about the relationship. *Process* information samples how the couple interacts in response to the various probes or tasks the therapist initiates. For example, if the couple is asked to discuss an issue of relevance to the relationship, the therapist may be particularly interested in the process of interchange between partners (e.g., the degree of effective listening to each other's perspective), rather than the actual content of the discussion.

Content information obtained from separate interviews with each spouse, or from individual spouse's self-report measures, is more reliable than similar information derived from conjoint interviews (Haynes, Jensen, Wise, & Sherman, 1981). Thus, reliance on conjoint interviews to gather content information is unwise. For example, reports of physical abuse are dramatically underreported in conjoint interview relative to either self-report inventories or individual interviews (O'Leary, Vivian, & Malone, 1992). In addition, in our experience, encouraging maritally distressed couples to recount lengthy lists of complaints about partners, in the presence of the partner, rarely promotes a collaborative set or moves therapy forward. For these reasons, we advise some combination of individual interviews and self-report assessments to gather content information.

Because a primary goal of assessment is to develop a shared perspective of the relationship that promotes change, conjoint interviews should focus on gathering and using process information. By combining process-focused conjoint sessions with individual assessment of content, it is possible to get reliable content information and also to achieve process goals.

A structure for an initial interview, which illustrates this combination of content and process-information gathering, is outlined in Table 13.1. We begin with a brief conjoint

Table 13.1. Summary of the Content of Initial Interview(s)

A. Joint session (10–15 minutes)
  Introductions
  Intentions in initial interview
  Confidentiality
B. Individual interviews (2 × 30 minutes each)
  Current Status of relationship problems
    Time course
    Separation
  Sources of difficulty
    Behavior
    Expectations
    Problem solving
    Typical week time use
    Sex
    External stressors
    Personal problems
C. Joint session (15–20 minutes)
  BCT approach
  Review individual material
  Suitability BCT
  Logistics of therapy

interview in which the agenda for the session is defined. The therapist then asks an open-ended question related to the reason for seeking assistance. This question is intended to assess process rather than content. To make the question effective, the therapist should engage eye contact with each partner while asking the question, but then look at a point midway between the partners (i.e., as the inflection occurs at the end of the question). Our interest at this point is the ability of the couple to collaborate in developing a coherent story to tell the therapist. If each partner shows respect toward the other and a shared view is presented, then a conjoint assessment of the content of the problems may be feasible. For example, a couple recently reported together that they each lacked the ability to stop conflict from being destructive, and they wanted help to improve this aspect of their relationship. A more typical response to a probe about conflict is an escalating disagreement about who has done what, who is to blame, and so forth. When this happens, the therapist should intervene early to prevent therapy from becoming another site for marital conflict. (Rarely in our experience do couples need to pay therapists money to practice destructive arguing; they usually have had considerable practice without professional charges.)

The second phase of the initial interview assesses content with one partner while the other partner fills out self-report measures in another room. The individual interview follows standard intake procedures of establishing key concerns and developing an empathic relationship between the therapist and client. Not all areas described in Table 13.1 necessarily will be covered in the first interview, but the most pressing immediate concerns of each partner should be identified. At the same time, probing certain of the areas described in Table 13.1 challenges clients to think about their relationship in new ways. For example, the question "What do you need to do differently to improve the relationship?" can move the client who is stuck in an exclusively partner-blaming mode to consider their own contribution to relationship problems.

The third phase of the interview rejoins the couple. The therapist frames expressed concerns in a manner consistent with the experience of the individual partners, while moving the couple toward a mutually acceptable problem definition. This is done by giving a relationship focus to the problems identified by the partners. For example, the therapist can restate concerns as the couple's having been unable to develop agreement on identified problem areas. Both partners can agree that these are issues that they need to resolve.

A key goal of the initial assessment interview(s) is to determine whether couple therapy is appropriate for the couple's problems. Appropriateness can be assessed at both a process and a content level. At a content level, one or both partners may explicitly state a firm intention to end the relationship. (Such clarity of intent is the exception, and, as noted earlier, more often there is ambivalence about the relationship.) At a process level, the primary interest is to observe how spouses deal with each other (not just how they talk about each other), and how they deal with therapist's probes. The objective here is to sample interaction behaviors that may be predictive of how they, as a couple and individually, are likely to deal with subsequent aspects of therapy. For example, if the conjoint phase of the initial sessions does not move from a starting point (e.g., the initial complaint) to some commitment to either terminate therapy or pursue further sessions, further assessment is needed to determine if the couple is ready to commit to therapy. A good rule of thumb states that the purpose of the first interview is to determine whether there will be a second interview.

Our approach explicitly labels *assessment* and *intervention* as two different forms of service. By doing so, we allow both parties (spouses and therapist) the option of deciding whether to continue in marital therapy. The purpose of the assessment phase, which can run for three or four sessions, is to provide a basis for observing couple interactions (process information) and to obtain useful thematic (content) information. These observations are made as couple and therapist attempt to move toward agreement about the goals of therapy. During this time, the couple also will be asked to complete assessment forms at home. The therapist receives, scores, and interprets these forms before each next scheduled conjoint session. The content of the forms provides the emphasis for the next assessment session. The last scheduled assessment session has a unique function; it is also a major decision point for committing to therapy. At this stage, the *findings* of the entire assessment process (interviews, forms, and observational data) are presented to the couple ("What do you think the various tests showed?" is a good way to begin). In this all-important "feedback" session, the therapist reveals what he or she has learned about the couple. It is at this point that a decision is made by therapist and couple whether therapy should continue. The operative here is a decision that rests in the hands of both parties. Just like the couple, the therapist may indicate an unwillingness to engage in marital therapy at this time. The assessment phase thus provides a message that therapy can only proceed under certain agreed upon conditions, that it is not provided automatically just for the asking.

At the content level, there are fairly straightforward questions that need to be addressed, although most of these can be more efficiently assessed by self-report measures. In couple therapy, one must be clear whether spouses or their children are in physical danger. (One must be familiar with local laws that govern reporting such dangers.) Clearly, if there is a present danger, it must take precedence over all other considerations. Similarly, one needs to be aware of concurrent problems, such as uncontrolled drinking, clinical depression, economic hardships, and possible conflict with ongoing individual therapy, among others.

On the process level, the concern is with how the couple deals with their issues right in the session and how they respond to therapist probes. Because assessment is intentionally different from the formal start of therapy, we can ask things during the assessment phase that would not be quite as fitting later on. For example, one can be incredulous at something the couple presents. Or one can raise the issue of separation or divorce when a couple has demonstrated considerable amounts of fighting (e.g., "Given the pain and problems you have caused for each other, I wonder why you haven't experimented with separation?"). One might choose to confront a couple with a realistic contradiction based on data: "Your forms are quite clear that you have a great deal of love for one another, and that you enjoy sex together; yet in our meetings you seem like terrorists, looking for opportunities to blast each other. How can you be both ways?"

It is somewhat less important that one get a meaningful answer to such an inquiry than merely having the opportunity to observe whether the couple takes the "bait" and reacts in a constructive manner (i.e., one that suggests there is hope for their relationship). For example, the couple might plead for help with the apparent contradiction (e.g., "That's the point! We can't seem to control ourselves. I feel unappreciated and I suspect she does too.") The therapist uses probes designed to move the couple from repetitive blaming cycles to a more forward-looking "We want it to be different; help us."

In a real sense, these assessment interviews (and especially the feedback session) are negotiations between the parties (couple and therapist) about the form that marital therapy will take. It allows for agreed-upon goals. It uses these initial contacts to inform what therapy will be like (e.g., therapist will not just let spouses emotionally beat each other up).

The use of probes serves still another function: It determines whether the spouses can move from partner blame (It's the other guy"), through a relationship focus ("We have a problem"), to self-directed change ("What is my contribution, and what can I do?"). People are unlikely to change if they are unaware of their contribution, and what is in it for them to change. Merely engaging in skill exercises is unlikely to be cost effective if one or the other person is "smoldering." By shifting the emphasis from him or her to "What can I do," we have a much better chance that skills training will be effective. Again, the skills feed back on personal effectiveness. For example, as we will describe later, certain communication exercises will foster personal assertiveness, which in turn increases the likelihood that one can influence outcomes (increased self-efficacy). We turn next to a description of some useful self-report measures that help in the planning for intervention.

Selected Self-Report Measures

A distinction can be drawn between measuring either level of "sentiment" or level of "relationship adjustment." *Sentiment* refers to the evaluation of the other (i.e., the extent to which one loves the other). *Adjustment* refers to emitting behaviors that roughly correspond to relationship competence. Self-report measures may focus more on sentiment than adjustment. Often the two are confounded, yielding an overall marital adjustment or satisfaction score. The cost-effectiveness of selecting specific assessment measures is important; one seeks to obtain maximally useful information quickly. The marital therapy area does not lack for self-report measures. In many cases, they seem to be measuring very similar constructs.

There are a number of highly similar self-report measures of "adjustment" or "satisfaction" that have received wide usage (see O'Leary, 1987; Sabatelli, 1988). The original marital-adjustment measure is the Locke–Wallace Marital Adjustment Scale (L-W; Locke & Wallace, 1959). Spanier extended the notion of relationship adjustment with his Dyadic Adjustment Scale (DAS; Spanier, 1976), which was intended to improve on the L-W, yet retained many of the same items. Both measures provide the sentiment- and adjustment-type items (although neither explicitly asks, "How much to do love your partner?"). Both are heavily weighted with items that assess spousal agreement on a host of areas (e.g., "How often do you and your partner agree on finances, religious matters, affection, friends, sex relations, etc."), and both utilize a rating scale that asks essentially, "All things considered, how happy are you in this relationship?" The DAS specifically asks how much effort one is willing to put into the relationship; the L-W asks whether one would marry the same person if one had it to do over again. The L-W is shorter, and despite its penchant for giving more credit (higher satisfaction score) when the woman is the one to make greater accommodation to the man, it has very good psychometric properties and provides a useful estimate of marital satisfaction. Scores below 100 on either test are indicative of increasing marital distress.

A different approach is represented by the Areas of Change Questionnaire (ACQ; Weiss, 1980b), based on the theory that the greater amount of change spouses desire, the greater their marital conflict. Here the emphasis is on the degree to which each partner desires more, less, or no change in the other's behavior. Each of 34 items begins with the stem: "I want my partner to...." The items cover affection, emotionality, communication, sex, aggression, finances, and so forth. Each item is rated on a scale ranging from *Very Much More*, through *No Change*, to *Very Much Less*. (Respondents also may check items as "critical" for their relationship.)

In the original form of the ACQ, each person also responded to the items by indicating his or her perception of what the other spouse desires. In this mode, for example, the stems read, "It would please my partner if I ... (engaged in behavior X) *Very Much More* and so forth. In a recent modification each person responds to the stem, "It would help my relationship if I ...". This latter variation focuses the person on his/her own possible contributions to making the relationship function more in the manner he or she desires. There are several ways of scoring these variations of the ACQ. For clinical purposes the sum of the absolute scores of suggested change gives a reasonable guide to the change requested of the partner and change believed necessary for the self (Halford & Sanders, 1989).

The third self-report measure, the Marital Status Inventory (MSI), provides an indication of how close the partners have come to seeking a divorce (Weiss & Cerreto, 1980). The MSI assesses which steps a couple has taken to end their relationship. Items range from "occasional thoughts of divorce" to more overt steps ("sought the advice of a close friend") to "filing for divorce." Several studies have reported on the use of the MSI (e.g., Arias & Beach, 1987; Griffin & Morgan, 1988). A score of 4 or greater (out of 14 possible items) is a major risk indicator for separation and predicts poorer prognosis in couple therapy.

The Conflict Tactics Scale (CTS; Straus, 1979) is a brief paper-and-pencil inventory assessing the reported frequency in the last 12 months of various verbal and physical acts of aggression by the respondent and his or her partner. There are reasonably high levels of agreement between partners' independent reports of the occurrence of marital aggression, and this instrument is very useful to screen for abuse (Langhinrichsen-Rohling & Vivian, 1994).

Couple functioning is influenced significantly by individual functioning. Given the frequency of occurrence of depression and alcohol abuse in distressed couples, we recommend routinely screening for these problems. The use of self-report measures such as the Beck Depression Inventory (BDI; Beck, Ward, Mendelson, Mock, & Erbaugh, 1961) and the Canterbury Alcoholism Screening Test (CAST; Elvy & Wells, 1984) is helpful.

Finally, it is often very helpful to allow the spouses an opportunity to respond in an open-ended fashion about perceived relationship strengths and weaknesses. This free format provides balance for those who find the specificity of items questionnaires too confining. Each person selects three areas (from a checklist of potential problems) that represent partner/relationship strengths and three that represent weaknesses. Each spouse writes something that is a partner strength and a weakness for each of the six areas (e.g., affection, children, finances, etc.). In this manner, each person is directed to find something positive to say, as well as complaining about annoying partner behaviors. Admittedly, the requirement to report the good along with the bad is difficult for some people, but the failure to identify positives in your partner is useful information as well. As with any open-ended self-reporting, people write all sorts of things in all sorts of detail, even though the instructions emphasize being behaviorally specific rather than generalizing vague assessments of the other.

This combination of self-report measures provides basic factual information about the couple. The data can be grouped according to class of information, degree of sentiment (DAS, L-W), amount of change desired (ACQ), individual problems (BDI, CAST), likelihood of terminating the relationship at this point in time (MSI), and occurrence of aggression (CTS). It is possible for a couple to have not only low DAS scores but also low MSI scores, suggesting that they are unhappy but not yet willing to separate. Or, a high level of depression in the male partner might be "coloring" all the other test scores (e.g., making relationship issues look worse than they are).

Quasi-Observation Measures

The process of monitoring either one's own or one's spouse's behavior is best thought of as a quasi-observational measure because, in addition to being participant observers, spouses are seldom trained observers. Although, in the strictest sense, reliability is questionable, such devices often are useful in allowing spouses to attend to the frequency, antecedents, and consequences of relationship events. For example, a couple instructed to track specific settings (situations) associated with conflict may come to recognize just how these settings trigger disruptive consequences for their relationship. In this manner, distressed couples can challenge one of their common assumptions, namely that it is all the partner's fault when arguments occur. Similarly, tracking instances of a spouse's pleasing behavior prompts attention to the positive-change efforts that person is making. Identifying actual setting events antecedent to conflict, or actual behavior exhibited during conflict, may have a desired effect. These monitoring systems can be used effectively to direct client attention to specific aspects of the ongoing stream of relationship behaviors.

An informative quasi-observational techniques is the Spouse Observation Checklist (SOC; Weiss et al., 1973; Weiss & Perry, 1983). Using this procedure, spouses individually record whether specific relationship events (some 480!) occurred during the immediate 24-

hour period, and whether each was "pleasing" or "displeasing." In its original form, the SOC was used to monitor spousal behaviors, but the same items have been used for self-monitoring of relationship behaviors (e.g., Halford et al., 1994). Events are grouped into three super relationship interaction categories that together subsume a total of 12 subcategories. The three major categories are Appetitive (relationship enhancing), Instrumental (maintenance functions), and By-Products (potential annoyances). The SOC represents a method for operationalizing relationships according to a behavior-exchange model based on costs and benefits. Thus, so-called appetitive events (the benefits of a committed relationship) comprise those behavioral exchanges that should enhance closeness, love, support, and good feelings generally. Among the appetitive subcategories are "affection," "sex," "consideration," "companionship," "communication process," and "coupling activities." Thus, items are included within each subcategory that reflect the intended function indicated by the category name. When couples engage in any of the behaviors listed, the result may be either pleasing or displeasing. For example, one "affection" item is "Spouse cuddled close to me in bed." Presumably that would be pleasing, but it could be quite displeasing in a distressed marriage.

Spouses can be asked to fill out the SOC, or the self-monitoring variation, daily, covering the previous 24 hours, for 1 to 2 weeks. They also record the level of their daily marital satisfaction on a 1 to 9 scale and the amount of time they spend together each day. The satisfaction ratings, when compared to category totals, give an indication of which events are associated with higher or lower marital satisfaction. Among its various uses, the SOC highlights relationship events that the spouses find desirable, and so can be used to set attainment goals; that is, once it is pinpointed by the SOC, the therapist can use this information to assist spouses in increasing the very behavioral exchanges that are most pleasing to them. The SOC has the advantage of being comprehensive but the disadvantage of being onerous for some clients to complete. The SOC can be customized by selecting items of particular relevance to a particular couple, thereby reducing the burden.

An offshoot of the SOC is the Cost–Benefit Exchange (C-B) which starts only with *a priori* positive SOC items. For each item, spouses separately rate how beneficial it would be if they engaged in that activity with their spouse. Using our example, "Spouse cuddled close to me in bed," we now ask how beneficial it would be if one engaged in that activity. Ratings are made on a 0 to 5 scale, with 0 being *No Benefit at All,* and 5 being a *High Degree of Benefit.* In order to assess the cost of these same behaviors, each spouse indicates on a 0 to 5 scale how costly it would be to provide that activity to the other. Thus, we obtain each individual's corresponding benefit and cost ratings for mutual comparison. Thus, for example, if husband rated the cuddling item a high (5) benefit but wife rated it a high (5) cost, there is the potential for serious rejection. Or, a person may rate an item as a high benefit to receive but also as a high cost to give to the other. From the various possible combinations of costs and benefits, both within and between persons, we can arrive at an inventory of what may be considered "good" and "poor" therapy items.

The distinction between good and poor therapy items is related to how one proceeds in encouraging partners to engage in specific behaviors (e.g., the cuddling item) intended to foster goodwill. One must always take into account the likelihood of success or failure of one's instructions. If we knew that a behavioral event was a high benefit and a high cost to the respective partner, we would be remiss to encourage that behavior until such time as the cost level changed. A good item to target for change would be one that both partners rate as high benefit (to receive) *and* low cost (to provide).

An added feature of the C-B analysis, in addition to assessing the amount of relationship-benefit potential, is being able to show those couples who complain of low mutual benefits that, in fact, they share many relationship benefits. According to our scoring convention, discussed earlier, an item that is high benefit and low cost for both partners is, by definition, a mutually good therapy item. Such an item is one that both partners desire and can readily provide. Whenever spouses disagree with regard to each person's respective benefits and costs on the same item, we can expect an unwillingness to engage in that behavior. Both the C-B and the SOC provide clear examples of how, in our model, there is a close relationship between assessment and intervention. The assessment choices are made with some intervention in mind.

Behavioral Observation

Last, we consider behavioral observation as another available assessment option. In the research domain, behavioral observation is the most extensively developed assessment strategy (cf. Weiss & Dehle, 1994; Weiss & Heyman, 1990b). Investigators usually assign couples an interactional task. The most frequently used task is discussion of a topic that is a source of conflict between the partners, because managing conflict is a problem for most distressed couples, although recent research shows distressed couples also have communication problems in low-conflict tasks such as reminiscing about past positive events in their relationship (Osgarby & Halford, 1995).

Researchers have developed various coding systems for analyzing communication behavior, most of which are intended to assess the couple's management of conflict (Markman & Notarius, 1987; Weiss & Dehle, 1994). In most systems, every observed partner behavior is classified into one of a series of explicitly defined content categories. For example, an utterance might be classified into categories such as criticism, suggestion of a problem solution, or agreement with the partner's previous utterance. Many systems also classify responses on the basis of affective expression, usually by focusing on nonverbal behaviors. The relevant research has identified several common patterns of interaction associated with marital distress (cf. Weiss & Heyman, 1990b).

These research-derived coding systems are very labor intensive, requiring reliably trained coders and videotaping facilities. However, it is possible to adapt the more formal, labor-intensive aspects of behavioral observation to the reality of service-oriented settings. As before, couples are asked to attempt to resolve a relationship issue (e.g., as derived from the ACQ, DAS, listings of strengths and weaknesses, etc.) without the therapist being present. An audiocassette recorder can be used if videotaping facilities are unavailable. Based on the research, it is possible to identify several common patterns associated with marital distress; these are summarized in Table 13.2. In essence, the process of effective communication can be divided into listener skills and speaker skills. Either partner may show deficits in these domains. In addition, it is possible to identify several maladaptive pairings of ineffective use of speaker and listener skills. For example, neither partner actively listens or sends (mutual avoidance), both partners send very negative messages (cross-complaining, usually accompanied by escalating anger), and one partner sends very negative messages and the other does not actively listen (demand for change by one partner leads to withdrawal by the other partner).

In the past, therapists have used communication-based coding systems to define targets for marital therapy: specifically, whether clients actually demonstrated all the specific skills identified in Table 13.2. Implicit in this approach is the assumption that each of these specific communication skills is necessary for good marital functioning. However,

Table 13.2.   Communication Behavior and Patterns Associated with Marital Distress

Behavior or pattern	Description
Ineffective listening	Deficits in active listening, such as minimal encouragers, open-ended questions, paraphrases, and summaries. Excesses of interrupts, disagreements, cross-complaining justification, and defensiveness.
Ineffective speaking	Deficits in assertive statements of concern, clear descriptions of events or behaviors. Excesses of angry accusations, rapid topic changes, sweeping generalizations, blaming.
Demand-withdraw	One partner does the majority of sending, demanding change, while the other attempts to close off discussion or withdraw.
Mutual escalation	Each partner engages in negative sending, with low rates of listening. The discussion tends to escalate in volume, and expressed negative affect.
Mutual avoidance	Partners are detached, with neither sending very much. Any issues raised are minimized and there is little exchange of information.

the extent to which couples use any specific communication skill bears little relationship to their response to marital therapy (Halford et al., 1993). Adaptive marital communication is likely to vary across relationships, times, and settings (Halford, Gravestock, Lowe, & Scheldt, 1992). Consequently, marital communication needs to be assessed ideographically for its functional impact within specific contexts, rather than being evaluated solely on its topographical match with a nomothetic template of adaptive communication. This is not to say that there are no general principles of good communication that the therapist can present to help clients self-select goals. For example, as noted earlier, presence of the demand–withdrawal pattern is associated with deterioration in relationship satisfaction (Gottman, 1993). As therapists, we often advise clients of this finding and suggest that therapy should seek to replace this pattern with healthier alternatives. This can be achieved in multiple ways, such as having the demander alter the manner in which he or she presents requests, and having the withdrawer seek further information about requested change, or develop strategies to cope with demands. We are unaware of any evidence that any specific communication skill is universally adaptive within relationships and prefer that clients self-select change goals within a broad framework of good communication developed conjointly with the therapist.

Integrating and Summarizing Assessment Information

As noted earlier, formal assessment aims to enable the therapist and clients to develop a shared conceptualization of the relationship and, collectively, to plan an appropriate intervention. To this end, we employ a guided-participation model of reviewing assessment information. The therapist presents results of the assessment to the couple, one assessment instrument at a time. He or she selects key findings and presents these to the couple. It is essential that findings are presented in a manner that ensures each partner will feel that his or her individual position is understood, yet, at the same time, the couple is drawn toward a collaborative relationship focus. The therapist continually checks with each partner that the descriptions and conclusion being reached are accurate according to that person's perception. After reviewing each instrument, the therapist summarizes findings and discusses with the couple the possible goals and logistics of therapy. Some general guidelines for making effective use of the feedback of assessment data are presented in Table 13.3. The most commonly identified goals for marital therapy are improving communication, controlling conflict, and improving shared quality time. Other common goals include renegotiating the sharing of household chores, working together to improve parenting difficulties, and enhancing the couple's sex life.

One question must be answered during this integrating session: Is this truly a marriage case? Is marital therapy an appropriate modality for the problems as presented? As a general rule, it is always better to assume that the couple's reasons for continuing the marriage may not always be apparent to an outsider. As therapists, we need to temper our expectations of a "good" marriage with the reality of any given couple's situation. If a couple has a distant relationship for 15 or more years, it is unlikely that marital therapy will turn them into "storybook" romantics. Oftentimes, if we look hard enough, we can see the basis for a marital *quid pro quo,* yet one that might not otherwise be apparent. Rule number one: Do not be overly hasty in encouraging the couple to separate!

Having cautioned against recommending termination of relationships, we now consider cases that may not bode well for starting marital therapy. From assessment, it should be clear whether the couple is likely to be responsive to new ideas. Among our less-than-optimistic marital therapy indicators, we include the following: The individuals do not seem to be able defocus past hurts; they have little sense of what their relationship may be like if it were to be closer to their ideal; initial sessions seem to have no discernible forward movement (e.g., one or both partners are still filling in details of past events as the session is ending); they repeatedly fail to hear the therapist. Similarly, if one person is commandeering relationship resources, for example, by insisting on continuing a sexual affair or being unwilling to curtail abusive behaviors, marital therapy is not likely to be appropriate.

Some examples may help to illustrate the issues involved in determining the appropriateness of marital therapy. The Howtens arrived at the second of their assessment sessions with Mrs. Howten bleeding from the lip. They reported they had argued heatedly on the way to the therapy session, and Mr. Howten had struck Mrs. Howten across the face as he was driving the car. In the CTS inventories that each had completed the week before, both partners had reported engaging in pushing, shoving, and slapping the other several times in the last year. The therapist spoke to each partner separately about the issue of violence and the need to prevent future assaults. Mr. Howten said he regretted that night's instance but refused to acknowledge that aggression was a problem, and became quite angry when challenged about this. He stated that he had never hurt his wife seriously and claimed that his aggression helped her to know he was serious about an issue. The therapist pointed out that assault is illegal, to which Mr. Howten replied that he doubted that the police would be interested in such a minor offense. Mrs. Howten reported feeling fearful and intimidated by her husband's anger and aggression, but said she did not want to upset him by making the aggression a focus of therapy. She suggested that her husband would

Table 13.3. Guidelines for Giving Assessment-Data Feedback to Couples

A. Goals of data presentation
1. Clear, logical, and comprehensible presentation of the relevant data.
2. To point out what the data say and what they mean, particularly how they relate to partner's current relationship practices.
3. To be aware of the possible emotional impact of the data.
4. To use the data to introduce treatment procedures and goals.

B. Notes on descriptive and interpretative comments
Descriptive comments: Present evidence/data on a partner's behavior or on the context of the behavior.
Interpretative comments provide judgments about what has been observed or reported. A therapist should provide the couple with the descriptive data/evidence on which his or her interpretations are based. This allows the couple to test the validity of the therapist's judgments.
Examples of interpretative comments and the descriptive evidence upon which they were based (allows a test of the "match" between the two types of statements):

Descriptive comment	*Interpretative comment*
Mrs. H. tells Mr. H. she would like him to take more responsibility for household chores.	She is a nag about housework.
Mr. H. goes to the pub every night.	He is an alcoholic, you know.

C. Problems in discussing assessment findings

Problems	*Possible solutions*
1. Failure to establish goals of session clearly.	1. Negotiate an agenda; establish time limits, etc.
2. Getting sidetracked by tangential issues.	2. Keep to agenda items, reschedule other business, use retrospective probes and transition probes to keep on track.
3. Being judgmental (e.g., offering premature interpretations of partner's behavior).	3. Present relevant descriptive data, one at a time, before offering interpretations; select meaningful/relevant examples to illustrate teaching points. Seek couple's view on your interpretations.
4. Being vague; overgeneralizing.	4. Be more specific; use clear examples.
5. Being too definitive, or overgeneralizing from inadequate database.	5. Be more tentative; acknowledge possible alternative interpretations; look to future data-collection tasks to test out alternative generated hypotheses.
6. Ignoring partner's views or becoming defensive when therapist's own views are challenged.	6. Encourage partners to present their own views of the problem. Reinforce them for mentioning their own ideas. Don't become defensive. Ask partners to become more specific, concrete, and to exemplify what they mean by statements. Point to future or existing data to clarify disagreements.
7. Partners not understanding your interpretations or conclusions about the nature of the problem.	7. Don't use jargon; use more straightforward examples and vocabulary (role-play examples if necessary). Probe to determine partners' understanding of what you have said.
8. Partners becoming defensive (e.g., self-condemning, upset, angry).	8. Use summarizing, reflection, rephrasing, and paraphrasing skills to identify source of partner concern. Be supportive. Challenge irrational assumptions by presenting alternative ways of conceptualizing the problem.
9. Using jargon.	9. Use everyday language. If you wish to teach a new concept, explain it clearly, exemplify it, and use it consistently.

Table 13.3.   *(Continued)*

10. The over talkative partner.	10. Use agendas. Use interviewing strategies to get partner back on track (e.g., closing-off summaries, transition probes, retrospective probes, interrupting partner); reschedule issue if it needs to be discussed.
11. The nonengaged partner.	11. Ask for partner's viewpoints/opinion. Reinforce partner for contributing by summerizing his or her viewpoint, being attentive, etc.

never really hurt her. The therapist brought the couple together and stated that controlling aggression would need to be a focus of therapy if marital therapy were to proceed, and restated concern for the safety of Mrs. Howten and the need for the couple to develop alternative means of managing conflict. Together, the couple restated their refusal to consider the issue and further therapy was terminated. In this instance, the couple and the therapist could not reach mutually acceptable goals.

The Olsons, a couple in their early 30s and without children, presented a challenge. They initially reported low levels of shared quality time, lack of affection, and sexual satisfaction. We soon learned that 6 months ago the husband had a brief homosexual affair while the wife was out of town on business. When he believed he acquired a sexually-transmitted disease (which turned out to be a minor infection), he told his wife about the affair. He had had a homosexual relationship as a teenager, which, together with the recent affair, made him feel uncertain about his sexual orientation (i.e., whether he was gay, bisexual, or heterosexual). He had been seeing a counselor regularly for 3 months to attempt to clarify his sexual preference, but he still felt uncertain. He has been unaffectionate and relatively disinterested in sex with his wife, except for the first few months of their relationship. She found all this very hurtful and upsetting. He had been depressed in the recent past, and now found his work life very demanding and unrewarding. The wife reported loving her profession and also reported being very active in her work. Since she had found out about the affair, she had become moderately depressed.

Attempts to elicit agreed-upon goals for therapy initially were difficult. The wife wondered whether the husband needed to decide his orientation before any work on the relationship could proceed, but felt angry at the idea of just waiting for him to make up his mind about whether he wished to be in a heterosexual relationship. The husband speculated that his homosexual feelings might be part of an unconscious need to avoid responsibility (the couple had discussed having a child, and he was very fearful of the responsibility and commitment this would involve.) "I guess we need to communicate better," the wife repeated, when the going got rough. The husband said he was conflict-avoidant and did not want to make waves or to hurt his wife. Both reported that they had discussed the issue repeatedly, but that no resolution had been reached on the future of the relationship.

Is this a case for couple therapy? Clearly the relationship is distressed, but there are individual issues that are relevant to the motivation to produce change. Therapy could focus on working with the husband to attempt to clarify his sexual orientation, with the wife to determine her feelings and desires about the relationship, or conjointly to work on the relationship. After three assessment sessions and discussion with the therapist, the couple decided that they needed to communicate better together; if they were to separate, they wanted to negotiate a low-conflict resolution, and if they were to stay together, they needed to rebuild their relationship. They also decided that each would attempt to make the relationship as good as they could over the next 2 to 3 months, with the goal of then deciding whether to stay together. Finally, it was agreed that the husband would undertake some behavioral tasks to attempt to clarify his sexual orientation, because simply thinking and talking did not seem to help him decide (e.g., he attended a series of self-help meetings of married, bisexual men to learn about their lifestyles). In this instance the couple and the therapist did develop goals that were relevant and acceptable to all parties.

Once the therapist and the couple have a common understanding of the relationship and the goals of therapy, then therapy can proceed by attempting to achieve those goals. We next describe the treatment procedures we use to achieve the most commonly negotiated goals of marital therapy.

DETAILED TREATMENT PROCEDURES

As noted earlier, behavioral approaches to couples' therapy promote partners being able to think about their problems within a relationship focus. At the end of therapy, it is intended that each partner will be able to self-identify changes needed to enhance their relationship, to be able to formulate strategies to self-direct change, and to self-evaluate the effects of that self-directed change. To achieve these terminal goals, we focus our treatment on enhancing each person's self-regulation skills within the relationship.

Behavior Change Procedures

Given that couples do not communicate by extrasensory perception, the key information they have about their partners is gained through partners' behavior, both verbal and nonverbal. Although the subjective impact of that behavior is mediated cognitively, behavior is still the medium through which a relationship occurs. Although such an observation may seem self-obvious, some approaches to couple therapy are so concerned with the processes occurring inside people's heads that they pay relatively little attention to the actual exchange of behaviors between partners. BCT, on the other hand, always places heavy emphasis on helping couples to identify and change behaviors in ways that promote their relationship.

In traditional approaches to BCT, behavior change usually is achieved through contracting. Typically, each partner is asked to identify behaviors that he or she would like the spouse to provide more often, and then a contract is drawn up between the spouses in an attempt to increase those behaviors. In the original formats, the contracts were in a *"quid pro quo"* form: If Partner 1 does X, then Partner 2 will do Y. A number of clinicians observed that these reciprocated contracts often led couples to disagreements about who should make the first change, and changes that did occur were often not perceived as being real changes in the relationship (Baucom & Epstein, 1990). Consequently, a number of clinicians advocate so-called parallel contracts: Each partner identifies change he or she wants from the spouse, but each then simply unilaterally agrees to change certain behaviors requested by the partner (cf. Weiss et al., 1974). Again, a number of clinicians reported problems with this approach. In essence, the approach often still leads partners to wait for their partner to make the first move to improve the relationship.

In our self-directed approach, we asked each partner to self-identify behaviors that they can do individually to benefit the relationship. Often this is quite highly structured initially. For example, we would use a variation on the "love days" procedure first described by one of us (Weiss et al., 1973). In a self-directed approach partners would be asked to identify those behaviors that they believe demonstrated caring for their partner. They would then be asked to select from this menu of self-defined behaviors particular behaviors thought to be helpful to change, and to make those changes on a given day. Here, persons are not responding directly to requests from the partner, but rather are taking responsibility for self-identifying things that they can do to enhance their own relationship.

We also seek to extend the ways in which individuals engage in relationship-enhancing behaviors by asking them to attend to a wide variety of areas in which they can make behavioral changes. Some of the most important areas that individuals might seek to change behaviors in their relationship are described in Table 13.4. For individuals who are finding it difficult to self-identify behaviors, we have generated a series of lists that provide clients with examples of behaviors that show classes of relationship activities such as partner support, caring, respect, and so forth. The C-B is an example of a highly structured means of guiding clients to self-identify behavior-change goals.

The self-directed approach does not prohibit a partner from seeking information from the spouse or others. However, we believe it is important for each person to view the act of asking one's spouse as a self-directing skill. Whenever individuals have difficulty with self-identifying behavior change, we encourage them to develop a menu of ways for identifying appropriate behaviors to improve. Thus, one strategy is simply to write down a list based on whatever thoughts or feelings occur at the time. Another strategy is to think back on past things that seemed to be helpful in the relationship, or to reflect on relationships whose members seemed to be successful and then to identify specific behaviors that were observed. Alternatively, clients may ask friends, relations, or other informants for suggestions of new behaviors to try. Clearly, the spouse is an important potential informant. The ultimate goal focusing on self-identification is to have each partner develop his or her skills in being creative within the relationship, and to take responsibility individually for producing change.

In subsequent therapy sessions, we place great emphasis on reviewing how partners went about implementing self-identified behavior changes. We recommend that each

Table 13.4. Classes of Behavior Most Strongly Related to Marital Satisfaction

Class of behavior	Example
Affection	Saying "I love you." Giving a hug or kiss. Enjoying a shared laugh or joke. Saying they enjoy partner's company.
Respect	Listening to the partner's opinion. Telling partner of admiration/respect. Saying/showing confidence in partner's abilities. Introducing partner to others with pride.
Support and assistance	Doing errands for partner. Making self available to do work for partner. Asking partner about his or her day. Doing something to save partner time/energy.
Communication of ideas	Telling partner about your day. Discussing topical events. Giving an opinion. Talking about mutual interest(s).
Shared quality time	Spending an hour or more just talking. Work together on a project. Take a drive or walk. Go out together, just the two of you. Discuss personal feelings.
Appreciation	Commenting on something the partner did. Saying "thank you." Telling a third party in the partner's presence about a positive action of the partner.

partner report on the positive actions he or she has undertaken, and the reactions that those behaviors elicited. Even when an intended positive behavior fails to bring about the desired result, there is useful information to be gained. For example, Nick had resolved to make Lyn an early morning cup of tea on the weekend. When he brought it in, she was a bit irritable with him. The therapist discussed this with Nick and noted that the couple had been out late the night before. Perhaps extra sleep would have been appreciated more than tea. The client is experimenting to see which behaviors under which circumstances produce the desired effect within the relationship. "Appreciation" is an especially important class of behavior: Noticing and supporting the efforts of the spouse, particularly in the early phases of therapy, are essential to progress. Hence, we would use tasks such as "catching your partner being nice." In this procedure, the individual is asked to identify what the partner did that was positive, and how he or she showed appreciation. Again, the emphasis is on being creative in how one expresses appreciation.

Self-directed changes must take the specifics of the problem area into consideration. For example, if there is a high degree of anger and hurt within the relationship, partners may not respond well to being asked to show affection or sexual playfulness toward one another, whereas they may be willing to show respect or civility. As therapy progresses, the therapist can encourage clients to extend the range and degree of effort they expend in promoting intimacy (e.g., one can ask clients to "shock their partner with pleasure"). The art in this process is being able to monitor the responses of the individuals and to make partners stretch by going a little further to rebuild their relationship.

The degree of structuring required in order to produce effective behavior change within different relationships varies considerably. For some couples, the process of going through a structured assessment, with feedback, identification, and mutual agreement on goals may be sufficient to allow them to make substantive changes in important relationship areas. Recent data suggest that for mildly distressed couples with DAS scores above 85, and MSI scores below 3, this minimal intervention can be quite effective (Halford, Osgarby, & Kelly, 1995). For other clients, particularly those with severe marital distress, the process of change is much more difficult. Often it requires the therapist to minimize the response cost for effort and to maximize the reinforcement of small gains. This can involve providing extensive lists of possible behavior changes, getting the partners to plan very carefully the precise behaviors that they will engage in at particular times and places in order to enhance their relationship, and carefully structuring reinforcement for those efforts.

In essence, we challenge all individuals in couple therapy to be more creative in the behaviors they engage in as a means of enhancing their relationship. Each partner is encouraged to experiment with different ways of being a partner in order to discover those unique relationship-enhancing behaviors (i.e., as each person wants it to be). Over the course of therapy, therapists should fade their influence over the identification and implementation of behavior change. By the end of therapy, it is desirable that clients should simply be able to report to the therapist on particular things that they have been engaging in, and other ideas that they have for implementing change.

Communication

Communication is the single, most commonly presented problem in marital therapy. Oftentimes, when people describe communication problems they are also referring to conflict management. Indeed, conflict management is very important, and in the next section of this chapter we include a description of therapeutic procedures to help couples manage conflict. Nonetheless, we are equally convinced that good communication is more than simply the absence of severe conflict. Good communication is about the couple being able to talk together in intimacy-enhancing ways.

Recent research highlights two important aspects of marital communication necessary for enhancing intimate communication. First is the extent to which couples engage in *validation*, which Markman, Floyd, Stanley, and Lewis (1986) define as any response that shows active listening, interest, or valuing of the partner's perspective on an issue. This can be achieved in a number of ways, such as effective attending behaviors, asking open-ended questions, paraphrasing, or adding content that follows on and is relevant to the perspective of the partner. A second characteristic of effective communication is partners' positive engagement in the discussion of topics. Numerous studies have shown that avoidance of topics (particularly those on which the couple disagrees), or withdrawing from discussions (by physically exiting, switching the topic, verbalizing refusal to discuss a particular issue further, or simply no longer attending to the partner), are both concurrently and prospectively associated with significant marital problems (e.g., Gottman, 1993; Heavey & Christensen, 1993). Positive engagement can be achieved by means of any of a number of enactive, positive speaker skills. The specific skills are not as important as their effectiveness for any given couple.

At the risk of belaboring the point, traditional BCT approaches to communication skills training often are based on the erroneous idea that specific skills must always be trained for all couples. Many approaches to BCT tend to focus on teaching couples a relatively fixed curriculum of skills (e.g., paraphrasing, asking open-ended questions, behavioral pinpointing). In our view, different styles of communication suit different couples and different circumstances; we can be reasonably confident, however, that the specific skills should provide a demonstration of validation and positive engagement. When we introduce communication skills training to couples, we stress the importance of achieving these two goals and proceed to assist partners in self-identifying particular skills that *they* think would enhance their marital communication.

The process of communication skills training might proceed as follows: The couple is asked to identify an appropriate topic for discussion. We try to focus on something initially that is unrelated to conflict, for example, asking the couple to talk to each other about what they have been doing over the last 7 or 8 hours, when they may have been apart. Having agreed that they will talk about their days, the couple is then asked to chat for 4 or 5 minutes. The ensuing conversation is audiotaped and then the tape is replayed to the couple. Each partner is asked to focus on his or her own communication. The instruction is to try and identify examples of particular things that each did that were helpful. To assist people who are less familiar with ways of describing their communication, the therapist often might provide a checklist of various communication skills, such as the one included in Table 13.5. (Many clients need some training to become familiar with the communication behaviors listed in the checklist.) Having self-identified a communication strength, clients are then asked to self-identify something they could do that would enhance their communication. For example, one partner might identify the fact that he or she could ask the other person to elaborate more by asking open-ended questions. The emphasis is on each partner's self-identifying goals for change. The couple is then asked to replay the discussion incorporating the skills that they have hypothesized will improve their communication. After the second run through the communication task, they are asked first to self-assess all their implementations of their stated goal, and second, to self-assess the impact their behaviors had on the relationship. Note that the emphasis is on each partner's self-

Table 13.5. Communication Skills Self-Evaluation Checklist

Name: _____ Date: _____

The aim of this form is for you to identify your strengths and weaknesses in communication and to specify goals for improvement. Rate each of the skills below using this code:

0—Very poor use of skill
1—Unsatisfactory use of skill
2—Satisfactory use of skill,
      but room for improvement
3—Good use of skill
N/A—Not applicable

Skill	0	1	2	3	N/A
1. Specific/concrete descriptors of behaviors and situation					
2. Self-disclosure of feelings					
3. Clear expression of positive					
4. Assertive expression of negatives					
5. Attending to partner					
6. Minimal encourages					
7. Reserving judgment					
8. Asking questions					
9. Summarizing content					
10. Paraphrasing feelings					

Self-identified strengths in communication: _____
_____
_____
_____

Self-identified weaknesses in communication: _____
_____
_____
_____
_____

identifying, appropriate self-change, and then self-evaluating the impact of that change on the relationship.

Many couples find it helpful to use an idea advocated by Notarius and Markman (1993) to separate out the listener and speaker roles. In this structure, one partner agrees to be the listener, and the other, the speaker. The listener may only use listening responses, (e.g., asking questions and paraphrasing), and may not use speaker responses (e.g., stating his or her own views). This structure can be particularly helpful when partners have a high rate of disagreements and interruptions, and low rates of positive listening.

There is a finite repertoire of important communication tasks that couples typically need to execute. Keeping each other up to date on what they are doing on a day-to-day basis is one example of something that happens reasonably often in good relationships. Couples in healthy relationships also tend to reminisce about important positive experiences that they have shared in their relationship history (Osgarby & Halford, 1995). These reminiscences are particularly likely to be elicited by particular events such as anniversaries, birthdays, and Christmas. Showing interest in your partner's interests and learning how you can be supportive of your partner are things that can be developed through positive communication. Based on their assessment results, we would work with couples to help them enhance their communication skills across these multiple areas.

Sequencing of communication tasks during therapy can have an important impact. Initially, focusing couples on tasks that are likely to elicit positive affect may enhance their chance of developing better communication. For example, asking the partners to discuss how they met and what first attracted them to each other is a task that often elicits positive feelings. Similarly, reminiscing about positive events also can be useful initially.

Communication skills training is not complete unless couples are able to engage in this improved communication at home. Routinely, throughout the course of therapy, we would ask couples to audiotape discussions they have at home. The task should be developed collaboratively with the couple; the therapist may define the general topic that the couple is to talk about and then each partner is asked to self-identify particular behaviors that he or she will try to engage in during the interaction. The tape is then reviewed in the next therapy session. The review proceeds with each partner individually monitoring his or her own behavior. This emphasis is very important, because it focuses partners on what they are able to change. In our experience, poor communication is often exacerbated by the tendency to blame the partner when things go wrong during communication.

Conflict Management

The most obvious sign of marital distress to most marital therapists is conflict that is evident in therapy sessions (cf. Weiss & Dehle, 1994). Most couples with marital problems will report difficulties in managing conflict. The expression of poor conflict management varies considerably. Some couples engage in a high frequency of repetitive, highly aversive, and escalating arguments. This pattern typically is accompanied by high levels of anger and very negative feelings toward the spouse for a period of time after the arguments (Gottman, 1993). A second pattern that is commonly evident is the so-called approach–withdrawal pattern. In this pattern, one partner seeks to discuss a conflictual topic while the other partner withdraws from the interaction. Such withdrawal is usually followed by further attempts by the person seeking change to raise additional concerns, which is then followed by further withdrawal. A third possible pattern is simply avoidance of discussion of difficult topics (Gottman, 1993), when couples have simply given up on discussing an issue. Couples tend to have a predominant pattern of conflict management, but clearly they may use some mixture of these different patterns over time and across topics.

In BCT approaches, *conflict management* means teaching couples rationally to problem-solve those areas that have been a source of conflict. Although rational problem solving can be useful in some cases, we feel that this is a very narrowly focused approach to managing conflict. In this section we consider a series of different methods couples might use better to manage conflict.

Couples who engage in repetitive, highly emotional arousal interactions feel a low sense of efficacy in being able to resolve the source of conflict (Notarius & Vanzetti, 1983), and one of the key goals of conflict management is to help partners to identify things that they may be able to do to contribute to more effective management of this conflict. To achieve this end, it is often helpful to use a structure that helps partners identify their own actions, and their cognitions about the interaction, during a conflictual interaction. The following is a procedure that relies heavily on affective expression.

Whenever a couple has had a recent aversive interaction, either one reported as having occurred at home, or something that may actually occur in the therapy session, the therapist then asks the partners to pause. Each is instructed about the importance of understanding what is happening from the other's perspective. The therapist selects one partner to talk to the therapist about that person's perception of the problem. The second partner is instructed not to talk or interrupt. The designated person is then asked a series of questions that help describe his or her actual behavior during the initial interaction, and then questions designed to elicit the subjective meaning of that interaction for the person. (This is a variation of McMullin and Gile's [1987] vertical arrow technique, which involves describing the cognitive processes occurring within the partner. The process is similar to that described by Christensen et al. [1995] and Greenberg and Johnson [1988], among others.) An example of this process is provided in the transcript following. Three things are important to note from the transcript: (a) The partner is able to express all of the anger and attacking feelings that he or she had towards the partner. (b) Over time, the person comes to describe other emotional responses such as fear of rejection, loneliness, and hurt. These have been described as "softer" or "cooler" emotions. The problem is framed in a way that the person acknowledges his or her vulnerability during a marital interaction; in so doing, the speaker phrases concerns in ways that may be easier for the partner to accept. (c) The therapist then integrates the perspective of the two partners to describe a pattern that is related to both of their subjective experiences, and describes the problem in a relationship focus.

Bill and Leanne: An Illustration

Bill and Leanne arrived in the session, each casting angry looks at the other. Leanne reported that they had had a heated argument about Bill's purchase of a compact disc. As she recounted this, Bill interrupted angrily, and they began to argue again.

T: Okay, Okay, I hear that both of you are angry with each other. I want us to understand why this conflict is such a problems for you two. I want to hear from each of you, but one at a time. I will try to understand what happened from each of your points of view. The other person is to keep quiet and listen. Bill, I wonder, would you listen first? I want you just to sit there and hear what Leanne has to say.

B: All right.

T: Leanne, I want to hear what happened as you saw and felt it. Bill, even if its hard, I just want you to listen, and your turn will come. Leanne, what happened that led up to the argument?

L: Well, I was cleaning out the cupboard when I came across this new CD. Bill knows this is an issue for us. We are short of money, and I ... well ... got so mad because we can't afford to be buying these things all the time. They are $20 or $25 (Australian), and he must have bought seven or eight in the last month. One, two hundred dollars ... just gone ... I felt so mad.

T: So you really felt angry that Bill had spent the money on the CD.

L: Yeah, so when he got home, I said "I really need to talk about this, you've blown more money on these things and we can't afford it." Well Bill didn't say much, and then flopped himself down in front of the TV—as usual—and I thought, "Well I can't take much more of this."

T: So you felt frustrated that Bill would not talk?

L: I was really mad as hell by this stage, and I said, "Bill we have to talk, I can't stand it when you ignore me like this." Well, he mumbled something about it being no big deal, and that he was tired. I felt so ..." *(sobs)*

T: What did you think when Bill said it was no big deal?

L: I felt like he wasn't taking me seriously, never takes me seriously.

T: When you think he is not taking you seriously, what does that mean to you?

L: I guess I feel like he isn't that interested in me. He walked out then, just left the room.

T: When he left, how did you feel?

L: Well, I got madder.

T: What was it about him leaving that mad you so mad?

L: Well it made me wonder if he wanted to talk to me at all.

T: And if you think he might not want to talk to you, what does that mean to you?

L: Well, if there is no communication, there is no marriage is there?

T: So, when you feel he does not want to talk, that makes you wonder about the future of the relationship?

L: Yeah.

T: And if you think there is no future to the relationship, how does that make you feel?

L: Kinda sick and hopeless, I guess.

T: So there are two feelings here; one is a hot, angry feeling of frustration that Bill won't talk; and a sadder, colder feeling that maybe Bill just isn't interested in you, and the marriage may fall apart.

L: Mmm hmm.

T: So is it the thought that he is not interested, and all that means to you, that makes this so important?

L: Yes, that is what hurts, makes me feel sick.

T: And that's why you feel you have to get him to talk, to find out if he does care, if he is interested?

L: That's it, I need to know. I don't want to be ignored.

T: *(turning to Bill)* Bill, Leanne was very distressed by the argument. From what she has just said, what was it that, from her point of view made you such a problem?

B: She seemed to think that I just don't want to talk to her, but that's not true I ...

T: Just before we move to your point of view, let's make sure we understand Leanne's perspective. So, she felt that you were not interested in talking. Why was that important to her?

B: Because, because ... er ...

T: Because she thinks this means you don't care about her. Rightly or wrongly, it feels to her like you may not love her, that the marriage is in real trouble.

B: Mmh.

T: Leanne, your turn to listen. Please do what Bill did, and just listen. You don't have to agree with what is said, but you do need to hear what Bill felt. Bill tell me about your experience of the interaction.

B: Well I got home, and wham! Leanne is in one of her moods. The new CD is waved around, as if it were evidence of a major crime, and I am Jack the Ripper. I was bushed, the kids in my class had been scrappy all afternoon, and I wanted to decompress. I wander over to the TV to unwind and let hurricane Leanne blow herself out. But there is no way I am going to get a break. We have to talk right now.

T: How did you feel when Leanne was pressuring you to talk?

B: Cornered.

T: So you feel trapped. What happens then?

B: Well, Leanne starts in about how I don't listen, and how she can't stand me ignoring her.

T: What were you thinking at this stage?

B: Here we go again. First the CD issue, and now I don't talk enough.

T: So you felt like you were doing lots wrong according to Leanne?

B: Yeah, sometimes I wonder if she sees any good in me at all.

T: Can you explain that to me.

B: Well, according to Leanne, I spend too much money, I don't talk enough, I don't do enough around the yard, I watch too much TV.

T: So you feels she sees lots of faults in you.

B: Yeah. And the CD was just one in a whole line of things at which I am no good.

T: So when you hear Leanne complain about the CD, it feels like just the latest in a whole series of complaints about you. How do you feel about that?

B: Well, I get mad. I think, hell, why do you bother with me if I'm so flawed?

T: So you wonder if Leanne really is committed to you?

B: Well, it stands to reason to me. If I'm so bad, how can she want to stay?

T: So what happens then?

B: Well, I thought about telling her to get the hell out, if that's how she felt. But then I stopped myself, I just had to get away before I blew my cool. But then she follows me into the bedroom.

T: So you are feeling overwhelmed by the criticism and want to get away, to prevent something bad happening.

B: Yeah.

T: What might happen Bill?

B: I might say "Get out," or throw things, or something.

T: And if you said "Get out"?

B: She might leave.

T: And if you think that she might leave, how does that make you feel?

B: Awful. I don't want Leanne and me to end. I am scared that might happen.

At this point the therapist then drew together the two versions of events. He highlighted that underlying each partner's anger was a fear for the relationship. It was because each did care about the other, and the marriage, that the interaction became so emotionally packed. Leanne's response to that feeling was to approach Bill, demanding to talk about the issues. Bill felt overwhelmed by these demands and withdrew in an attempt to prevent damage. On completion of the task, the couple agreed that the problem of the conflict was due to this demand–withdraw pattern. The next step then was to help them identify what they could do differently to control the conflict.

This approach uses conflict to assist each partner in identifying his or her own cognitive and emotional processes and the communication behaviors that they exhibit. The therapist and each individual client then negotiate self-change goals. Appropriate self-change goals would be trying to use a particular communication skill, taking a small break from the interaction when arousal becomes overwhelming, or challenging directly some of the person's cognitions that elicit the extreme distress.

Another aspect of conflict management is helping couples identify how particular settings may impede the likelihood of successful conflict resolution. For example, Halford et al. (1992) have shown that when certain settings are associated with many competing demands, when there is considerable distraction, and/or either partner has experienced significant, general, extrarelationship stress, there are much higher levels of conflict. Couples can be taught to self-monitor where, when, and about what they have high levels of conflict. Couples can be taught how to restrict potential conflict topics to non-high-risk settings. Simple strategies such as agreeing to talk about money problems or differences about parenting at quiet times, with minimal chance of interruption, often produces substantially better interaction than when these same interactions occur while the other person is distracted (e.g., watching a favorite TV program, or trying to get children ready for school).

Couples who typically avoid conflictual topics usually do so because previous conflictual discussions have escalated into unproductive arguments. Thus, for the avoidant couple, the very process of therapy can instigate further attempts at conflict discussions, which in turn may actually increase the frequency of arguments. Thus, for some couples the initial phases of therapy seem to indicate that things are getting worse. On the one hand, we have an obligation to acknowledge increased conflict as one of the risks of therapy for couples who are identified during the assessment phase as conflict avoidant. On the other hand, it is also important to emphasize that once a conflict ensues, it is then possible to identify what factors are responsible for maintaining it and thereby to do something about it. Sometimes, however, one or both partners may be so concerned about the possible negative effects of conflict that they continue to withdraw or avoid any form of discussion of difficult topics.

Couples usually develop implicit rules about how they manage conflict. These rules are rarely spelled out; sometimes it can be helpful to get couples to identify the sorts of rules that they use to manage conflict, and to self-determine whether as a couple they wish to continue with those rules. In Table 13.6 we describe some of the common rules that couples apply to their conflicts. It is often useful to discuss the implicit rules being used and to solicit suggestions from spouses about possible alternative rules. For example, an implicit rule may be that it is acceptable for someone to raise a discussion about any topic at any time, regardless of the circumstances. Obviously such open access may not be a useful method for managing conflict. It may be more preferable for the individual who has a troublesome, yet important issue, to select an appropriate time and place to talk it through with his or her partner. Then we ask partners to consider the implicit rules in their relationship for handling conflict, what they see as desirable rules, and what they as individuals can do to enhance their current patterns of conflict management.

Finally, we consider the role of problem-solving training, formerly recognized as the cornerstone of conflict management from a behavioral-marital perspective. We now believe that problem solving is one element of a much broader continuum of methods of conflict management. Originally, in teaching problem solving, the goals were to apply a rational, logical approach to providing the couple a range of options, and have them jointly decide on a mutually acceptable course of action. In keeping with our self-management focus, we do not arbitrarily teach people these problem-solving steps. Rather, we suggest to people that each of these general steps are things that some couples have found helpful. We ask the couple to self-evaluate the way in which they currently solve one of their problems, for example, getting them to discuss how they are going to handle a current conflict. If the interaction is unsuccessful, we then ask the couple to identify which of the various steps in problem solving they did and did not implement. In keeping with our self-management focus, we ask partners individually to self-assess their performance at various steps along the way. In other words, we ask partners to consider: "Did they listen to and validate the other person's perspective? Did they clearly state, in a nonattacking way, their own perspective of the problem. Did they allow the conversation to continue until each partner's perspective had been validated? Did they generate a full range of options of what was available to them, and consider each of the options from each partner's perspective? Was a specific option considered for implementation?" We then ask the people to identify specific skills that they could use to try to produce change. If a couple had been unsuccessful in their discussions of a topic, they are asked to discuss it again, emphasizing the techniques just listed.

Robert L. Weiss and
W. Kim Halford

Table 13.6.   Rules for Managing Conflict[a]

The purpose of this guide is to help you decide which rules may be helpful in managing conflict in you relationship. Place a tick beside those rules you wish to implement

1. Either person can raise a topic for discussion at any time

2. If the other person doesn't want to talk, he or she can say "no," but must suggest another time within a day or so.

3. If either person feels the conversation is not working he or she can either (a) suggest a brief time-out or (b) ask to reschedule the discussion.

4. Regularly (at least once a month) do some relationship planning.

5. A partner who wishes to raise a topic that has been a source of repeated conflict in the past should pick a good time to raise that difficult issue. Good times for discussion:

> —Alone together
> —No distractions
> —With time

6. If an argument occurs, use the speaker–listener strategy to restart the conversation.

[a]Adapted from Notarius and Markman (1993).

The benefit of the classical problem-solving approach may be most apparent when people are faced with making complex decisions. However, many of the sources of conflict that couples report are not complex, but rather mundane and repetitive. Who will drop a child off at school, or who should make the bed in the morning, are not difficult decisions, yet they are often a source of major conflict. In our view, these conflicts are due to the thoughts, feelings, and poor conflict-management skills that people have acquired, rather than a deficit in rational problem-solving abilities. Consequently, we recommend the rational problem-solving approach toward the end of therapy, when the problems seem to be particularly complex and difficult.

GENERALIZATION AND MAINTENANCE

Therapists' contacts with couples are limited to interactions held over a period of time in consulting rooms. Often it is presumed that those changes observed in marital inter-actions in this setting predict to more widespread and sustained gains. For example, therapists may assume that observed changes in marital problem solving noted in therapy are associated with equivalent changes at home, or we may assume that as couples report more constructive attributions about each other's behavior in therapy sessions, they are making similar attributions at home. Perhaps more to the point, we assume that such changes are maintained after termination of therapy. Unfortunately, research shows that such changes often do not generalize from therapy to other settings, and that they do not maintain for long periods (Jacobson, 1989; Drabman, Allen, Tarnowski, & Simonian, 1990; Stokes & Baer, 1977).

Even if couples successfully generalize the effects of therapy during the time they are attending sessions, it still may be difficult to maintain these effects. A variety of changes over time may lead to diminished marital satisfaction and functioning. Couples' inter-actions may be influenced by major stressors, such as ill health or financial problems. Other factors having a major negative effect on relationship satisfaction include lifestyle changes produced by having children, having children grow up, changing jobs, and changes in leisure activities. These developmental changes may either prevent the maintenance of interactional patterns acquired in therapy, or they may make the acquired interactional patterns inappropriate.

Settings and Marital Interaction

Too often, both research and practice have adopted a restricted view of the effects of the role of situational variables on marital interaction. In clinical practice, many therapists rely on global reports by the partners to evaluate the progress of therapy (e.g., "How have things been in the past week?"). Such reports rarely attend to the impact of situational variables. Research assessing marital interaction often utilizes self-report inventories that implicitly require the respondent to disregard situational variables by making generalizations about their relationship. For example, Broderick and O'Leary (1986) assessed people's feelings about their partner by having them rate how positively they feel about their partner as a friend, confidant, and so forth. Similarly, Eidelsen and Epstein's (1982) Relationship Beliefs Inventory rates general endorsement of beliefs about relationships such as "Disagreement is destructive," without reference to context. It is one thing to state that "disagreement can be healthy in a relationship" when filling in a form in the therapist's office, and quite another to hold that same belief when confronting a seemingly belligerent spouse.

The crucial variable in assessing marital interactions, naturally enough, is assumed to be the presence of the spouse. By default, it would seem that the variety of household and community settings in which marital interactions occur comprise a relatively homogeneous class of environments. Alternatively, settings can impact communication in significant ways. The concept of "high-risk" settings has grown out of the work on drug abuse and parenting. *High-risk settings* are defined as a complex of setting variables that increase the probability of problematic behavior. Parenting, for example, suggests being in physical settings with competing demands (e.g., in the kitchen preparing a meal and attending to a child), which in turn have been shown to constitute a high-risk setting for poor parenting (Sanders & Christensen, 1985). For people with alcoholism, interpersonal conflict, and interpersonal pressure to drink are high-risk settings for relapse to inappropriate drinking (Marlatt & Gordon, 1985).

Description of high-risk settings for marital communication problems has significant implications for marital therapy; clients may be trained during therapy in skills to cope with high-risk settings. For instance, couples might be taught to recognize some situations as having too many competing demands, or to recognize their own or their partner's mood state as too negative for effective problem solving. Under such circumstances couples could be taught to agree to an immediate solution where required, and to schedule a discussion to negotiate an acceptable permanent solution at an alternative time and situation.

Halford et al. (1992) asked couples to self-monitor occurrence of stressful marital interactions across a 2-week period. Couples recorded times, places, topics of discussion, and prior activities associated with occurrence of stressful interactions. They found that certain times, places, and activities were associated with increased risk for stressful interaction, including being in the kitchen, a weekday, and subjects' rating their day as having been stressful. The topics about which stressful interactions occurred were related to ongoing activities of the partners. In other words, disagreements about child care often developed when one or both partners were engaged in child care; disagreements about household chores often developed in association with doing household chores.

As with antecedents, consequences of distressed marital interaction in natural settings are important. The consequences of assertively confronting one's spouse about a perceived problem may be quite different when done in therapy than when done in front of friends at a social gathering. Clinical practice of marital therapy has paid insufficient attention to the impact of situational variables on marital interaction. The self-regulation approach encourages each partner to experiment with different behaviors in particular settings, thereby determining which behaviors have the desired effects in which settings.

As already noted, when discussing certain topics, many distressed couples encounter failure, which teaches them to simply avoid future discussions about those topics. Partners frequently report that they have "given up talking about that," "found talk never gets any where," and "We just go over the same things time after time." Avoidance of discussion of difficult issues can occur for lengthy periods until situational demands force the couple to attend to that particular issue. For example, a couple who disagrees about shared parenting responsibilities may avoid the topic until one of their children is sick and one of the two working partners needs to stay home to care for the child. Similarly, financial difficulties may not be discussed until unpaid bills have reached a point where they can no longer be ignored (e.g., threats of utility shutoff). Discussions that are thus forced on the couple in this way often occur under time pressure and considerable stress. These factors decrease the chances of effective communication and conflict resolution. Couples need to establish prompts to initiate discussion at times likely to promote effective conflict management, and to develop skills to control destructive conflict in high-risk situations.

A frequent high-risk setting worthy of mention is the very next interaction a couple has after a disagreement. Many distressed couples report that unresolved conflict often leads to repeated arguments about the same topic. Frequently, partners will ruminate about the disagreement, focusing their thoughts on the perceived injustices of the situation, or the blameworthiness of their spouse. It is these very cognitions that maintain their anger. When the topic is raised again, the chance of a repeat argument is high. In contrast, nondistressed couples will often view an argument as a cue to rethink the problem and try to approach their partner in a constructive manner.

Promoting Generalization

Marital therapy usually is arranged so that only the couple and the therapist are present; there are no interruptions, no distractions or competing demands. Discussion time is not pressured, and the therapist has solicited each partner's agreement as to the topic to be discussed. Yet, the settings identified as high risk for stressful interactions are completely different, usually involving discussion of an issue prompted by ongoing activities and multiple competing demands. Given these very different circumstances, we should not be surprised that some couples experience difficulties in applying at home the skills they learn in therapy.

There have been a number of reviews of existing knowledge of how to promote generalization of positive therapeutic effects (e.g., Edelstein, 1989; Stokes & Baer, 1977; Stokes & Osnes, 1988). In order to illustrate the application of these principles to marital therapy, we have extracted some basic guidelines for promoting generalization.

To enhance generalization, we need only to maximize the similarity of therapy and target settings. However, doing therapy in people's homes is often impractical, even though sometimes this can be helpful. Alternatively, it is possible to incorporate crucial elements of the target setting into therapy. Thus, for example, we have children attend some sessions with parents if negative interactions often arise in the presence of the couple's children. If distractions increase the likelihood of negative interaction, then we arrange for distractions. One couple had frequent disagreements when the husband was engrossed in television and unresponsive to his wife. The couple brought a videotape of the husband's favorite football team's last game to the session. While this was being played, the couple practiced various strategies they could use in that setting (e.g., the wife agreed only to interrupt if the topic was urgent, and to do so by standing in front of the television, while the husband agreed to listen when his wife took that step). They were then asked to practice the application of these same strategies at home.

A major difference between therapy and home settings is that most interactions in therapy are signaled, whereas those at home are not. Interactions at home can be signaled by having couples contract to discuss issues at prearranged times and to agree beforehand on the topic. Conversely, unsignaled interactions can be arranged in therapy. For example, toward the end of therapy, we often say that we will ask each of them to raise an issue in a negative manner during a session without warning the other (e.g., being very critical of the other person). Each person's in-session task is now to respond constructively to the "ambush" (unsignaled interaction). The therapist can then observe and assist the respondent to react constructively. Perhaps the metaphor of creating "battle conditions" makes the point even more cogently.

Training across multiple problem areas and settings requires that couples practice new skills in an array of problematic interactions. Successfully applying problem-solving skills to issues with finances during a therapy session does not assure that they will be able to do this for other problems; that is, it is unhelpful to dichotomize couples according to those who do, and those who do not, have particular communication skills. Rather, couples can apply certain skills to some problems in some settings. To be maximally beneficial, therapists and couples need to apply skills across many problem areas and settings.

Throughout this chapter we have emphasized the importance of therapeutic homework tasks. Such tasks promote the application of changed modes of behaving, thinking, and feeling in the settings in which couples interact. By systematically reviewing therapy homework, the therapist gauges the extent to which therapeutic gains are being applied outside the therapy setting. Reviews also prompt therapist and couple to problem-solve further about ongoing problems in particular settings.

We also promote generalization by extracting and emphasizing the general principles underlying specific examples. For example, we might point out a couple's pervasive pattern of withdrawal from conflictual interaction followed by reengagement, followed by withdrawal (a not uncommon pattern in our experience). Once a successful method for breaking this cycle is found, the couple is invited to apply these coping strategies across diverse examples. Each partner is asked to state to the other when he or she thinks the troublesome pattern is happening, and to arrange for a signaled interaction on the problematic topic once the pattern is identified.

This discussion of general principles is not limited to problems in conflict resolution. For one couple, the pattern consisted of their making considerable effort to increase shared activities whenever their relationship was in trouble, yet they made little effort if no relationship problems were evident. The net effect was that the relationship would take repeated nosedives in quality, even though the couple was unaware of this pattern of reduced shared activities. The therapist highlighted the pattern, and time was spent on how the couple could maintain their shared positive activities at a level that was satisfactory to them. (Their solution, albeit a bit lean, was to schedule a monthly dinner during which they discussed the previous month's activities and formulated plans for future activities).

Another important way to promote generalization requires therapists to decrease the degree to which they structure client marital interactions, while increasing the couple's control over the process and content of sessions. Initially, therapists will need to be fairly directive in order to break down heavily overlearned habits and to promote new modes of interaction (e.g., making recommendations about behavior between sessions), but as therapy progresses, it is necessary to ensure that the prompts and consequences that elicit new interactional patterns are present in the couple's day-to-day lives. In other words, each partner needs to be initiating change attempts and identifying solutions.

The following case is an example of how one might decrease therapist control. A husband, Rick, had difficulty in managing his anger; he would break household objects during arguments. Both partners were concerned that he could further lose control and physically abuse his wife. Rick reported that he used to ruminate about the couple's disagreements for days afterwards. During these ruminations, he would attribute the blame to his wife, Maria, and repeatedly tell himself that she had been unreasonable. This would culminate in his attempts to "force his wife to see reason." The therapist and Rick developed a series of anger-reducing self-statements, which were written on a card. The therapist instructed him to read the card out loud to himself three times after any marital argument, and not to initiate any subsequent discussion of the topic until the next therapy session. In the next session, Rick was directed to read the card again, and then to reopen discussion under the guidance of the therapist. The rationale was to arrange an antecedent that would maximize the opportunity for constructive engagement of the couple, and reduce the chance of unhelpful anger or abuse. Over time, several settings in which anger was a problem were dealt with in a similar manner. At a later point in therapy, the following exchange took place between the couple.

> **T:** Rick, both you and Maria are saying that your anger is under better control than before, which is a major gain you have worked hard to achieve.
> **R:** I certainly feel more in control of myself. … I don't let arguments replay in my head and torture me, and feel like I can approach Maria in a more reasonable frame of mind.
> **T:** Maria?
> **M:** I agree, Rick starts much better when we talk. But he still loses his cool and starts shouting sometimes when we argue. He does not let me have my say.
> **R:** Well, you're not perfect on that either, and I'm trying, you know.
> **T:** You both seem to be identifying the anger as a problem in your discussions. I would like you to discuss what could you do about that, okay?
> **M:** Rick, I think we should have a cool-off signal. You know, like a raised hand which says "This is getting out of hand," and we pause for a minute.
> **R:** Okay, yeah. Maybe we could say again what we are discussing at that point. We often get onto all sorts of stuff when we're steamed.

The discussion continued, with the couple developing several strategies for dealing with anger in conflict-resolution discussions. The therapist asked how they would implement these ideas, and again the couple discussed this issue and arrived at a solution. In this example, the therapist prompted the discussion, but then left the development and implementation of solutions to the couple. Through the course of marital therapy, the extent of therapist structuring of process and content needs to decrease, allowing the couple to take increasing responsibility for setting the goals of the session and for identifying the solutions to their difficulties.

Ultimately, our goal is to empower couples to monitor and change their interactions in the settings in which they choose to interact. The whole process of therapy needs to focus on the optimal methods of increasing couples' independence of the therapist in achieving their relationship goals. Clearly, the promotion of generalization is central to the process of therapy.

Maintenance

Maintenance refers to the persistence of the effects of therapy after the end of treatment, although when termination is gradual, defining the end point is difficult. Thus, if initially the therapist sees the couple on a weekly basis, then fades to monthly sessions, and finally only has 6-month follow-up sessions, the point at which treatment was "completed" is somewhat arbitrary. Perhaps there is a better method to express the maintenance question: To what extent do the partners continue to exhibit their new behavioral, cognitive, and affective patterns after contact with the therapist is significantly reduced or stopped entirely?

Jacobson (1989) found that, over a 5-year period, the effects of marital therapy on marital satisfaction gradually dissipated after termination until the satisfaction scores of those who had received therapy were no longer significantly different from scores when they first presented. This might be interpreted as an indication that therapy had failed, since marital problems had not been "cured." However, the couples have enjoyed a period of years in which their marital satisfaction was higher than it otherwise would have been. Does a period of improved quality of marital life count as a success, or should the therapy have produced a permanent effect in order to be of value?

Kendall (1989) argues that expecting permanent behavior change from psychotherapy is an unreasonable expectation, resulting from a misapplication of a metaphor with physical illness. More specifically, he suggests that many people think of therapy only in terms of a permanent removal of the cause of the problem. Just as penicillin may kill bacteria, therapy might be expected to alter personality or produce other immutable intrapsychic changes. However, Kendall argues that a social-learning analysis of behavior problems attributes the cause of clinical problems largely to environmental factors. Therapy at one time cannot be expected to permanently modify the client's environment. Rather, therapy aims to alter crucial aspects of the current environment and the clients' response to that environment. As time passes, other influences modify the environment and clients' functioning. This is analogous to how medical treatment really works, in that we expect the doctor to treat the current problems, but not to guarantee we will never get sick again.

Optimal marital therapy aims not only to improve current functioning, but also to reduce the chance of recurrence of problems. We would be justifiably dissatisfied if the effects of marital therapy disappeared as soon as the couple terminated therapy. However, a significant improvement in marital functioning—sustained over a period of years—would seem a worthwhile achievement even if permanent, high marital satisfaction were not achieved.

There has been little systematic empirical research on the determinants of maintenance of marital therapy effects. Many behavioral marital therapists have suggested that booster sessions may help maintenance effects (e.g., Beach et al., 1990; Stuart, 1980). Booster sessions are additional sessions held after the initial course of therapy, usually

Table 13.7. High-Risk Settings for Future Relationship Problems

Marriage and Life Stress Inventory

The idea of this inventory is to assess how different life stressors may impact on your marriage in the future. For each item, rate how likely as a percentage (0–100%) each event is to happen to you in the next 6 months. Then rate how much stress this would put on your marital relationship from 0—*No Effect* to 100—*Devastating*.

Event	Likelihood this will occur in next 6 months (0–100%)	Stress on marriage if it happened (0–100)
Illness or injury that kept you in bed a week or more, or took you to hospital	_____	_____
Major change in your sleeping habits	_____	_____
Change to a new type of work	_____	_____
Change in your responsibilities at work:		
(a) More responsibilities	_____	_____
(b) Less responsibilities	_____	_____
(c) Promotion	_____	_____
(d) Transfer	_____	_____
Experiencing troubles at work		
(a) With your boss	_____	_____
(b) With your co-workers	_____	_____
(c) With people you supervise	_____	_____
Change in residence		
(a) A move within the same town or city	_____	_____
(b) A move to a different town, city or state	_____	_____
Major change in your living conditions (home improvements or a decline in you home or neighborhood)	_____	_____
In-law problems	_____	_____
Spouse beginning or ceasing work outside the home	_____	_____
Wife becoming pregnant	_____	_____
Wife having a miscarrige or abortion	_____	_____
A major personal achievement	_____	_____
Sexual difficulties	_____	_____
Beginning or ceasing school or college	_____	_____
Change of school or college	_____	_____
Vacation	_____	_____
Change in your social activities (clubs, movies, visiting)	_____	_____
A minor violation of the law	_____	_____
A new, close, personal relationship	_____	_____
A "falling out" of a close, personal relationship	_____	_____
Taking on a moderate purchase, such as TV, car, freezer, etc.	_____	_____

Table 13.7. (*Continued*)

Taking on a major purchase or a mortgage loan, such as a home, business property, etc.	_____	_____
Experiencing a foreclosure on a mortgage or loan	_____	_____
Experiencing a major change in finances		
(a) Increased income	_____	_____
(b) Decreased income	_____	_____
(c) Credit-rating difficulties	_____	_____

spaced further apart than those during the regular course of therapy; booster sessions also focus on the maintenance of gains achieved by the end of treatment. Whisman (1990) reviewed the use of booster sessions across a number of different areas of clinical problems. He concluded that booster sessions were moderately successful in improving the maintenance of therapy gains with problems such as weight loss, alcohol abuse, treatment of depression, and smoking cessation. Whisman found common characteristics in the more successful booster sessions: sessions focused on the subject's self-reinforcing for positive gains that had been made over the course of therapy; identification of possible high-risk settings that might promote relapse; training people in specific skills to cope with such high-risk settings; and encouraging clients to put themselves in environments that promoted maintenance.

Application of these general principles to marital therapy provides us with a number of important strategies to help maintain gains. It is essential that clients reinforce themselves for positive gains they have made. Assessment of outcome at the end of therapy should not only tell the therapist and client about the degree of success of therapy, but it should also serve as a reinforcer of the positive gains made. For example, whenever a couple reports substantially improved communication skills and substantially increased marital satisfaction, they must also recognize the association between these two gains. The importance of continuing to use their newly acquired communication skills cannot be overemphasized.

One way to promote continuing use of newly acquired skills is to plan ahead for implementing maintenance. For example, the couple may schedule regular reviews of how they are doing in their relationship. We would ask couples regularly to set aside a time on a weekly or fortnight basis, during which they would discuss the positive aspects of their relationship as noted over the last couple of weeks. Particular problem areas that had arisen also would be discussed at this time. Prior to such a discussion, partners could be encouraged to read through a card reminding them of the sorts of steps that they wish to follow in trying to solve the problem together. For example, if husband has often had difficulty with active listening skills, there could be a specific instruction to actively listen and to attempt to paraphrase his wife's comments. These regular schedulings of events with specific built-in antecedents are intended to help maintain the behavior changes achieved.

Identifying potential circumstances that might lead to relapse is another important maintenance strategy. Toward the end of therapy we ask couples to fill out the future high-risk settings inventory (presented in Table 13.7). Situations listed are those we have found often associated with relapse after the end of marital therapy. We ask couples to fill out how likely it is that these events will happen to them and the probability that, if such events were to occur, they would cause relapse. The couple then engages in problem-solving discussion to identify what they could do should these situations arise. The rationale is not only to prepare people for the most likely events that might precipitate relapse, but also by getting people to have such discussions across a range of possible future high-risk settings, they will generalize this learning to almost all of the possible high-risk situations that may develop in the future.

When should couples return to therapy? In our experience it is often difficult for couples to decide that problems have reached a point at which they should seek further help. It is often useful to make explicit that this is a difficult decision, and to highlight how the couple may make such a decision in the future. The healthiness or positive aspect of seeking additional assistance when required should be emphasized. If the couple's quality of marital functioning diminishes somewhat, it should be seen as a lapse, rather than a loss of all their previous progress. Couples need to be reminded that they have the necessary skills for increasing relationship satisfaction. Ultimately, our goal is to help people to make changes in a variety of home settings, and for those changes to be long lasting.

PROBLEMS IN IMPLEMENTATION

Therapists should be optimistic about their effectiveness and their potential for effecting change. Nonetheless, there are reality constraints to that optimism, constraints that should be evident before one launches a treatment plan. This section discusses some of these impediments to successful treatment planning. Ultimately, all marital therapy is elective: One cannot mandate that a couple improve their relationship. Realistically, marital therapy requires a considerable commitment, and conjoint therapy is not appropriate simply because the couple arrives at therapy together. If a partner has mostly "left" the relationship, expressing more than mere ambivalence, it is questionable whether marital therapy can (or should) attempt to turn that around. This is different from helping resolve ambivalence, which may be responsive to new evidence that things can be different. To this end, we recommend reviewing the assessment results: An MSI score of 4 or greater, a DAS score of less than 70, and an ACQ total score greater than 24 indicate a low probability of successful therapy outcome if one defines success as a revitalized marriage. In such instances, clients should be informed of the amount of work required and the likelihood of success.

From a different perspective, conjoint therapy can be the treatment of choice even when initially only one partner presents. Often the presenting partner expresses doubts about the other's willingness to engage in therapy, although this conclusion may be based on unreliable data (e.g., she or he refused to go to therapy at an earlier time). The better test would be for the therapist and presenting client to problem-solve where, when, and with what words the client might extend an invitation to the partner to join therapy to improve the relationship. In addition, or alternatively, the therapist could contact the nonpresenting spouse, (with the presenting client's permission), and invite attendance at therapy. A useful approach by the therapist may follow along these lines: "Your partner has seen me because she (or he) is concerned about the relationship between you two. She (or he) cares about you and what happens to your relationship. I would find it very helpful to hear your view of the relationship. Without your help, I am frankly quite limited in what I can do for either one of you. Would you be willing to come and see me so I can better understand your relationship?" Often an invitation from a third party (i.e., not one of the spouses) decenters the stalemate sufficiently to allow the necessary change.

Sometimes marital therapy cannot be accomplished because individual psychopathology predominates the clinical picture. For example, if alcohol abuse, depression, or other disorders severely affect one partner, individual therapy may be more appropriate. We suggest three considerations that should influence the decision about whether to proceed with individual or couple therapy. First is the couple's stated beliefs about the relationship between individual and marital problems: A positive predictor of the appropriateness of couple therapy is a shared view that individual problems are a consequence of relationship problems. Second, consider the priorities the partners attach to resolving different aspects of the problem. If one partner is very ill from alcohol abuse, reducing the harm from drinking may need to be a first priority. Third, can the individual with significant psychopathology engage in couple therapy? Severe alcohol abuse, depression, psychosis, or other problems may require treatment before conjoint couple therapy is realistic. In the not uncommon instance of the partners and therapist being unable initially to clarify the three issues described earlier, the clinical assessment can be used to guide decision making. The relative timing of the onset of individual problems and marital problems can generate hypotheses about causal connections between individual and couple problems (e.g., "She only became depressed after we started having so many problems"). A functional analysis of the interrelationship of problems within the current relationship is essential. For example, when alcohol and marital problems coexist, does marital conflict initiate drinking binges, or does drinking initiate marital conflict? In many instances the relationship between individual and couple problems is reciprocal and couple therapy can be very useful in such cases. Depression and alcohol abuse have been treated within the context of marital-therapy models similar to the one being documented here, although with some modifications to address the individual problems of one of the partners (e.g., Beach et al., 1990; O'Farrell, 1993).

Should we agree to marital therapy if violence has been, and continues to be, an issue? Spousal abuse has become so politicized that one hardly dares make recommendations. Unquestionably, the safety of the target of abuse is foremost. In assessing the risks associated with violence, it is important to establish the frequency, severity, and predictability of violence in the relationship. CTS offers a reliable means for doing that assessment. One episode of mutual pushing and shoving in the context of a marital argument should not preclude marital therapy. On the other hand, repeated, violent wife beating by a male who has convictions for assault, and who is heavily abusing alcohol, would contraindicate couple therapy. Men who batter their wives are a very heterogeneous group in terms of the frequency and severity of violence, and the extent to which men's violence is directed exclusively toward their partners versus being more generally assaultive (Holtzworth-Munro & Stuart, 1994). It is likely that as our knowledge of the causes and consequences of these different patterns increases, we will be better able to predict the risks of further violence and the appropriateness of conjoint therapy. In the meantime, we counsel caution in using couple therapy in instances in which assault has resulted in injury.

In cases of marital violence, we need to address short-term versus long-term solutions to violence: by *short-term* we mean immediate safety concerns, such as seeking shelter if necessary. This is different from having to decide whether a nonviolent relationship is possible and/or amenable to intervention. We recommend that unless there can be positive assurances that the target person (almost always the wife) will be safe from harm, we should not proceed with marital therapy. In our experience, abusing spouses are well versed in making verbal promises of change without actually changing; in cases of severe violence, the perpetrator's simple (repeated) assurances fail to persuade us that the victim is safe.

Last, we consider some process issues in which the focus is on managing the rules or boundaries of marital therapy. Spouse A calls between sessions with vital "information" about spouse B. ("I think you should know that Henry hates my kids and always has"; "I think you need to know that my wife has a long history of having affairs.") These one-side disclosures, although certainly newsworthy, can create the appearance of unintended coalitions: As therapist, you now know something that heretofore has not been made public ("So Henry, I understand you're not fond of Mary's kids?").

Many so-called process issues are better dealt with before they appear as problems. Having explicit rules before agreeing to a treatment regimen as to how "confidences" will be handled is a must. Yet, one does not wish to cut off important information (e.g., that Joe's drinking is rapidly undermining the family finances). One facilitative move early on would be to say something along these lines:

> **T:** From time to time, one or both of you may choose to tell me something that you didn't say in front of the other person or in our sessions. If you do that, I will assume that your intent is for me to do or say something that will bring the issue to a head in order to make it less of a problem. In other words, you are asking me to bring it up, because you don't feel able to do so yourself. I will do that, but I will do that in a way that I feel will be most helpful. You may not want to hear about it, but I will decide how best to use the information. So, if you hear me mention some family secret, you can assume that this is something I believe we need to look at, even if it means embarrassment or risks making one of you feel the other guy has done you dirty.

In this way the therapist is acting as a temporary message conduit; eventually the partners will have to establish their own rules.

CASE EXAMPLE

Assessment

The following case example is a little unusual in that the couple was not married and had lived together in the same household only some of the time when they presented. However, this case illustrates why it is that therapists must avoid preconceptions about how mutually satisfying relationships can develop and be sustained. Because during the initial conjoint session the couple collaboratively told the story of their relationship and their reasons for coming in, the first interview was conducted conjointly.

Nancy (age 37) was a postgraduate fine arts student and Mark (age 29) was a social worker at a local counseling service. They had a 4-year relationship and a daughter Angela (age 3). They were not married and reported they had no intention of getting married, but stated they were committed to the relationship. At the time of presentation, Nancy and Angela were living together in a house. Mark shared a house with his sister, and visited Nancy and Angela every night after work, and stayed with them on weekends. This living arrangement had existed for the last 2 years; prior to that time the couple had lived in the house now occupied by Nancy.

Nancy and Mark met each other at a party about 4 years ago. At the time, each had recently ended long-term relationships, and neither saw themselves as being interested in a long-term relationship. They were strongly attracted to each other and had a passionate sexual affair that each reported they expected to be brief. Mark was planning an extended overseas holiday, and Nancy was planning a return to study that might have meant changing states. Nancy forgot the low-dose contraceptive pill she had been taking and became pregnant. She felt she could not undergo an abortion and decided she would have the child. When she told Mark, he accepted her decision and undertook to share responsibility for the child.

Mark took his planned holiday but cut it short to be with Nancy in the last stages of her pregnancy. They moved in together with the intention of living as a couple. They reported that the last stages of pregnancy and early phases of childrearing were quite difficult; they did not know each other all that well and the transition to parenthood required changes in lifestyle they had not anticipated. About 1 year after Angela was born, they found they were arguing frequently, each felt stressed, and there was little positive feeling between them. Mark moved out to live with his sister but continued to share parenting roles with Nancy. Both reported this separation reduced frequency of their arguments, but there was still considerable tension between them.

At the end of the first session the couple stated that they wanted to improve their ability to communicate effectively together. Their reason was that, if they were to stop being a couple, they still felt a need to share parenting of Angela and to negotiate a good arrangement for her. If they were to remain a couple, then resolving conflict with less acrimony was important.

Between sessions the partners completed and mailed to the therapist the Dyadic Adjustment Scale (DAS), the Marital Status Inventory (MSI), the Conflict Tactics Scale (CTS) and the Areas of Change Questionnaire (ACQ). Mark scored 95 and Nancy 92 on the DAS, indicating mild distress for both partners. The version of the MSI they completed was an adaptation for couples in committed but unmarried relationships. Each scored 4 on this scale, indicating that each was giving some active consideration to ending the relationship. The mild level of the distress is prognostic of good outcome, but the steps taken toward separation and the limited time spent together were seen as predictive of poorer outcome for the relationship. The CTS reports indicated that physical aggression was not occurring in the relationship, which each partner confirmed individually.

On the ACQ, Mark's most requested changes were for Nancy to argue less, accept praise more, and express her emotions more clearly. He reported that in order to improve the relationship, he felt he needed to argue less, spend more time with Angela, and work late less often. Nancy requested most change in Mark's having sex more often, arguing less, and being less disciplinarian with Angela. She felt that she needed to pay more attention to her appearance, argue less, and express her emotions more clearly.

In Week 2, I (WKH) spoke with each partner individually and discussed the desired changes each sought in the relationship. While one partner was being interviewed, the other completed the Communication Patterns Questionnaire (CPQ; Christensen & Sullaway, 1984), which assesses use of patterns such as mutual avoidance of conflict, demand–withdraw, and mutual negative escalation. In individual interviews, each partner verbally confirmed the written reports; reducing destructive conflict and improving communication were seen as the most important goals by each partner. Both identified that they often disagreed about the amount of time they were spending together, and how to parent Angela.

In his interview, Mark reported that Nancy wanted him to spend more time at their house and to be more active in parenting. Mark felt pressured by these demands. He also reported that he often felt stressed by his counseling duties, and found going home to Nancy and Angela stressful when he was very tired. Finally, Mark raised concern about his ability to sustain a relationship. He reported having felt very constricted when he and Nancy were living together full time. He felt unsure about whether his ambivalence about his commitment to Nancy was because he found it difficult to make a commitment to anyone, or if it was problem about how he felt about Nancy. On the one hand, he felt she was a very special, warm person, but he was unsure if he felt passionate about her.

Nancy reported some resentment at the fact that she was doing the majority of the parenting of Angela. This had slowed down her study, and she felt Mark was not really sharing the burdens of parenting. Nancy also expressed concern at the relative infrequency with which she and Mark had fun times together, and the infrequency with which they had sex together. She wondered about Mark's attraction to her and was concerned that perhaps she should pay more attention to her appearance.

At the beginning of the third session, the couple was asked to discuss the issue of parenting Angela, which they both agreed was a key problem. As the partners had verbalized an appreciation of their own contribution to the relationship problems in the earlier individual and conjoint interviews, I asked them to self-assess their communication skills at the completion of this discussion using the checklist in Table 13.5. Unfortunately the discussion became fairly heated, and they were unable to focus their attention on the self-evaluation task. When asked to identify their own communication weaknesses, each tended to blame the partner for what went wrong. Much of the rest of the session focused on debriefing the couple on the process.

In Session 4, the therapist described the assessment information to the couple. Beginning with the interview reports, I noted that their relationship history was not ideal for developing a sense of voluntary engagement in a relationship. Each had felt somewhat trapped initially, and a sense of responsibility had overwhelmed a sense of fun between them. The need to develop more fun was identified during this discussion as another goal for therapy. Based on the DAS and ACQ self-report measures, it was suggested that the partners saw therapy as fine tuning a relationship that was mildly unsatisfactory. This perception was endorsed by both partners. The key targets for change were identified as improved communication and conflict management, negotiating the sharing of parenting and household tasks, and improving the quality time the couple had together. I then reviewed the communication task from the previous week, noting how the couple had been unable during "battle conditions" to identify constructive actions to change their poor conflict management. Enhancing each partners' ability to self-correct destructive conflict management was defined as a goal. Commitment was a final issue of discussion. It was resolved by each partner to work together to enrich the relationship as much as possible in the next 4 weeks, and then to review whether they wished to remain in the relationship and therapy at that time.

Therapy

Sessions 5 to 8 occurred weekly and targeted two areas: (1) increasing positive, fun relationship activities, and (2) communication skills training. Two strategies were employed to encourage greater quality time together. The couple completed the Inventory of Rewarding Activities (IRA; Birchler & Weiss, 1977). This is a 100-item inventory of specific activities in which the partners report on the frequency with which these activities have been undertaken in the last 4 weeks, with whom the activity was done (alone, with spouse, with spouse and others, with others but not spouse), and whether the partner wanted to do more of that activity. Each partner then read the other person's list and was asked to select and organize at least one activity per week that he or she believed would be fun for both of them.

The second activity was the organization of a planned date, as described by Annon (1976). In this activity, one partner takes responsibility for organizing a couple date. The organizer sets the mood and tone of the activity, and can request the other person to fit in with the activity (e.g., wearing particular clothing to suit the activity). All aspects of the activity are the responsibility of the organizer, including child-care arrangements. The activity does not have to be expensive or difficult to organize, but must be selected to be fun and to extend the couple's current range of pleasurable activities. Mark chose to go to a bookstore together and then to coffee, and Nancy prepared a special dinner to eat at home while Angela was out at her mother's home. Both of these activities went well, and the couple was asked to identify extra activities each could take responsibility for organizing.

Communication skills training consisted of the couple discussing low-conflict topics in the session, using the communication skills checklist to self-assess their own communication skills. In the process of this training, Nancy mentioned that she felt Mark did not know much about the course she was taking, or show much interest in her study. After negotiation, the couple was set the task of Mark asking Nancy about the course, how she was doing in it, and how she felt about where it was leading. They did this task between sessions and reviewed the tape in the next session. In subsequent weeks, each partner talked to the other about their days as assigned tasks, and the couple became more confident about their communication skills.

In Week 7, the couple came in reporting an argument about parenting. Together they reported that Mark had been late getting home (about 9:00 P.M.) one night, and he criticized Nancy for allowing Angela to be up so late. Nancy was angry that he was late, and that he was criticizing her parenting. An affect-exploration procedure, as described earlier in the chapter, was used. In this process, Nancy stated that she questioned Mark's commitment to the relationship and felt that they needed to be living together full time if the relationship was to work. She described that she felt burdened by her parenting responsibilities and felt Mark was not doing his fair share.

Mark responded to the affect exploration, acknowledging his difficulty in making a firm commitment to the relationship. Mark noted that he had not ever really committed to any relationship, and described his fear of being truly committed and it not working out. A combination of the vertical arrow technique and gentle challenging led him to conclude that if he were ever to have a really close relationship, he would need to take the risk of putting his all into the relationship, but it still might not work out. Mark made a statement that he would increase his involvement, with responsibility for the care of Angela as a first step toward making this commitment. Following on from this process with Mark and Nancy, Mark suggested that the two of them discuss other ways in which he could support Nancy in her study. The discussion about that issue had helped him to realize the importance of the study to Nancy, and that he wished to help her achieve her goals.

In Week 8, the couple reviewed the tape of their discussion, and each felt very positive about the improvements in their communication. Noting the increasing rate of pleasurable activities, the couple together queried how much more therapy might be necessary. It was agreed to have a session 2 weeks later to review the maintenance of progress. In the intervening time, each partner agreed to organize at least one pleasurable couple activity. They also wanted to discuss the issue of whether Mark would move in with Nancy and Angela full time.

In Week 10, the couple reported that they had an argument in the first few days after the previous session, and that each had felt hurt by the interaction. Following that argument, neither partner had organized a pleasant couple activity, and they had not had the discussion as to whether Mark would move in full time. They were discouraged about the relationship and how they had fallen back to old habits in just 2 weeks. The argument occurred at the evening meal. Angela had refused to come to the table when called by Nancy for dinner, saying she wanted to see the end of a TV program. Mark had said that was all right, and Nancy had felt this was unreasonable. They argued in front of Angela, who became upset, and Mark had left. Again an affect exploration procedure was followed. Mark, in his recount of his experience, reported that he had had a very stressful day at work, and that Angela was whining when she asked to watch TV, and he just wanted her to stop. It was noted that many of the couple's arguments occurred in the late afternoon and evening. Nancy recounted how for her, Angela's delaying the mealtime meant it would be later before her chores for the day were completed. She also noted how in the morning, if Angela had been late to bed, she was hard to get up in time to get to child care while Nancy went to study.

We noted the importance of the couple developing some agreed on rules for child management. We also noted that when Mark was stressed by work it was a high-risk time for relationship arguments. Mark and the therapist problem-solved specific steps he could take to prevent work stress impacting on the relationship with Nancy. Mark identified playing relaxing music in the car as a way to prevent him from worrying about work during the commute home, and the importance of focusing on being positive in his initial greeting to Nancy and Angela. He also felt he would enjoy playing with Angela when he first got home, which would free Nancy from child supervision while she prepared the evening meal. (Nancy did almost all food preparation in the household, while Mark cleared up after the meals. Both reported this was a satisfactory arrangement for them.)

The therapist discussed the postargument phase with the couple as a high-risk time for further relationship deterioration. Nancy described how she had been angry at Mark for just leaving, because she felt that he was avoiding commitment. Mark agreed that leaving was not always helpful. They identified some positive coping self-statements that each could use after an argument during a period of time-out from each other (e.g., "Was that really all that important?" "What did I contribute to the problem?" "It will help if I calm myself so that I can decide what to do next." "What can I do to repair the damage we have done?"). The importance of making an effort to do positive things with each other when the relationship is strained was emphasized. By avoiding being positive during that time they ensured that relationship interactions would be negative.

Based upon the this analysis of the problem, I asked each partner to set some goals for themselves in terms of behaviors that would reduce the chance of arguments leading to major reductions in relationship enjoyment. Mark and Nancy independently each resolved to (1) apologize after an argument for his or her contribution, and (2) utilize the speaker–listener technique to discuss the issue about which the argument occurred, offering to be the listener first. The couple resolved to discuss issues about parenting in terms of when each thought Angela should be going to bed, and how to respond to noncompliance by Angela to an instruction. They were asked to bring back a brief set of written rules they agreed to, and to tape their discussion. In addition one of them was to organize a couple activity (the therapist did not specify who). It was agreed to have three more weekly sessions and then review progress.

In Week 11, the couple brought back their written parenting agreement. The therapist reviewed the rules and suggested the couple add the rule that each would support the other in their instructions to Angela, even if they disagreed with the instruction at the time. They were then to discuss the issue later in private. Each person saw the importance of supporting the other's parenting efforts. The discussion itself went well, and they self-evaluated their communication skills as improving again. Nancy had organized a brief outing to a coffee shop on the weekend, which they both enjoyed, and Mark volunteered that he had a couple of ideas for activities to surprise Angela with in the next week.

In Weeks 12 and 13, the couple negotiated rules for managing conflict as a homework task. They agreed to make use of brief time-out periods when the arguments became heated, to make use of the speaker–listener strategy to recommence the discussion, and to attempt to select quiet times to raise discussion of major concerns. During this time, Nancy reported that she was no longer seeking an increase in the time she and Mark were together during the week. She reported that, with the increased support from Mark for her study, she had extra time to see her friends. She reported that the nontraditional nature of their relationship had its attractions.

Toward the end of the session in Week 13, the couple reported that they felt their need for therapy was diminishing but were concerned things might go wrong once therapy ended. In Session 14, therapy focused on events that might lead to deterioration in their relationship. Factors such as increased work stress, difficulties with Angela, and competing demands for their time outside the relationship were mentioned. The couple was asked to problem-solve what they could do to prevent these factors from interfering with the progress they had made in their relationship. In one example, Nancy noted that Mark's longtime male friend was coming to town, whom she did not like that much. Last time this man had visited she had felt Mark paid little attention to her and Angela. Nancy had examinations coming up with her course, and was concerned that she might lose Mark's support at an important time to her. The couple was asked to discuss this issue at home and to report back on what they resolved.

In Session 14, the couple reported they had worked out an arrangement for the time when Mark's friend was in town. Mark agreed to see him only on a particular weekend, and to see him without Nancy. The therapist asked each partner to review the changes he or she had made across the course of therapy, and what each felt had made the most important difference. Each partner was then asked to identify concrete steps each would take to sustain these behavior changes. In so doing, the therapist faded the level of prompts and reinforcers used to promote self-regulation within the relationship, thereby enhancing maintenance.

A follow-up session was scheduled in Week 18. In this session, the couple again completed the DAS and mailed this to the therapist prior to the sessions. The DAS scores for Mark and Nancy were 123 and 118, respectively. The therapist then completed a second feedback session in which he summarized the changes the couple had made individually and conjointly. In essence, the couple had achieved most of the goals they had set for themselves. Nancy reported that, even if the relationship had a limited duration, she felt good about what existed now and felt Mark was committed to being a good parent with her. Mark reported feeling comfortable with the existing arrangement. Three months later, a follow-up session was scheduled. The couple canceled the 3-month session, with Nancy reporting that they were fine and did not feel the need to come in. Mark called 6 months after therapy terminated and requested a conjoint session. In that session, the couple reported that they felt they had let the couple activities slip a bit and were concerned. The therapist prompted the couple to problem-solve what to do immediately, and how to prevent a recurrence of the problem. The couple resolved to hold at least fortnightly planning sessions. The goal of those sessions was to plan joint activities and to ensure the pleasure quotient was maintained. In a subsequent 6-month telephone follow-up call, the couple reported that they were getting on well. They had retained their living arrangement.

The case is atypical, in that the couple had an unusual relationship history and unconventional living arrangement. The case is typical, in that therapy did not proceed smoothly from assessment-to-goal definition to goal attainment. Rather, the couple experienced both therapy highs when progress seemed rapid, and therapy lows when the relationship had recurrent difficulties. The case also illustrates how couples can negotiate difficult issues, such as the level of relationship involvement and independence, in creative ways. It is noteworthy that the partners' seemingly disparate initial goals (Nancy wanting to live together full time, and Mark not wanting to do this) were resolved not by rational problem solving but by changes in the partners' stated goals. Nancy lost the wish to live with Mark full time when their relationship was changing in other ways.

SUMMARY

There are a number of features that, by way of summary, distinguish the approach to couple therapy described in this manual. Perhaps most noteworthy are the extensive references to the empirical literature that run throughout these pages. Whenever possible, we have tried to demonstrate that our approach to marital and couple therapy interacts greatly with what we know empirically at this time about relationships. In this regard, we, ourselves, have changed direction from what earlier was a much more direct attempt to teach couples how to change one another, to one that now emphasizes self-regulation. Nonetheless, this newer formulation—focusing on what the individual can do to achieve his or her own relationship ends—is still very much based on what we consider to be sound behavioral ideas. For example, therapies of all sorts seek not only to alleviate current distress but we hope also to engender new coping skills. However, as noted earlier, the evidence for unplanned generalization is weak at best. Therefore, we deem it essential to provide therapists with techniques that are designed to increase the likelihood that skills acquired in therapy will be functional after therapy. Nor have we abandoned the central role that situations play in determining behavior. Based on current research on settings, we have pinpointed some very specific techniques for helping couples manage their own affective, behavioral, and cognitive processes.

The approach presented here rests quite heavily on assessment. In our experience, practitioners generally are loath to spend time on systematic assessment. Couples present sufficient complexity to warrant our taking the time to develop an understanding of these relationship patterns. Perhaps given unlimited time, anyone could develop a comprehensive understanding. But to do so in a reasonable length of time is the hallmark of the marital assessment approach we offer. Assessment, although burdensome, is the key to effective planning. Assessment, as discussed here, encourages therapists to generate testable hypotheses about relationship dysfunction. Someone once said that there is nothing as practical a good theory. Not only has practice stimulated theory in this area, but theory has generated studies of many of the intervention techniques we recommend.

In one sense, behavioral couple therapy must be realistic in order to be serviceable. Thus, we emphasize giving careful thought to which couples, under what circumstances, we can realistically hope to help. We have argued that not every couple presenting for "marital therapy" is appropriate for that modality. We have enumerated some of the limiting conditions.

Finally, we present a case that certainly cannot be considered an artificial textbook example. Part of the challenge of marital therapy is that there are no textbook cases! As clinicians, we have broader or narrower repertories of intervention techniques. Our case example demonstrates how marital therapy is an accommodation between what we might like to accomplish and what the couple would like to accomplish (or perhaps is capable of accomplishing). Motivation for change is always an issue in deciding about therapy. By encouraging individuals to set their own relationship goals, but asking them to design intervention tactics, we put the motivational ball in their court, so to speak. A danger of BCT is also one of its very successes; with such an active form of therapy, with so much emphasis on innovation, therapists run the risk of working harder than the clients. By engaging spouses as we do, encouraging them to set and monitor their own goals, we guard against the risk of "doing too much" for the client. It is perhaps worth reminding ourselves that the true functional control in the relationships we consult with lies with the partners themselves; we are only a very small part of the drama of relationship intimacy.

APPENDIX: AVAILABILITY OF ASSESSMENT INSTRUMENTS

The following information lists availability of assessment instruments described in the manual. Some are copyrighted and not available in the public domain.

I. *Areas of Change Questionnaire (ACQ)*: Individual forms as well as computer-administered formats, available through MultiHealth Systems.
   See also:
   Margolin, G., Talovic, S. & Weinstein, C. D. (1983). Areas of Change Questionnaire: A practical approach to marital assessment. *Journal of Consulting and Clinical Psychology, 51*, 920–931.

II. The following copyrighted instruments are available from the Oregon Marital Studies Program (OMSP), Department of Psychology, University of Oregon, Eugene, OR 97403
   A. *Inventory of Rewarding Activities (IRA)*: An extensive listing of activities done alone, with spouse, with others; indicates present frequencies as well as desired frequencies.
   B. *Cost–Benefit Exchange (C-B)*: Computer scoring and item printout also available through OMSP.
   C. *Spouse Observation Checklist (SOC)*: Behavior checklist covering 400-plus items for 7-day periods.
   D. *Marital Status Inventory (MSI)*: 14-item steps to divorce scale.

III. An alternative to the CAST for alcohol screening is the *Self-Administered Short Michigan Alcoholism Screening Test (SMAST)*.
   See also:
   Selzer, M. L., Vinokur, A., van Rooijen, L. A. (1975). A self-administered short Michigan Alcoholism screening test (SMAST). *Journal of the Study of Alcohol, 36*, 117–126.

REFERENCES

Annon, J. (1976). *Behavioral treatment of sexual problems*. New York: Harper & Row.

Arias, I., & Beach, S. R. H. (1987). Validity of self-reports of marital violence. *Journal of Family Violence, 2,* 139–149.

Azrin, N. H., Naster, B. J., & Jones, R. (1973). A rapid learning-based procedure for marital counselling. *Behaviour Research and Therapy, 11,* 365–382.

Baucom, D. H., & Epstein, N. (1990). *Cognitive behavioral marital therapy*. New York: Brunner/Mazel.

Baucom, D. H., & Lester, G. W. (1986). The usefulness of cognitive-restructuring as an adjunct to behavioral marital therapy. *Behavior Therapy, 17,* 385–403.

Beach, S. R. H., Arias, I., & O'Leary, K. D. (1986). The relationship of marital satisfaction and social support to depressive symptomatology. *Journal of Psychopathology and Behavioral Assessment, 8,* 305–316.

Beach, S. R. H., & O'Leary, K. D. (1986). The treatment of depression occurring in the context of marital discord. *Behavior Therapy, 17,* 43–49.

Beach, S. R. H., Sandeen, E. E., & O'Leary, K. D. (1990). *Depression in marriage*. New York: Guilford Press.

Beck, A. T., Ward, C. H., Mendelson, M., Mock, J. E., & Erbaugh, J. K. (1961). An inventory for measuring depression. *Archives of General Psychiatry, 4,* 451–571.

Behrens, B. C., Sanders, M. R., & Halford, W. K. (1990). Behavioral marital therapy: An evaluation of treatment effects across high and low risk settings. *Behavior Therapy, 21,* 423–433.

Birchler, G. B., & Weiss, R. L. (1977). *Inventory of Rewarding Activities*. Eugene, OR: Oregon Marital Studies Program, University of Oregon.

Bloom, B., Asher, S., & White, S. (1978). Marital disruption as a stressor: Review and analysis. *Psychological Bulletin, 85,* 967–880.

Broderick, J., & O'Leary, K. D. (1986). Contribution of affect, attitudes, and behavior to marital satisfaction. *Journal of Consulting and Clinical Psychology, 54,* 514–517.

Cascardi, M., Langhinrichsen, J., & Vivian, D. (1992). Marital aggression: Impact, injury, and health correlates for husbands and wives. *Archives of Internal Medicine, 152,* 1178–1184.

Christensen, A., Jacobson, N. S., & Babcock, J. (1995). Integrative behavior couple therapy. In N. S. Jacobson & A. S. Gurman (Eds.), *Clinical handbook of couple therapy* (pp. 31–64). New York: Guilford Press.

Christensen, A., & Sullaway, M. (1984). *Communication Patterns Questionnaire*. Unpublished questionnaire, University of California, Los Angeles.

Dadds, M. R., Schwartz, S., & Sanders, M. R. (1987). Marital discord and treatment outcome in the treatment of child conduct disorders. *Journal of Consulting and Clinical Psychology, 55,* 396–403.

Drabman, R. S., Allen, S., Tarnowski, K. J., & Simonian, S. J. (1990). Behavior modification with children: The generalisation trap. *Behaviour Change, 7,* 63–171.

Edelstein, B. (1989). Generalization: Terminology, methodological and conceptual issues. *Behavior Therapy, 20,* 357–364.

Eidelsen, R. J., & Epstein, N. (1982). Cognition and relationship maladjustment: Development of a measure of dysfunctional relationship beliefs. *Journal of Consulting and Clinical Psychology, 50,* 715–720.

Elvy, G. A., & Wells, J. E. (1984). The Canterbury Alcoholism Screening Test (CAST): A detection instrument for use with hospitalised patients. *New Zealand Medical Journal, 97,* 111–115.

Emery, R. E., Joyce, S. A., & Fincham, F. D. (1987). The assessment of child and marital problems. In K. D. O'Leary (Ed.), *Assessment of marital discord* (pp. 223–262). Hillsdale, NJ: Erlbaum.

Fincham, F. D., & Bradbury, T. D. (1990). *The psychology of marriage*. New York: Guilford Press.

Glenn, N. D., & Weaver, C. N. (1981). The contribution of marital happiness to global happiness. *Journal of Marriage and the Family, 43,* 161–168.

Glick, P. C. (1989). Remarried families, stepfamilies and stepchildren: A brief demographic profile. *Family Relations, 38,* 24–27.

Gottman, J. M. (1993). The role of conflict engagement, escalation, and avoidance in marital interaction: A longitudinal view of five types of couples. *Journal of Consulting and Clinical Psychology, 61,* 6–15.

Greenberg, L. S., & Johnson, S. M. (1988). *Emotionally focused therapy for couples*. New York: Guilford Press.

Griffin, W., & Morgan, A. R. (1988). Conflict in maritally distressed military couples. *American Journal of Family Therapy, 16,* 14–22.

Grych, J. H., & Fincham, F. D. (1990). Marital conflict and children's adjustment: A cognitive-contextual framework. *Psychological Bulletin, 108,* 267–290.

Hahlweg, K., Reissner, L., Kohli, G., Vollmer, M., Schindler, L., & Revenstorf, D. (1984). Development and validity of a new system to analyze interpersonal communication: Katagoriensystem fur partnershaftliche interaktion (Interactional Coding System). In K. Hahlweg & N. Z. Jacobson (Eds.), *Marital interaction: Analysis and modification* (pp. 182–198). New York: Guilford Press.

Halford, W. K., Gravestock, F., Lowe, R., & Scheldt, S. (1992). Toward a behavioral ecology of stressful marital interactions. *Behavioral Assessment, 13,* 135–148.

Halford, W. K., & Osgarby, S. (1993). Alcohol abuse in individuals presenting for marital therapy. *Journal of Family Psychology, 11,* 1–13.

Halford, W. K., Osgarby, S., & Kelly, A. (1995). Brief behavioral couples therapy: A preliminary quasi-experimental evaluation. Manuscript submitted for publication.

Halford, W. K., & Sanders, M. R. (1989). Behavioral marital therapy in the treatment of psychological disorders. *Behaviour Change, 6,* 165–177.

Halford, W. K., Sanders, M. R., & Behrens, B. C. (1993). A comparison of the generalization of behavioral marital therapy and enhanced behavioral marital therapy. *Journal of Consulting and Clinical Psychology, 61,* 51–60.

Halford, W. K., Sanders, M. R., & Behrens, B. C. (1994). Self-regulation in behavioral couples therapy. *Behavior Therapy, 25,* 431–452.

Haynes, S. N., Jensen, B. J., Wise, E., & Sherman, D. (1981). The marital intake interview: A multimethod criterion validity assessment. *Journal of Consulting and Clinical Psychology, 49,* 379–387.

Heavey, L. H., Layne, C., & Christensen, A. (1993). Gender and conflict structure in marital interaction: A replication and extension. *Journal of Consulting and Clinical Psychology, 61,* 16–27.

Holtzworth-Munroe, A., & Stuart, G. L. (1994). Typologies of male batterers: Three sub-types and the differences among them. *Psychological Bulletin, 116,* 476–497.

Hooley, J. M., & Teasdale, J. D. (1989). Predictors of relapse in unipolar depressives: Expressed emotion, marital distress and perceived criticism. *Journal of Abnormal Psychology, 98,* 229–235.

Jacobson, N. S. (1989). The maintenance of treatment gains following social learning-based marital therapy. *Behavior Therapy, 20,* 325–336.

Jacobson, N. S., Dobson, K., Fruzetti, A. E., Schmaling, K. B., & Salusky, S. (1991). Marital therapy as treatment of depression. *Journal of Consulting and Clinical Psychology, 59,* 547–557.

Jacobson, N. S., & Margolin, G. (1979). *Marital therapy: Strategies based on social learning and behavior exchange principles.* New York: Guilford Press.

Jaffee, P., Wolfe, D. A., Wilson, S., & Zak, L. (1986). Emotional and physical health problems of battered women. *Canadian Journal of Psychiatry, 31,* 625–629.

Kendall, P. (1989). The generalization and maintenance of behavior change in behavior therapy. Commentary. *Behavior Therapy, 20,* 311–324.

Koop, C. E. (1985). *The Surgeon General's workshop on violence and public health.* Washington, DC: Government Printing Office.

Langhinrichsen-Rohling, J., & Vivian, D. (1994). The correlates of spouses' incongruent reports of marital aggression. *Journal of Family Violence, 9,* 265–283.

Levinger, G., & Huston, T. L. (1990). The social psychology of marriage (pp. 19–58). New York: Guilford Press.

Locke, H. J., & Wallace, K. M. (1959). Short marital adjustment and prediction test: Their reliability and validity. *Marriage and Family Living, 21,* 251–255.

Markman, H. J., Floyd, F., Stanley, S. M., & Lewis, H. C. (1986). Prevention. In N. S. Jacobson & A. S. Gurman (Eds.), *Clinical handbook of marital therapy* (pp. 173–195). New York: Guilford Press.

Markman, H. J., & Notarius, C. I. (1987). Coding marital and family interaction: Current status, In T. Jacob (Ed.), *Family interaction and psychopathology* (pp. 329–390). New York: Plenum Press.

Marlatt, G. A., & Gordon, J. R. (Eds.). (1985). *Relapse prevention.* New York: Guilford Press.

McMullin, R. E., & Giles, T. R. (1987). *Cognitive behavior therapy: A restructuring approach.* New York: Grune & Stratton.

Millward, C. (1990). What marriage means to young adults. *Family Matters, 29,* 26–28.

Notarius, C. I., & Markman, H. J. (1993). *We can work it out.* New York: Perigee.

Notarius, C. I., & Vanzetti, N. A. (1983). The marital agenda protocol. In E. Filsinger (Ed.) *Marriage and family assessment: A source book for family therapy* (pp. 209–227). Beverly Hills: Sage.

O'Farrell, T. J. (1986). Antabuse contracts for married alcoholics and their spouses: A method to maintain antabuse ingestion and decrease conflict about drinking. *Journal of Substance Abuse and Treatment, 3,* 1–8.

O'Farrell, T. J. (1989). Marital and family therapy in alcoholism treatment. *Journal of Substance Abuse and Treatment, 6,* 23–29.

O'Farrell, T. J. (1993). Conclusions and future directions in practice and research on marital and family therapy. In T. J. O'Farrell (Ed.) *Treating alcohol problems: Marital and family interventions* (pp. 403–434). New York: Guilford Press.

O'Leary, K. D. (1987) *Assessment of marital discord*. Hillsdale, NJ: Erlbaum.

O'Leary, K. D., Barling, J., Arias, I., Rosenbaum, A., Malone, J., & Tyree, A. (1989). Prevalence and stability of physical aggression between spouses: A longitudinal analysis. *Journal of Consulting and Clinical Psychology*, *57*, 263–268.

O'Leary, K. D., & Beach, S. R. H. (1990). Marital therapy: A viable treatment for depression and marital discord. *American Journal of Psychiatry*, *147*, 183–186.

O'Leary, K. D., & Vivian, D. (1990). Physical aggression in marriage. In F. D. Fincham & T. N. Bradbury (Eds.), *The psychology of marriage* (pp. 323–348). New York: Guilford Press.

O'Leary, K. D., Vivian, D., & Malone, J. (1992). Assessment of physical aggression against women in marriage: The need for multimodal assessment. *Behavioral Assessment*, *14*, 5–14.

Osgarby, S., & Halford, W. K. (1995). *Positive intimacy skills and marital distress*. Manuscript submitted for publication.

Sabatelli, R. M. (1988). Measurement issues in marital research: A review and critique of contemporary survey instruments. *Journal of Marriage and the Family*, *50*, 891–915.

Sanders, M. R., & Christensen, A. P. (1985). A comparison of the effects of child management and planned activities in five parenting environments. *Journal of Abnormal Child Psychology*, *13*, 101–117.

Schindler, L., & Vollmer, M. (1984). Cognitive perspectives in behavioral marital therapy: Some proposals for bridging theory, research, and practice. In K. Hahlweg & N. S. Jacobson (Eds.), *Marital Interaction: Analysis and Modification*. New York: Guilford Press.

Selzer, M. L., Vinokur, A., & van Rooijen, L. A. (1975). A self-administered short Michigan Alcoholism screening test (SMAST). *Journal of the Study of Alcohol*, *36*, 117–126.

Spanier, G. B. (1976). Measuring dyadic adjustment: New scales for assessing the quality of marriage and similar dyads. *Journal of Marriage and the Family*, *38*, 15–28.

Stark, E., & Flitcraft, A. (1988). Violence among intimates. In V. B. Van Hasselt, R. L. Morrison, A. S. Bellack, & M. Hersen (Eds.), *Handbook of family violence* (pp. 293–318). New York: Plenum Press.

Steinmetz, S. K., & Lucca, J. S. (1988). Husband battering. In V. B. van Hasselt, R. L. Morrison, A. S. Bellack, & M. Hersen (Eds.). *Handbook of family violence* (pp. 233–246). New York: Plenum Press.

Stets, J. E., & Straus, M. A. (1990). The marriage license as a hitting license: A comparison of dating, cohabiting and married couples. In M. A. Straus & R. J. Gelles (Eds.), *Physical violence in American families: Risk Factors and adaption to violence in 8,415 families*. New Brunswick, New Jersey: Transaction Press.

Stokes, T. R., & Baer, D. M. (1977). An implicit technology of generalization. *Journal of Applied Behavioral Analysis*, *10*, 349–367.

Stokes, T. R., & Osnes, P. G. (1988). An operant pursuit of generalization. *Behavior Therapy*, *20*, 337–355.

Straus, M. A. (1979). Measuring intrafamily conflict and violence: The Conflict Tactics Scale. *Journal of Marriage and the Family*, *41*, 75–88.

Straus, M. A., & Gelles, R. (1986). Societal change and change in family violence from 1975 to 1985 as revealed by two national surveys. *Journal of Marriage and the Family*, *48*, 465–479.

Stuart, R. B. (1969). Operant-interpersonal treatment of marital discord. *Journal of Consulting and Clinical Psychology*, *33*, 675–682.

Stuart, R. B. (1980). *Helping couples change: A social learning approach to marital therapy*. New York: Guilford Press.

Terman, L. M. (1938). *Psychological factors in marital happiness*. New York: McGraw-Hill.

Vanicelli, M., Gingerreich, S., & Ryback, R. (1983). Family problems related to the treatment and outcome of alcoholic patients. *British Journal of Addiction*, *78*, 193–204.

Weiss, R. L. (1978). The conceptualization of marriage from a behavioral perspective. In T. J. Paolino & B. S. McCrady (Eds.), *Marriage and marital therapy: Psychoanalytic, behavioral and systems theory perspectives* (pp. 165–239). New York: Brunner/Mazel.

Weiss, R. L. (1980a). Strategic behavioral marital therapy: Toward a model for assessment and intervention. In J. P. Vincent (Ed.), *Advances in family intervention, assessment and theory* (Vol. 1, pp. 229–271). Greenwich, CT: JAI Press.

Weiss, R. L. (1980b). *The Areas of Change Questionnaire*. Eugene, OR: Oregon Marital Studies Program, University of Oregon.

Weiss, R. L. (1984). Cognitive and strategic interventions in behavioral marital therapy. In K. Hahlweg & N. S. Jacobson (Eds.), *Marital interaction: Analysis and modification* (pp. 337–355). New York: Guilford Press.

Weiss, R. L., Birchler, G. R. & Vincent, J. P. (1974). Contractual models for negotiation training in marital dyads. *Journal of Marriage and the Family*, *36*, 321–330.

Weiss, R. L., & Cerreto, M. C. (1980). The Marital Status Inventory: Development of a measure of dissolution potential. *American Journal of Family Therapy, 8,* 80–85.

Weiss, R. L., & Dehle, C. (1994). Cognitive–behavioral perspectives on marital conflict. In D. D. Cahn (Ed.), *Conflict in intimate relationships* (pp. 95–115). Hillsdale, NJ: Erlbaum.

Weiss, R. L., & Heyman, R. E. (1990a). Marital distress. In A. Bellack & M. Hersen (Eds.) *International handbook of behavior modification* (pp. 475–501). New York: Plenum Press.

Weiss, R. L., & Heyman, R. E. (1990b). Observation of marital interaction. In F. D. Fincham & T. N. Bradbury (Eds.), *The psychology of marriage* (pp. 87–117). New York: Guilford Press.

Weiss, R. L., Hops, H., & Patterson, G. R. (1973). A framework for conceptualizing marital conflict: A technology for altering it, some data for evaluating it. In L. D. Handy & E. L. Mash (Eds.), *Behavior change: Methodology concepts and practice* (pp. 309–342). Champaign, IL: Research Press.

Weiss, R. L., & Perry, B. A. (1983). The Spouse Observation Checklist. In E. E. Filsinger (Ed.), *A sourcebook of marriage and family assessment.* Beverly Hills: Sage.

Whisman, M. A. (1990). The efficacy of booster maintenance sessions in behavior therapy: Review and methodological critique. *Clinical Psychology Review, 10,* 155–170.

Widom, C. S. (1989). Does violence beget violence? A critical examination of the literature. *Psychological Bulletin, 106,* 3–28.

Wolcott, I., & Glazer, H. (1989). *Marriage counselling in Australia: An evaluation.* Melbourne: Institute of Family Studies.

Zimmer, D. (1983). Interaction patterns and communication skills in sexually distressed, maritally distressed, and normal couples: Two experimental studies. *Journal of Sex and Marital Therapy, 9,* 251–266.

14

Insomnia

David L. Van Brunt, Brant W. Riedel, and Kenneth L. Lichstein

> He that can take rest is greater than he that can take cities.
> —BENJAMIN FRANKLIN

Although most people occasionally suffer from disturbed sleep, to the person suffering from chronic or severe insomnia the bed may become a battlefield; a nightly struggle ensues in which the sufferer attempts to force what comes naturally to others. As a biological imperative, sleep's absence may result in physical, cognitive, and emotional consequences. In this volume covering various types of psychological disorders, it is evident that few problems exist in isolation. Insomnia is a prime example of how physical, behavioral, and cognitive factors can interact to produce distressing symptoms. As we shall see, insomnia can co-occur with other disorders as one of several symptoms, or it can stand alone as a presenting problem of substantial magnitude. We begin by describing insomnia and its correlates and then review methods for distinguishing it from related disorders. We then review several treatment options that may be used to improve sleep, as assessed by both objective measures of sleep duration and the subjective experience of the patient. We conclude with a case example in hope of clarifying the use of the methods described.

DESCRIPTION OF INSOMNIA

Clinical Features

Insomnia can be broadly classified as either difficulty initiating sleep (sleep-onset insomnia) or difficulty maintaining sleep (sleep-maintenance insomnia). The latter can be further subdivided into either frequent or lengthy nocturnal awakenings, or early morning

David L. Van Brunt, Brant W. Riedel, and Kenneth L. Lichstein • Department of Psychology, University of Memphis, Memphis, Tennessee 38152.

Sourcebook of Psychological Treatment Manuals for Adult Disorders, edited by Vincent B. Van Hasselt and Michel Hersen. Plenum Press, New York, 1996.

awakenings with an inability to return to sleep (terminal insomnia). Sufferers may present with one or any combination of the aforementioned difficulties. The actual degree of sleep disturbance varies greatly among insomniacs and is not necessarily correlated with the intensity of subjective dissatisfaction. For example, among three sleepers who each have 40-minute sleep latencies, one may complain of severe insomnia, another of only mild insomnia, and the other may remain completely unconcerned with or unaware of any significance of this sleep-onset delay. The frequency of insomnia also varies widely. Some insomniacs report difficulty sleeping nearly every night, while others complain of more sporadic sleep disturbance.

Associated Features

Although some insomniacs report significant levels of daytime impairment, many do not. Researchers have generally found no significant difference between insomniacs and noninsomniacs on traditional measures of daytime sleepiness (Mendelson, Garnett, Gillin, & Weingartner, 1984; Seidel et al., 1984). Mendelson et al. also found that daytime measures of psychomotor functioning, attention, vigilance, and episodic memory did not reliably distinguish insomniacs from normal sleepers. However, insomniacs did exhibit significantly poorer long-term semantic memory at each measurement point during the day. In addition, there is evidence that insomniacs subjectively identify daytime impairment resulting from their nighttime sleep difficulties. Insomniacs score high on the Insomnia Impact Scale, a self-report questionnaire that assesses subjects' perception of the effect of insomnia on physical, cognitive, emotional, social, and occupational aspects of daytime functioning (Hoelscher, Ware, & Bond, 1993).

Despite a general absence of studies showing reliable differences between insomniacs and normal sleepers, one recent study found striking evidence for higher levels of daytime alertness among primary insomniacs (i.e., insomnia not secondary to another disorder). Regestein, Dambrosia, Hallett, Murawski, and Paine (1993) studied the hyperarousal of subjects using an innovative methodology. Twenty chronic primary-insomnia patients (average length of disorder was 13.6 years) and 20 normal control subjects completed a hyperarousal scale consisting of 26 Likert-type items and the physiological measure of auditory evoked potentials to assess daytime arousal levels. Although previous studies have failed to distinguish primary insomniacs from normal subjects, the hyperarousal scale used by Regestein and colleagues distinguished them sharply. The authors characterized the measure as an indicator of "tenacious thoughtfulness and attentiveness that often involved increased emotion" (p. 1532). This is congruent with the Minnesota Multiphasic Personality Inventory (MMPI) profiles seen among insomniac patients, which typically reflect rumination, depression, and tension (to be discussed). In addition to the hyperarousal scale, the electrophysiological evidence suggested a stable nervous system response pattern of increased daytime alertness. The authors hypothesized that increased daytime alertness may predispose individuals to insomnia. Although promising, this study was only preliminary in nature and used a highly specialized subgroup of the insomniac population. Therefore, the generalizability of the findings are as yet unknown.

Epidemiology

In epidemiological studies investigating the prevalence and severity of sleep disturbance in the general population, insomnia is the most prevalent sleep disorder (Bixler, A.

Kales, Soldatos, J. D. Kales, & Healey, 1979). Occasional insomnia has been estimated to afflict approximately 35% of the adult population (Mellinger, Balter, & Uhlenhuth, 1985), and surveys suggest that about 10% to 20% of adults suffer from insomnia that is severe or chronic (Buysse & Reynolds, 1990). Older insomniacs predominantly suffer from sleep maintenance problems, whereas younger insomniacs more frequently complain of difficulty falling asleep. Insomnia is reported more commonly among females than males, and the incidence of insomnia symptoms increases with age (Ford & Kamerow, 1989).

Etiology

Insomnia can emanate from several diverse sources, including psychological or psychiatric determinants, poor sleep hygiene, and medical or drug-related factors. Each of these is reviewed here.

Psychological Factors

Insomnia often includes a learning component. Transient insomnia (duration less than 1 month) resulting from a particular stressor (lifestyle changes, interpersonal difficulties) may evolve into chronic insomnia as a person begins to associate going to bed with insomnia rather than sleep. The anxiety associated with the impending poor night's sleep creates an arousal that is incompatible with sleep. Thus, the bedroom, the bed itself, and rituals associated with going to bed may become conditioned stimuli that continue to elicit insomnia long after the original stressor is removed. In addition, a person who experiences transient insomnia may develop fears connected with his or her inability to sleep and paradoxically attempt to force sleep onset, producing further physiological and cognitive arousal. A vicious cycle is established in which a person's fears concerning sleep and overzealous attempts to promote sleep serve to maintain current sleep difficulties and perhaps engender chronic insomnia.

In addition to the conditioning that can occur during insomnia's development, cognitions unrelated to sleep concerns may play a formative role. Intrusive cognitions may include problem solving, planning future activities, brooding over the day's events, or other thoughts that tend to arouse rather than relax the insomniac. In two separate investigations, insomniacs have identified cognitive factors as more frequent sources of sleep disruption than somatic variables, such as bodily tension or restlessness (Espie, Brooks, & Lindsay, 1989; Lichstein & Rosenthal, 1980). In addition, Gross and Borkovec (1982) demonstrated that an experimental manipulation intended to increase cognitive arousal led to lengthier sleep latencies in a sample of normal sleepers. Other studies of insomniac subjects, however, have failed to demonstrate such a relationship between cognitive arousal and sleep initiation difficulties (Haynes, Adams, & Franzen, 1981; Sanavio, 1988).

Unrealistic sleep goals may also generate an insomnia complaint. People who require little sleep may covet superfluous sleep. Similarly, older sleepers may strive to sleep as well as they did when younger, despite their changing sleep needs. In such cases, dissatisfaction exists, although no detrimental effects result directly from the individual's sleep pattern (Lichstein, 1988b).

Psychiatric Factors

Insomnia is often associated with affective disorders, although the causal relationship between them can be ambiguous. For example, researchers have detected a relationship between insomnia and depressive symptomatology (Levin, Bertelson, & Lacks, 1984; Mendelson et al., 1984), but which problem preceded or contributed to the other is not clear. In addition, insomniacs tend to produce high scores on scales associated with anxiety such as the MMPI's Psychasthenia Scale (Levin et al., 1984). Whereas this may indicate some form of psychopathology, it also may reflect a general ruminative style that correlates with complaints of intrusive cognitions mentioned earlier.

Poor Sleep Hygiene

Sleep hygiene is a general category that encompasses a diverse group of behaviors and environmental variables that tend to promote sleep. A lack of attention to any of these behavioral factors may produce or at least contribute to the maintenance of insomnia. Table 14.1 lists several sleep-promoting or sleep-harming behaviors that are of common concern. Behaviors associated with physical activity, diet, and sleep scheduling, as well as environmental factors, can all have a bearing on a person's ability to achieve a satisfying quality and quantity of sleep. A more detailed discussion of the relationship between sleep-hygiene violations and poor sleep will be presented in the section on behavioral treatments for insomnia.

Medical Status

Complaints of insomnia can co-occur with some medical disorders and may even be a presenting problem that ends in a diagnosis of another medical condition. Medical problems commonly associated with insomnia include neurological disorders (e.g., dementia,

Table 14.1. Sleep Hygiene Guidelines

Drug use	1. Decrease the use of caffeine 4–6 hours before bed, and if possible eliminate it from the diet altogether (sources include coffee, tea, colas, chocolate, and some over-the-counter medications).
	2. Eliminate the use of nicotine (a stimulant) near bedtime.
	3. Avoid the use of alcohol to induce sleep. Although as a depressant it may facilitate sleep onset, the ensuing sleep is fragmented and less satisfying.
Dietary factors	4. A *light snack* may help induce sleepiness.
	5. A heavy *meal* too close to bedtime may interfere with sleep.
Daily behaviors	6. Avoid vigorous exercise within 3–4 hours of sleep.
	7. *Regular* exercise in the later afternoon may deepen sleep (sporadic exercise as an attempt to "wear yourself out" has not been shown to be effective.)
	8. Establish a regular time for retiring and rising each day to strengthen circadian cycling.
	9. Do not nap.
Environmental factors	10. Minimize light.
	11. Minimize noise, using earplugs if necessary or a white noise generator to produce soporific noise.
	12. Keep sleep area at a comfortable temperature, avoiding extremes of heat and cold.

parkinsonism), chronic obstructive pulmonary disease, asthma, gastroesophageal reflux, peptic ulcer disease, sleep apnea, and pain syndromes such as fibrositis. See American Sleep Disorders Association (1987) for a more thorough discussion.

Drugs

Many prescribed and over-the-counter medications can produce insomnia. As an example, some analgesics contain caffeine and many types of bronchodilators, steroids, and some antihypertensive drugs may produce insomnia as a side effect (Espie, 1991). Also, whereas one drug may not cause insomnia by itself, interactions between drugs may lead to sleep disturbance. Ironically, sleeping pills can play a role in insomnia exacerbation. Benzodiazepines, the most widely used class of sleeping pills, may cause a "rebound insomnia" when discontinued, often resulting in insomnia that is more severe than the original insomnia for which the pill was taken (Kales, Soldatos, Bixler, & Kales, 1983b). Insomnia is often associated with the use of alcohol, nicotine, and certain illegal drugs. Alcohol may provide the illusion of improved sleep due to a decreased sleep latency, but tends to increase wakefulness during the second half of the sleep period (Kay & Samiuddin, 1988). Nicotine can also contribute to sleep disturbance (Soldatos, J. D. Kales, Scharf, Bixler, & A. Kales, 1980), and users of other stimulants (such as cocaine and amphetamines), may also find sleep elusive.

DIFFERENTIAL DIAGNOSIS AND ASSESSMENT

DSM-III-R Categorization

The third revised edition of the *Diagnostic and Statistical Manual of Mental Disorders* (DSM-III-R; American Psychiatric Association, 1987) divides insomnia into three categories. The first of these, *insomnia related to another mental disorder,* includes insomnia that results from mental disorders such as major depression, generalized anxiety disorder, or adjustment disorder with anxious mood. The second, *insomnia related to a known organic factor,* is given to insomnia that is produced by physical disorders (e.g., pain syndromes, sleep apnea) or the use of medication or other drugs. The third category is *primary insomnia.* This label refers to insomnia complaints that are not encompassed by the first two categories, and is what is usually meant by the term *insomnia.* This expansive category includes a wide range of psychological causes of poor sleep.

The International Classification of Sleep Disorders (ICSD; American Sleep Disorders Association, 1987) provides a more detailed description of sleep syndromes and divides primary insomnia into several categories (see Table 14.2). Psychophysiological insomnia is the most prevalent ICSD diagnosis for patients presenting with insomnia. Disorders that would fall under the DSM-III-R's broad categories of *insomnia related to a known organic factor* (e.g., apnea) and *insomnia related to another mental disorder* are listed as distinct sleep disorders.

Differential Diagnosis

Because other sleep disorders may produce symptoms similar to those associated with primary insomnia, the process of differential diagnosis can prove challenging for the clinician. Many clues for differential diagnosis can be extracted from an interview, but

Table 14.2. The International Classification of Sleep Disorders (ICSD) Categorization of Insomnia[a]

Psychophysiological insomnia	"Disorder of somatized tension and learned sleep-preventing associations that results in a complaint of insomnia and associated decreased functioning during wakefulness" (p. 28).
Sleep-state misperception	"Disorder in which a complaint of insomnia or excessive sleepiness occurs without objective evidence of sleep disturbance" (p. 33)
Idiopathic insomnia	"A lifelong inability to obtain adequate sleep that is presumably due to an abnormality of the neurological control of the sleep–wake system" (p. 35).
Inadequate sleep hygiene	"A sleep disorder due to the performance of daily living activities that are inconsistent with the maintenance of good quality sleep and full daytime alertness" (p. 73).
Environmental sleep disorder	"A sleep disturbance due to a disturbing environmental factor that causes a complaint of either insomnia or excessive sleepiness" (p. 77). Examples included noise, uncomfortable temperature, or bed-partner movements.
Altitude insomnia	"An acute insomnia, usually accompanied by headaches, loss of appetite, and fatigue, that occurs following ascent to high altitudes" (p. 80).
Adjustment sleep disorder	"Sleep disturbance temporally related to acute stress, conflict, or environmental change causing emotional arousal" (p. 83).

[a]Insomnia types that are primarily associated with childhood are not included in this table.

referral of a patient for nocturnal polysomnography (PSG) may be imperative. PSG involves all night monitoring of brain activity (EEG), eye movement (EOG), muscle tension (EMG), respiration during sleep (and awake time), and other physiological variables, and is necessary for the definitive diagnosis of certain sleep disorders. Some of these disorders are described here, along with the features that the cautious clinician can use to differentiate them from insomnia.

One opportunity for misdiagnosis is present in the case of narcolepsy. Narcolepsy is characterized by excessive daytime sleepiness (EDS), which often results in an inability to stay awake during tasks requiring substantial vigilance (e.g., driving a car). In addition to sudden sleep attacks, narcoleptics may also report cataplexy (loss of muscle tone induced by strong emotions), hypnagogic hallucinations (vivid, dream-like images seen while falling asleep), and sleep paralysis (an inability to move while falling asleep or immediately after awakening). Insomnia and narcolepsy can be confused by the lay observer because of the nighttime sleep difficulties and EDS that may be associated with both disorders. However, many insomniacs do not experience EDS (especially not to the degree found among narcoleptics), and some narcoleptics will not complain of nocturnal sleep disturbance. Other symptoms of narcolepsy (i.e., cataplexy and sleep paralysis) are not reported by insomniacs. The critical tests in diagnosing narcolepsy are PSG and multiple sleep latency tests (MSLTs). MSLTs consist of PSG monitoring during four 20-minute daytime nap opportunities, a requirement for identifying the two narcoleptic earmarks of excessive daytime sleepiness and sleep onset rapid eye movements (REM).

Another area of potential confusion lies with circadian rhythm disorders. Many biological functions, including body temperature and the sleep–wake system, follow a rhythmic cycle that lasts about 25 hours (circadian rhythm). Circadian rhythm disorders result when a person's circadian rhythm does not match the demands of his or her environment. The circadian disorders often confused with insomnia are delayed sleep-phase syndrome (DSPS) and advanced sleep-phase syndrome (ASPS). DSPS involves the inability to fall asleep until much later than conventional times (as governed by the person's environment and social expectations). People suffering from DSPS often cannot fall asleep until sometime early in the morning (2:00–6:00 A.M.) yet will be forced to awaken only a few hours later in order to fulfill daytime responsibilities. Students and night-shift workers are likely to develop this disorder. Patients with ASPS show the opposite pattern, falling asleep and awakening earlier than is desired. One sharp distinction, however, is that for ASPS patients the total sleep duration is not shortened. For example, an individual with ASPS may be unable to stay awake past 6:00 P.M., despite a desire to do so, and will awaken for the last time the next morning at 1:00 A.M.. Thus, DSPS mimics sleep-onset insomnia, while ASPS may imitate terminal insomnia if total sleep duration is not considered.

Despite their similarities, some features of DSPS enable discrimination from insomnia without the use of PSG. A sleep-history assessment with DSPS patients will often reveal a pattern of sleeping unusually late on weekends and holidays when early morning arising is not required. Sleep length is also a key indicator, because many DSPS patients are able to sleep for a normal length of time when social/environmental constraints are removed. A consistent sleep-onset time favors a diagnosis of DSPS, as it suggests a problem with the time that one is trying to fall asleep rather than a general inability to initiate sleep. Stability of the complaint can also be a clue to differential diagnosis; insomniacs typically have sporadic (though often frequent) difficulties initiating sleep, whereas DSPS patients experience difficulty nearly every night.

ASPS and insomnia differ in that individuals with ASPS are unable to stay awake past a very early hour in the evening. Despite this circadian impairment, sleep duration is unaffected. In distinguishing ASPS from terminal insomnia, it is important to note that the terminal insomniac will be able to stay awake later in the evening but will then have an abbreviated sleep duration. As is the case with DSPS, ASPS is manifested nearly every night, whereas terminal insomnia may occur only a few times per week.

When speaking of obtaining a "proper amount" of sleep, it is important to remember that this amount varies greatly between individuals. Someone sleeping less than 8 hours per night is defined as an insomniac only if he or she is consistently unable to get adequate rest from those hours of sleep. *Short sleepers* are individuals who sleep for only a short period of time each night but exhibit no consequent impairment of functioning during the day. They may complain of insomnia because they view their sleep pattern as abnormal, have unsuccessfully attempted to increase sleep length, or fear that dire consequences may result from limited sleep. Some short sleepers attempt to solve their perceived problem by spending more time in bed. Unfortunately, this strategy may pair anxious awake time with the bed and result in an increase in awake time; a sleep pattern resembling insomnia is then established. An assessment of sleep history will often distinguish a short sleeper from a sleep-maintenance insomniac. Short sleepers usually report a long history of obtaining a small amount of high-quality sleep (even on weekends and holidays when allowed to "sleep in") while experiencing no impairment in daytime functioning. Insomniacs, by comparison, describe significantly lengthier sleep time prior to their insomnia complaint. The short sleeper who complains of insomnia should be assured that acquiring a limited amount of sleep is not necessarily dangerous or "abnormal," and treatment should involve the establishment of more realistic sleep goals.

A health problem that may lead to a complaint of insomnia is sleep apnea. Although apneics do not typically have difficulty initiating sleep, they may complain of sleep-maintenance problems. Clues that suggest a diagnosis of apnea rather than primary insomnia include bed-partner report of heavy snoring, breathing irregularities, obesity, morning headaches, and sleeping better when sitting upright. Although the prototypical sufferer of obstructive sleep-apnea syndrome is a middle-aged obese male, anyone can develop this problem. Polysomnography is required for a definitive diagnosis of this disorder.

Periodic limb movements during sleep (PLMS) may also be mistaken for primary insomnia. Patients with PLMS who complain of sleep maintenance difficulties are often unaware of the cause of their problem. Because of this lack of awareness, the observations of a bed partner can provide valuable information to the clinician during the process of differential diagnosis. Another indicator of PLMS is the presence of restless legs syndrome (RLS). RLS consists of uncomfortable, "crawling" sensations in one's legs that interfere with sleep onset, and nearly every person suffering from RLS also suffers from PLMS (although the converse is not true). As with sleep apnea, PSG is required to investigate the role of PLMS in a patient's sleep concerns.

Primary insomnia may also be confused with insomnia resulting from an underlying mental disorder. Psychiatric testing and diagnostic interviews will provide important information to the clinician, and there is some evidence that PSG may be useful for diagnosing insomnia due to a psychiatric disorder. In one study, primary insomniacs, subjects with generalized anxiety disorder, and patients with major depression experienced similar sleep-continuity problems, but depressed patients could be distinguished from the other two groups on the basis of shortened REM latency and increased eye movements during REM (Reynolds et al., 1984).

Assessment Strategies

When presented with a sleep-related complaint, a clinician will first want to conduct a thorough interview with the patient. If possible, a bed partner of the patient should be consulted about the patient's sleep habits as well. Bed partners are often a source of information that can give clues about nocturnal behavior of which the patient is unaware, such as apnea or limb movements. An initial interview should investigate the following areas of interest:

1. The nature and severity of the problem (i.e., "6 months of initial insomnia").
2. Frequency of occurrence: Although the initial response may be global and diffuse (i.e., "all the time"), it is important to follow up for specifics. When pressed ("There hasn't been a *single* night in the last 6 months when you have fallen asleep?"), patients can provide more meaningful information.
3. Date of onset and circumstances surrounding that time: This includes any emotional, social, or economic factors or stresses at the time of onset. If the problem is sporadic rather than chronic, determine what circumstances are likely to exacerbate the condition.
4. Detailed sleep history: Assess what "normal" sleep is for the patient by getting a description of sleep habits preceding the current symptoms (e.g., number of hours slept, number of awakenings).

5. Daytime sequelae: This includes an evaluation of sleepiness, fatigue, performance, and mood. Do these factors fluctuate with the quality of the previous night's sleep?

6. The patient's emotional and behavioral reactions during a bad night of sleep: What fears (possibly irrational) are associated with not being able to sleep? What does the patient do when unable to sleep?

7. Sleep hygiene: The regularity of sleep schedule, exercise, dietary habits, and napping can all affect sleep (see Table 14.1).

8. Psychiatric factors: Is the patient experiencing depressive symptomatology or feeling anxious? If psychiatric factors are uncovered during the initial interview, a more detailed psychiatric diagnostic interview is recommended.

9. Medical factors: Check for the existence of breathing irregularities, limb twitches, and pain.

10. Medication and other drugs: What medication is being taken, and does the patient smoke, drink alcohol, or use other drugs of abuse? Frequency and quantity of usage should be investigated.

11. Treatment history: This should include a history of treatment types, treatment response, and compliance with treatment procedures.

12. Patient perspectives: Ask the patient to theorize about the etiology of his or her complaint. Also, what goal (possibly unrealistic) is the patient hoping to attain through treatment?

After the initial interview, several assessment options are available. PSG is indispensable for the assessment of sleep apnea and periodic limb movements, but its usefulness for primary-insomnia assessment is questionable for several reasons. First, insomnia may be setting-specific, and an overnight study in a sleep laboratory might not fairly represent a patient's insomnia. Although often patients sleeping in a lab for assessment will demonstrate a "first-night effect" of disrupted sleep, a "reverse first-night effect" could occur in some primary insomniac patients due to a proclivity to sleep better outside of the usual environment. In such a case, a PSG would overestimate the quality of the patient's typical sleep. PSG assessment in a person's natural environment has been developed to compensate for this problem, but obviously the intrusiveness of the procedure is not totally removed. Second, a major contributor to some insomnias, trying too hard to sleep, could be eliminated because insomniacs may feel less pressure to sleep at the laboratory and may actually want to prove their inability to sleep. A third disadvantage of PSG is that a single overnight study might not detect insomnia that is not present every night. Although multiple overnight studies might solve this problem, their use is impractical due to the substantial expense associated with PSG. Finally, PSG does not measure subjective sleep perception (e.g., satisfaction, patient's estimates of sleep variables), an important aspect of any insomnia complaint.

Edinger et al. (1989) have suggested an alternative perspective on the value of PSG in diagnosing insomnia. They point out that sleep apnea, periodic limb movements, and other sleep disorders that may have a similar clinical presentation to insomnia occur at increasing rates with advancing age. Edinger and colleagues suggest that for patients 40 years of age and older, PSG assessments of "insomniacs" have a substantial likelihood of altering the initial diagnosis of insomnia.

If PSG is not pursued, other objective sleep-measurement instruments that are less expensive and intrusive than PSG have been developed. The Sleep Assessment Device

(SAD) monitors patients' responses to faint tones during the night and provides estimates of sleep latency, duration of awakenings, total sleep time, and sleep efficiency that closely match PSG measurements (Lichstein, Nickel, Hoelscher, & Kelley, 1982). Wrist actigraphy offers estimates of sleep and wake time, but may exhibit substantial disagreement with PSG results (Hauri & Wisbey, 1992). In contrast to PSG, neither device provides information about sleep stages.

Objective measurements notwithstanding, the most readily available source of information is the patient's self-report. Sleep diaries are the most popular method of self-report. Sidebar 14.1 contains the sleep questionnaire that we utilize for clinical and research purposes. Diaries are completed daily and should at minimum include estimation of the following sleep parameters: (1) time entering and leaving bed, (2) latency to sleep, (3) number of awakenings and total awake time, (4) time of final awakening, (5) napping, (6) subjective sleep quality ratings, (7) daytime sleepiness, and (8) medication–alcohol usage. From these self-report data, additional variables such as total time in bed, total sleep time, and sleep efficiency percentage (100 × total sleep time/time in bed) can be calculated. The clinician will probably also want insomniacs to monitor other sleep-related variables, such as caffeine consumption and exercise.

Obviously, self-report measures are subject to inaccuracy. The use of a daily diary for tracking the problem as it occurs is extremely important; however, recollection of this information may blur over time and be subject to exaggeration by the desperate patient in search of help. Despite a lack of precision, insomniacs' self-reports tend to correlate significantly with PSG measures (Carskadon et al., 1976; Haynes, Fitzgerald, Shute, & Hall, 1985) and therefore can be useful for tracking treatment progress. In addition to assessment of subjective sleep perception, sleep diaries offer several advantages over objective measures including reduced intrusiveness, greater availability, and lowered expense. They may also provide clinicians with an index of treatment compliance, as the unwillingness to complete daily monitoring may foreshadow other forms of patient resistance.

TREATMENT

Evidence for Prescriptive Treatments

The following section concentrates on treatment of primary insomnia. When insomnia results from medical or psychiatric factors, the focus of treatment becomes the underlying disorder rather than the insomnia itself. Possible treatment approaches for medical or psychiatric contributors to insomnia are numerous and beyond the scope of the present discussion, and some are covered elsewhere in this volume.

Behavior Therapy

Relaxation Techniques. Several relaxation strategies have been proposed as treatments for insomnia. Popular relaxation methods are briefly described here, along with pertinent empirical evidence for their effectiveness. A more detailed discussion of various relaxation techniques is provided elsewhere (Lichstein, 1988a).

Progressive relaxation (PR) is the most widely researched treatment for insomnia (Lichstein & Fischer, 1985) and involves sequentially tensing and relaxing the body's major muscle groups while concentrating on and contrasting somatic sensations of tension and

---

Sidebar 14–1a

Sample Sleep Diary Used to Collect One Week of Data (Front)

Name _____

Please answer the following questionnaire *When you awaken in the morning.* Enter the date you are filling it out and provide the information to describe your sleep the night before. Definitions explaining each line of the questionnaire are given on the back side.

	Example								
This morning's date	10/16/93								
1. Nap (yesterday)	70								
2. Bedtime (last night)	10:55								
3. Time to fall asleep (last night)	65 min or 12:00 am								
4. Number of awakenings (last night)	4								
5. Total time spent awake (last night)	110 min or 1:50								
6. Final wake-up time (this morning)	6:05								
7. Out of bed time (this morning)	7:10								
8. Quality rating (of last night's sleep)	2								
9. Sleepiness (yesterday afternoon)	6								
10. Medication, caffeine, or alcohol (include amount & hour)	wine 1 @ 8p Halcion .25 mg bedtime								

Sidebar 14–1b

Reverse Side of Sleep Diary

ITEM DEFINITIONS

1. If you napped yesterday, enter total time napping in minutes.
2. What time did you enter bed for the purpose of going to sleep; or, if you were reading or engaging in other activites in bed, at what time did you wish to fall asleep?
3. Counting from the time you wished to fall asleep, how many minutes did it take you to fall asleep?
4. How many times did you awakan during the night?
5. What is the total amount of time you were awake during the night? This does not include time to fall asleep at the beginning of the night or awake time in bed before the final morning arising.
6. What time did you wake up this morning?
7. What time did you actually get out of bed this morning?
8. Enter *one* of the numbers below to indicate your overall *quality rating*, or the general level of satisfaction of your sleep last night:
    1. Very poor
    2. Poor
    3. Fair
    4. Good
    5. Excellent
9. Enter *one* of the numbers below to indicate the greatest amount of sleepiness you felt yesterday afternoon
    1. Feeling active and vital; alert; wide awake.
    2. Functioning at a high level, but not at peak; able to concentrate.
    3. Relaxed; awake; not at full alertness; responsive.
    4. A little foggy; not at peak; let down.
    5. Fogginess; beginning to lose interest in remaining awake; slowed down.
    6. Sleepiness; prefer to be lying down; fighting sleep; woozy.
    7. Almost in reverie; sleep onset soon; lost struggle to remain awake.
10. List any sleep medication, alcohol, or caffeine taken within a few hours of bedtime. Indicate time used.

relaxation. About 16 muscle groups are tensed and released, with a greater amount of time spent on the relaxation phase (45 sec) than in the tension phase (7 sec). Numerous studies have demonstrated its superiority to no treatment for diminishing sleep-onset latency (Lick & Heffler, 1977; Nicassio, Boyland, & McCabe, 1982; Turner & Ascher, 1979). In studies involving a placebo intervention, however, PR performance is less impressive. Some investigations showed greater sleep latency improvement for PR subjects (Freedman & Papsdorf, 1976; Lick & Heffler, 1977), whereas other researchers found no significant outcome differences between PR and placebo (Lacks, Bertelson, Gans, & Kunkel, 1983; Nicassio et al., 1982).

Guided imagery may also offer some relief from insomnia. During guided imagery, patients are encouraged to focus their attention on an image, such as a pleasant nature scene or a particular object. Retaining patients' attention on the image is essential, and this may be aided by having them concentrate on particular sensations associated with the nature scene or various details of a neutral object. The employment of imagery training as a method for combating intrusive cognitions is intuitively appealing, and its usefulness is empirically supported (Woolfolk & McNulty, 1983).

There is evidence that traditional relaxation strategies are less effective for older insomniacs. Lick and Heffler (1977) observed a poorer treatment response to PR among older subjects, and Morin and Azrin (1988) found no significant outcome difference between imagery training (IT) and no treatment in a sample whose average age was 67.4 years. Lichstein and Johnson (1993) developed a hybrid relaxation procedure that is designed to be less physically demanding and complex than traditional methods and therefore may be better suited for older insomniacs. The procedure involves concentration on relaxed somatic sensations, but the muscle tension–release cycles of PR are omitted. Breathing exercises and the repetition of an autogenic phrase are also included. In a recent empirical investigation involving subjects 60 years and older, the hybrid procedure led to significant sleep improvement for insomniacs not using hypnotic medications and reduced hypnotic usage without sleep deterioration for medicated insomniacs (Lichstein & Johnson, 1993).

In addition to the type of relaxation procedure employed and the number of practice opportunities provided by treatment sessions, the extent of practice between sessions may heavily influence outcome. Therapists should encourage daily practice of relaxation techniques, monitor compliance with this assignment, and if necessary, investigate reasons for noncompliance.

Stimulus Control.   Bootzin (1972) was the first to present an operant analysis of insomnia. In this view, falling asleep is viewed as a behavior meant to elicit positive reinforcement (rest). In insomnia, the bedtime routine begins to be associated instead with a negative consequence, namely sleeplessness and anxiety. Stimulus-control therapy is derived from this viewpoint, and the following six instructions are given to the patient:

1. Do not use your bed or bedroom for anything (at any time of the day) but sleep (or sex). Examples of activities that patients may have to avoid include eating, watching television, and working in the bedroom.
2. Go to bed only when sleepy.
3. If you do not fall asleep within about 15 to 20 minutes, leave the bed and do something in another room. Go back to bed only when you feel sleepy again. Clock-watching with regard to the 15 to 20 minute rule is not recommended, as this may result in undue pressure and tension as the minutes march by.
4. If you do not fall asleep quickly upon returning to bed, repeat the above instruction as many times as necessary. Also, if you do not fall asleep rapidly after an awakening, follow item 3 again. Do not be discouraged if at first you find yourself "up all night." Remember, you were awake before anyway, just lying in bed. Since you are awake, acknowledge that fact by leaving the bed and bedroom entirely.
5. Establish a routine time to get out of bed. Use your alarm to leave bed at the same time every morning, *regardless of the amount of sleep obtained*. This will aid your body in establishing a consistent sleep rhythm.
6. Do not nap.

Stimulus control has a consistently shown itself to be more effective than no treatment for sleep latency reduction (Ladouceur & Gros-Louis, 1986; Puder, Lacks, Bertelson, & Storandt, 1983; Turner & Ascher, 1979). In addition, most investigations that have compared stimulus-control to placebo interventions have demonstrated superior sleep-latency curtailment for the stimulus-control subjects (Espie, Lindsay, Brooks, Hood, & Turvey, 1989; Lacks et al., 1983; Turner & Ascher, 1979). Researchers have also provided evidence that stimulus control leads to significantly greater improvement of sleep-maintenance insomnia than no treatment or placebo interventions (Morin & Azrin, 1987, 1988; Turner & Ascher, 1979).

Sleep Restriction. A relatively new behavioral approach to insomnia involves limiting a patient's time in bed. Sleep-restriction therapy was developed in response to the proposal that excessive time in bed perpetuates insomnia (Spielman, Saskin, & Thorpy, 1987). The term *sleep restriction* may actually be somewhat misleading, because it is actually the patient's time in bed and not sleep time *per se* that is restricted during this type of therapy. Sleep-restriction therapy consists of the following steps:

1. Patients complete 2 weeks of sleep diaries, and the therapist uses these questionnaires to calculate average total subjective sleep time.
2. The amount of time patients are allowed to spend in bed is initially restricted to this average total sleep time. However, no patient is asked to limit time in bed to less than 4.5 hours, regardless of baseline total sleep time. Napping or lying down during periods outside of the prescribed time limits is prohibited throughout treatment.
3. Patients choose fixed times to enter and leave bed. For example, a patient prescribed 6 hours in bed may choose either an 11:00 P.M. to 5:00 A.M. schedule or a 1:00 to 7:00 A.M. schedule. As with stimulus control, the importance of a consistent awakening time is stressed.
4. Mean sleep efficiency is calculated by the following simple formula:

$$\frac{\text{Time spent sleeping}}{\text{Total time in bed}} \times 100$$

   If sleep efficiency is $\geq$ 90% over a period of 5 days, a patient's time in bed is increased by allowing the patient to enter bed 15 minutes earlier. Five days of unaltered sleep schedule always follows an increase of time in bed.
5. If sleep efficiency drops below an average of 85% for a period of 5 days, time in bed is reduced to the mean total sleep time for those 5 days. No curtailment of time in bed occurs during the first 10 days of treatment or for 10 days following a sleep-schedule change.
6. If mean sleep efficiency falls between 85% and 90% during a 5-day period, a patient's sleep schedule remains constant.

Spielman et al. (1987) tested the effectiveness of sleep-restriction therapy with a group of 35 chronic insomniacs whose average age was 46. After an 8-week treatment program, subjects showed significant improvement in sleep latency, total wake time, sleep efficiency, and total sleep time. Lichstein (1988b) recognized the usefulness of bed-time restriction in treating "insomnoids," patients who experience nocturnal sleep disruption without corresponding daytime sleepiness. Insomnoid states may be particularly prevalent among older patients who frequently experience reduced total sleep time and increased awake time but no daytime sleepiness. Lichstein's sleep-compression therapy differs from sleep restriction in that sleep compression does not immediately reduce time in bed to the baseline total sleep-time average. Instead, the patient's time in bed is reduced by gradually delaying the time entering bed and advancing morning arising time. Lichstein (1988b) treated a 59-year-old insomnoid with sleep-compression therapy and observed substantial improvement in sleep latency, total awake time, sleep efficiency, and sleep-quality ratings. Hoelscher and Edinger (1988) successfully reduced sleep latency and wake time after sleep onset in a small group of older insomniacs by utilizing a treatment package that included bed-time restriction, stimulus control, and sleep education. Friedman, Bliwise, Yesavage, and Salom (1991) applied a modified version of sleep restriction to a group of 10 geriatric insomniacs. Subjects experienced significant reductions in sleep latency and wake time after sleep onset at posttreatment, and sleep latency remained significantly shortened at 9-month follow-up. Unfortunately, none of the aforementioned studies included a control group.

Sleep-Hygiene Instruction. Sleep hygiene refers to behaviors and environmental conditions that promote sleep (see Table 14.1). For example, general daytime activity level and exercise may influence sleep. A survey by Marchini, Coates, Magistad, and Waldum (1983) indicated that insomniacs were less active during the day than normal sleepers. It has also been suggested that exercise increases delta (deep) sleep. Torsvall (1981) reviewed 20 studies and concluded that the hypothesis of a relationship between deep sleep and exercise was usually supported in physically fit subjects but was less often upheld in untrained participants. Thus, long-term commitments to exercise that result in physical fitness are more likely to improve sleep quality than short-term increases in exercise. A few studies included in the review suggested additional benefits such as extended sleep length and decreased sleep latencies in response to increased exercise. However, Torsvall reports that exercise close to bedtime and increases in physical activity by untrained subjects appear to increase wakefulness and restless sleep.

Poor dietary habits may also contribute to insomnia. For example, caffeine is derived from several sources in one's diet, including coffee, tea, and soft drinks, and can produce insomnia. A recent study found that nocturnal sleep following caffeine consumption was characterized by significantly less total sleep time, less Stages 2 and 4 sleep, and significantly greater sleep latencies and total awake time than sleep preceded by caffeine-free days (Bonnet & Arand, 1992). However, tolerance to the effects of caffeine (with the exception of reduced Stage 4 sleep) developed after a week, suggesting that regular users of caffeine may be less at risk for sleep disturbance than sporadic consumers. In addition, the effects of caffeine differed substantially across individuals. Because sensitivity to the effects of caffeine varies greatly, its role in perpetuating insomnia should be considered even in patients with low to moderate consumption rates.

Napping may also detract from nighttime sleep, but empirical investigations have produced mixed results. One group of researchers found that an afternoon nap was followed by significantly longer sleep latencies and reduced total sleep time at night (Feinberg et al., 1985). However, in another study, no significant nocturnal sleep impairment was observed after a short daytime nap (Aber & Webb, 1986). The effect of a daytime nap probably varies significantly across individuals, and differences in duration and timing of the naps may have contributed to discrepant results. Aside from possible effects on nocturnal sleep duration, there is evidence to suggest that naps affect the quality of the ensuing night's sleep. Afternoon naps often rob the subject of restful Stage 4 sleep the following night, an effect that may lead to complaints about sleep quality (see Morin, 1993 for a more thorough description). Insomniacs should be advised to experiment with eliminating naps, and long naps late in the day should especially be discouraged.

A treatment study that compared sleep-hygiene instruction, stimulus-control, and a meditation technique showed improvements by all groups but no significant differences between groups on the outcome variables wake time after sleep onset, duration of awakenings, and number of awakenings, although self-reported compliance with treatment instructions was significantly lower among stimulus-control subjects in comparison to the remaining two groups (Schoicket, Bertelson, & Lacks, 1988). Despite comparable sleep-maintenance improvement, sleep-hygiene subjects were significantly more likely than stimulus-control and meditation participants to still consider themselves insomniacs at posttreatment. A survey of noninsomniacs and insomniacs suggested that insomniacs possess more sleep hygiene knowledge but actually practice sleep hygiene less than noninsomniacs (Lacks & Rotert, 1986). Because knowledge and practice were generally high for both groups, investigators concluded that poor sleep hygiene is not likely to be a primary cause of insomnia but nevertheless should be addressed in treatment due to its potential for perpetuating poor sleep.

Pharmacotherapy

In working with insomniacs, the question of medications frequently arises. Patients often will have already received medication from their primary physician or have enlisted the use of over-the-counter sleep aids. In addressing patients' concerns about pharmacological therapy, two things are to be considered. First, the potential costs and benefits of medication use must be addressed for both long- and short-term gains. Second, the interaction between psychological interventions and pharmacotherapy should be considered.

Benzodiazepines are the most popular pharmacological intervention for insomnia. Despite their demonstrated ability to reduce sleep latency and improve sleep maintenance, benzodiazepines have some significant disadvantages. The first disadvantage is drug tolerance. Tolerance appears to develop after only a few weeks of nightly benzodiazepine use, resulting in a return to baseline-level insomnia symptoms (Gillin & Byerly, 1990). The second problem is adverse daytime effects, including performance deficits and increased sleepiness (Roth, Roehrs, & Zorick, 1988). Benzodiazepines with a long elimination half-life, such as flurazepam (Dalmane), are particularly likely to produce "carryover effects," a problem potentially amplified in older patients who metabolize drugs more slowly. Third, withdrawal from benzodiazepines may produce a rebound insomnia and heightened anxiety (Kales et al., 1983b) that leaves patients in as bad or worse condition than when they originally sought treatment. Rapidly eliminated benzodiazepines, such as triazolam (Halcion), appear to be more likely to cause rebound insomnia and may lead to increased morning wakefulness (Kales, Soldatos, Bixler, & Kales, 1983a, 1983b). Rebound insomnia and rebound anxiety can produce an additional problem by fostering psychological dependence on benzodiazepines as insomniacs attempt to avoid adverse withdrawal effects through the chronic use of sleeping pills. Finally, benzodiazepines are typically associated with altered sleep stages. Stage 2 sleep is increased, while Stages, 3, 4, and REM sleep are significantly reduced (Roth et al., 1988). Due to the aforementioned undesirable effects associated with benzodiazepines, they are usually only recommended for short-term treatment of transient sleep difficulties and are contraindicated for long-term use with chronic insomnia.

The interaction between pharmacotherapy and behavior therapy has not been heavily researched. In a comparison between behavior therapy and triazolam therapy, McClusky, Milby, Switzer, Williams, and Wooten (1991) noted that triazolam treatment showed superior immediate treatment effects, whereas behavior therapy (stimulus control) showed superior effects at a 9-week follow-up. They suggested that a combination of triazolam, to gain short-term effects, and behavior therapy, for long-term effects beginning when the triazolam lost effectiveness, might be beneficial. Milby et al. (1993) examined the issue by comparing patients receiving a combination of stimulus control–relaxation therapy and triazolam to patients receiving triazolam alone. They noted significant improvement in sleep latency and total sleep time for both groups but also noted a significant treatment by time interaction. The interaction suggested better results for the combined therapy on measures of total sleep and subjective restedness ratings, and the authors concluded that the combination of sedative therapy with behavioral therapy is superior to drugs alone in the treatment of insomnia.

Another study resulted in very different conclusions. Hauri and Wisbey (1993) examined the effectiveness of Halcion combined with sleep-hygiene instruction to that of sleep hygiene alone or a wait-list control. They observed that both treated groups improved sleep time and sleep efficiency when compared to wait-list controls. Additionally they noted no difference between the two treatment groups immediately following treatment. However, a 1-year follow-up showed that whereas sleep-hygiene patients retained their improved sleep, subjects receiving the combination therapy had reverted back to their pretreatment sleep patterns. Hauri and Wisbey concluded that behavioral therapies such as sleep hygiene and relaxation should *not* be combined with drug use.

Unfortunately, comparing these studies for purposes of generalization is difficult because each used different forms of behavior therapy and drug treatment. It is worth bearing in mind that drug interactions do exist with behavioral therapy, and clinicians may need to consider this in the event of treatment difficulties. There is clearly a need for more definitive research in this domain.

Alternative Treatments

Unlike most treatment strategies that require insomniacs to take specific steps to induce sleep, paradoxical-intention (PI) therapy suggests that patients attempt to remain awake. Supporters of PI propose that sleep is an involuntary physiological reaction and therefore cannot be fully controlled by conscious effort. Attempts to control the sleep process (i.e., trying to make oneself fall asleep) result in arousal that prevents sleep onset. The repeated failures at achieving sleep onset produce a sleep-incongruous performance anxiety that is reframed as a successful attempt at remaining awake. Specifically, patients are asked to assume a comfortable position in bed, turn out the lights, and attempt to stay awake as long as possible. Patients are encouraged to try to keep their eyes open, although more active methods for maintaining wakefulness (e.g., physical activity, reading, or watching television) should be avoided.

Despite the success of PI in earlier studies, Espie and Lindsay (1985) demonstrated that it may be a poor treatment choice for some insomniacs. In a study of 6 patients treated with PI, 3 subjects exhibited favorable sleep-latency changes, but 2 participants experienced sleep-latency exacerbation to such a degree that PI treatment was discontinued. The average sleep latency of a sixth subject increased during the first 3 weeks of treatment but dropped below baseline levels for weeks 4 to 8.

Selecting Psychological Treatment Strategies

When choosing an optimal treatment strategy, two approaches are appropriate. First, a clinician can select an intervention that has proven to be more effective in treatment-comparison studies. Second, a treatment package could be tailored to meet the perceived needs of a particular client. Each of these approaches are discussed here.

A recent review of insomnia-treatment studies suggests that bed-time restriction strategies and stimulus control (SC) will lead to greater improvement by posttreatment than PI and PR (Lacks & Morin, 1992). However, the differences between treatment approaches were less substantial by short-term follow-up ($M = 2$ months). Three studies have directly compared PR, SC, and PI. Turner and Ascher (1979) found that PR, SC, and PI were equally effective for sleep latency and number of awakenings, but performed significantly better than no treatment or placebo on the same measures. Conflicting results were reported by Lacks et al. (1983), who observed that SC led to significantly greater sleep-latency reduction at posttreatment and follow-up than PR, PI, and placebo, which were comparably potent. In a third investigation, SC and PI subjects showed more substantial sleep-latency amelioration than PR, placebo, and no-treatment groups (Espie et al., 1989). Sleep-latency reduction was comparable for SC and PI, but SC achieved its effect more quickly than PI. In comparison to both SC and PI, however, PR produced superlative increases in sleep-quality variables such as "restedness after sleep" and "enjoyment of sleep." In summary, these studies suggest that SC, PR, and PI are useful treatments for insomnia. Stimulus control appears to be the quickest route to improving the quantitative measure of sleep latency; however, progressive relaxation may produce greater qualitative improvement. An evaluation of the nature of the insomnia complaint may have some guiding value in choosing from among these strategies.

Another research group conducted two studies that compared SC to imagery training (IT). The first investigation included subjects with an average age of 57, and sleep-maintenance difficulties were the focus of treatment (Morin & Azrin, 1987). At posttreatment, SC reduced nocturnal awake time significantly more than IT (65% and 16%, respectively). By 3-month follow-up, IT subjects had significantly reduced awake time but still lagged significantly behind SC subjects. By 1-year follow-up, no significant differences for awake time existed between the two groups. A second investigation by the same authors (Morin & Azrin, 1988) treated subjects with an average age of 67 and found a significant reduction in the duration of awakenings for both SC and IT groups at posttreatment, but only SC was significantly more effective than no treatment. At 1-year follow-up, there were no significant differences in duration of awakenings between the SC and IT groups. SC produced a significantly greater increase in total sleep time from baseline to posttreatment than IT and no treatment. In addition, SC subjects reported greater satisfaction with treatment progress than IT subjects.

Friedman et al. (1991) compared sleep-restriction therapy (SRT) to relaxation training (RT) in a group of older insomniacs. The RT protocol consisted of a slightly modified form of progressive relaxation and unspecified visualization exercises. Subjects treated with RT and SRT showed significant shortening of sleep latency and wake time after sleep onset (WASO) by posttreatment, and significant latency gains were maintained for both groups at 3-month follow-up. Although no significant differences for WASO or sleep latency were observed between groups, the percentage decrease of WASO in SRT subjects (32.7%) was twice that of RT participants (15.9%).

In examining the various treatment options available, it seems intuitively sound to tailor the treatment approach to the nature of the insomniac's complaint. However, little research has been conducted to validate this claim, and the evidence to date is equivocal at best. Two studies have explored the efficacy of tailored treatments. Sanavio (1988) hypothesized that patients demonstrating high cognitive arousal when trying to fall asleep would respond more favorably to a cognitively based intervention in contrast to biofeedback. Such was not the case. Although patients receiving the cognitive treatment reported a reduction in presleep cognitive intrusions, and patients receiving biofeedback reported a decrease in presleep tension, the groups did not differ from each other for shortening sleep latency. Both groups had significant improvement in total sleep time through a 12-month follow-up period. Surprisingly, Sanavio observed a treatment type by cognitive-intrusion-level interaction on measures of sleep quality, with subjects complaining of high cognitive intrusion levels showing more quality improvement from biofeedback therapy and those with low intrusion levels benefiting more from the cognitive intervention. As mentioned earlier, this seems to represent the sometimes sharp distinction between quantity of sleep as often assessed in the laboratory, and quality measures that may also have a large bearing on the perceived success of treatment.

Another study examining the value of tailored treatment (TT) was conducted by Espie et al. (1989) using subjects randomly assigned to either PI, PR, or SC. Assignment to a particular treatment in the TT group was based on a questionnaire that attempted to identify significant causal factors. Ironically, posttreatment sleep latency improvement was greater for random therapy (49%) than for TT (35%). These researchers reanalyzed their results from the perspective of clinical significance, defined as a 50% sleep-latency reduction and a final sleep latency $\leq$ 30 minutes. Tailored training was compared on both criteria to random assignment to PR, PI, or SC. Stimulus control was the best treatment by both criteria, with 64% of SC subjects abbreviating sleep latency by 50% or more and 71% ending treatment with mean latencies $\leq$ 30 minutes. Tailored treatment finished second in both categories (50%, 43%), PI was a close third (47%, 40%), and PR was last (21%, 7%). Although the results of this particular study offer strong support for SC being an optimal treatment strategy, it must be remembered that sleep-latency reduction does necessarily correlate with subjective sleep quality.

Despite the paucity of evidence in favor of TT approaches, some matches between treatment strategies and insomnia complaints are intuitively appealing and should be given consideration. For example, relaxation strategies seem appropriate for the insomniac who complains of significant anxiety or muscle tension during the day or while attempting to fall asleep. Similarly, bed-time restriction strategies appear especially suited for the insomniac who complains of disrupted sleep but little daytime impairment. Much research has yet to be done examining not only nighttime benefits of tailored approaches, but the effects on daytime correlates to insomnia complaints as well. At the very minimum, providing a treatment program that corresponds to the presenting complaint lends face validity that may reassure the wary patient that the therapy is "on the mark."

Problems in Carrying Out Interventions

Difficulties with pharmacotherapy have been detailed in a previous section. Administration of behavioral interventions can also prove problematic. Even the most potent treatment plan can be rendered ineffective by client noncompliance. Clients prescribed stimulus control may find it difficult to use their bedrooms only for sleeping, and relaxation patients may not faithfully practice between sessions. Compliance with stimulus-control and bed-time restriction approaches require discipline and resourcefulness, as patients must carefully regulate entering and leaving bed, and develop strategies for filling additional out-of-bed time.

Patient compliance may also be impeded by initial discouragement when sleep-related difficulties increase during early phases of behavioral treatment. Higher levels of exercise may increase wakefulness in the unfit subject, and PI could produce lengthier sleep latencies. Decreases in total sleep time and daytime fatigue may accompany the early stages of therapies that restrict time in bed (Spielman et al., 1987). Friedman et al. (1991) altered the standard protocol of sleep-restriction therapy in an effort to increase compliance. Although the modified intervention allowed for greater tolerance of patient sleep-schedule preferences, the attrition rate for the sleep-restriction group was greater than that of a relaxation condition. Education about possible negative treatment side effects and an emphasis on long-term benefits that should result from short-term sacrifices may fortify patients against initial skepticism and discouragement, while increasing the therapist's perceived credibility.

Relapse Prevention

It should be kept in mind also that many of the interventions reviewed earlier can be conceptualized not only as interventions to correct faulty sleep patterns, but also as wellness behaviors to be carried forward as a part of daily living. A stimulus-control regimen, for example, will not often need to be invoked consciously once a normal sleep pattern is established. If, however, patients find themselves lying awake in bed and unable to sleep, they should revert back to the guidelines of removing themselves from the bedroom and returning only when ready for sleep (lest old associations re-form). In a similar vein, relaxation-training exercises can be practiced daily whether sleep is disturbed or not. Education regarding sleep hygiene might need to be refreshed in the insomniac suffering a lapse, but the behaviors described can certainly be lived with routinely.

To our knowledge, there are no empirical investigations of methods for preventing insomnia relapse. However, clues can be drawn from work in other health-psychology domains. Marlatt and George (1990) proposed a relapse-prevention model that was originally developed for addictive behaviors (e.g., smoking, alcoholism) but can be applied to any therapeutic program that requires behavior change. First, the patient is provided with skills to recognize and effectively cope with "high-risk situations." Weekends and holidays would be high-risk situations for the insomniac whose sleeping difficulties stem mainly from excessive time in bed. Successfully coping with the situation might involve scheduling early morning activities to motivate a timely departure from bed. Second, the patient is encouraged to cognitively reframe initial relapses as "lapses" or isolated slips that do not necessarily imply a full-blown relapse to baseline levels of a disorder. Such an intervention is particularly appropriate for insomniacs, as they may overreact to a single night of poor sleep. Disputing the importance of one bad night and stressing the *normality* of an occasional sleep difficulty should dampen the fears and catastrophic predictions that might impair future efforts to sleep. In addition to the suggestions of Marlatt and George, therapists may employ other relapse-prevention strategies, such as enlisting the aid of the patient's social-support system and establishing a reward system contingent on sleep-enhancing behavior.

CASE EXAMPLE

Case Description

Mrs. W., a 59-year-old woman, came to the sleep disorders center with a complaint of persistent difficulty initiating sleep nearly every night. The initial interview revealed the following background information:

- Mrs. W.'s sleep problem began approximately 6 years ago, following a severe illness. She described the illness as a viral infection that lasted for about 6 weeks, during which time she felt "wiped out," ran a consistently high fever, and was unable to sleep (she stated that she was drifting in and out of consciousness but never felt as though she was asleep). She also stated that she began hallucinating, at which point she was prescribed medications (she could not recall the name) that helped her to sleep.
- She remained on the sleep medications for about 9 weeks, then discontinued their use when her illness subsided. At that point, the insomnia first noted during her illness rapidly returned.
- She described her sleep habits prior to this illness as typically involving a 5- to 10-minute sleep latency, followed by 6 to 8 hours of uninterrupted sleep. She attributed the variation in sleep duration to daytime demands and routinely woke up to an alarm. She denied any early morning awakenings.
- She has smoked cigarettes for most of her life, except for two brief quit attempts during the past 4 years. She reported modest improvement in her sleep when not smoking. She denied the use of alcohol and drank a modest amount of regular coffee in the mornings and early afternoons.
- She reported an irregular sleep routine. She stated that she would sometimes go to bed at night with her husband around midnight and lie awake in bed until about 4:00 A.M. At other times, she would stay up and listen to radio broadcasts in another room until 3:00 or 4:00 A.M. She would awaken without an alarm at varied times, ranging from 6:00 A.M. to 7:30 A.M. When asked if she ever "lapsed" back into her old sleep pattern, she admitted that on two occasions (recreational-vehicle vacation trips into the mountains) she was able to fall asleep much earlier, sleep a full 5.5 hours, and awaken refreshed.
- Aside from initial fatigue in the early morning, she denied any daytime sleepiness.
- She denied any daytime napping.
- Although not involved in a rigorous exercise plan, she would take nightly 1- to 2-mile walks with her husband in the early evening. At the time of the initial interview, she was in good physical health.
- Her initial goals for therapy were to return to her "old, normal" sleep pattern of 6 to 7 hours of uninterrupted sleep, with a sleep latency of less than 20 minutes.

Differential Diagnosis and Assessment

The interview did not suggest any psychiatric factors contributing to the current symptomatology, although Mrs. W. did report being very anxious about her unusual "sleep disability." She did not report any chronic pain, and neither she nor her husband had noticed breathing irregularities or limb twitches during sleep. Delayed sleep-phase syndrome was unlikely for two reasons: first, her awakening time was consistent regardless of environmental demands to sleep or awaken at a particular time. Second, on her vacations, she was able to temporarily reestablish a bedtime closer to her previous norm. The information gathered suggested a diagnosis of primary insomnia in addition to some age-related sleep changes and sleep-hygiene problems.

When scheduling our appointment for the following week, Mrs. W. was given a week's sleep dairy along with instructions for its completion (Sidebars 14.1a and 14.1b). It was stressed that she complete them upon awakening on a daily basis. In addition, she was asked to monitor the frequency, timing, and quantity of caffeine use, and the timing and duration of exercise. The Stanford Sleepiness Scale (Hoddes, Dement, & Zarcone, 1972) was used to monitor daytime sleepiness.

The first part of the second session was spent reviewing Mrs. W.'s sleep diary. Consistent with her global report, Mrs. W.'s diary indicated a very erratic sleep routine. She had an average sleep latency of 76 minutes, based on a few nights of several hours' latency and a couple nights of a very short sleep latency (when she would stay up listening to radio in the living room until sleepy). She got out of bed shortly after awakening, typically around 6:30 A.M. Her average sleep efficiency was 65%. She used caffeine moderately, usually in the mid-afternoon. Once asleep, she rated her sleep as "fair" on most nights and did not report high levels of daytime sleepiness.

At one point during the second meeting, she remarked that she felt completing the diaries made her sleep worse. She elaborated by stating that she felt "pressured" to sleep, and knowing that her performance was being watched made her more mindful of what she might be doing to make herself sleep badly. She reported that she got out of this pattern of self-blame by reassuring herself that it was a sickness that caused the insomnia and not her own behavior. This led to a new line of questioning in the interview, one examining the nature of her thoughts about the bedroom. She stated that although she had no particular feelings about it, she was reminded of "the sickness that started this whole mess" every time she looked forward to "another rotten night's sleep." In addition, she described a pessimistic attitude about getting better but wanted to try therapy as a last resort before turning back to medications.

Case Conceptualization and Treatment Selection

At this point in the treatment process, several issues had been identified. Following an intense illness in which severe insomnia was a side effect, she received temporary relief through the use of sleep medication. Upon its discontinuation, she experienced a rebound insomnia that she attributed to the original illness. She began to associate the bedroom with frustration and dissatisfaction, a factor that started a cycle of self-fulfilling prophecies of disrupted sleep. In addition, she had unrealistic sleep goals in light of her changing sleep needs. Whereas she used to need 6 to 7 hours of sleep to feel rested, she now felt rested after 5 or 6 hours (as observed from her vacation sleep schedule). In light of these goals, even a good night's sleep was seen as another failure.

With these potential problem areas, the following treatment plan was selected:

- *Education*: Mrs. W. was to be educated about the changing sleep needs that occur with age, in order to set more realistic sleep goals.
- *Stimulus Control*: Some of these rules were already being followed by Mrs. W. She did not do other activities in her bedroom and did not take naps. However, she would sporadically spend as many as 3 hours lying in bed feeling frustrated about her wakefulness and had a slightly irregular awakening time.
- *Relaxation Training*: Mrs. W. was to be trained in and practice relaxation techniques involving mental imagery and passive-relaxation methods.
- *Sleep Hygiene*: Mrs. W. noticed that her sleep improved when she quit smoking, but she had only succeeded in abstaining for a month at a time. She was encouraged to eliminate caffeine use and to reduce smoking in the evening hours (or, if possible, quit smoking altogether). Increased daily exercise in the earlier part of the day was also recommended.

Treatment Course and Difficulties

The remainder of the second session was devoted to training Mrs. W. to use a hybrid-relaxation procedure (Lichstein & Johnson, 1993) and imagery. It was explained to Mrs. W. that the imagery and relaxation strategies were to help her with the "performance anxiety" that she felt as bedtime approached, but that to be effective they would need to be practiced every day. A time was set for daily practice, and she received a handout that summarized the relaxation procedures. She was also instructed to record the date and time of each practice session, along with a rating on a scale of 1 to 10 of how relaxed she felt before and after each practice session. Stimulus-control guidelines and rationale were discussed.

At the start of the third session, Mrs. W. presented a half-finished sleep diary and announced that treatment was not working. She reported practicing the relaxation program for three nights, but that she was still not falling asleep as before. Because her only other experience with treatment had been with sleeping pills, she had hoped for similarly rapid results with psychological interventions. Acknowledging her concerns, the therapist inquired about her expectations for treatment and explained that a permanent solution to this chronic problem would require a careful, well-thought-out therapy program. In addition, an analogy was drawn to the process of physical therapy after a difficult surgery, in which full function is restored only after weeks of difficult work. The real frustration, she (P) explained to the therapist (T), came in finding herself out of the bedroom more often than she had been before.

P: It drives me crazy! I feel like I'm taking a test when I go in there, and that I'll get thrown out of the room if I fail! You said it would be hard at first, but I had no idea.

T: Sounds like the performance anxiety you described earlier....

P: I'd rather just forget about the darned clock and watch the ceiling! At least if I'm in bed I'm relaxing, even if I *am* awake.

T: Well, two things about that; first, remember we said that clock watching is counterproductive. It would be better to turn the clock away and not worry about it. If you happen to notice that some time has passed, then acknowledge that you are not yet ready to sleep by going somewhere else in the house. Second, you said you're relaxing when you lie there? I don't remember you describing it that way before.

P: Well—relaxing?—no, not really. It's just such an awful feeling to know that I was only in bed for 2 hours.

T: Isn't that how much time you were spending asleep anyway? Even if you were lying there for 4 hours to get those 2?

P: Yeah, I guess that's right. It's just so discouraging. Do you think I'll ever get back to sleeping like I was before that virus hit me?

T: I'm sure your sleep can improve, though you may not need to sleep as much as you did at that time.

P: What makes you say that?

T: You said you sleep more "normally" on your RV trips, right?

P: Yes, but I still don't get 7 hours.

T: The number of hours you sleep isn't the best gauge of sleep adequacy. A better measurement is how satisfied you are with the sleep you get, and how you feel the next day. On vacations, don't you awaken refreshed after just over 5 hours?

P: Actually, I do. I don't really feel too horribly tired much of the time anyway, but those times I feel especially good.

T: Exactly. And you've never been one to sleep a really long time anyway. You may be one of those fortunate souls that can be rested on fewer than average hours of sleep.... We just need to find what *your* normal duration is. Bear in mind our conversation about how sleep needs change with age.

The remainder of the third session largely was spent rehearsing the relaxation strategies. She felt more encouraged after the session, noting that her relaxation skills appeared to be improving. Some time was also spent reviewing the sleep-hygiene issues, her goals and progress, and discussing the no-win nature of trying to "force" sleep.

By the fourth session she had caught a glimpse of encouragement from a couple of decent nights' sleep. In reviewing the week's diaries, she noted that on two nights she was able to fall asleep shortly after entering bed. One new piece of information that she added at this point was that being sleepy allowed her to let sleep happen, increasing confidence that sleep onset was imminent by the time she entered the bed. There were a couple of times that she "couldn't catch herself in time," and she fell asleep in the living room. Mrs. W. and the therapist discussed the importance of pairing the sleepy feelings with the bedroom and together generated alternatives that would help get her back to the bedroom rather than establish a pattern of sleeping on the couch. She seemed more involved and committed to therapy during this session. Relaxation was practiced again, this time with Mrs. W. speaking the instructions aloud as she performed them. She reported growing satisfaction with the relaxation exercises, explaining that in addition to physically relaxing her, it gave her something pleasant to think about.

When Mrs. W. came for her fifth session, she reported that she had been reducing her evening cigarette use. She reported heightened nervousness during the day but recalled that this was her usual withdrawal symptom. She was delighted to find that she could use her relaxation practice as a way to help her feel less nervous during the daytime. Her husband was urging her to quit smoking altogether. She was beginning to see greater sleep lengths, although she still went to bed 2 or 3 hours after her husband. At this point, however, she was beginning to notice a reduction in her anxiety on entering the bedroom. She had successfully revised her expectations and goals to achieving a satisfying sleep, of whatever length. Mrs. W. stated that keeping this attitude "took the pressure off," and coincidentally increased her sleep time.

Mrs. W. returned a few weeks later to share her progress. She reported an average of 5 hours asleep each night, but said she felt as though that was enough sleep for her. She had found a couple of activities she enjoyed doing while her husband slept, and came to view those hours as "private time." She attributed some of her success to the fact that she quit smoking, noting other physical benefits as well. She was continuing to use her relaxation exercises, although not on a daily basis. Mrs. W. stated that she still occasionally spent more time awake than she would like but adhered to the stimulus-control guidelines to avoid picking up old habits.

Mrs. W. never reached her original goal of "6 to 7 hours" of sleep but came to realize that she really did not need that much sleep to feel satisfied. Based on her satisfaction with her improved sleep pattern, she and the therapist mutually agreed to discontinue the sessions. She agreed, however, that therapy itself was ongoing and that she was in charge. Mrs. W. also reflected the understanding that some nights may not be satisfactory, but that an occasional "lapse" was normal for anybody. Of course, an invitation was extended to contact the therapist again if needed. A follow-up phone call 1 month later confirmed that her bedtime and sleep-onset pattern was becoming more stable, and that she continued to be satisfied with the sleep she was receiving.

In summary, Mrs. W.'s sleep complaint stemmed from a combination of anxiety about the bedroom coupled with unrealistic sleep goals. Although initially discouraged by the initial decrease of time in bed, she eventually came to view the bed as a place for sleep rather than worry. Education about changing sleep needs with age also helped her to set more realistic sleep goals, and the definition of a good night's sleep was changed from a simple measure of sleep duration to a more functional definition of sleep quality as measured by daytime functioning. The relaxation served not only to assist her in combating the physical tension and anxiety of bedtime but also served as a useful tool for daytime stresses as well.

Mrs. W.'s case also demonstrates the importance of enlisting the patient as an ally and partner in treatment, and establishing the credibility of the treatment plan. Her early reaction following the implementation of stimulus-control methods almost discouraged her to the point of terminating therapy. A prediction of the difficulties on the front end, and acknowledgment and examination of her difficulties as they arose, gave her confirmation that she was on the right track. In addition, problem solving what to do with her time awake made her a more active agent of change and gave her the methods and practice for solving similar problems in the future.

SUMMARY

Insomnia is a prevalent sleep disorder that can occur in conjunction with other health problems or exist in isolation. In general, insomnia is particularly common among females and older adults. The use of the unitary term *insomnia* is somewhat deceptive, because it is a heterogeneous disorder with etiology and symptoms that vary widely between individuals. The diversity of symptoms and overlap with other disorders makes careful assessment and differential diagnosis essential for treatment planning. Assessments should include objective measures when possible but should not ignore the patient's subjective perceptions of the disorder. Self-report measures are an effective tool in the assessment process. Although such reports may appear to sacrifice precision, it is the person's subjective experience that prompted the complaint, and therefore subjective reports should not be dismissed lightly. Sleep-quality variables may be as important in assessment and treatment planning as sleep-quantity variables, and increased sleep length does not necessarily imply increased satisfaction.

Many patients have either already explored pharmacological interventions or may wish to do so in the future. Although pharmacotherapy has demonstrated some short-term gains, it is contraindicated for the treatment of chronic insomnia. Several behavioral treatments are effective at reducing symptoms, but their success is depended on patient compliance. Despite the intuitive attraction of tailoring treatments to the nature of patients' complaints, there is little research evidence to support this so far. However, there may be gains due to tailoring treatments (such as bolstering face validity and client confidence in treatment) that have not yet been examined through empirical research. Closer examinations of this method are still needed to aid therapists in maximizing the probability of successful interventions.

REFERENCES

Aber, R., & Webb, W. B. (1986). Effects of a limited nap on night sleep in older subjects. *Psychology and Aging, 1*, 300–302.

American Psychiatric Association. (1987). *Diagnostic and statistical manual of mental disorders* (3rd ed., rev.). Washington, DC: Author.

American Sleep Disorders Association. (1987). *International classification of sleep disorders: Diagnostic and coding manual.* (Diagnostic Classification Steering Committee, M. J. Thorpy, Chairman). Rochester, MN: Author.

Bixler, E. O., Kales, A., Soldatos, C. R., Kales, J. D., & Healey, S. (1979). Prevalence of sleep disorders in the Los Angeles metropolitan area. *American Journal of Psychiatry, 136*, 1257–1262.

Bonnet, M. H., & Arand, D. L. (1992). Caffeine use as a model of acute and chronic insomnia. *Sleep, 15*, 526–536.

Bootzin, R. R. (1972). Stimulus control treatment for insomnia. *Proceedings of the American Psychological Association, 7*, 395–396.

Buysse, D. J., & Reynolds, C. F. (1990). Insomnia. In M. J. Thorpy (Ed.), *Handbook of sleep disorders* (pp. 375–433). New York: Dekker.

Carskadon, M. A., Dement, W. C., Mitler, M. M., Guilleminault, C., Zarcone, V. P., & Spiegel, R. (1976). Self-reports versus sleep laboratory findings in 122 drug-free subjects with complaints of chronic insomnia. *American Journal of Psychiatry, 133*, 1382–1388.

Edinger, J. D., Hoelscher, T. J., Webb, M. D., Marsh, G. R., Radtke, R. A., & Erwin, C. W. (1989). Polysomnographic assessments of DIMS: Empirical evaluation of its diagnostic value. *Sleep, 12*, 315–322.

Espie, C. A. (1991). *The psychological treatment of insomnia.* Chichester, UK: Wiley.

Espie, C. A., Brooks, D. N., & Lindsay, W. R. (1989). An evaluation of tailored psychological treatment of insomnia. *Journal of Behavior Therapy and Experimental Psychiatry, 20*, 143–153.

Espie, C. A., & Lindsay, W. R. (1985). Paradoxical intention in the treatment of chronic insomnia: Six case studies illustrating variability in therapeutic response. *Behaviour Research and Therapy, 23*, 703–709.

Espie, C. A., Lindsay, W. R., Brooks, D. N., Hood, E. M., & Turvey, T. (1989). A controlled comparative investigation of psychological treatments for chronic sleep-onset insomnia. *Behaviour Research and Therapy, 27*, 79–88.

Feinberg, I., March, J. D., Floyd, T. C., Jimison, R., Bossom-Demitrack, L., & Katz, P. H. (1985). Homeostatic changes during post-nap sleep maintain baseline levels of delta EEG. *Electroencephalography and Clinical Neurophysiology, 61*, 134–137.

Ford, D. E., & Kamerow, D. B. (1989). Epidemiologic study of sleep disturbances and psychiatric disorders. *Journal of the American Medical Association, 262*, 1479–1484.

Freedman, R., & Papsdorf, J. D. (1976). Biofeedback and progressive relaxation treatment of sleep-onset insomnia: A controlled all-night investigation. *Biofeedback and Self-Regulation, 1*, 253–271.

Friedman, L., Bliwise, D. L., Yesavage, J. A., & Salom, S. R. (1991). A preliminary study comparing sleep restriction and relaxation treatments for insomnia in older adults. *Journal of Gerontology, 46*, P1–P8,

Gillin, J. C., & Byerly, W. F. (1990). The diagnosis and management of insomnia. *New England Journal of Medicine, 322*, 239–248.

Gross, R. T., & Borkovec, T. D. (1982). Effects of a cognitive intrusion manipulation on the sleep-onset latency of good sleepers. *Behavior Therapy, 13*, 112–116.

Hauri, P. J., & Wisbey, J. (1992). Wrist actigraphy in insomnia. *Sleep, 15*, 2393–301.

Hauri, P. J. & Wisbey, J. (1993). Can we mix behavioral therapy and hypnotics? *Sleep Research, 22*, 207.

Haynes, S. N., Adams, A., & Franzen, M. (1981). The effects of presleep stress on sleep-onset insomnia. *Journal of Abnormal Psychology, 90*, 601–606.

Haynes, S. N., Fitzgerald, S. G., Shute, G. E., & Hall, M. (1985). The utility and validity of daytime naps in the assessment of sleep-onset insomnia. *Journal of Behavioral Medicine, 8*, 237–247.

Hoddes, E., Dement, W. C., & Zarcone, V. (1972). The development and use of the Stanford Sleepiness Scale. *Psychophysiology, 9*, 150.

Hoelscher, T. J., & Edinger, J. D. (1988). Treatment of sleep-maintenance insomnia in older adults: Sleep period reduction, sleep education, and modified stimulus control.–*Psychology and Aging 3*, 258–263.

Hoelscher, T. J., Ware, J. C., & Bond, T. (1993). Initial validation of the insomnia impact scale. *Sleep Research, 22*, 149.

Kales, A., Soldatos, C. R., Bixler, E. O., & Kales, J. D. (1983a). Early morning insomnia with rapidly eliminated benzodiazepines. *Science, 220*, 95–97.

Kales, A., Soldatos, C. R., Bixler, E. O., & Kales, J. D. (1983b). Rebound insomnia and rebound anxiety: A review. *Pharmacology, 26*, 121–137.

Kay, D. C., & Samiuddin, Z. (1988). Sleep disorders associated with drug abuse and drugs of abuse. In R. L. Williams, I. Karacan, & C. A. Moore (Eds.), *Sleep disorders: Diagnosis and treatment* (pp. 315–371). New York: Wiley.

Lacks, P., Bertelson, A. D., Gans, L., & Kunkel, J. (1983). The effectiveness of three behavioral treatments for different degrees of sleep onset insomnia. *Behavior Therapy, 14*, 593–605.

Lacks, P., & Morin, C. M. (1992). Recent advances in the assessment and treatment of insomnia. *Journal of Consulting and Clinical Psychology, 60*, 586–594.

Lacks, P., & Rotert, M. (1986). Knowledge and practice of sleep hygiene techniques in insomniacs and good sleepers. *Behaviour Research and Therapy, 24*, 365–368.

Ladouceur, R., & Gros-Louis, Y. (1986). Paradoxical intention vs. stimulus control in the treatment of severe insomnia. *Journal of Behavior Therapy and Experimental Psychiatry, 17*, 267–269.

Levin, D., Bertelson, A. D., & Lacks, P. (1984). MMPI differences among mild and severe insomniacs and good sleepers. *Journal of Personality Assessment, 48*, 126–129.

Lichstein, K. L. (1988a). *Clinical relaxation strategies.* New York: Wiley.

Lichstein, K. L. (1988b). Sleep compression treatment of an insomnoid. *Behavior Therapy, 19*, 625–632.

Lichstein, K. L., & Fischer, S. M. (1985). Insomnia. In M. Hersen & A. S. Bellack (Eds.), *Handbook of clinical behavior therapy with adults* (pp. 319–352). New York: Plenum Press.

Lichstein, K. L., & Johnson, R. S. (1993). Relaxation for insomnia and hypnotic medication use in older women. *Psychology and Aging, 8*, 103–111.

Lichstein, K. L., Nickel, R., Hoelscher, T. J., & Kelley, J. E. (1982). Clinical validation of a sleep assessment device. *Behaviour Research and Therapy, 20*, 292–297.

Lichstein, K. L., & Rosenthal, T. L. (1980). Insomniacs' perceptions of cognitive versus somatic determinants of sleep disturbance. *Journal of Abnormal Psychology, 89*, 105–107.

Lick, J. R., & Heffler, D. (1977). Relaxation training and attention placebo in the treatment of severe insomnia. *Journal of Consulting and Clinical Psychology, 45*, 153–161.

Marchini, E. J., Coates, T. J., Magistad, J. G., & Waldum, S. J. (1983). What do insomniacs do, think, and feel during the day? A preliminary study. *Sleep, 6*, 147–155.

Marlatt, G. A., & George, W. H. (1990). Relapse prevention and the maintenance of optimal health. In S. Shumaker, E. B. Schron, & J. Ockene (Eds.), *The handbook of health behavior change* (pp. 44–63). New York: Springer.

McClusky, H. Y., Milby, J. B., Switzer, P. K., Williams, V., & Wooten, V. (1991). Efficacy of behavioral versus triazolam treatment in persistent sleep-onset insomnia. *American Journal of Psychiatry, 148*, 121–126.

Mellinger, G. D., Balter, M. B., & Uhlenhuth, E. H. (1985). Insomnia and its treatment. *Archives of General Psychiatry*, *42*, 225–232.

Mendelson, W. B., Garnett, D., Gillin, J. C., & Weingartner, H. (1984). The experience of insomnia and daytime and nighttime functioning. *Psychiatry Research*, *12*, 235–250.

Milby, J. B., Wooten, V., Williams, V., Hall, J., Khuder, S., & McGill, T. (1993). Efficacy of combined triazolam–behavioral therapy in chronic sleep onset insomnia. *Sleep Research*, *22*, 237.

Morin, C. M. (1993). *Insomnia: Psychological assessment and management*. New York: Guilford Press.

Morin, C. M., & Azrin, N. H. (1987). Stimulus control and imagery training in treating sleep-maintenance insomnia. *Journal of Consulting and Clinical Psychology*, *55*, 260–262.

Morin, C. M., & Azrin, N. H. (1988). Behavioral and cognitive treatments of geriatric insomnia. *Journal of Consulting and Clinical Psychology*, *56*, 748–753.

Nicassio, P. M., Boylan, M. B., & McCabe, T. G. (1982). Progressive relaxation, EMG biofeedback and biofeedback placebo in the treatment of sleep-onset insomnia. *British Journal of Medical Psychology*, *55*, 159–166.

Puder, R., Lacks, P., Bertelson, A. D., & Storandt, M. (1983). Short-term stimulus control treatment of insomnia in older adults. *Behavior Therapy*, *14*, 424–429.

Regestein, Q. R., Dambrosia, J., Hallett, M., Murawski, B., & Paine, M. (1993). Daytime alertness in patients with primary insomnia. *American Journal of Psychiatry*, *150*, 1529–1534.

Reynolds, C. F., Taska, L. S., Sewitch, D. E., Restifo, K., Coble, P. A., & Kupfer, D. J. (1984). Persistent psychophysiologic insomnia: Preliminary research diagnostic criteria and EEG sleep data. *American Journal of Psychiatry*, *141*, 804–805.

Roth, T., Roehrs, T., & Zorick, F. (1988). Pharmacological treatment of sleep disorders. In R. L. Williams, I. Karacan, & C. A. Moore (Eds.), *Sleep disorders: Diagnosis and treatment* (pp. 373–395). New York: Wiley.

Sanavio, E. (1988). Pre-sleep cognitive intrusions and treatment of onset-insomnia. *Behaviour Research and Therapy*, *26*, 451–459.

Schoicket, S. L., Bertelson, A. D., & Lacks, P. (1988). Is sleep hygiene a sufficient treatment of sleep-maintenance insomnia? *Behavior Therapy*, *19*, 183–190.

Seidel, W. F., Ball, S., Cohen, S., Patterson, N., Yost, D., & Dement, W. C. (1984). Daytime alertness in relation to mood, performance, and nocturnal sleep in chronic insomniacs and noncomplaining sleepers. *Sleep*, *7*, 230–238.

Soldatos, C. R., Kales, J. D., Scharf, M. B., Bixler, E. O., & Kales, A. (1980). Cigarette smoking associated with sleep difficulty. *Science*, *207*, 551–553.

Spielman, A. J., Saskin, P., & Thorpy, M. J. (1987). Treatment of chronic insomnia by restriction of time in bed. *Sleep*, *10*, 45–56.

Torsvall, L. (1981). Sleep after exercise: A literature review. *Journal of Sports Medicine and Physical Fitness*, *21*, 218–225.

Turner, R. M., & Ascher, L. M. (1979). Controlled comparison of progressive relaxation, stimulus control and paradoxical intention therapies for insomnia. *Journal of Consulting and Clinical Psychology*, *47*, 500–508.

Woolfolk, R. L., & McNulty, T. F. (1983). Relaxation treatment for insomnia: A component analysis. *Journal of Consulting and Clinical Psychology*, *51*, 495–503.

15

Cognitive–Behavioral Treatment of Body-Image Disturbances

Thomas F. Cash and Jill R. Grant

> We are bound to our bodies like an oyster is to its shell.
> —PLATO

INTRODUCTION

The human condition is inherently one of embodiment. Mind–body controversies aside, the function and appearance of the body is life shaping. This is true both in terms of others' reactions to our bodies as we develop and interact with our social world and in terms of how we perceive and react to our own conditions of embodiment. The psychology of physical appearance (Cash, 1990; Jackson, 1992) considers both perspectives—the "outside view" concerning the social effects of appearance and the "inside view" that pertains to our highly personalized experiences of our own looks. The latter, in a broad sense, is what psychologists have come to call *body image*. This distinction is crucial because in appearance, as in other respects, we do not see ourselves as others see us (Cash, 1990).

For many people in our society, body experiences are fraught with discontent, self-conscious preoccupation, fruitless yet persistent attempts to alter appearance, and struggles to manage resultant negative emotions. Body-image problems are difficulties in their own right, and they contribute to a range of other psychological difficulties.

The central purpose of this chapter is to enhance the understanding of body image, its dysfunctions, and their assessment and treatment. The first half of the chapter provides essential conceptual and empirical foundations for clinicians working with a range of clients experiencing body-image problems. The chapter's second half delineates a step-by-step program of cognitive–behavioral body-image therapy (Cash, 1991b, 1995).

Thomas F. Cash • Department of Psychology, Old Dominion University, Norfolk, Virginia 23529. **Jill R. Grant** • Virginia Consortium for Professional Psychology, Norfolk, Virginia 23529.

Sourcebook of Psychological Treatment Manuals for Adult Disorders, edited by Vincent B. Van Hasselt and Michel Hersen. Plenum Press, New York, 1996.

**Thomas F. Cash and
Jill R. Grant**

As Fisher (1986, 1990) articulately documented, the body-image construct has long history. Early in this century, body-image concepts and studies focused on neurologically impaired patients. Although this brought the study of body image to the scientific arena, little heed was paid to psychological aspects of body experience. Mid-century scholars, such as Schilder, Scheerer, Witkin, Fisher, and Shontz, went beyond the neuropathological realm to develop diverse psychological perspectives on body-related experiences in everyday life.

In the past 15 years, much of the research on body image has emanated from a burgeoning interest in clinical eating disorders. As reviewed by Garner and Garfinkel (1981), Cash and Brown (1987), and Thompson (1990), this literature has largely conceived of body image in two relatively distinct ways. First is the *perceptual* construct that pertains to the accuracy or distortion of persons' estimates of their physical size (i.e., body width). To assess this dimension, a plethora of methods has emerged—from simple silhouette drawings to elaborate video-distortion techniques. Second is the *attitudinal* body-image construct reflected in people's affective, cognitive, and behavioral dispositions *vis-à-vis* their physical attributes, especially their appearance (Cash, 1990). A blended approach uses perceptual methods to assess body dissatisfaction as the magnitude of discrepancies between self- and ideal-percepts (Keeton, Cash, & Brown, 1990; Williamson, 1990).

Much has been gained from this marriage of body image and eating-disorders research, but there are detrimental consequences as well (Cash & Brown, 1987; Hsu, 1982; Pruzinsky & Cash, 1990a). Body image has become narrowly synonymous with either distorted body-width estimates or a discontent with (over)weight. Ignored in this research genre are attributes unrelated to weight (e.g., facial features, chest size, height, hair loss), people with disfigurements, women over 30, and men. Akin to the proverbial three blind men who selectively grope to identify an elephant, researchers exploring body image only from an eating-disorders vantage point will conclude that the body-image elephant is an adolescent female who misperceives her hated hips and thighs.

Most apparent from the rich and diverse history of the construct is the complexity of body image. In their book, *Body Images: Development, Deviance, and Change*, Cash and Pruzinsky (1990) concluded by delineating seven integrative themes from the body-image literature (pp. 337–347). We wish to expand on these themes here in laying the foundation for the assessment and treatment of dysfunctional body-image experiences:

1. *Body images are multifaceted.* Despite our use of the conventional singular term, there is no unitary entity "body image." Body image cannot be defined adequately by a single modality, such as the degree of contentment with one's weight. Clinicians and researchers must seek to understand the complex interplay among the constituent elements of body image.

2. *Body images refer to perceptions, thoughts, and feelings about the body and bodily experience.* The percepts include appraisals of one's actual physical attributes and internalized standards or ideals. Cognitive elements range from superordinate assumptions or schemas about one's body to discrete thoughts in specific contexts. Body-image affect goes beyond mere evaluative satisfaction or dissatisfaction with one's body to encompass a full range of associated positive and dysphoric emotions.

3. *Body-image experiences are intertwined with feelings about the self.* The nonphysical self and the "body self" are developmentally and reciprocally interrelated (Cash,

1990; Krueger, 1989, 1990). Just as events that undermine body image can threaten one's personal sense of self, a vulnerable self-concept can attenuate one's body-image integrity.

4. *Body images are socially determined.* Interpersonal experiences and cultural socialization define the social meanings of physical aesthetics and the personal meanings of one's own physical characteristics. Over the life span, social and societal messages convey standards of attractiveness and offer formative feedback about one's goodness of fit with the standards (Fallon, 1990; Lerner & Jovanovic, 1990).

5. *Body images are not entirely fixed or static.* Body images operate on both trait and state levels. Although there are dispositional proclivities to experience one's body in certain perceptual, cognitive, and affective ways, situational or contextual events serve to activate mediated body-image states with considerable variability between and within persons. An understanding of the contextuality of negative body-image states is of paramount clinical importance (Cash, 1994c).

6. *Body images influence information processing.* People who are schematic for (i.e., cognitively and emotionally invested in) their appearance attend to and process implicit information about their appearance differently than aschematic persons (e.g., Labarge, Cash, & Brown, in press; Markus, Hamill, & Sentis, 1987). Appearance-schematic persons with negative body-image attitudes are particularly susceptible to distorted perceptions of events which, in turn, promulgate dysphoric affect.

7. *Body images influence behaviors.* Body-image cognitions and affect motivate behavioral patterns, both approach and avoidant patterns. Approach patterns include appearance-enhancement or maintenance activities (e.g., grooming and exercise) because they produce self- or socially reinforcing consequences that one is attractive or matches physical ideals. Patterns of avoidance—whether of specific people, activities, poses, or situations—are negatively reinforced to the extent that they provide immediate relief from body-image dysphoria.

EPIDEMIOLOGY OF BODY DISSATISFACTION

In 1985, Cash, Winstead, and Janda conducted a national research survey on body image in *Psychology Today* magazine. Over 30,000 readers responded, and a stratified random sample of 2,000 was taken to represent the Sex × Age distribution in the U. S. population. The results revealed that about two of every five women and about one in three men were dissatisfied with their overall looks. Thus, a sizable percentage of both sexes indicated having trouble accepting their appearance.

Table 15.1 provides a breakdown of the specific foci of body-image discontent. Weight was the most disliked physical attribute—55% of women and 41% of men were displeased with their weight. Data from the survey as well as from other studies to be discussed later (see Cash, 1990) have shown that whereas women are mostly worried about being too fat, men are as concerned about being skinny as they are about being fat. The survey also revealed 57% of women and 50% of men to be dissatisfied with their waist/stomach area. Furthermore, although rounded hips are the biologically natural expression of womanhood, half of the women (yet only 21% of the men) disliked their lower torso—their hips, thighs, and buttocks. Being too flabby was a common concern, evidenced by the fact that muscle tone was a focus of discontent for 45% of women and 32% of men. About 30% of both sexes disliked their chest or breast area. The two physical attributes with which people

Table 15.1. Sources of Body-Image Discontent[a]

Disliked physical attributes	1972 survey		1985 survey	
	Men	Women	Men	Women
Height	13%	13%	20%	17%
Weight	35%	48%	41%	55%
Muscle tone	25%	30%	32%	45%
Face	8%	11%	20%	20%
Upper torso	18%	27%	28%	32%
Mid torso	36%	50%	50%	57%
Lower torso	12%	49%	21%	50%
Overall appearance	15%	23%	34%	38%

[a]Adapted from Cash, Winstead, and Janda (1986).

seemed most satisfied were their face and height. Roughly 20% of men and women were not content with these characteristics.

The vast majority of the survey respondents were people dissatisfied with at least one aspect of their appearance. In fact, only 28% of men and 15% of women expressed satisfaction with *all* body areas listed in the survey. Thus, total contentment is more the exception than the rule.

Table 15.1 also includes the results of an identical *Psychology Today* survey done 13 years earlier (Berscheid, Walster, & Bohrnstedt, 1973). A comparison of the percentages of dissatisfaction between the two surveys indicates that body images are not getting any better. In most respects, both men and women reported more dissatisfaction in the 1980s than in the 1970s. Furthermore, a just-completed representative survey of American women (Cash & Henry, in press) suggests that they now possess even less body satisfaction than was observed in 1985.

BODY IMAGES AND PSYCHOPATHOLOGY

A number of psychological disorders have body-image disturbances as a primary defining feature. For other disorders, body-image dysfunctions represent important secondary or associated difficulties. Pruzinsky (in Cash & Pruzinsky, 1990) provided an excellent overview of body image and psychopathology.

Eating Disorders

Bruch (1962) is credited as being the first to recognize negative body image as a central feature of eating disorders. In the past decade, anorexia nervosa, bulimia nervosa, and milder forms of eating disturbance, which are prominent among women, have received much empirical study and public attention (Rosen, 1990; Schlundt & Johnson, 1990; Williamson, 1990). The revised third edition of the *Diagnostic and Statistical Manual of Mental Disorders* (DSM-III-R; American Psychiatric Association, 1987) and the fourth edition (DSM-IV; American Psychiatric Association, 1994) posit body-image concerns among the diagnostic criteria for both anorexia and bulimia nervosa. Dozens of studies have revealed consistent connections between a range of body-image disturbances and problematic eating behavior and attitudes (see Rosen, 1990; Thompson, 1990). There is considerable evidence that negative body-image experiences predict severity of problematic eating patterns, and studies are beginning to point to body-image disturbances as precursors of eating-disordered behavior (Rosen, 1992; Striegel-Moore, Silberstein, Frensch, & Rodin, 1989; Thompson, 1992).

A key controversy concerns the specific nature of body-image disturbances among persons with eating disorders (Cash & Brown, 1987; Hsu, 1982; Hsu & Sobkiewicz, 1991; Huon & Brown, 1986). To provide some resolution to this issue, Cash and Deagle (1995) conducted a meta-analysis of 65 studies that compared either anorexic or bulimic patients and normal controls on various indices of body image. The results offered evidence that these clinical groups perceptually overestimate their body size more than do controls. Perceptual distortion of the average eating-disordered patient exceeded 73% of controls. Perceptual methods that used whole-body estimates yielded somewhat stronger effects than were found with multiple-site estimation procedures. More striking, however, were the differences on attitudinal body image—on both weight/shape attitudes and global appearance evaluations. The level of body dissatisfaction among the average eating-disordered person surpassed that of 91% of controls. Comparable clinical–control differences occurred for perceptual self-ideal discrepancies. Whereas anorexics and bulimics did not differ in their degree of perceptual distortion, bulimics displayed significantly more negative body-image attitudes than did anorexics.

Thus, this meta-analytic research clearly demonstrates a stronger link of attitudinal body image with eating disorders than is the case for perceptual distortion indices. Given the multidimensionality of the attitudinal body-image construct, its most salient components require closer examination. Cash and colleagues (Brown, Cash, & Mikulka, 1990; Cash, 1994b; Muth & Cash, 1995) distinguish among three attitudinal dimensions—evaluation (e.g., satisfaction, cognitive appraisals), cognitive–behavioral investment (e.g., schemas, strength of ideals, appearance-management behaviors), and affect (i.e., body-image dysphoria). A number of scholars (Fairburn, 1987; Garfinkel, 1992; Wilson & Smith, 1989) have proposed that the primary distinctive feature of eating-disordered individuals is the investment they make in weight and body shape for self-worth. In fact, Brown, Cash, and Lewis (1989) compared adolescent female binge–purgers and weight-matched controls and found that the former not only reported less favorable body-image evaluations but they also had more cognitive–behavioral investment in their looks.

As Bruch (1962) originally argued, amelioration of negative body experiences is necessary for effective treatment of eating disorders. Rosen's (1990) review highlights the crucial role of body-image disturbances as prognostic, maintaining factors in eating disorders, both in anorexia nervosa and bulimia nervosa. Although not all findings are consistent, substantial evidence suggests that body-image disturbances may engender attrition from treatment, and that the persistence of such disturbances following otherwise successful treatment outcomes is a powerful predictor of relapse (Rosen, 1990). Despite this evidence, there exists little systematic research to ascertain the additive efficacy of body-image treatment to the therapeutic regimens for eating disorders.

Body Dysmorphic Disorder

Body dysmorphic disorder (BDD) is a form of psychopathology with body-image disturbance as a primary defining feature. This somatoform disorder, newly listed in the

DSM-III-R, was historically referred to as "beauty hypochondria" and "dysmorphophobia" (for review see Phillips, 1991). DSM-III-R and DSM-IV descriptions of BDD include an individual's preoccupation with an imagined or exaggerated flaw in physical appearance. Such preoccupation in an essentially normal-appearing person or exaggerated concern in someone with a minor physical anomaly is usually not of delusional proportion (i.e., is a mostly ego-dystonic, overvalued idea rather than a somatic delusion) and does not occur exclusively during the course of other disorders (e.g., transsexualism or eating disorders).

Many have raised questions about the diagnostic utility of BDD as defined in the DSM-III-R (Phillips, 1991; Pruzinsky, 1990; Rosen, 1992; Thompson, 1992). Boundaries between BDD and somatic delusional disorder are clinically difficult to discern. In fact, the DSM-III-R states that delusional and nondelusional beliefs about perceived bodily defects may represent variations of the same disorder, a proposition also argued by McElroy, Phillips, Keck, Hudson, and Pope (1993). The DSM-IV dropped the nondelusional criterion, permitting an additional diagnosis of delusional disorder, somatic type, if applicable. Adding to the confusion about diagnosis is the difficulty distinguishing between a pathological condition and "normal concerns" with appearance. For these reasons, the DSM-IV added the criterion that the preoccupation must be sufficiently severe to cause "clinically significant distress" or functional impairment. More problematic, however, is that persons with substantial body-image distress who have more than a "minimal defect" in their appearance are diagnostically excluded. Alternatively, Thompson (1992) has reasonably proposed a spectrum of "Body-Image Disorders" with various subtypes.

Researchers differ in their conceptualizations of BDD. It has been described as an obsessive–compulsive disorder (OCD; Hollander, Liebowitz, Winchel, Klumker, & Klein, 1989; Phillips, 1991) and as a social phobia (Marks & Mishan, 1988; Rosen, 1992). Vitiello and de Leon (1990) disagree that BDD is linked to OCD, due to differential pharmacotherapeutic response of the two disorders. Moreover, the lifetime comorbidity of BDD and OCD is only 25%. Likewise, McKenna (1984) states that although the disorder is characterized by strong irrational beliefs that can dominate the individual's life, the beliefs are overvalued ideas that are not truly obsessional in nature. BDD's lifetime comorbidity with social phobia is 54% (McElroy et al., 1993). In her review of the literature, Phillips (1991) found that depression is the most frequently mentioned associated disorder. The lifetime comorbidity with any mood disorder is 96% for BDD patients, and nearly 40% have a history of suicide attempts (McElroy et al., 1993). Phillips (1991) adds that although several researchers have implied that depression is actually caused by BDD, it is difficult to determine causality without prospective studies.

Because the research literature on BDD is still in its infancy, the disorder's prevalence is unknown. Contributing to lack of knowledge about this disorder is the fact that individuals may suffer silently due to embarrassment about their preoccupation. Those who do seek treatment likely present in medical rather than mental health settings (Phillips, 1991), as they pursue dermatological or surgical correction of their "defect." Many people with BDD spend inordinate time and effort checking their appearance in a mirror, grooming in ways to conceal or camouflage the perceived defect, comparing their appearance to others, and avoiding situations in which their appearance may be subject to social scrutiny. A subset of people with BDD actually becomes homebound (Phillips, McElroy, Keck, Pope, & Hudson, 1993). Some severe BDD patients may engage in facial picking (i.e., "neurotic excoriation") and exacerbate the initially minor flaw (Stein & Hollander, 1992).

As Pruzinsky (1990) has discussed in greater length than we will here, several other psychiatric disorders are characterized by body-image disturbances. As mentioned earlier, delusional disorder of the somatic type may be a psychotic variant of BDD. Sometimes termed "monosymptomatic hypochondriacal psychosis" (Munro, 1988), the delusions typically focus on either body odors, bodily infestation, or body dysmorphia. Gender-identity disorders, such as transsexualism, involve a perceived discrepancy between biological sex and gender identity (American Psychiatric Association, 1987, 1994). Koro, a rare and largely culture-bound syndrome that occurs in males in south and east Asia, is his belief that the penis is retracting into the body and will lead to death (American Psychiatric Association, 1994; Rubin, 1982). Walsh and Rosen (1988) argued that self-mutilation may represent an extreme expression of body dissatisfaction. Conversion, depersonalization, somatization, and hypochondriacal disorders have also been considered to reflect body-image distortions of somatic sensation and function (Fisher, 1986; Kellner, 1986; Lacey & Birtchnell, 1986).

BODY-IMAGE DISTURBANCES AND OTHER PSYCHOLOGICAL DIFFICULTIES

Researchers report moderate associations between body dissatisfaction and poor psychological adjustment in general for men and women across the life span (Cash, 1985, 1990; Cash & Pruzinsky, 1990; Cash et al., 1986; Thompson, 1990). Numerous correlational studies reveal that evaluative body image accounts for about one-fourth to one-third of variation in global self-esteem (see Cash, 1990; Thompson, 1990). Furthermore, linkage between body esteem and self-esteem is especially strong among persons who are more psychologically invested in physical appearance (e.g., Cash, 1993b; Pliner, Chaiken, & Flett, 1990; Rosen & Ross, 1968).

The literature also confirms a relationship between body dissatisfaction and depression (e.g., Archer & Cash, 1986; Fabian & Thompson, 1989; Marsella, Shizuru, Brennan, & Kaneoka, 1981; Noles, Cash, & Winstead, 1985; Thompson & Psaltis, 1988). Noles et al. (1985) observed that whereas nondepressed individuals overestimate their actual level of physical attractiveness, those with moderate or higher depression have a negatively distorted view of their attractiveness. Pruzinsky (1990) adds that there is often a presentation of depression in conjunction with requests for cosmetic surgery.

Despite surprisingly little research on the topic, evidence does point to a positive relationship between body image and social functioning (e.g., Cash, 1985; Cash & Soloway, 1975; Mitchell & Orr, 1976; Pruzinsky & Cash, 1990b; Tiggemann & Rothblum, 1988). In Cash's (1993b) prescreening of 279 college women on multiple indices of body image and psychosocial adjustment for a body-image therapy study (Grant & Cash, 1995), body satisfaction showed consistently moderate positive correlations with social confidence and negative correlations with public self-consciousness and social-evaluative anxiety. Moreover, self-consciousness and social anxiety were higher for body-dissatisfied women who were appearance-schematic and invested in their appearance than those who were not.

Another potentially important consequence of a negative body image concerns sexual functioning. If one is self-consciously dissatisfied with one's body, then an intimate sharing of this self-perceived "naked truth" with another person can elicit apprehension and avoidance. Such anxious self-focus (Barlow, 1986), or "spectatoring," vis-à-vis how one's disliked body looks can interfere with sexual arousal and performance. The few studies conducted on this topic support these propositions. Links between body image and feelings about and engagement in sexual activity have been found (Cash et al., 1986; Faith, Schare, & Cash, 1993; Hangen & Cash, 1991; Kelley, 1978; MacCorquodale & DeLamater, 1979). Hangen and Cash (1991) found that body dissatisfaction was related to a narrower range of sexual experiences and lower sexual satisfaction among male and female college students. For women, a generally negative body image was related to less frequent orgasmic experiences. Women reporting a high frequency of sexual difficulties rated their appearance more negatively and reported more avoidance of and self-consciousness about body exposure in sexual situations. In both sexes, body-exposure anxiety in sexual contexts was associated with lower sexual drive and less sexual experience.

BODY-IMAGE DISTURBANCES AMONG OBESE AND OTHER PHYSICALLY STIGMATIZED POPULATIONS

Being overweight or obese is a highly stigmatized condition in our society throughout the life span. Attributes representing negative physical, personal, and social characteristics are assigned by children and adults to people with endomorphic physiques (for review, see DeJong & Kleck, 1986). The unfavorable social stereotyping of fat persons may adversely affect their vocational (Larkin & Pines, 1979) and educational opportunities (Canning & Mayer, 1966). The stigma is lessened, albeit not eliminated, if people attribute such obesity to medical causes beyond the person's control; otherwise, the person's weak character is regarded as responsible (DeJong, 1980; Lewis, Cash, Jacobi, & Bubb-Lewis, 1995). Obesity is related to downward social mobility among women (Goldblatt, Moore, & Stunkard, 1965; Gortmaker, Must, Perrin, Sobol, & Deitz, 1993) and seems to be more detrimental to women's social relationships than those of men (Tiggemann & Rothblum, 1988). Stake and Lauer (1987) observed that overweight women date less often, have less date or mate satisfaction, and experience more peer criticism than overweight men or average-weight men and women. In a recent longitudinal study, Gortmaker et al. (1993) documented progressive impairments in the income and marriageability of obese women relative to lighter cohorts, independent of health-related factors. The social prejudice and discrimination against overweight persons is so powerful that organizations such as the National Association to Advance Fat Acceptance have been established for social action and support on their behalf.

It is no wonder that obesity often entails a negative body image (Cash, 1990; Cash & Green, 1986; Friedman & Brownell, 1995). The overweight condition, however, may be as much a state of mind as it is a state of body. One survey (Seligman, Joseph, Donovan, & Gosnell, 1987) queried nearly 500 children and found that over half of the girls regarded themselves as overweight, despite the fact that only 15% actually were, and that 31% of 10-year-olds reported "feeling fat." Among college students, Klesges (1983) found that 58% of women and 20% of men who were of average weight classified themselves as over-weight. In the previously discussed national body-image survey (Cash et al., 1986), 47% of women and 29% of men who were average weight considered themselves overweight. In contrast, 40% of underweight women judged themselves as normal weight, compared to only 10% of underweight men. Thus, although our culture directs most of its weight-related messages toward females, males are not immune to the effects of such messages (Cash & Hicks, 1990; Drewnowski & Yee, 1987). One difference is that men are fairly equally divided between those who feel they are too heavy and those who feel they are too thin (Muth & Cash, 1995; Silberstein, Striegel-Moore, Timko, & Rodin, 1988).

In their controlled study, Cash and Hicks (1990) discovered that how an average-weight person classifies his or her weight has a strong bearing on attitudinal body image, eating behaviors, and psychosocial well-being. Objectively average-weight adults of either sex who proclaimed themselves overweight evaluated their bodies more negatively, having greater dissatisfaction not only with appearance but also with their bodily fitness and health. Underscoring the importance of cognitive factors in body image, there were greater psychological differences as a function of *self-classified* weight among truly average-weight persons than there were between *actual* weight groups (i.e., average-weight versus overweight persons) who thought of themselves as overweight. Thus, the label a person assigns to his or her weight has strong implications for the person's body-image affect and self-esteem (see also DelRosario, Brines, & Coleman, 1984; Tucker, 1982). Once this label has been self-assigned, the veridical presence of the overweight condition exerts few additional differences. Cash and Hicks (1990) further confirmed that being overweight, whether in distorted self-perception or in reality, is more detrimental to the well-being of women than men.

Obese people do not represent a psychologically homogeneous population (Brownell & Wadden, 1991). All fatness "is not created equal." Heavy women with a "pear-shaped" distribution of fat reported stronger weight concerns and eating disturbance than did women with an "apple-shaped" distribution of fat (Radke-Sharpe, Whitney-Saltiel, & Rodin, 1990). Two other subgroups seem to have especially disparaging body images. Relative to obese controls, those who enroll in very-low-calorie diet programs for weight loss are more invested in their appearance yet have more negative body-image evaluations (Cash, 1993a). Another subgroup consists of those who have a binge-eating disorder (BED), a new diagnostic category proposed in the DSM-IV. About 30% of overweight or obese persons in weight-loss programs exhibit BED, in which they eat large amounts of food in a short time period, feel out of control of their eating, but do not engage in compensatory behaviors, as is the case for bulimia nervosa (American Psychiatric Association, 1994; Fairburn & Wilson, 1993). These binge eaters often show greater psychological maladjustment on a variety of measures (see Friedman & Brownell, 1995; but also see Brody, Walsh, & Devlin, 1994, who found no differences). Even with psychological adjustment controlled, obese bingers report more overweight preoccupation, body dissatisfaction, and stronger appearance investment relative to nonbingers (Cash, 1991a; Grilo, Wilfley, Jones, Brownell, & Rodin, 1994).

Unfortunately, weight loss carries no assurance that body-image dysphoria is lost as well. Consistent with Stunkard's original proposition (Stunkard & Burt, 1967; Stunkard & Mendelson, 1967), Cash, Counts, and Huffine (1990) observed that formerly overweight women (relative to never-overweight controls) may persist in their negative "vestigial" body-image thoughts, feelings, and concerns about weight—a phenomenon that Cash (1994a) has termed "phantom fat." Even though body-image improvements do follow substantial weight reductions among obese persons, these improvements appear to be as fragile as the weight losses themselves (Cash, 1994a). Indeed, substantial weight regain occurs for most initially successful dieters, and retrospective studies indicate diminished body satisfaction is a salient effect of regaining weight (Kayman, Bruvold, & Stern, 1990; Wadden, Stunkard, & Liebschutz, 1988).

Another physically stigmatized population consists of people with congenital or traumatic disfigurements. Disfigurements often alter more than what people look like. Scholarly reviews document the social and psychological adversities that facial disfigurements can entail (Bernstein, 1990; Bull & Rumsey, 1988). As Pruzinsky (1992) has articulated, people with disfigurements face two formidable tasks. First, they must cope with the strain of their social interactions with nondisfigured persons, who may stare, avoid contact, or make unkind remarks. Such difficulties may foster social withdrawal by those with disfigurements, who seek refuge with family members or a few familiar friends (Macgregor, 1990). The second challenge concerns development of a satisfactory body image. Cash (1992b) compared adults with and without some type of self-perceived disfigurement. Whereas 46% of those without a disfigurement had a generally positive body image, this was true for only 29% of people with a disfigurement. Furthermore, 69% and 58% these two groups, respectively, reported a favorable overall sense of psychosocial well-being. Thus, although disfigurements certainly pose considerable challenges for coping, many persons cope well with the accompanying personal, medical–surgical, and social stressors (Macgregor, 1979, 1990; Shontz, 1990).

Once again, an appreciation of the diversity of this population is essential. Although the psychological sequelae are not linearly related to the degree of disfigurement, congenital anomalies generally have a more favorable psychological prognosis than acquired deformities (e.g., accidents, burns, or other traumas; Pruzinsky & Edgerton, 1990). Disfigurements that alter facial features central to interpersonal communication (e.g., eyes or mouth) may exert the most stigmatic effects (Bull & Rumsey, 1988). Moreover, Breslau (1992) suggested that burn victims with "hidden" disfigurements may have the greatest adjustment difficulties. People with a visible defect are forced to cope with and ultimately accept its social noticeability. On the other hand, less publicly visible defects may instigate avoidant, concealment behaviors that reinforce untested beliefs that others' seeing the defect would engender mutual distress.

DEVELOPMENT OF A NEGATIVE BODY IMAGE

The causal factors in the emergence of dysfunctional body experiences may be divided into two basic categories. First are the historical, developmental influences that shape the acquisition of particular body-image attitudes. Second, there are the current, proximal influences that direct the flow of body experiences in everyday life. Articulated from a cognitive–social learning framework, these past and present forces are shown graphically in Figure 15.1.

Historical, Developmental Determinants

One's sense of self is rooted in the experience of being embodied (Krueger, 1990; Mahoney, 1990). The body is the boundary that separates a person from all that is not the person—from the outside world. Humans, like certain other higher primates, have the capacity of self-awareness. By 2 years of age, most children can recognize their bodily self in the mirror (e.g., Schulman & Kaplowitz, 1977). Increasingly, this physical reality becomes a self-representation.

Historical influences:

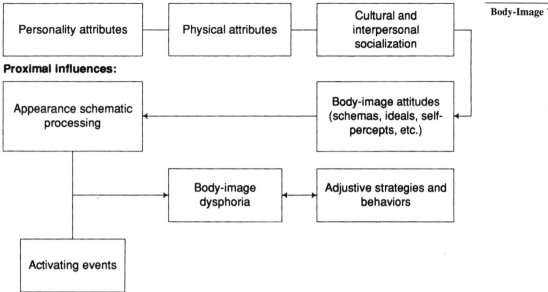

Figure 15.1 The causes of a negative body image.

Developmental psychologists have discovered that body image takes shape as pre-schoolers internalize the messages and physical standards of society and then judge themselves against them (Lerner & Jovanovic, 1990). In this way, children develop conceptions of what is good (how one *should* look) and what is bad (how one should *not* look) with respect to height, weight, muscularity, hair color, and even the style or brand name of clothing. From childhood on, people evaluate their appearance in terms of how well it matches the "shoulds" (Cash & Jacobi, 1992; Jacobi & Cash, 1994). Likewise, they form self-expectations and judge self-worth based on these internalized standards.

Thus, body image develops in a cultural context (see Fallon, 1990; Silverstein, Perdue, Peterson, & Kelly, 1986). Western society teaches that thinness for women and muscularity for men are desirable. Unlike earlier periods, the past several decades of this century has heralded a thinner, not-so-curvaceous body type as the standard of feminine beauty. Fashion models, film stars, and beauty pageant contestants have become thinner, even as the female population has gotten heavier. Recent social pressures require that women not only be slender but also that they be well-toned. In contrast, among societies in which food is scarce, corpulence is often a sign of success and survival.

Although less demanding than standards for women, there clearly are appearance expectations for men in our society. Growing up male means encountering pressures to look tough and be tough. Men are "supposed" to be tall, have broad shoulders, a muscular chest and biceps, small buttocks, strong facial features, and a full head of hair. In record numbers, men today seek cosmetic surgery, including hair transplants, pectoral implants, face-lifts, and liposuction (American Society for Plastic and Reconstructive Surgery, 1993).

Various studies have examined people's physical standards for the other sex and the accuracy of people's assumptions concerning these ideals (e.g., Fallon & Rozin, 1985;

Thomas F. Cash and
Jill R. Grant

Jacobi & Cash, 1994). Evidence attests to distorted beliefs about what the other sex truly finds most attractive. People seem to equate others' standards with their own personal ideals, although others' expectations are seldom as extreme or stringently held. For example, men are often more appreciative of a heavier female body type than women *believe* men are. Nor do men idealize blonde beauty and large breasts to the degree women think. Similarly, women do not necessarily hold the same narrow standards of "macho" male attractiveness that men assume women hold.

The process of socialization about the meaning of the human body goes beyond media messages. Families also model values pertaining to appearance (Rieves & Cash, 1995). The parent who spends lots of time, effort, and money trying to make the kids look perfect is modeling the attitude that good looks are crucial to acceptance in the "outside world." Growing up with a family member who constantly frets about his or her looks may convey that looks are something to worry about. Having a sibling doted on for being attractive may lead to implicit social comparisons that diminish one's body satisfaction and foster resentment and envy (Rieves & Cash, 1995).

Being taunted or teased about appearance during childhood can have an enduring effect on body image (e.g., Cash et al., 1986; Fabian & Thompson, 1989; Grilo, Wilfley, Brownell, & Rodin, in press; Thompson & Psaltis, 1988). Indeed, appearance is the most common content of social teasing in childhood (Shapiro, Baumeister, & Kessler, 1991). In a survey of college women (Cash, 1995a), 72% revealed that they had been repeatedly teased or criticized about some aspect(s) of their appearance (especially facial features and weight) earlier in their lives. Among these, nearly half said the teasing occurred moderately to very often, especially by peers during mid-childhood to early teen years. Almost half reported having had an unappealing nickname. Moreover, 71% said these experiences had permanently marred their body image. In fact, more frequent and upsetting teasing/criticism was significantly associated with greater current body dissatisfaction and distress. These findings have been recently replicated by Rieves and Cash (1995).

Puberty brings dramatic changes in appearance. It can also bring an intense preoccupation with these changes and with how they will be perceived by others (Pruzinsky & Cash, 1990b). The timing of physical maturation can be pivotal in the emotional meaning that teenagers attach to their changing bodies (e.g., Brooks-Gunn & Warren, 1985, 1988; Downs, 1990; Lerner & Jovanovic, 1990). Girls whose breasts and hips develop earlier than those of their peers may receive unwanted attention and become self-conscious. Rather than welcoming their new shape as a sign of emergent womanhood, many girls view it as unappealing fat. Boys with lagging growth in stature and muscularity experience concern about their bodies and whether they will ever "grow up." Teenagers' sense of acceptability—whether they expect to be popular, especially in dating—revolves partly around how they *believe* their looks are regarded by their peers.

Changes in one's appearance are a natural part of aging and development. People have control over some aspects of their appearance and can make choices, such as a new haircut or style, that either can enhance their body image *or* lead to a gnawing concern that they've ruined their looks. Other aspects are beyond one's control: the result of heredity or life's misfortunes. For example, *androgenetic alopecia,* or hereditary hair loss, can have a deleterious effect on men's and women's body images (Cash, Price, & Savin, 1993; Cash & Pruzinsky, in press). People may also have body-image difficulties as the result of traumatic alterations of appearance (e.g., severe facial injuries or mastectomy).

A final source of influence on body-image development pertains to certain moderating personality traits (Cash, 1990). Most prominent, of course, is the extent to which persons are appearance schematic, defining much of their selfhood in terms of their physical attributes. Self-esteem and social confidence are also crucial moderator variables. The child, adolescent, or adult who has acquired a positive sense of self is less vulnerable to societal "shoulds" or assaults on his or her physical acceptability. Public self-consciousness can also lay the foundation for a negative body image. This attentional predisposition to view oneself as would an audience can potentiate self-scrutiny and preoccupation with one's appearance.

Proximal Determinants

Cultural socialization, interpersonal experiences, physical traits and changes, and personality factors serve as predisposing causes of positive or negative body-image attitudes. However, how these attitudes affect day-to-day body experiences depend on precipitating, cognitive-mediational, and maintaining factors. Figure 15.1 summarizes these current causal influences.

From the first author's (TFC) perspective (Cash, 1994b, 1994c, 1995b; Grant & Cash, 1995; Pruzinsky & Cash, 1990a), specific contextual events serve to activate schema-driven processing of information about, and self-appraisals of one's body appearance. The activating events typically involve body exposure, social scrutiny, social comparisons, wearing certain clothing, looking in the mirror, eating, weighing, exercising, or some unwanted change in one's appearance. The self-evaluations draw on extant body-image attitudes and discrepancies between self-perceived and idealized physical characteristics. Implicit or explicit *internal dialogues* (i.e., automatic thoughts, interpretations, and conclusions), here termed "private body talk," reflect habitual and faulty patterns of reasoning—namely, the commission of specific cognitive errors (e.g., dichotomous thinking, selective abstraction, arbitrary inference, emotional reasoning, etc.). These cognitions potentiate various body-image affects, which in turn motivate adjustive, emotion-regulating actions. Among the "defensive" actions are avoidant and concealment behaviors, compulsive appearance-correcting rituals, social-reassurance seeking, and compensatory actions. Such patterns function as maintaining causes via negative reinforcement to the extent that they enable the person to escape, reduce, or regulate dysphoric cognitive and affective experiences.

The cognitive–behavioral body-image treatment program delineated later is based on this conceptual model of body-image development. The assessments used in the program measure the variables, both historical and proximal, specified in the model. The components of body-image therapy are similarly tied to this explanatory framework.

REVIEW OF BODY-IMAGE TREATMENT STUDIES

Prior to the mid-1980s, only a handful of studies had examined the effectiveness of psychotherapeutic body-image treatments. Moreover, all of these studies had some basic methodological shortcoming (e.g., nonrandom assignment, absence of a control group, no specification of intervention techniques, or no follow-up assessment). Although the quantity and quality of body-image treatment research have increased within the last decade, the limited research remains surprising in view of the clinical significance and widespread prevalence of a negative body image in the general population.

An overview of body-image treatment studies with clinical (particularly eating-disordered) populations is presented, followed by a more detailed examination of studies of cognitive–behavioral body-image therapies (body-image CBT) expressly for persons with clinical or subclinical body-image disturbances.

Body-Image Outcomes with Eating-Disorder Treatments

Despite the importance of body-image disturbances in the development, maintenance, and relapse of anorexia nervosa and bulimia nervosa, until recently few published treatment studies with these patients have incorporated body-image interventions and measurements. Many studies that have examined body-image variables were flawed by failures to explicate the focal body-image treatment procedures, to employ control groups, to use adequate, standardized body-image assessments, and to examine body image before and after treatment (see Rosen, 1990, for review). Given these problems, few firm conclusions can be drawn regarding the effectiveness of body-image interventions with eating-disordered populations. To our knowledge, no study has compared the *same* treatment with and without a systematic body-image treatment component. Rather, comparisons have been made between two *different* treatments, one of which gave body image some (albeit usually brief) therapeutic attention (e.g., Fairburn et al., 1991; Garner et al., 1993). Nevertheless, there are several noteworthy observations from these studies.

Psychoeducational approaches to the treatment of bulimia nervosa have produced varied results in altering body image. Berry and Abramowitz (1989) concluded that education was not especially effective in decreasing body dissatisfaction. Similarly, in a controlled study, Conners, Johnson, and Stuckey (1984) found only a nonsignificant trend for improved body satisfaction from a multifaceted program that included education, behavioral, and cognitive techniques. Wolchik, Weiss, and Katzman (1986) found that clients participating in an educational and experiential treatment reported less body dissatisfaction at the end of treatment but were not more improved than untreated controls. In an uncontrolled study, Davis, Olmsted, and Rockert (1990) found that a psychoeducational program led to significant changes in eating disturbance but not in body dissatisfaction. Subsequently, Olmsted et al. (1991) treated bulimics with cognitive-behavioral and brief psychoeducational treatments, both having sessions to address body-image concerns. Although the former treatment surpassed the latter in reduction of binge–purge behaviors, the researchers found equivalent and significant improvement on the study's sole body-image index (i.e., the Body Dissatisfaction subscale of the Eating Disorders Inventory).

Behavioral and cognitive–behavioral therapies may lead to favorable body-image changes in bulimic individuals (Leitenberg, Rosen, Gross, Nudelman, & Vara, 1988; Ordman & Kirschenbaum, 1985; Wilson, Rossiter, Kleinfield, & Lindholm, 1986; Wolf & Crowther, 1992). Leitenberg et al. (1988) concluded, however, that the positive outcome in their study was far from optimal. In a uncontrolled study, Wooley and Kearney-Cooke (1986) incorporated psychoeducational, experiential, and cognitive–behavioral techniques and found significant gains in bulimics' body satisfaction and decreases in their appearance preoccupation at posttreatment and 1 year later.

Fairburn and his colleagues (1991) at Oxford compared behavioral, interpersonal, and cognitive–behavioral therapies for bulimia nervosa. Only the latter included educational and procedural interventions focusing on body weight/shape concerns. The cognitive–behavioral program did produce more efficacious outcomes on weight and shape attitudes, especially relative to behavior therapy. Fairburn, Peveler, Jones, Hope, and Doll (1993) then conducted a 12-month follow-up to discern predictors of relapse. Congruent with other findings discussed earlier (see Rosen, 1990), patients with the greatest residual body-image discontent were clearly prone to relapse. The authors stressed the "need to reduce the degree of [body-image] attitudinal disturbance to minimize the risk of relapse" (p. 698).

Wolf and Crowther's (1992) results were partially consistent with those of Fairburn et al. (1991). They found that body satisfaction increased more for subjects participating in cognitive–behavioral *or* behavioral group therapy than for a wait-list control group, and that this increase was maintained at short-term follow-up. Only the cognitive–behavioral group displayed less dieting preoccupation after treatment.

Recently, Garner and his colleagues (1993) compared psychodynamic (supportive–expressive) and cognitive–behavioral therapies for bulimia nervosa. The clients verified that, as intended, the latter treatment dealt more with weight/shape preoccupations. Such body-image concerns were indeed more improved for having received cognitive–behavioral therapy.

Collectively, these treatment studies suggest that bulimics' body images are unlikely to improve without direct body-image interventions. Even when body image is targeted in the treatment programs, typically it is for only one or two sessions, and little focus is given in terms of ongoing extratherapeutic assignments. When included, body-image outcome measures are usually limited to a single weight/shape dissatisfaction scale.

There is little doubt that cognitive–behavioral therapy can significantly reduce the constituent symptoms of bulimia nervosa, including weight/shape concerns (Wilson & Fairburn, 1993; Wilson & Pike, 1993). However, the *clinical* significance (Jacobson & Truax, 1991) of the observed body-image improvements is seldom examined. A statistically significant improvement by no means yields a functionally normal or adaptive body image (Grant & Cash, 1995). Rosen (1990) has argued that treatment studies with bulimics have focused too much on eating behavioral changes (i.e., abstinence from bingeing and purging) as the defining criteria for improvement. Such behavioral changes are not necessarily indicative of body-image changes. Few body-image treatment studies have been conducted with anorexic patients. The primary focus of their treatment has been eating and weight regulation, which again offers no guarantee of body-image improvement.

Psychotherapy Outcome Studies for Body Dysmorphic Disorder

Controlled psychotherapy outcome studies of BDD are practically nonexistent. Phillips (1991) states in her review that published case studies (which have used behavioral, psychodynamic, or supportive interventions) yield mixed results. Of those BDD case studies incorporating cognitive or behavioral techniques, most patients were also receiving pharmacotherapy. Munjack (1978) and Giles (1988) found that desensitization techniques were successful in reducing BDD symptoms. Likewise, in their treatment of five BDD patients, Marks and Mishan (1988) reported improvement in maladaptive beliefs and social avoidance through the use of *in vivo* exposure and cognitive techniques. In contrast, Braddock (1982) found that assertiveness training and differential-reinforcement techniques were effective in increasing social behavior but not in changing dysfunctional beliefs in an adolescent inpatient with BDD. Similarly, Solyom, DiNicola, Phil, Sookman, & Luchins (1985) were unsuccessful in treating 2 patients with thought stopping and aversion-relief but were successful using a flooding procedure with one patient. Vitiello and de Leon (1990) reported a case study in which unspecified behavioral therapy plus pharmacotherapy was ineffective.

Recently, Neziroglu and Yaryura-Tobias (1993) briefly treated 5 BDD patients with exposure and response prevention. The authors observed clinical improvements in 4 patients, none of whom were receiving pharmacotherapy. Unfortunately, no standardized body-image assessments were included, but ratings of the patients' extent of overvalued ideation of ugliness declined following treatment and were maintained 1 year later.

Standing alone in the literature is Rosen, Reiter, and Osoran's (1995) controlled treatment-outcome study in which 54 BDD patients were assigned to either a no-treatment condition or body-image CBT. The latter consisted of eight 2-hour sessions to modify intrusive and dysfunctional body-image thoughts, expose patients to avoided body-image situations, and reduce excessive appearance-checking behaviors (see Rosen, 1995). Standardized body-image measures, including Rosen and Reiter's (1994) structured diagnostic interview for BDD, were administered at pretest, posttest, and 4-month follow-up. Results indicated a significant decrement of BDD symptoms and improvement in evaluative body image for treated versus control patients. These changes generalized to global psychological well-being and were sustained at follow-up.

The literature is largely negative or silent regarding the effectiveness of alternative treatments. The caveat of some psychodynamic therapists in treating BDD is to "focus on the underlying disturbance and not to become distracted by the patient's potential preoccupation with body image" (Bloch & Glue, 1988, p. 274). Sundry pharmacotherapies have mostly yielded unsuccessful outcomes. Although one possible exception (Hollander et al., 1989) may be the use of serotonin reuptake blockers (i.e., fluoxotine) or clomipramine, controlled trials with proper assessments have not be conducted. Body-image CBT appears to hold the greatest promise for the treatment of BDD.

Body-Image Therapy with Obese Persons

Most clinicians probably regard dieting and weight loss as the appropriate route to a better body image among obese people. Moreover, most weight-management programs focus on eating and exercise, and virtually ignore body image. The notion of body acceptance without weight reduction is seldom a consideration, although some professionals (Brownell, 1991; Brownell & Wadden, 1991; Cash, 1992a; Garner & Wooley, 1991) now argue for such alternative treatments in view of the biogenetic determinants of obesity and the rather poor long-term maintenance of weight loss. Antidieting educational programs are emerging to help people replace unhealthy dieting with "natural" eating and healthy exercise (e.g., Ciliska, 1990; Polivy & Herman, 1983, 1992). There is little evidence, however, that such programs alone foster meaningful improvements in body image.

Body-image CBT appears promising for obese persons (Rosen & Cash, 1995). Rosen, Orosan, and Reiter (1995) randomly assigned 51 body-dissatisfied, obese women to this treatment or to a wait-list control condition. Clients received eight weekly 2-hour sessions of body-image CBT, based on Rosen, Saltzberg, and Srebnik (1989) and including the assignment of Cash's (1991b) audiocassette program (described later in detail). Immediately after treatment and at a 4.5-month follow-up, CBT-treated clients, relative to controls, reported significantly improved weight/shape satisfaction, reduced size overestimation, fewer body dysmorphic symptoms, enhanced global adjustment and self-esteem, and less dysfunctional eating patterns. Furthermore, these changes occurred without significant weight modification, and individual client's weight changes were uncorrelated with their body-image changes.

Given the prevalence of body-image discontent among women, most body-image therapy outcome studies have been conducted with "nonclinical," body-dissatisfied women who were neither obese nor met diagnostic criteria for eating disorders (Freedman, 1990). Typically, however, the women did manifest subclinical symptoms associated with their very negative body images—namely, poor self-esteem, anxiety, depression, and eating disturbances. Those studies comparing body-image CBT with a control or alternative treatment condition are now presented.

In 1987, Dworkin and Kerr compared efficacy of cognitive, cognitive-behavioral, and reflective therapies relative to a wait-list control group in increasing body satisfaction and self-concept in 79 college women. Participants reported moderate to severe body-image disparagement on the Body-Cathexis Scale. Student therapists conducted individually administered, structured treatments consisting of three 30-minute sessions. Cognitive therapy entailed administration of a self-report inventory of body-image beliefs, cognitive restructuring of automatic thoughts, homework assignments, and generalization strategies. The cognitive–behavioral treatment was similar except for addition of self-reinforcement and imagery exercises focusing on assertiveness and body acceptance. In reflective therapy, therapists used minimal verbal following, paraphrasing, and reflection in exploring subjects' body-image feelings during specific developmental phases of their lives. Journal-keeping homework was also incorporated into the reflective therapy condition. To assess body satisfaction and self-esteem, the Body-Cathexis and Self-Cathexis Scales were administered on the same schedule for all four conditions.

Dworkin and Kerr's (1987) results revealed that whereas all subjects showed improved body satisfaction and self-concept, gains for those participating in treatment were significantly greater than was true for the wait-list group. Cognitive therapy was most effective in producing positive body-image changes, and the other two treatments were comparably effective. Cognitive–behavioral and cognitive therapy were equally effective in enhancing self-concept, and both were superior to reflective therapy. Thus, Dworkin and Kerr concluded that short-term therapy can be effective in increasing body satisfaction and self-esteem. In explaining the differential body-image outcomes for cognitive and cognitive–behavioral treatments, the authors speculated that certain exercises in the latter condition (e.g., subjects' imagining growing larger) may have weakened positive effects of other techniques and that therapist reinforcement in the cognitive treatment may have been more effective than self-reinforcement in the cognitive–behavioral treatment.

The authors pointed out several limitations of their study. The most noteworthy shortcomings were the reliance on only two, rather global outcome measures, and the lack of a follow-up assessment. Because treatment was quite minimal in terms of the number and duration of sessions, determining the maintenance of the therapeutic outcomes is crucial.

Concurrent with the Dworkin and Kerr (1987) study, Butters and Cash (1987) were independently examining the effectiveness of a more extensive body-image CBT program. They compared a 6-week individual-treatment program with a wait-list control group, who were subsequently treated with a brief 3-week version of the program. Subjects were college women who were within 25% of desirable weight and reported substantial body dissatisfaction (i.e., scored below the 25th percentile on the Appearance Evaluation subscale of the Multidimensional Body–Self Relations Questionnaire). These 31 women were randomly assigned to treatment or control conditions. Four trained clinical psychology doctoral students (two men and two women) served as therapists. The 1-hour structured, individual-treatment sessions consisted of direct therapist contact, audiotaped written information, and homework exercises. The 6-week program used body-image education, relaxation training, desensitization, identification and restructuring of negative body-image cognitions, enhancement of positive body-image activities, generalization training, relapse prevention, and stress inoculation. The 3-week program, for the subsequent treatment of control subjects, was primarily cognitive in nature (e.g., desensitization was omitted) and was identical to the last three sessions of the longer treatment. Multiple measures of body-image and psychological adjustment were administered in the 6-week program at pretreatment, posttreatment, and a 7-week follow-up; controls were assessed twice before their 3-week treatment and once again at posttreatment. Body-image assessments included self-appraisals of appearance, body dissatisfaction, cognitive investment in appearance, dysfunctional body-image beliefs, and dysphoria during mirror exposure. Other standardized outcome measures included social self-esteem, self-evaluations of physical fitness and sexuality, and a global symptom index.

Butters and Cash (1987) confirmed significant affective and cognitive body-image improvements from pre- to posttreatment for the 6-week treatment group relative to the untreated controls, and these changes were maintained at follow-up. Improvements entailed more favorable and satisfying body-image evaluations, less appearance investment, reductions in dysfunctional body-image cognitions, and less mirror-exposure distress. In addition, self-evaluations of fitness, sexuality, social self-esteem, and global functioning were significantly better for the 6-week treatment group compared to the control group at posttest. A comparison of the 6-week and 3-week treatments revealed no reliably different outcomes on any of the dependent variables.

To expand and improve on the two previous controlled investigations, Rosen et al. (1989) examined efficacy of body-image CBT compared to minimal treatment. By using a minimal therapy condition as opposed to a wait-list control group, the researchers were better able to control for demand characteristics and to determine the effectiveness of the active ingredients of body-image CBT relative to various nonspecific treatment elements. Unlike previous studies, Rosen and his colleagues also extended the control treatment condition to a 2-month follow-up assessment to determine the comparative maintenance of the outcomes of both treatments.

Selection criteria among female college students included average weight status, the absence of an eating disorder, and a score one standard deviation above the mean on the Body Shape Questionnaire (P. J. Cooper, Taylor, Z. Cooper, & Fairburn, 1987). The final subject sample consisted of 23 women averaging 19 years of age, who were randomly assigned to minimal treatment or body-image CBT. Sessions in each condition were conducted in small groups of 3 or 4 clients. The two female-student therapists conducted both treatment types and were blind to subjects' data. Treatment manuals and supervision after each session were used to standardize treatments. Subjects' treatment credibility ratings were equivalent for the two conditions.

For both treatments, 2-hour group sessions lasted 6 weeks. Body-image CBT consisted of education, homework exercises, identification and restructuring of maladaptive body-image cognitions and behaviors, and body-size and weight-estimation exercises to correct perceptual distortions. The minimal therapy condition was similar in format to CBT, except that it did not include structured exercises to correct maladaptive cognitions, behavior, and perceptions. Outcome measures tapped perceptual, cognitive-evaluative, and behavioral domains of body image. To assess perceptual distortion, subjects' combined width estimates of body areas were compared with actual measurements. The Body Shape Questionnaire and the Body Dissatisfaction subscale of the Eating Disorders Inventory provided cognitive-evaluative body-image measures. The Body Image Avoidance Questionnaire (Rosen, Srebnik, Saltzberg, & Wendt, 1991) was used to measure subjects' reported behavioral avoidance related to body-image discontent.

Subjects' pretreatment perceptual-size distortions were comparable to women with eating disorders. For clients in body-image CBT, their estimates became significantly more accurate, fell within the normal range, and were maintained after treatment. In contrast, the minimal therapy group did not show significant changes in their perceptual distortions over time. Although clients in both conditions reported significant decrements in body-image discontent from pre- to posttreatment, only those who had received CBT changed from a clinical to normal range. At follow-up, the same between-group difference was evident. On body-image avoidance, only the cognitive–behavioral group made significant changes.

Thus, Rosen et al. (1989) concluded that group cognitive–behavioral treatment was effective in producing positive changes in perceptual, evaluative, and "behavioral" aspects of body image. Unlike Dworkin and Kerr (1987), they found this treatment to be more effective than minimal, nondirective therapy. These discrepant results may be due to differing treatment intensities and techniques used in the two studies. Unlike Butters and Cash (1987), Rosen et al. (1989) did not examine generalization of body-image changes to other facets of psychosocial functioning.

In a subsequent dismantling study, Rosen and his colleagues (1990) compared two versions of body-image CBT to determine whether the correction of perceptual distortion was necessary to produce body-image changes. Selection criteria were similar to the Rosen et al. (1989) study, and clients were 26 very body-dissatisfied college women of average weight, without present or past eating disorders. Subjects were randomly assigned to one of the two equally credible treatment conditions, which again consisted of small-group sessions lasting 2 hours each for 6 weeks. The supervised therapists were three advanced clinical psychology graduate students who were blind to clients' data and used treatment manuals. As in the earlier study, structured sessions focused on perceptual, cognitive-evaluative, and behavioral aspects of negative body image. The two treatments differed only in that one included exercises to facilitate clients' realistic appraisals of body size and weight.

At pretreatment, posttreatment, and 3-month follow-up, body-image indices assessed multiple domains, and psychological adjustment was measured with the Global Severity Index of the Symptom Checklist-90-Revised (SCL-90-R) and the Rosenberg Self-Esteem Scale. The researchers also assessed eating attitudes and behaviors, using the Eating Disorder Examination and self-monitored eating records.

Results revealed no differences between the two treatment groups at the three assessment phases. Both groups made significant improvements in all measured aspects of body image, psychological adjustment, and dysfunctional eating patterns. The only variable that did not show reliable change after treatment was average caloric intake. Improvements were maintained at follow-up, except that meal frequencies and binge episodes did not differ from pretreatment levels.

These findings reaffirm the efficacy of a short-term body-image CBT administered in a group format. Rosen and his colleagues (1990) also inferred from their findings that significant decreases in perceptual-size distortion may have resulted from cognitive-evaluative changes, because the inclusion or exclusion of explicit exercises to alter size perception did not produce differential outcomes. Rosen et al. (1990) were the first to demonstrate that positive body-image changes were also linked to changes in eating attitudes and behaviors that were not directly addressed in treatment.

Fisher and Thompson (1994) recently carried out an interesting investigation in which body-dissatisfied college women received either body-image CBT in groups or a physical exercise program. After mass testing and screening, 54 women were chosen to participate. Selection criteria required a score of at least 1.5 standard deviations below the normative mean on the Multidimensional Body–Self Relations Questionnaire (MBSRQ) Appearance Evaluation subscale, the absence of severe psychiatric or medical disorders, weight within 12.5% of the actuarial norm, and denial of excessive eating restraint, bingeing, or purging. After being matched on body mass (kg weight/m² height), subjects were randomly assigned to body-image CBT, exercise training, or a no-treatment control group. There were two 6-week therapy waves of each treatment type. Multiple dependent measures were used to assess cognitive, affective, perceptual, and behavioral body-image dimensions.

Both the psychological and exercise treatments consisted of weekly 1-hour sessions and homework assignments, over the course of 6 weeks. Credibility and expectancy ratings were comparable for both conditions. In conducting body-image CBT, senior female psychology undergraduates were trained, supervised, and used a treatment manual (from Butters & Cash, 1987). The exercise treatment consisted of body-image and exercise education, low-impact aerobics emphasizing weight-relevant body sites, and weight-lifting activities. In addition to the one scheduled exercise session each week, participants were assigned the exercise regimen as homework two more times weekly.

Attrition left 46 subjects at posttest. Results revealed that the two treatments produced significant decreases from pre- to posttreatment in body-image anxiety and dissatisfaction; untreated controls remained unchanged. For treatment *and* control groups, however, significant and equivalent decreases occurred in body-image avoidance behaviors and size overestimation. Unfortunately, an attrition rate in excess of 50% at the 3-month follow-up prevented conclusions about the stability of outcomes.

While Fisher and Thompson (1994) concluded that the cognitive–behavioral and exercise treatments produced comparable positive outcomes on several facets of body image, they expressed concern that the observed improvements might not be clinically significant. They cautioned that although fitness training may hold promise for body-image enhancement, it may also risk reinforcing beliefs that body acceptance requires body alteration (e.g., weight loss or better muscle definition). Although their point is well taken, a recent quasi-experimental study by Hensley and Cash (1994) indicated that, relative to a sedentary control group, women who completed a semester-long aerobic dance class showed favorable changes in both state and trait body satisfaction. Exercisers improved their cardiorespiratory fitness, albeit without changes in weight. As Fisher and Thompson (1994) aptly recommended, the additive efficacy of cognitive–behavioral and fitness interventions is worthy of empirical evaluation.

The final, published investigation of body-image CBT to be described here is a comparative outcome study conducted by Grant and Cash (1995). The primary purpose of their study was to evaluate this therapy in two formats—a group therapy modality versus a largely self-directed format with modest therapist contact. Recent meta-analytic evidence reveals that, for a variety of psychological problems, largely self-administered, structured interventions with only minimal therapist contact can produce therapeutic outcomes that are often as favorable as therapist-administered treatments (Gould & Clum, 1993; Scogin, Bynum, Stephens, & Calhoun, 1990).

Grant and Cash (1995) utilized Cash's (1991b) published audiocassette program *Body Image Therapy: A Program for Self-Directed Change,* which consists of eight 30-minute cassette sides, a client workbook, and a clinician's manual. The program is a much-expanded version of Butters and Cash's (1987) treatment. Clients were 23 college women who met the following criteria: negative body image on the MBSRQ Appearance Evaluation subscale; no current or past-year clinical eating disorder; body-mass index within 25% of the norm; Beck Depression Inventory score less than 24, and no suicidal ideation; and not in concurrent psychological treatment. Clients were assessed at pretreatment, posttreatment, and 2-month follow-up on state, trait, and situational measures of body-image attitudes and on self and ideal body-size percepts. Generalization measures included self-esteem, social anxiety, self-consciousness, depression, and eating disturbance.

Clients were randomly assigned to modest-contact and group treatments. Both completed the audiocassette program. The modest-contact group ($n = 11$) met for 15 to 20 minutes weekly with one of two trained female assistants. The assistant explained the assigned tapes and homework procedures, answered questions, reviewed homework, reinforced compliance, and facilitated problem solving of difficulties with homework compliance. In the group therapy condition, clients ($n = 12$) met for 90 minutes weekly in one of two therapy groups, each led by one of two female therapists. As well as assigning and reviewing homework, therapists solicited participants' discussion of their body-image experiences, goal setting, behavioral rehearsal, and problem solving. Both treatment conditions entailed 11 sessions over a 4-month period. Sessions involved the following procedures, respectively:

1. Self-assessment of historical and contextual influences on negative body-image development.
2. Self-monitoring (diary-keeping) of body-image experiences—antecedents, cognitions, and consequences.
3. Multimodal relaxation training.
4. Systematic body-image desensitization (imaginal and then with actual mirror exposure).
5. Identifying and monitoring of cognitive body-image errors.
6–7. Cognitive restructuring to dispute cognitive errors and to alter dysfunctional internal dialogues.
8. Self-assessment of self-defeating body-image behaviors.
9. Exposure, response prevention, stress inoculation, self-regulation, and mastery-and-pleasure activities to decrease avoidant/compulsive patterns and to increase positive body-image behaviors.
10. Review and integration of cognitive–behavioral skills and problem solving/assertion with "difficult" people and situations.
11. Development of relapse-prevention strategies.

Grant and Cash (1995) found equivalent therapeutic outcomes for the two cognitive–behavioral treatments. All outcomes were sustained at the 2-month follow-up and included significant improvements in body-image evaluation and satisfaction and reductions in negative body-image affect across a range of situational contexts (including mirror exposure). Clients further reported reduced schematic investment in their appearance, fewer cognitive body-image errors and negative body-image thoughts, and less body-image focus and avoidance during sexual relations. They became less preoccupied with and anxious about their weight and reported more congruence between self- and ideal-body-size percepts. Gains generalized to improvements in self-esteem, social-evaluative anxiety, self-consciousness, depression, and eating disturbance.

Unlike all previous studies, Grant and Cash (1995) systematically examined the clinical significance of body-image changes, using the statistical procedures recommended by Jacobson and Truax (1991). Results confirmed that the degree of reliable and/or functional improvements in body image were generally quite favorable for both group and modest-contact modalities.

Recently, Cash and Lavallee (1995) compared Grant and Cash's (1995) data with those of an equally body-dissatisfied sample ($n = 12$) treated via Cash's (1995b) CBT self-help book, *What Do You See When You Look in the Mirror?*, which was administered without face-to-face professional contact. The latter program produced significant improvements in body image and adjustment. The levels of compliance and outcomes were equivalent to those that Grant and Cash had found under conditions involving greater degrees of professional contact. Partial support was also found for the proposition that greater compliance yields better outcomes.

In summary, the collective results of these controlled or comparative outcome studies attest to the efficacy of cognitive–behavioral procedures in the amelioration of negative body image among women of average weight who do not manifest clinical eating disorders. As all these investigations used what would typically be referred to as nonclinical populations, it is important to note that all subjects in these studies reported extreme levels of body dissatisfaction, and many were experiencing associated psychosocial difficulties. Body-image CBT appears effective in meaningfully improving cognitive, evaluative, affective, perceptual, and self-reported behavioral aspects of body image. This treatment has been found to be successful when implemented by relatively inexperienced therapists in group, individual, and supervised self-directed formats. Furthermore, body-image changes have been consistently shown to generalize to other areas of psychosocial functioning that are associated with a negative body image. Most changes from body-image CBT are maintained at least 2 or 3 months after therapy; however, longer follow-ups have never been conducted.

A COGNITIVE–BEHAVIORAL BODY-IMAGE THERAPY PROGRAM

The remainder of this chapter is devoted to a detailed, practitioner-oriented description of a body-image CBT program, largely based on Cash's (1995b) most recent version of the program. Practitioners are urged to be familiar with Cash's (1995b) "self-help" book and/or Cash's (1991b) earlier audiocassette version of the program (for which transcripts are also available from the author). In view of the aforementioned evidence on the efficacy of the program in which clients used such taped and written materials, clinicians may wish to consider their assignment to clients as an economical, informative, and structuring complement to therapy. This strategy may be of particular value when body-image problems are a secondary focus of treatment, and the clinical priorities of therapy sessions require working on other areas.

Caveats for the Clinical Practice of Body-Image Cognitive—Behavioral Therapy

Body-image CBT requires that practitioners possess specific clinical skills and be alert to certain important issues:

1. The program assumes that the clinician has the requisite conceptual and technical competencies in CBT, as well as the essential skills in developing and maintaining a therapeutic relationship. Even in highly structured programs such as this, professional problem solving and decision making are always needed in maximizing the outcomes of individual clients. Trainees should conduct the program only with proper supervision.

2. In clinical practice, clients with a negative body image typically present with a range of other psychological disorders or difficulties. A thorough assessment of clients' functioning and principal complaints is mandatory, and the clinician must acquire an accurate understanding of the functional significance of the body-image disturbances in relation to other aspects of the clients' psychosocial problems. There is no substitute for sound professional judgment in discerning the priorities for intervention. Body-image CBT should not be offered as the sole treatment for clients who, for example, are clinically depressed or anxious, exhibit eating disorders, or have sexual dysfunctions. Treatment strategies for these associated disorders are elaborated in other chapters of this volume. Body-image CBT can be effectively integrated with these treatments.

3. Body-image CBT can be conducted in either individual or group therapy. The latter requires professional acumen in the management of group processes, structure, and contents to harness their utility for the benefit of individuals. Accordingly, practitioners should be familiar with the use of CBT in groups, as described, for example, by Sank and Shaffer (1984).

4. Although the program is structured as eight discrete steps, these are carried out in a manner that cumulatively builds skills and integrates therapeutic techniques. Clinical priorities should dictate the introduction of components of the program.

Step 1: A Comprehensive Body-Image Assessment

Soon after the initial interview(s) in which the clinician and client have decided that body image will be a significant target of therapy, an extensive battery of body-image measures should be administered. These serve as (1) baseline indices of multiple facets of the client's body experiences; (2) information for feedback to educate the client about his or her strengths and vulnerabilities, and as evidence of the causal processes in the client's body experiences; and (3) crucial data for treatment planning. Most are self-report inventories that can be given clients to complete and return the following session. Thompson (1990; Thompson, Penner, & Altabe, 1990) has provided excellent "consumer guides" to many of these instruments; however, additional measures have emerged more recently. A description of psychometrically reliable and valid body-image assessments used often and suggested by the present authors follows.

One set of measures enables the clinician to determine clients' basic body-image evaluation, body-image affect, and cognitive–behavioral investment in, and reactions to appearance.

Multidimensional Body–Self Relations Questionnaire

The 69-item MBSRQ provides a standardized, attitudinal assessment of body image (Cash, 1994d; Cash et al., 1986) and consists of three groups of reliable and valid subscales: (1) the factor scales (Brown et al., 1990), (2) the Body Areas Satisfaction Scale (BASS; Cash, 1989), and (3) the Weight Attitude scales. Appearance Evaluation assesses evaluative attitudes regarding one's overall physical appearance. Appearance Orientation measures the degree of importance of and attention paid to one's appearance, as well as behavioral efforts to maintain and improve appearance. Additional factor scales assess evaluation and orientation regarding physical health and fitness. The BASS taps dissatisfaction with specific body areas or aspects (e.g., weight, height, face, lower torso, muscle tone, etc.). Finally, there are two weight-related subscales: (1) Overweight Preoccupation (Cash et al., 1991) reflects fat anxiety, weight vigilance, current dieting, and eating restraint and (2) Self-Classified Weight refers to how persons label their bodies, from "very underweight" to "very overweight."

Body-Image Automatic Thoughts Questionnaire (BIATQ)

The BIATQ (Cash, Lewis, & Keeton, 1987; Rucker & Cash, 1992) is a 52-item index of persons' reported "automatic" thoughts about their appearance, rated from never (1) to very often (5). Two relatively independent subscales reliably assess positive and negative thoughts (alphas > .90). The BIATQ may be scored as the ratio of negative thoughts relative to positive plus negative thoughts (Grant & Cash, 1995).

Appearance Schemas Inventory (ASI)

The ASI (Cash & Labarge, in press) assesses specific assumptions regarding the salience and meaning of one's appearance in one's life. Its 14 statements are rated on a 1 to 5, disagree–agree scale (e.g., "The only way I could ever like my looks would be to change what I look like"; "To be feminine, a woman must be as pretty as possible"). ASI scores are reliable (alpha = .84) and have been found to predict dysfunctional body-image thoughts and affect.

Situational Inventory of Body-Image Dysphoria (SIBID)

The SIBID (Cash, 1994c) lists 48 situations for which subjects indicate their frequency of negative body-image emotions, from *Never* (0) to *Always or Almost Always* (4). The items include social and nonsocial contexts, activities related to exercising, grooming, eating, intimacy, and physical self-focus, as well as appearance alterations (e.g., changes in weight or hairstyle). The SIBID is a reliable (alphas > .90), stable (1-month $r = .86$), and convergently valid index of negative body-image affect.

Body-Image Avoidance Questionnaire (BIAQ)

The BIAQ is a 19-item inventory of behaviors performed to control and conceal one's appearance, especially weight-related aspects (Rosen et al., 1991). Subjects rate frequencies from *Always* (5) to *Never* (0). The authors report satisfactory internal consistency and stability, as well as factor scoring.

Body-Shape Questionnaire (BSQ)

This popular measure consists of 34 items pertaining to concerns about body weight and shape (Cooper et al., 1987). Subjects rate items on a frequency scale from *Never* (1) to *Always* (6). The BSQ possesses good reliability and validity.

Body-Image Ideals Questionnaire (BIQ)

This specialized measure reliably assesses the strength of and perceived discrepancy from personal ideals on 11 physical attributes, such as weight, muscularity, complexion, etc.

(Cash & Szymanski, 1995; Szymanski & Cash, 1995). The BIQ's composite sum of strength × discrepancy scores correlates well with other body-satisfaction measures and indices of psychological adjustment.

These clinician-administered procedures should also be considered:

Body Dysmorphic Disorder Examination (BDDE)

Rosen and Reiter (1992) developed and validated this structured clinical interview to facilitate the diagnosis of BDD. Requiring about 30 minutes to administer, the BDDE assesses body-image discontent and preoccupation, self-consciousness and avoidance of social situations due to appearance-related concerns, restriction of physical activities and movements, body checking and camouflaging, comparing self to others, and reassurance seeking. The BDDE is psychometrically sound and useful in guiding the clinician through multiple facets of clients' body experience and identifying targets of body-image CBT.

Body Image Assessment (BIA) Procedure

To provide a perceptual index of body dissatisfaction, Williamson and colleagues (1989) constructed nine cards with female-body silhouettes ranging from *Very Thin* (1) to *Obese* (9). Subjects first choose a card to depict perceived (current) body size and then, after cards are reshuffled, choose one to convey ideal size. A difference score quantifies self-ideal discrepancy. Williamson et al. (1989) and Keeton et al. (1990) have substantiated the BIA's reliability and validity. Tabular conversions of self-percepts to distortion scores are possible (Williamson et al). Clinical use of the BIA may involve additional administrations using instructions to elicit "how you *feel* you look," "how *others* think you look," and so forth.

In Vivo *Distress Ratings*

In a weigh-in distress assessment, clients rate their level of discomfort (from 0 to 100) while being weighed on a scale (without receiving weight feedback). For the mirror-exposure distress procedure, clients stand 3 feet from a full-length, preferably tri-fold mirror, view their image for 30 seconds, and rate their discomfort from 0 to 100. Several studies have confirmed these procedures' validity (e.g., Butters & Cash, 1987; Cash et al., 1990; Grant & Cash, 1995; Keeton et al., 1990; Rucker & Cash, 1992).

Adjustment/Generalization Measures

The clinician should select pertinent measures of psychosocial functioning known to be associated with a negative body image. Among these might be (1) a global functioning index (e.g., the SCL-90-R or the Brief Symptom Inventory); (2) self-esteem (e.g., the Rosenberg Scale or the Texas Social Behavior Inventory; (3) social-evaluative anxiety (e.g., the Self-Consciousness Scales or the Fear of Negative Evaluation Inventory); (4) depression (e.g., the Beck Depression Inventory); (5) dimensions of eating disturbance (e.g., the Eating Disorder Inventory or the Bulimia Test–Revised). Most of these and other possible measures are contained in the second edition of Fischer and Corcoran's (1994) helpful sourcebook of *Measures for Clinical Practice*.

Step 2: Body-Image Education and Self-Discoveries

Early in therapy, the clinician should explain the tenets of CBT in terms of unlearning and relearning patterns of thinking, feeling, and behaving. Clients must come to see their role as active participants in change, increasingly taking control over their own experiences. The therapist should be viewed as catalyst and teacher, helping guide clients' development of competencies and corrective experiences. Therapy is to be construed as a collaborative process of creating and building changes. To strengthen further the credibility of body-image CBT, the scientific support for its efficacy should be stressed.

The aim of the next couple of sessions is to enhance a client's understanding of the origins and elements of his or her individual body-image experiences. This objective is pursued by carrying out several psychoeducational activities:

1. The client is given information on the psychology of physical appearance by means of a "bibliotherapeutic" assignment (e.g., Chapter 1 of Cash, 1995, or Tape Side 1 of Cash, 1991b). This information promotes rational knowledge of the truths and myths about the effects of objective appearance on people's lives and demonstrates the stronger effects of subjective body image. It "normalizes" the client's body-image concerns. It provides the client with a framework (from Figure 15.1) to understand the components and causes of a negative body image.

2. Through discussions, the therapist and client begin to apply this information to personalize the client's self-knowledge in terms of both the predisposing, developmental determinants (e.g., cultural messages, physical changes, teasing, etc.) and the proximal influences. With respect to the former, the client is asked to start keeping a "body-image diary" and write down critical events and experiences, from early childhood to the present, regarded as formative in his or her body-image development.

3. Drawing on the results of the body-image assessments (from Step 1) and an A-B-C model of the systematic unfolding of the client's current body-image experiences, the therapist and client begin to articulate the proximal influences. They collaborate to discover "Activators"—salient, precipitating events and situations, "Beliefs"—thoughts, assumptions, perceptions, and interpretations in the internal dialogues of the client's "Private Body Talk", and "Consequences"—the resultant emotions and adjustive behaviors. The therapist instructs the client in self-monitoring and assigns diary-keeping for his or her A-B-C sequences. Body-image emotions are self-rated (e.g., 0 to 10) in terms of their intensity and duration. First, the client records these sequences for typical past episodes of body-image distress. These are brought in and reviewed with the therapist, who collaborates in the revelation of apparent themes. Next, the client is asked to make diary entries for ongoing body-image experiences and to bring the diary to each session for discussion.

4. From these increasingly precise discoveries of patterns and processes, the therapist (T) and client (C) begin to set more explicit therapeutic goals. The client is asked to articulate these goals by completing a "Body-Image Needs Sheet." This session excerpt illustrates some of the discoveries and goals stated by Doris, a 19-year-old, nonobese, weight-worried client:

> **T:** Let's take some time now, Doris, so you can tell me the key things you've discovered so far and what you believe you really need to change in order to feel better about your body.
>
> **C:** Well, mostly I can see the path from my past—things that weren't my fault. You know, how my mother hassled me so much for being a fat kid, and how the other kids were so cruel.

What I realize is that, in my own head, I still give myself the same grief about my weight that they did. It's hard not to feel all the social pressures, from the media on down to other people's comments. It's hard being anything but tall, thin, blonde, and beautiful. But those women have their pressures too. Besides, I'm not them, and I need to stop hating myself for not being them.

T: So one of your goals is to start letting go of all those unfair experiences from when you were growing up and begin looking at and treating yourself differently?

C: I've got to! I just don't know how.

T: Well, learning how is exactly what therapy is for. Based on the questionnaires you answered and on the A-B-Cs in your diary, what would be different in your everyday life if you *were* treating yourself better?

C: Lots! First, I'd throw away the damned scales. I'd quit giving myself a hard time for gaining 1 pound or for not losing 10. I'd go to aerobics class and have a good workout instead of worrying whether the people there think I look fat. I'd quit telling myself that my boyfriend secretly hates my body. I'd stand up to my mother instead of being humiliated by her nagging me about my weight. I'd trash all those baggy sweaters and wear anything I want.

T: I agree, Doris. If you were doing those things, you would definitely have a much happier relationship with your body. During the week, I'd like you to write these goals down. Be as specific as you can. I want you to list all the other goals you can think of that would enable you to have a more positive body image. Next week we'll review these and begin working toward your accomplishing them.

Step 3: Body-Image Exposure and Desensitization

The goal of this step is to facilitate clients' exposure to the bodily foci and situational events that provoke discontent and dysphoria. This step is conducted procedurally as self-control desensitization (Goldfried & Davison, 1976), as opposed to its conception as passive, reciprocal inhibition. Clients actively use acquired relaxation skills to reduce and manage negative body-image emotions. The following procedures are carried out:

1. Termed *body-and-mind relaxation* (Cash, 1991b, 1995b), training includes progressive muscle relaxation, diaphragmatic breathing, imagery exercises, and self-instructional and autogenic techniques (for cued relaxation). After an initial in-session induction, clients are given a 30-minute tape (e.g., Tape Side 3 from Cash, 1991b) or a transcript with instructions for making their own tape (see Cash, 1995b). They are to practice relaxation daily for a week, rating the effects on both mental and physical relaxation and noting any problems, as well as those components that seem most effective.

2. In the next session, the therapist guides the client toward cue-controlled relaxation, without a tape, and begins hierarchy development. Two hierarchies are created, with 6 to 12 items each. The first consists of body areas or features that are the focus of varying degrees of discontent. Inspection of results from the BASS assessment is helpful here. The second hierarchy concerns situations or events that trigger body-image distress. Consulting the body-image diary and results from the SIBID are useful. Table 15.2 exemplifies each hierarchy, with items ordered as 0 to 10 SUDS ratings of discontent or discomfort.

3. In the initial desensitization trials, clients use relaxation skills to manage discomfort as they progressively "picture" disaffected body areas, from least to most disliked. The goal each time is *not* to be anxiety-free but to control and reduce discomfort. Clients begin in-session and continue as daily homework, noting progress and difficulties. Each item is imagined for 15 seconds, then 30 seconds, and then 1 minute, moving up the hierarchy with reasonable control of discomfort.

Table 15.2.   Exemplary Hierarchies for Body-Image Desensitization

Sharon's hierarchy of body areas and features

Area/Feature	SUDS rating
My thighs	10
My buttocks	9
My chipped front tooth	7
The birthmark on my right shoulder	5
My hair texture	3
My eyes	1
The size and shape of my breasts	0

Sharon's hierarchy of distressing situations

Situation	SUDS rating
My boyfriend seeing my lower body during sex	10
Being on the beach or at the pool in a swimsuit	9
Wearing snug slacks or shorts	8
Having a photograph taken of me (and having to smile broadly)	7
Weighing myself	7
Trying on clothes at the mall	6
Somebody asking about my birthmark	5
Others seeing me with my hair wet	4
Being around thin, attractive women	3
Exercise class	2
When people comment on how fat somebody is	1
Wearing my favorite colors and clothes	0

4. The next set of trials involve the client's completing the hierarchy during *in vivo*, full-length mirror confrontation while fully dressed. Again, in-session trials can initiate the procedure, which the client completes as homework and records problems and progress for discussion with the therapist.

5. Next, mirror desensitization is carried out privately at home, while the client is entirely or mostly undressed. For obvious professional reasons, this should *never* be conducted as an in-session exercise. Even in total privacy, many clients will experience substantial distress and resistance to this procedure. Clinical judgment is essential regarding whether these trials should be attempted at this time.

6. A final, imaginal-desensitization procedure targets the contexts of body-image distress. Again, most trials can be a self-directed homework assignment, with the instructional set of controlling rather than eliminating discomfort. Clients' records of their experiences should be examined and discussed in order to reinforce successes and suggest solutions to difficulties.

Our clinical experiences and research data (Grant & Cash, 1995) indicate that although clients will indeed gain a greater sense of emotional control from these exercises, they resist such exposure, especially mirror exposure, as quite aversive. Spending several weeks solely on exposure and desensitization is unwise. Instead, we recommend that, after imaginal body-areas desensitization, the practitioner introduce Step 4 of the program. The remaining trials can be done gradually, concurrent with other, cognitive interventions over the next several sessions. These interventions build particularly effective skills for managing body-image dysphoria. Nevertheless, the mirror exercises remain important among the situations that, from the perspectives of coping and extinction, clients must learn to confront rather than avoid.

Step 4: Identifying and Questioning Appearance Assumptions

Cognitive therapy draws on the techniques of Ellis (1977) and Beck (1976) to identify and alter maladaptive cognitive phenomena at various interdependent levels—from automatic thoughts to cognitive errors to underlying beliefs, assumptions, or schemas. "A schema is a structure for screening, coding, and evaluating the stimuli that impinge on the organism" (Beck, 1967, p. 283). Markus (1977) described self-schemas as

> cognitive generalizations about the self, derived from past experience, that organize and guide the processing of self-related information contained in an individual's social experience ... and make individuals resistant to counter-schematic information. (p. 63)

People vary in the cognitive investments and meanings they place on their physical appearance. Most persons with a negative body image are highly appearance-schematic, having an elaborate array of emotion-laden, implicit beliefs or assumptions that tie their looks to their basic sense of self.

This phase of therapy targets the assumptions, listed in Table 15.3, that clients endorsed previously on the ASI. The goal is for clients to discover the personal maladaptivity and tenuous veracity of their assumptions, which serve as a basis of their body-image distress.

The therapist and client engage in a dialogue to identify, elaborate, and examine the client's core appearance assumptions that serve to guide dysfunctional thoughts, feelings, and behaviors. Homework assignments support this process of discovery and questioning

Table 15.3. The Appearance Schemas Inventory[a]

1	2	3	4	5
Strongly disagree	Mostly disagree	Neither disagree nor agree	Mostly agree	Strongly agree

Clients will have rated these beliefs on a 1 to 5 scale:

1. What I look like is an important part of who I am.
2. What's wrong with my appearance is one of the first things that people will notice about me.
3. One's outward physical appearance is a sign of the character of the inner person.
4. If I could look just as I wish, my life would be much happier.
5. If people knew how I really look, they would like me less.
6. By controlling my appearance, I can control many of the social and emotional events in my life.
7. My appearance is responsible for much of what has happened to me in my life.
8. I should do whatever I can to always look my best.
9. Aging will make me less attractive.
10. For women: To be feminine, a women must be as pretty as possible.
    For men: To be masculine, a man must be as handsome as possible.
11. The media's messages in our society make it impossible for me to be satisfied with my appearance.
12. The only way I could ever like my looks would be to change what I look like.
13. Attractive people have it all.
14. Homely people have a hard time finding happiness.

[a]Adapted from Cash and Labarge (in press).

Thomas F. Cash and
Jill R. Grant

that Cash (1995b) refers to as establishing "reasonable doubt." The sequence of procedures, with illustrative therapeutic dialogue, are as follows:

1. The therapist reintroduces the explanatory framework that regards cognitive processes as pivotal in body-image difficulties. The aim of unearthing potential "sources of fuel" for distress is emphasized.

2. From the ASI, items that the client had rated as a 4 or 5 are targeted. The client is asked to expand briefly upon his or her personal belief in each.

3. Drawing on occasions in which the client felt body-image dysphoria, the therapist helps make connections between one or two particular assumptions and their experiential effects.

4. The therapist selects one or two of these that are espoused less vehemently. A Socratic dialogue ensues in which the therapist guides the client to explore the evidence for the truth and falsity of the belief. In effect, questions concern "What's wrong with this picture?" "Can you think of instances that contradict this?" "If you didn't believe this, how would you have reacted differently?"

5. The therapist reiterates the importance of the client's questioning these underlying assumptions. A homework assignment asks the client to write, for each endorsed assumption, "When I assume ———, then I think ———, and I feel ———." The client is then to write down possible exceptions, contradictions, flaws, and so forth, with each assumption.

6. In the next session, the therapist reviews the homework, reinforcing and elaborating (a) evidence of the body-image implications of the client's assumptions, and (b) instances of effective challenges of these assumptions. The client and therapist collaborate in developing more rational, accurate statements, which the client will write down and rehearse. Of course, the assumptions on the ASI are not exhaustive. The therapist should listen for and ferret out other implicit beliefs. Throughout, the therapist must understand the "kernel of truth" in some of the assumptions and not take incredulous positions. Exploring the necessity for and consequences of the assumption is more effective than attacking its absurdity.

The following excerpt illustrates the dialogue between the therapist (T) and Debbie (C), a 20-year-old college student who strongly agreed with Assumptions 3 and 7: "One's outward physical appearance is a sign of the inner person" and "My appearance is responsible for much of what has happened to me in my life."

T: Debbie, you say that you believe that one's outward physical appearance is a sign of the inner person. Can you think of an exception to this? Maybe you've met someone and developed a first impression based on their looks but found out later that their outward appearance didn't reflect what they were really like.

C: Yeah, that's happened a few times. I remember meeting a beautiful woman once at a party and immediately thinking that she was probably stupid or stuck-up, you know, the stereotype. Later she and I talked for a while when we were in the food line and I really liked her— she seemed like an intelligent and warm person. Obviously, I was wrong about her "inner person."

T: Good! So judging books by their covers can be inaccurate. I'll bet if you think about it you'll come up with lots more examples. The important thing is that you do have evidence of exceptions to this belief. Now I want you to think of how the belief may apply to you and your looks. Is your outward appearance necessarily a reflection of who you are on the inside?

C: (*Smiles*) I get it. I need to start questioning myself when I make these sweeping assumptions. One problem with this assumption as applied to me is that I'm a spiritual person and my looks don't convey anything about that.

T: Exactly! You are much more than what you look like. Now let's break this appearance assumption down so that you have a better idea of how it can lead to emotional distress. In your diary, you can list what you focus on, what you are thinking, and how you feel when that assumption kicks in. This will give you a good idea about how the assumption works against you. Also, make a list of statements that question and challenge the belief. I want you to become familiar with them by saying them aloud to yourself.

Debbie constructed the following challenging statements: "My personality has nothing to do with what I look like." "The real me is on the inside and I express the real me in my actions; this is what people actually notice." For her second appearance assumption, she asked herself, "Have bad things happened in my life that had nothing to do with my appearance?" "Are there times when my appearance was actually linked to success?" followed by assertions such as "My behavior is more responsible than my appearance for what happens to me." "If I stand in a corner and don't talk to anyone, it's likely that I appear unapproachable. If someone doesn't talk to me or notice me, it's probably because I am self-conscious and don't act interested, not because of my looks." "I can change my behavior to change the social outcome."

Debbie supplemented and reviewed her "reasonable doubts" each morning as she sipped coffee before school and again in the evening before dinner. She kept a diary of these challenges and revisions to her assumptions and how she felt after saying them aloud. With practice, she came to believe more in her revised beliefs, and she was able to forestall distress when recognizing the old, faulty assumptions at work in specific life situations.

Step 5: Discovering and Correcting Cognitive Errors

The next level of cognitive therapy focuses on the client's problematic private body talk during particularly distressing episodes of body dissatisfaction. This step flows logically from the previous one, and a number of cognitive strategies are employed to help the client "capture" and correct faulty thoughts and inferences concerning his or her appearance.

1. The client learns to identify specific, cognitive body-image errors (Cash, 1992c) and develops strategies to correct these errors with more rational internal dialogues. The therapist gives the client a description and examples of each of 12 errors from Cash's (1991b) Tape Side 5 or the pertinent chapter in Cash (1995b). As summarized in Table 15.4, the errors are given mnemonically useful names instead of technical labels (e.g., the "Beauty or Beast" error rather than *dichotomous reasoning*). The client reviews his or her body-image diary (i.e., the A-B-C sequences) for examples of private body talk that reflect each error and rates each from 0 to 4 according to its match with the client's thought patterns.

2. The therapist coaches and models to help the client develop corrective thinking strategies for typically faulty private body talk. The client is also encouraged to link his or her cognitive errors to the higher order appearance assumptions identified earlier. Before working on corrective thinking strategies *in vivo,* the client first expounds them on homework sheets for representative episodes of body-image dysphoria—adding a "D" for "disputing" to the A-B-C sequence. The client writes down the self-statements and interpretations that reflect each error, followed by disputational counterarguments to each.

3. During the next session, the client and therapist elaborate and rehearse these disputations, which Cash (1995b) characterizes metaphorically as a "New Inner Voice."

Table 15.4. Cognitive Body-Image Errors[a]

1. *Beauty or beast*: Dichotomous thinking about one's appearance (either attractive or ugly, thin or fat, short or tall, well-dressed or a slob, etc.) instead of viewing one's physical attributes on a continuum.
2. *Unreal ideal*: Comparing one's appearance against standards of perfection (i.e., lofty self-expectations, models, etc.).
3. *Unfair-to-compare*: Same as item 2, except that comparisons are made with real people encountered who have desired physical attributes.
4. *Magnifying glass*: Excessive focus on self-perceived flaws.
5. *Blind mind*: Minimization of one's physical assests.
6. *Ugly-by association*: Generalization of discontent, in biased fault-finding with various facets of one's looks.
7. *Blame game*: Arbitrary inference that one's appearance was the cause of some unwanted event or outcome.
8. *Mind misreading*: Projection of one's own negative body-image thoughts by assumptions about what others must think.
9. *Misfortune telling*: Inferences that one's looks will lead to particular negative consequences in the future.
10. *Beauty bound*: Conclusions that one's looks prohibit or prevent one from engaging in certain activities.
11. *Feeling ugly*: Emotional reasoning that feeling ugly is evidence that one must in fact be ugly.
12. *Moody mirror*: Generalization of negative thoughts and mood states from nonappearance events to body experience.

[a]Adapted from Cash (1995b).

The therapist has the client read aloud his or her new counterarguments for corrective thinking. To prepare the client for *in vivo* self-monitoring and cognitive restructuring, the therapist introduces a thought-stopping strategy, the "Stop, Look, and Listen" technique, which refers to (a) *stopping* the negative self-talk in midstream; (b) *looking* at the activating events and the maladaptive private body talk to discern the inherent cognitive errors that are operating and producing body-image emotional reactions; and (c) *listening* to more rational, accurate, corrective self-statements that dispute the errors.

4. The client is asked to audiotape corrective thinking dialogues and listen to them daily to facilitate their acquisition. The client continues to keep a body-image diary to record the application of corrective thinking in the daily management of dysfunctional body-image experiences. Now the client adds entries for *in vivo* disputations and their emotional *effects*. The latter completes an A-B-C-D-E sequence.

5. During this phase of therapy, the therapist may encounter several sources of client resistance. Creative ways to simplify diary keeping may be needed for noncompliant clients (e.g., taping instead of writing, limiting entries to a fixed number per day or week, using preprinted notecards). In addition, some clients may object that this is "just positive thinking" and is too simplistic to be effective. The therapist must help them (a) to see that cognitive restructuring is more personalized and complex than merely "thinking happy thoughts"; (b) to discover and weaken the cognitive–affective underpinnings of their resistance (e.g., "I'm too unhappy with my looks to change how I think"); (c) to understand that cognitive changes lead to gradual body-image emotional changes, not immediate, dramatic shifts from bad to good; and (d) to suspend their "understandable" skepticism for a while to allow themselves a "well-deserved and overdue" opportunity to have more satisfying body experiences. Intensively focused, in-session cognitive interventions that produce positive shifts in state affect may be valuable instigators of compliance. Finally, of course, therapists should never take compliance for granted by neglecting to reinforce clients' completion of and learning from homework.

Consider a case example of some of the procedures in this phase of therapy. Andy is a 40-year-old male with considerable distress about his balding. He (C) indicated to the therapist (T) that the Ugly-by-Association, Unfair-to-Compare, Magnifying Glass, and

Blind Mind errors occur often in his thinking and lead to feelings of dejection and disgust about his looks.

T: Andy, can you think of instances of your private body talk that reflect an Ugly-by-Association error?

C: I stare in the mirror at my bald spot and feel depressed because I think it makes me look older. I wonder how old I look. So I zoom in on the wrinkles under my eyes and then the gray in my eyebrows, and I think about how old or unattractive all these areas look. The more I find wrong with my body, the older, uglier, and more depressed I feel.

T: That's sure a perfect example of Ugly-by-Association thinking. You begin at the top of your head and then literally start "looking for trouble"—looking for any signs anywhere on your body that you might appear old. You really do a number on yourself. Now tell me, what's wrong with this pattern of thought? What are some reasonable arguments against it?

C: Well, like you said, it's just looking for trouble, looking for anything I can find to help make me miserable. It can go nowhere but to convince me I'm over the hill. It's pointless. It's stupid. I hate it. I guess I should try to stop myself before I go too far and feel bad about practically every aspect of my body. But that's hard.

T: I know it's hard, Andy, but you've got the right goal. You want to put the mental brakes on your runaway train of thoughts because you really don't like the direction the train is taking you. In your mind's eye, put up the big red sign that stays STOP! Then, look at what happening: You're being really unfair to yourself, picking apart your body, searching for whatever you dislike. Then, if you listened to the arguments you just mentioned, could you head in the direction you'd rather go?

C: It would help. I do need to realize that it is unfair. Like we talked about earlier with my Blind-Mind thinking, I need to focus on the fact that like my physique because I work out regularly. Just because I'm balding doesn't mean I'm an old man. I hate losing my hair and I should just leave it with that and walk away from the damned mirror.

During the session, the therapist had Andy stand in front of the mirror, verbalize the dysfunctional thoughts reflecting this error, and rehearse aloud the corrective thinking. He was asked to write this in his diary when he got home and then to write out corrective dialogues for his other main cognitive errors.

Regarding the Unfair-to-Compare error, for example, Andy reported that he would often compare himself to men his age who have thick hair and think: "They make me look bad. I'm so envious of them. How can I ever feel okay about myself when I'm up against people who look like that?" As a result, he felt self-conscious and resentful. He decided to use the following counterarguments to dispute this error: "Here I go again, comparing myself with someone else and feeling bad. The truth is, everybody is better looking than some folks and less attractive than others. Their looks have nothing to do with the way I look. They don't make me look bad; my own biased thoughts and comparisons do." He would then shift his focus to something he really likes about himself that someone with plenty of hair may not have, such as his sense of humor, being a decent golfer, or the fact that he's 6 feet tall and has good upper body definition. He also made himself look around and notice that lots of guys, even ones younger than he, have hair loss: "Some are a lot balder than I am. I remind myself I'm not so abnormal."

Step 6: Modifying Self-Defeating Body-Image Behaviors

This part of therapy targets clients' maladaptive behavior patterns associated with a negative body image. Although these defense maneuvers may offer temporary emotional relief, they serve to perpetuate body dissatisfaction and body-image dysphoria. Two classes of such self-defeating patterns are avoidant behaviors and obsessive–compulsive patterns. Both types are motivated by desires to escape, reduce, or manage negative body experiences (e.g., anxiety, self-consciousness, embarrassment). According to Cash (1995b), body-image avoidance may include avoidance of specific *practices* (e.g., weighing, wearing certain "revealing" clothing), particular *people* (e.g., attractive individuals, those who match one's physical ideals), various *places* (e.g., exercise class, the beach or pool), or certain *poses* (i.e., that accentuate one's disliked features). In addition, there are "grooming to hide" behaviors in which clothing, cosmetics, or hairstyling are used inflexibly to conceal or camouflage perceived flaws. The compulsive patterns are *appearance-preoccupied rituals* of two types: Time-consuming "fixing" behaviors are perfectionistic efforts to manage, repair, or alter one's appearance, usually by elaborate grooming regimens. Relatedly, there are "checking" rituals that include frequent mirror checking, weighing, social reassurance seeking, and so forth. This phase of therapy applies a range of behavioral and cognitive strategies to decrease the avoidant and compulsive patterns and strengthen clients' control over them.

1. Drawing on the cognitive–behavioral conceptual model (Figure 15.1), the therapist helps the client understand the function and maladaptivity of the aforementioned behavior patterns. Using the client's assessments (e.g., body-image diary entries, the BIAQ, etc.), the therapist and client collaborate in identification of the client's maladaptive body-image behaviors of each type. A homework assignment asks the client to develop an inventory of his or her self-defeating patterns.

2. The therapist helps the client to construct hierarchies of each type of pattern. There are two hierarchies of avoidant behaviors—one for practices, persons, poses, and places avoided; and another for "grooming to hide." Items are arranged in order of the client's efficacy expectations (from 0 = *No Confidence* to 100 = *Complete Confidence*) that he or she will be able to confront or execute whatever is avoided. Similarly, a third hierarchy arranges compulsive patterns in order of efficacy expectations that he or she can refrain from performing the ritual under cued or high-probability circumstances.

3. Before attempting to alter these behaviors, the client is taught a strategy derived from stress-inoculation training (Meichenbaum, 1985). This "PACE yourself" strategy (Cash, 1995b) entails four steps—*Prepare* (and rehearse an exact plan for confronting the avoidance or resisting the ritual), *Act* (on the plan), *Cope* (using relaxation, imagery, corrective thinking to manage any discomfort), and *Enjoy* (predetermined self-rewards).

4. One item at a time, the client develops a detailed PACE strategy for confronting each item on the avoidance and "grooming to hide" hierarchies, mentally rehearses the plan, and then carries out the strategy. After each attempt at changing a self-defeating pattern, the client notes the results in his or her diary and makes changes in the strategy as needed. In this manner, the client moves up the hierarchy, from easiest to most difficult activities.

5. A similar step-by-step procedure is followed in developing and implementing graduated exposure and response prevention strategies (Foa & Wilson, 1991; Steketee & White, 1990) for reducing appearance-preoccupied, compulsive rituals. The therapist and client creatively tailor plans that include controlling the rituals by means of delay tactics, time restriction, frequency rationing, obstruction, or scheduling of the specific fixing and checking behaviors (see Cash, 1995b). Throughout this process, the client uses the PACE strategy, incorporates previously learned skills in coping and corrective thinking, and records the plans and results in the diary.

This phase of body-image CBT is illustrated by the case of Sarah, an attractive 37-year-old woman who had a mastectomy less than a year ago. Although her cancer was successfully removed, she developed a negative body image after the surgery. She opted to postpone reconstructive surgery, and she purchased a prosthetic bra that she seldom wears. Her body-image distress was accompanied by several avoidant behaviors and frustrating rituals that she identified. Table 15.5 shows her three hierarchies, organized in terms of her self-efficacy of not engaging in each self-defeating pattern. This excerpt is from a session with the therapist (T) in which she (C) worked on particular items from her hierarchies.

T: Sarah, now let's work out a strategy for you to take on the avoidant behavior that will be easiest to confront—your avoiding profile poses in public. Can you think of how to confront this? Pick a time and place to start facing it, and anticipate what negative thoughts and feelings are likely to crop up.

C: I could try standing so that my co-workers see my body's side profile when I'm in the break-room at work. This is one place where I am very aware of how I appear to others. Usually there are several people socializing in that area. I already know what I'll be thinking: "Betty is looking at my flat chest and feeling sorry for me. She'll probably go talk to our other co-workers about how I should get reconstructive surgery to improve my image." I'll be tempted to pick up a book or paper and hold it to my chest.

T: Good. Your goal would be to maintain that profile without avoiding it or covering your chest. Now, think about how you can prepare for this and how you can handle any of the discomfort you expect may occur.

C: Beforehand, I could picture myself doing this and imagine feeling confident, like I used to feel. I could use the breathing techniques I've learned. To stop my Mind-Misreading error, I could tell myself, "It's silly to think that other people are looking at my chest. They have better things to do. Besides, even if they notice, so what? It's not like it's a big secret that I had a mastectomy." Instead of standing there dwelling on being self-conscious, I need to lighten up and enjoy people's stories and jokes. If I participate like I used to, then work will be more fun.

Table 15.5. Exemplary Hierarchies of Self-Defeating Body-Image Behaviors

	Self-efficacy ratings
Sarah's Avoided Practices, Places, People, and Poses:	
Sexual activity with husband	5
Having others ask me about the mastectomy	10
Going to the swimming pool	15
Participating in dance aerobics	20
Trying on tops at the clothing store	25
Hugging or being hugged	45
Sustaining profiles poses in public	60
Sarah's "Grooming to Hide" Behaviors:	
Wearing a flannel gown to bed	20
Wearing only loose blouses and sweaters	30
Sarah's Fixing and Checking Rituals:	
Checking appearance excessively in mirror at home	10
Checking appearance excessively in mirrors away from home	20
Repeatedly changing tops before going out in public	30

[a]Self-efficacy ratings refer to the client's expectancy (from 0 = *No Confidence* to 100 = *Complete Confidence*) that she will be able to confront and engage in the avoided item or to refrain from engaging in the grooming, fixing, or checking behaviors.

T: Great! I can tell that you've been practicing your new corrective thinking to take control over your private body talk. Using imagery and relaxation sounds like a really good idea. But I wonder if you can see an appearance assumption lurking here.

C: You're right. I'm assuming that what's wrong with my looks is the most noticeable thing about me. And, of course, it's not. Plus they know how I look, and they still like me. If they're uncomfortable, it's probably because I am. If I were able to talk to them about my mastectomy, we'd all probably be less tense. But that's something I'm not ready for. For now I think I'll start with not avoiding the break-room for 5 minutes each day.

T: It takes a little while Sarah. Let's just do this one step at a time. Socializing in the break-room for 5 minutes each day will certainly help you be ready. I want you to rehearse your plan mentally for a couple of days and then set a start date. You might want to add some more self-statements about accepting any discomfort you may feel as you stand in profile around your co-workers and knowing the discomfort will pass. So how will you reward yourself for tackling this situation?

C: I'll tell myself, "Hurray, I did it, and it wasn't that bad." I also could get one of my favorite snacks from the machine or buy a magazine after work.

T: Good! That's a specific plan to deal with avoiding profile poses. Now, walk through your plan aloud with me and imagine yourself actually doing it. How does it feel?

Sarah developed similar PACE strategies for her other avoidant and "grooming-to-hide" behaviors, using corrective thinking strategies, positive coping imagery, and relaxation skills. She also shared her sexual avoidance problem with her husband and asked him to help her with gradual exposure experiences that would help her relax and enjoy his intimate touching. For her rituals, Sarah chose to limit herself to two blouse changes before leaving the house and to progressively limit her total mirror-checking time from 30 to 5 minutes. She also decided to delay 5 minutes before searching out a mirror in public whenever she felt the urge to check her appearance. She found that if she distracted herself with something to read, her urge to check would usually subside. After several weeks of rehearsing and implementing her plan for each hierarchy item, Sarah felt more in control of her behavior and reported enjoying life more because she was less self-conscious and less restrictive of her social activities. She joined a support group to talk with and help other women who recently had a mastectomy.

Step 7: Body-Image Enhancement with Physical Mastery and Pleasure Activities

Therapeutic steps thus far have targeted negative cognitive and behavioral patterns. In Step 7, the client engages in exercises to increase positive body experiences. Introducing this phase of therapy, the therapist uses a *dysfunctional relationship* metaphor for framing how the client relates to his or her body (Cash, 1995b). The goal is to improve the relationship by expanding the client's experiences of "treating his or her body right." The client increases sensate, health/fitness, and appearance-related activities to produce a sense of mastery and pleasure—and positive body-self relations. Many people with a negative body image overemphasize their appearance and fail to derive rewarding experiences from aspects of bodily functioning. For example, they exercise but focus on weight loss rather than on the mastery and pleasure of the experience (Cash, Novy, & Grant, 1994). In this step, the client also carries out creative *affirmative actions* (Cash, 1991b, 1995b) to enhance favorable body-image thoughts and feelings.

1. The client completes a survey (Cash, 1991b, 1995b) to specify the frequency of various body-related activities over the past year. The client rates the mastery (i.e., goal-related accomplishment) and pleasure (i.e., fun or enjoyment) derived from each. Table 15.6 lists a sample of these activities. For activities that have provided (or could provide) at least a moderate sense of mastery or pleasure, the client categorizes them into appearance, health/fitness, and sensate domains.

2. The therapist points out that people differ in terms of how they may view particular activities (e.g., going for a brisk walk may entail health/fitness goals, an appearance-related goal of weight control, or sensate experiences). The client selects two or three activities for mastery and for pleasure in each of the three categories, and then begins scheduling and engaging in one or two per day. In his or her diary, the client records the mastery or pleasure experienced with each activity.

3. The therapist reviews with the client the results of these activities, reinforcing the client's self-regulatory abilities to expand the sources of his or her positive body-related experiences. If the client has difficulty carrying out an activity, the therapist helps develop appropriate cognitive and behavioral strategies to overcome resistance.

4. Next, the therapist and client develop additional experiential exercises (Cash,

Table 15.6. Sample Items from the Survey of Positive Physical Activities[a]

Rate how often you engaged in each activity during the past year. Then rate how much mastery and pleasure you felt. If you did not engage in the activity, rate the mastery and pleasure you'd expect.

Frequency (Freq):
  0 = never; 1 = once or only a few times; 2 = fairly often; 3 = often.
The experience of Mastery (M) refers to your sense of accomplishment or achievement felt when engaging in the activity.
  0 = none; 1 = somewhat; 2 = moderate; 3 = a lot.
The Experience of Pleasure (P) refers to feeling enjoyment or having fun when engaging in the activity.
  0 = none; 1 = somewhat; 2 = moderate; 3 = a lot.

Freq	M	P	
___	___	___	Taking a long or brisk walk
___	___	___	Swimming
___	___	___	Playing tennis or racquetball
___	___	___	Taking a relaxing shower or bath
___	___	___	Wearing favorite casual clothes
___	___	___	Brushing hair in a soothing manner
___	___	___	Sitting in a spa or hot tub
___	___	___	Putting on makeup
___	___	___	Social dancing
___	___	___	Riding a bicycle
___	___	___	Having a manicure
___	___	___	Getting a body massage or backrub
___	___	___	Getting a facial or a cosmetic makeover
___	___	___	Lifting weights or using exercise machines
___	___	___	Wearing cologne or perfume
___	___	___	Doing calisthenics

[a]Adapted from Cash (1995b).

1995b) to promote a positive body image. For example, the client can engage in a "Writing Wrongs" exercise to help change his or her attitude toward the body. In this exercise, the client writes his or her body a letter in an effort to improve the "relationship." The therapist can provide examples and explain that the client should think of the letter as writing to an estranged friend with whom she or he wants to renew contact and start fresh.

5. Brief mirror affirmations can also facilitate a client's positive body image. In practicing these affirmations, the client can draw on compliments that he or she receives or desires to receive from others.

6. Another exercise, "I Am Becoming," requires that the client discern how he or she would think, feel, and act differently if his or her body-image ideals were actually possessed. Then, the client spends a day enacting this body-image "script." In a related exercise, the client gives special treatment one day each week to a particular, liked aspect of his or her body.

Kathy is a 30-year-old graduate student who feels that she has neglected her body during the past year due to long hours spent studying, reading, and writing papers. In completing the physical activity survey, she discovered that during the past year she had engaged in few body-related activities that gave her a sense of mastery or pleasure. She decided to increase the frequency of the following fitness/health activities: taking long walks, playing tennis, and participating in an aerobics class. The sensate activities on her list were dancing, taking a relaxing bath, wearing her favorite fragrance, and rubbing her body with lotion. Her appearance-related activities included applying nail polish, getting a new hairstyle, and wearing more colorful clothing.

> **T:** Kathy, last week, you made lists of the physical activities you thought would give you a sense of mastery and pleasure. How successful were you with these?
> **C:** Well, as you can see from my schedule and my new haircut, I did several of the things on my list. I felt really good during and afterward; I rated my sense of mastery or pleasure quite high for most. But I had trouble carrying out some of the health/fitness exercises.
> **T:** You really did a lot of the things you scheduled, and your new haircut looks terrific. Why do you think you had trouble with the physical exercise activities?
> **C:** I planned to go to aerobics class one night but talked myself out of it, because I didn't have a decent outfit to wear. I knew that everyone there would be dressed in cute little workout clothes and that I would look dumpy.
> **T:** Your private body talk sounds familiar, doesn't it?
> **C:** Yeah, it goes along with my old belief that I always have to look my best and my tendency to compare my looks to others. I can see that the Beauty-Bound error kept me at home that night.
> **T:** So, Kathy, if your beliefs and thoughts are preventing you from doing what you want to do, what's the solution?

When Kathy incorporated corrective thinking strategies into her body-enhancement plans, she found that she was able to engage in all of the activities on her list. She wrote a letter to her body, in which she apologized for neglecting it over the past year and promised to pay more attention to the positive things it had to offer her. Despite feeling a bit silly at first, she practiced a few mirror affirmations that addressed the appearance assumptions she found were interfering with her activity schedule. She also decided to give herself a manicure every Sunday night while she watched her favorite television program. Kathy found that her body-enhancement exercises became important ways for her to enjoy her body and expand her body image beyond appearance.

Step 8: Relapse Prevention and Maintenance of Body-Image Changes

In this final step of the program, the client evaluates his or her progress in making positive body-image changes, identifies goals for future work, and develops specific preventative-maintenance strategies to deal effectively with high-risk situations and potential setbacks (Marlatt & Gordon, 1984; Meichenbaum, 1985).

1. It is expected that the therapist will have continuously monitored the client's cognitive, affective, and behavioral progress during the program, using diary records and selected assessments that had been given prior to treatment. Nevertheless, at this stage, the therapist readministers all of the pretreatment assessments. To facilitate a sense of accomplishment, the therapist reinforces the areas of greatest improvement that were tied to specific goals the client had set. Together, the client and therapist then identify any lingering problem areas and set new body-image goals, such as feeling better about certain body areas or gaining more control over particularly distressing thoughts, feelings, and situations.

2. Often, clients mention troublesome interactions with certain individuals that precipitate body-image distress. For example, nagging or critical comments of friends and relatives can be chronic sources of difficulty. Accordingly, with therapist modeling and with role playing, the client learns interpersonal problem-solving and assertiveness skills in managing these "difficult people" (Alberti & Emmons, 1974; S. A. Bower & G. H. Bower, 1976; Cash, 1995b). If these interpersonal precipitants become apparent earlier in therapy, the therapist should intervene at that time to enable the client to resolve the situation. For example, the client must acquire the means to "neutralize" a lover or spouse who hurls daily insults that undermine the client's body image.

3. The therapist helps the client use the PACE strategy in anticipating and developing preventative plans that take into account current vulnerabilities and areas of potential setbacks. Through a collaborative effort, the therapist and client plan for high-risk situations by drawing upon cognitive–behavioral strategies that the client previously found to be helpful. The therapist further normalizes temporary setbacks as "lapses not relapses" and as signals to use the skills imparted in the program. An important attitude to instill in the client is, "Don't give yourself a hard time for having a hard time!"

Jim is a 30-year-old salesman who sought body-image therapy because he was preoccupied with his acne-scarred skin and large nose. With the help of his therapist, he learned to recognize and change problematic cognitive and behavioral patterns that contributed to his distress. He completed body-image assessment again after 12 weeks of therapy and realized that he had accomplished a great deal. However, he discovered that he was still somewhat uncomfortable viewing his face in the mirror. He set a new goal to become more at ease with his mirror image and identified some of the problematic thought patterns that needed further change. In addition, he wanted to learn to deal better with a co-worker who often made wisecracks about his appearance.

T: Jim, what kinds of things does Bill say to you at work, and how do you feel?

C: He says stuff like, "You're gonna scare away the customers with that face." Sometimes he calls me "pizza face." He always laughs, says he's just kidding and that I shouldn't be so sensitive. I used to feel hurt, but now I just get mad. I usually try to stuff my feelings and walk away, but I'm still angry hours later.

T: Well, obviously Bill can be pretty rude. Let's come up with a plan for you to deal with him. Like you did with the PACE technique, it's important that you think about the situation and plan ahead of time exactly what you want to say. When would be the best time to approach him?

C: Not when other people are around. Probably during mid-morning break. I could invite him to my office for coffee.

T: That's good. Now it's important that you first tell Bill exactly what he does and says that you dislike. Use "I" statements to let him know how you feel. Can you think of what you would like to say?

C: Of course I'd like to tell him to go to hell, but then he'd just say I'm overreacting. So I could say, "Bill, I feel pretty annoyed when you make fun of my complexion by calling me 'pizza face' or saying that I will scare away customers. I know that you see this is as just good-natured kidding, but to me it feels disrespectful and offensive."

T: Okay, Jim, now think about a specific solution you can offer. Tell Bill precisely what do you want from him.

C: I could say, "Bill, as a friend, I'm asking that from now on you not call me names or make references to my complexion, whether you are only kidding or not."

T: That's great! The last step is to get Bill to agree to the solution by pointing out mutual benefits. Maybe you could say something like, "If you stop calling me names, I'd be happy to help you get your display together on Monday mornings." Something like that, but be sure that whatever you offer feels acceptable to you.

C: That sounds like a good deal to me. I'll write out these steps so I'll be prepared and feel more in control.

Jim also incorporated relaxation skills and cognitive strategies into his plan. After practicing aloud, anticipating what Bill was going to say, and visualizing himself succeeding in the situation, he carried out the plan. Because Bill complied with Jim's assertive request, Jim did not have to escalate his assertion to the point of stating negative sanctions for noncompliance. Jim also reported generalization of his assertiveness to several other social situations.

Termination and Follow-up Issues

The sessions of Step 8 serve to consolidate gains, set future goals and strategies for reaching them, and establish plans for relapse prevention and maintenance. At this point, as throughout therapy, the therapist should articulate and encourage the generalization of cognitive and behavioral skills from body image to other areas of the client's life. The therapist should also promote the view that the end of therapy is not the end of change. Attributing improvements to the client's efforts and skills is important to prevent the client's leaving with a "What will I do without you" view of the therapist. The therapist may wish to "keep the door open" for booster sessions to attend any problems the client has with respect to attainment of the new goals. Furthermore, as a bridge to foster continued change, the therapist may wish to schedule a 3- to 6-month follow-up session.

CONCLUSIONS AND FUTURE DIRECTIONS

The past decade has witnessed conceptual and empirical advances in our understanding of body image and its dysfunctions. An important part of this progress is the apparent clinical utility of body-image assessments and treatments derived from a cognitive–behavioral perspective. Yet there are many gaps to be filled. The body-image therapy program described here incorporates an extensive array of cognitive and behavioral interventions. Dismantling studies are needed to determine the most efficacious elements of the treatment. The evaluation of body-image CBT as an addition to extant treatments for obesity and eating disorders is essential (Rosen & Cash, 1995). Its continued evaluation as a treatment for body dysmorphic disorder remains a priority (Rosen, 1995). Its efficacy as an adjunct or alternative to elective cosmetic surgery should be examined. Clinicians and researchers should also assess the helpfulness of body-image CBT to persons challenged by physical disfigurements (Cash, 1992a). Finally, in view of the known social and developmental risk factors that lead to prevalent body-image disturbances, there is potential value in a psychoeducational adaptation of the program for the prevention of body-image problems among children and early adolescents.

REFERENCES

Alberti, R. E., & Emmons, M. (1974). *Your perfect right* (rev. ed.). San Luis Obispo, CA: Impact Press.

American Psychiatric Association. (1987). *Diagnostic and statistical manual of mental disorders* (3rd ed., rev.). Washington, DC: Author.

American Psychiatric Association. (1994). *Diagnostic and statistical manual of mental disorders* (4th ed.). Washington, DC: Author.

American Society for Plastic and Reconstructive Surgery. (1993). *Data on the frequency of various cosmetic procedures.* Arlington Heights, IL: Author.

Archer, R., & Cash, T. F. (1985). Physical attractiveness and maladjustment among psychiatric inpatients. *Journal of Social and Clinical Psychology, 3,* 170–180.

Barlow, D. H. (1986). Causes of sexual dysfunction: The role of anxiety and cognitive interference. *Journal of Consulting and Clinical Psychology, 54,* 140–148.

Beck, A. T. (1967). *Depression: Causes and treatment.* Philadelphia: University of Pennsylvania Press.

Beck, A. T. (1976). *Cognitive therapy and the emotional disorders.* New York: International Universities Press.

Bernstein, N. R. (1990). Objective bodily damage: Disfigurement and dignity. In T. F. Cash & T. Pruzinsky (Eds.), *Body images: Development, deviance, and change* (pp. 131–148). New York: Guilford Press.

Berry, D. M., & Abramowitz, S. I. (1989). Educative/support groups and subliminal psychodynamic activation for bulimic college women. *International Journal of Eating Disorders, 8,* 75–85.

Berscheid, E., Walster, E., & Bohrnstedt, G. (1973, November). Body image. The happy American body: A survey report. *Psychology Today, 7,* 119–131.

Bloch, S., & Glue, P. (1988). Psychotherapy and dysmorphophobia: A case report. *British Journal of Psychiatry, 152,* 271–274.

Bower, S. A., & Bower, G. H. (1976). *Asserting your self.* Reading, MA: Addison-Wesley.

Braddock, L. E. (1982). Dysmorphophobia in adolescence: A case report. *British Journal of Psychiatry, 140,* 199–201.

Breslau, A. (1992). The beauty of disfigurement. In R. E. Bochat (Ed.), *Special faces: Understanding facial disfigurement* (pp. 34–39). New York: National Foundation for Facial Reconstruction.

Brody, M. L., Walsh, B. T., & Devlin, M. J. (1994). Binge eating disorder: Reliability and validity of a new diagnostic category. *Journal of Consulting and Clinical Psychology, 62,* 381–386.

Brooks-Gunn, J., & Warren, M. P. (1985). Effects of delayed menarche in different contexts: Dance and nondance students. *Journal of Youth and Adolescence, 14,* 285–300.

Brooks-Gunn, J., & Warren, M. P. (1988). The psychological significance of secondary sexual characteristics in nine- to eleven-year-old girls. *Child Development, 59,* 1061–1069.

Brown, T. A., Cash, T. F., & Lewis, R. J. (1989). Body-image disturbances in adolescent female binge-purgers: A brief report of the results of a national survey in the U.S.A. *Journal of Child Psychology and Psychiatry, 30,* 605–613.

Brown, T. A., Cash, T. F., & Mikulka, P. J. (1990). Attitudinal body-image assessment: Factor analysis of the Body-Self Relations Questionnaire. *Journal of Personality Assessment, 55,* 135–144.

Brownell, K. D. (1991). Dieting and the search for the perfect body: Where physiology and culture collide. *Behavior Therapy, 22,* 1–12.

Brownell, K. D., Wadden, T. A. (1991). The heterogeneity of obesity: Fitting treatments to individuals. *Behavior Therapy, 22,* 153–177.

Bruch, H. (1962). Perceptual and conceptual disturbances in anorexia nervosa. *Psychosomatic Medicine, 24,* 187–194.

Bull, R., & Rumsey, N. (1988). *The social psychology of facial appearance.* New York: Springer-Verlag.

Butters, J. W., & Cash, T. F. (1987). Cognitive–behavioral treatment of women's body-image dissatisfaction. *Journal of Consulting and Clinical Psychology, 55,* 889–897.

Canning, H., & Mayer, J. (1966). Obesity—Its possible effect on college acceptance. *New England Journal of Medicine, 275,* 1172–1174.

Cash, T. F. (1985). Physical appearance and mental health. In J. A. Graham & A. Kligman (Eds.), *Psychology of cosmetic treatments* (pp. 196–216). New York: Praeger Scientific.

Cash, T. F. (1989). Body-image affect: Gestalt versus summing the parts. *Perceptual and Motor Skills, 69,* 17–18.

Cash, T. F. (1990). The psychology of physical appearance: Aesthetics, attributes, and images. In T. F. Cash & T. Pruzinsky (Eds.), *Body images: Development, deviance, and change* (pp. 51–79). New York: Guilford Press.

Cash, T. F. (1991a). Binge-eating and body images among the obese: A further evaluation. *Journal of Social Behavior and Personality, 6,* 367–376.

Cash, T. F. (1991b). *Body-image therapy: A program for self-directed change.* New York: Guilford Press.

Cash, T. F. (1992a). Body images and body weight: What is there to gain or lose? *Weight Control Digest, 2*(4), 169ff.

Cash, T. F. (1992b). Body-image therapy for persons with facial disfigurement: A cognitive–behavioral approach. In R. E. Bochat (Ed.), *Special faces: Understanding facial disfigurement* (pp. 25–33). New York: National Foundation for Facial Reconstruction.

Cash, T. F. (1992c). *The Private Body Talk Questionnaire: An instrument for the assessment of cognitive body-image errors.* Unpublished research, Old Dominion University, Norfolk, VA.

Cash, T. F. (1993a). Body-image attitudes among obese enrollees in a commercial weight-loss program. *Perceptual and Motor Skills, 77,* 1099–1103.

Cash, T. F. (1993b). *Multiple measures of body image and their psychosocial correlates.* Unpublished research, Old Dominion University, Norfolk, VA.

Cash, T. F. (1994a). Body image and weight changes in a multisite comprehensive very-low-calorie diet program. *Behavior Therapy, 25,* 239–254.

Cash, T. F. (1994b). Body-image attitudes: Evaluation, investment, and affect. *Perceptual and Motor Skills, 78,* 1168–1170.

Cash, T. F. (1994c). The Situational Inventory of Body-Image Dysphoria: Contextual assessment of a negative body image. *The Behavior Therapist, 17,* 133–134.

Cash, T. F. (1994d). *The users' manual for the Multidimensional Body-Self Relations Questionnaire.* Available from the author, Old Dominion University, Norfolk, VA.

Cash, T. F. (1995a). Developmental teasing about physcial appearance: Retrospective descriptions and relationships with body image. *Social Behavior and Personality, 23,* 123–130.

Cash, T. F. (1995b). *What do you see when you look in the mirror?: Helping yourself to a positive body image.* New York: Bantam Books.

Cash, T. F., & Brown, T. A. (1987). Body image in anorexia nervosa and bulimia nervosa: A review of the literature. *Behavior Modification, 11,* 487–521.

Cash, T. F., Counts, B., & Huffine, C. E. (1990). Current and vestigial effects of overweight among women: Fear of fat, attitudinal body image, and eating behaviors. *Journal of Psychopathology and Behavioral Assessment, 12,* 157–167.

Cash, T. F., & Deagle, E. (1995). *Body-image disturbances in anorexia nervosa and bulimia nervosa: A meta-analysis.* Manuscript submitted for publication.

Cash, T. F., & Green, G. K. (1986). Body weight and body image among college women: Perception, cognition, and affect. *Journal of Personality Assessment, 50,* 290–301.

Cash, T. F., & Henry, P. (in press). Women's body images: The results of a national survey in the U.S.A. *Sex Roles.*

Cash, T. F., & Hicks, K. L. (1990). Being fat versus thinking fat: Relationships with body image, eating behaviors, and well-being. *Cognitive Therapy and Research, 14,* 327–341.

Cash, T. F., & Jacobi, L. (1992). Looks aren't everything (to everybody): The strength of ideals of physical appearance. *Journal of Social Behavior and Personality, 7,* 621–630.

Cash, T. F., & Labarge, A. (in press). The development and validation of the Appearance Schemas Inventory. *Cognitive Theory and Research.*

Cash, T. F., & Lavallee, D. M. (1995). *Cognitive–behavioral body-image therapy: Extended evidence of the efficacy of a self-directed program.* Manuscript submitted for publication.

Cash, T. F., Lewis, R. J., & Keeton, P. (1987, March). *Development and validation of the Body-Image Automatic Thoughts Questionnaire.* Paper presented at the annual meeting of the Southeastern Psychological Association, Atlanta, GA.

Cash, T. F., Novy, P., & Grant, J. (1994). Why do women exercise? Factor analysis and further validation of the Reasons for Exercise Inventory. *Perceptual and Motor Skills, 78,* 539–544.

Cash, T. F., Price, V., & Savin, R. (1993). The psychosocial effects of androgenetic alopecia among women: Comparisons with balding men and female controls. *Journal of the American Academy of Dermatology, 29,* 568–575.

Cash, T. F., & Pruzinsky, T. (Eds.). (1990). *Body images: Development, deviance, and change.* New York: Guilford Press.

Cash, T. F., & Pruzinsky, T. (in press). The psychosocial effects of androgenetic alopecia and their implications for patient care. In D. Stough (Ed.), *Surgical and medical hair restoration.* St. Louis: Mosby.

Cash, T. F., & Soloway, D. (1975). Self-disclosure correlates of physical attractiveness: An exploratory study. *Psychological Reports, 36,* 579–586.

Cash, T. F., & Szymanski, M. (1995). The development and validation of the Body-Image Ideals Questionnaire. *Journal of Personality Assessment, 64,* 466–477.

Cash, T. F., Winstead, B. W., & Janda, L. H. (1985, July). Your body, yourself: A *Psychology Today* reader survey. *Psychology Today, 19,* 22–26.

Cash, T. F., Winstead, B. W., & Janda, L. H. (1986, April). The great American shape-up: Body image survey report. *Psychology Today, 20,* 30–37.

Cash, T. F., Wood, K. C., Phelps, K. D., & Boyd, K. (1991). New assessments of weight-related body image derived from extant instruments. *Perceptual and Motor Skills, 73,* 235–241.

Ciliska, D. (1990). *Beyond dieting: Psychoeducational interventions for chronically obese women, a nondieting approach.* New York: Brunner/Mazel.

Conners, M., Johnson, C. L., & Stuckey, M. K. (1984). Treatment of bulimia with brief psychoeducational group therapy. *American Journal of Psychiatry, 141,* 1512–1516.

Cooper, P. J., Taylor, M. J., Cooper, Z., & Fairburn, C. G. (1987). The development and validation of the Body Shape Questionnaire. *International Journal of Eating Disorders, 6,* 485–494.

Davis, R., Olmsted, M. P., & Rockert, W. (1990). Brief group psychoeducation for bulimia nervosa: Assessing the clinical significance of change. *Journal of Consulting and Clinical Psychology, 58,* 882–885.

DeJong, W. (1980). The stigma of obestiy: The consequences of naive assumptions concernign the causes of physical deviance. *Journal of Health and Social Behavior, 81,* 75—87.

DeJong, W., & Kleck, R. (1986). The social–psychological effects of overweight. In C. P. Herman, M. P. Zanna, & E. T. Higgins (Eds.), *Physical appearance, stigma, and social behavior: The Ontario symposium* (Vol. 3, pp. 65–87). Hillsdale, NJ: Erlbaum.

DelRosario, M. W., Brines, J. L., & Coleman, W. R. (1984). Emotional response patterns to body-weight related cues: Influence of body weight image. *Personality and Social Psychology Bulletin, 10,* 369–375.

Downs, A. C. (1990). The social–biological constructs of social competency. In T. P. Gullotta, G. R. Adams, & R. Montemayor (Eds.), *Developing social competency in adolescence* (pp. 43–94). New York: Sage.

Drewnowski, A., & Yee, D. K. (1987). Men and body image: Are males satisfied with their body weight? *Psychosomatic Medicine, 49,* 626–634.

Dworkin, S. H., & Kerr, B. A. (1987). Comparison of interventions for women experiencing body image problems. *Journal of Counseling Psychology, 34,* 136–140.

Ellis, A. (1977). *Techniques for disputing irrational beliefs.* New York: Institute for Rational Living.

Fabian, L. J., & Thompson, J. K. (1989). Body image and eating disturbance in young females. *International Journal of Eating Disorders, 8,* 63–74.

Fairburn, C. G. (1987). The definition of bulimia nervosa: Guidelines for clinicians and research workers. *Annals of Behavioral Medicine, 9,* 3–7.

Fairburn, C. G., Jones, R., Peveler, R. C., Carr, S. J., Solomon, R. A., O'Connor, M. E., Burton, J., & Hope, R. A. (1991). Three treatments for bulimia nervosa: A comparative trial. *Archives of General Psychiatry, 48,* 463–469.

Fairburn, C. G., Peveler, R. C., Jones, R., Hope, R. A., & Doll, H. A. (1993). Predictors of 12-month outcome in bulimia nervosa and the influence of attitudes to shape and weight. *Journal of Consulting and Clinical Psychology, 61,* 696–698.

Fairburn, C. G., & Wilson, G. T. (1993). *Binge eating: Nature, assessment, and treatment.* New York: Guilford Press.

Faith, M., Schare, M. L., & Cash, T. F. (1993, November). *The Body Exposure in Sexual Activities Questionnaire: Psychometrics and sexual correlates.* Paper presented at the Association for Advancement of Behavior Therapy, Atlanta, GA.

Fallon, A. E. (1990). Culture in the mirror: Sociocultural determinants of body image. In T. F. Cash & T. Pruzinsky (Eds.), *Body images: Development, deviance, and change* (pp. 80–109). New York: Guilford Press.

Fallon, A. E., & Rozin, P. (1985). Sex differences in perceptions of body shape. *Journal of Abnormal Psychology*, *94*, 102–105.

Fischer, J., & Corcoran, K. (1994). *Measures for clinical practice: A sourcebook* (2nd ed.). New York: Free Press.

Fisher, E., & Thompson, J. K. (1994). A comparative evaluation of cognitive–behavioral therapy (CBT) versus exercise therapy (ET) for the treatment of body image disturbance: Preliminary findings. *Behavior Modification*, *18*, 171–185.

Fisher, S. (1986). *Development and structure of the body image*. Hillsdale, NJ: Erlbaum.

Fisher, S. (1990). The evolution of psychological concepts about the body. In T. F. Cash & T. Pruzinsky (Eds.), *Body images: Development, deviance, and change* (pp. 3–20). New York: Guilford Press.

Foa, E. B., & Wilson, R. (1991). *Stop obsessing!: How to overcome your obsessions and compulsions*. New York: Bantam.

Freedman, R. (1990). Cognitive–behavioral perspectives on body-image change. In T. F. Cash & T. Pruzinsky (Eds.), *Body images: Development, deviance, and change* (pp. 272–295). New York: Guilford Press.

Friedman, M. A., & Brownell, K. D. (1995). Psychological correlates of obesity: Moving to the next research generation. *Psychological Bulletin*, *117*, 3–20.

Garfinkel, P. E. (1992). Evidence in support of attitudes to shape and weight as a diagnostic criterion of bulimia nervosa. *International Journal of Eating Disorders*, *1*, 321–325.

Garner, D. M., & Garfinkel, P. E. (1981). Body image in anorexia nervosa: Measurement, theory and clinical applications. *International Journal of Psychiatry in Medicine*, *11*, 263–284.

Garner, D. M., Rockert, W., Davis, R., Garner, M. V., Olmsted, M. P., & Eagle, M. (1993). Comparison of cognitive–behavioral and supportive–expressive therapy for bulimia nervosa. *American Journal of Psychiatry*, *150*, 37–46.

Garner, D. M., & Wooley, S. C. (1991). Confronting the failure of behavioral and dietary treatments for obesity. *Clinical Psychology Review*, *11*, 729–780.

Giles, T. R. (1988). Distortion of body image as an effect of conditioned fear. *Journal of Behaviour Therapy and Experimental Psychiatry*, *19*, 143–146.

Goldblatt, P. B., Moore, M. E., & Stunkard, A. J. (1965). Social factors in obesity. *Journal of the American Medical Association*, *192*, 97–102.

Goldfried, M., & Davison, G. C. (1976). *Clinical behavior therapy*. New York: Holt, Rinehart & Winston.

Gortmaker, S. L., Must, A., Perrin, J. M., Sobol, A. M., & Dietz, W. H. (1993). Social and economic consequences of overweight in adolescence and young adulthood. *New England Journal of Medicine*, *329*, 1008–1012.

Gould, R. A., & Clum, G. A. (1993). The meta-analysis of self-help treatment approaches. *Clinical Psychology Review*, *13*, 169–186.

Grant, J., & Cash, T. F. (1995). Cognitive–behavioral body-image therapy: Comparative efficacy of group and modest-contact treatments. *Behavior Therapy*, *26*, 69–84.

Grilo, C. M., Wilfley, D. E., Brownell, K. D., & Rodin, J. (in press). Teasing, body image, and self-esteem in a clinical sample of obese women. *Addictive Behaviors*.

Grilo, C. M., Wilfley, D. E., Jones, A., Brownell, K. D., & Rodin, J. (1994). The social self, body dissatisfaction, and binge eating in obese females. *Obesity Research*, *2*, 24–27.

Hangen, J. D., & Cash, T. F. (1991, November). *Body-image attitudes and sexual functioning in a college population*. Paper presented at the meeting of the Association for Advancement of Behavior Therapy, New York.

Hensley, S., & Cash, T. F. (1994). *Effects of aerobic exercise on state and trait body image*. Unpublished manuscript, Old Dominion University, Norfolk, VA.

Hollander, E., Liebowitz, M. R., Winchel, R., Klumker, A., & Klein, D. F. (1989). Treatment of body-dysmorphic disorder with serotonin reuptake blockers. *American Journal of Psychiatry*, *146*, 768–770.

Hsu, L. K. (1982). Is there a disturbance in body image in anorexia nervosa? *Journal of Nervous and Mental Disease*, *170*, 305–307.

Hsu, L. K., & Sobkiewicz, T. A. (1991). Body-image disturbance: Time to abandon the concept for eating disorders? *International Journal of Eating Disorders*, *10*, 15–30.

Huon, G. F., & Brown, L. B. (1986). Body images in anorexia nervosa and bulimia nervosa. *International Journal of Eating Disorders*, *5*, 421–439.

Jackson, L. A. (1992). *Physical appearance and gender: Sociobiological and sociocultural perspectives*. Albany: SUNY Press.

Jacobi, L., & Cash, T. F. (1994). In pursuit of the perfect appearance: Discrepancies among self- and ideal-percepts of multiple physical attributes. *Journal of Applied Social Psychology*, *24*, 379–396.

Jacobson, N. S., & Truax, P. (1991). Clinical significance: A statistical approach to defining meaningful change in psychotherapy research. *Journal of Consulting and Clinical Psychology, 59*, 12–19.

Kayman, S., Bruvold, W., & Stern, J. S. (1990). Maintenance and relapse after weight loss in women: Behavioral aspects. *American Journal of Clinical Nutrition, 52*, 800–807.

Keeton, W. P., Cash, T. F., & Brown, T. A. (1990). Body image or body images? Comparative, multidimensional assessment among college students. *Journal of Personality Assessment, 54*, 213–230.

Kelley, J. (1978). Sexual permissiveness: Evidence for a theory. *Journal of Marriage and the Family, 40*, 455–468.

Kellner, R. (1986). *Somatization and hypochondriasis*. New York: Praeger.

Klesges, R. C. (1983). An analysis of body-image distortions in a nonpatient population. *International Journal of Eating Disorders, 2*, 35–41.

Krueger, D. W. (1989). *Body self and psychological self: Developmental and clinical integration in disorders of the self*. New York: Brunner/Mazel.

Krueger, D. W. (1990). Developmental and psychodynamic perspectives on body-image change. In T. F. Cash & T. Pruzinsky (Eds.), *Body images: Development, deviance, and change* (pp. 255–271). New York: Guilford Press.

Labarge, A. S., Cash, T. F., & Brown, T. A. (in press). Use of a modified Stroop task to examine schematic processing of appearance-related information among college women. *Cognitive Therapy and Research*.

Lacey, J. H., & Birtchnell, S. A. (1986). Body image and its disturbances. *Journal of Psychosomatic Research, 30*, 623–631.

Larkin, J. C., & Pines, H. A. (1979). No fat persons need apply: Experimental studies of the overweight stereotype and hiring preferences. *Sociology of Work and Occupations, 6*, 312–327.

Leitenberg, H., Rosen, J. C., Gross, J., Nudelman, S., & Vara, L. (1988). Exposure plus response prevention treatment of bulimia nervosa. *Journal of Consulting and Clinical Psychology, 56*, 535–541.

Lerner, R. M., & Jovanovic, J. (1990). The role of body image in psychosocial development across the life span: A developmental contextual perspective. In T. F. Cash & T. Pruzinsky (Eds.), *Body images: Development, deviance, and change* (pp. 110–127). New York: Guilford Press.

Lewis, R. J., Cash, T. F., Jacobi, L., & Bubb-Lewis, C. (1995). *Prejudice toward fat people: Development and validation of the Anti-Fat Attitudes Test*. Manuscript submitted for publication.

MacCorquodale, P., & DeLamater, J. (1979). Self-image and premarital sexuality. *Journal of Marriage and the Family, 41*, 327–339.

Macgregor, F. C. (1979). *After plastic surgery: Adaptation and adjustment*. New York: Praeger.

Macgregor, F. C. (1990). Facial disfigurement: Problems and management of social interaction and implications for mental health. *Aesthetic Plastic Surgery, 14*, 249–257.

Mahoney, M. J. (1990). Psychotherapy and the body in the mind. In T. F. Cash & Pruzinsky (Eds.), *Body images: Development, deviance, and change* (pp. 316–333). New York: Guilford Press.

Marks, I., & Mishan, J. (1988). Dysmorphophobic avoidance with disturbed bodily perception: A pilot study of exposure therapy. *British Journal of Psychiatry, 152*, 674–678.

Markus, H. (1977). Self-schemata and processing information about the self. *Journal of Personality and Social Psychology, 35*, 63–78.

Markus, H., Hamill, R., & Sentis, K. P. (1987). Thinking fat: Self-schemas for body weight and the processing of weight relevant information. *Journal of Applied Social Psychology, 17*, 50–71.

Marlatt, G. A., & Gordon, J. (1984). *Relapse prevention: A self-control strategy for the maintenance of behavior change*. New York: Guilford Press.

Marsella, A. J., Shizuru, L., Brennan, J., & Kaneoka, V. (1981). Depression and body image satisfaction. *Journal of Cross-Cultural Psychology, 12*, 360–371.

McElroy, S. L., Phillips, K. A., Keck, P. E., Hudson, J. I., & Pope, H. G. (1993). Body dysmorphic disorder: Does it have a psychotic subtype? *Journal of Clinical Psychiatry, 54*, 389–395.

McKenna, P. J. (1984). Disorders with overvalued ideas. *British Journal of Psychiatry, 145*, 579–585.

Meichenbaum, D. (1985). *Stress inoculation training*. Elmsford, NY: Pergamon Press.

Mitchell, K. R., & Orr, F. F. (1976). Heterosexual social competence, anxiety, avoidance, and self-judged physical attractiveness. *Perceptual and Motor Skills, 43*, 553–554.

Munjack, D. J. (1978). The behavioral treatment of dysmorphophobia. *Journal of Behavior Therapy and Experimental Psychiatry, 9*, 53–56.

Munro, A. (1988). Monosymptomatic hypochondriacal psychosis. *British Journal of Psychiatry, 153*(Suppl. No. 2), 37–40.

Muth, J. L., & Cash, T. F. (1995). *Gender differences in body-image attitudes: Evaluation, investment, and affect.* Manuscript submitted for publication.

Neziroglu, F. A., & Yaryura-Tobias, J. A. (1993). Exposure, response prevention, and cognitive therapy in the treatment of body dysmorphic disorder. *Behavior Therapy, 24*, 431–438.

Noles, S. W., Cash, T. F., & Winstead, B. A. (1985). Body image, physical attractiveness, and depression. *Journal of Consulting and Clinical Psychology, 53*, 88–94.

Olmsted, M. P., Davis, R., Rockert, W., Irvine, M. J., Eagle, M., & Garner, D. M. (1991). Efficacy of a brief group psychoeducational intervention of bulimia nervosa. *Behavior Research and Therapy, 29*, 71–83.

Ordman, A. M., & Kirschenbaum, D. S. (1985). Cognitive–behavioral therapy for bulimia: An initial outcome study. *Journal of Consulting and Clinical Psychology, 53*, 305–313.

Phillips, K. A. (1991). Body dysmorphic disorder: The distress of imagined ugliness. *American Journal of Psychiatry, 148*, 1138–1149.

Phillips, K. A., McElroy, S. L., Keck, P. E., Pope, H. G., & Hudson, J. I. (1993). Body dysmorphic disorder: 30 cases of imagined ugliness. *American Journal of Psychiatry, 15*, 302–308.

Pliner, P., Chaiken, S., & Flett, G. L. (1990). Gender differences in concern with body weight and physical appearance over the life span. *Personality and Social Psychology Bulletin, 16*, 263–273.

Polivy, J., & Herman, P. (1983). *Breaking the diet habit.* New York: Basic Books.

Polivy, J., & Herman, P. (1992). Undieting: A program to help people stop dieting. *International Journal of Eating Disorders, 11*, 261—268.

Pruzinsky, T. (1990). Psychopathology of body experience: Expanded perspectives. In T. F. Cash & T. Pruzinsky (Eds.), *Body images: Development, deviance, and change* (pp. 170–189). New York: Guilford Press.

Pruzinsky, T. (1992). Social and psychological challenges for individuals with facial disfigurement. In R. E. Bochat (Ed.), *Special faces: Understanding facial disfigurement* (pp. 15–24). New York: National Foundation for Facial Reconstruction.

Pruzinsky, T., & Cash, T. F. (1990a). Integrative themes in body-image development, deviance, and change. In Cash, T. F., & Pruzinsky, T. (Eds.), *Body images: Development, deviance, and change* (pp. 337–349). New York: Guilford Press.

Pruzinsky, T., & Cash, T. F. (1990b). Medical interventions for the enhancement of adolescents' physical appearance: Implications for social competence. In T. P. Gullotta, G. R. Adams & Montemayor (Eds.), *Developing social competency in adolescence* (pp. 220–242). New York: Sage.

Pruzinsky, T., & Edgerton, M. (1990). Body-image change in cosmetic plastic surgery. In T. F. Cash & T. Pruzinsky (Eds.), *Body images: Development, deviance, and change* (pp. 190–236). New York: Guilford Press.

Radke-Sharpe, N., Whitney-Saltiel, D., & Rodin, J. (1990). Fat distribution as a risk factor for weight and eating concerns. *International Journal of Eating Disorders, 9*, 27–36.

Rieves, L., & Cash, T. F. (1995). *Reported social developmental factors associated with women's body-image attitudes.* Manuscript submitted for publication.

Rodin, J., Silberstein, L., & Striegel-Moore, R. (1984). Women and weight: A normative discontent. *Nebraska Symposium on Motivation, 32*, 267–307.

Rosen, G. M., & Ross, A. O. (1968). Relationship of body image to self-concept. *Journal of Consulting and Clinical Psychology, 32*, 100.

Rosen, J. C. (1990). Body-image disturbances in eating disorders. In T. F. Cash & T. Pruzinsky (Eds.), *Body images: Development, deviance, and change* (pp. 190–214). New York: Guilford Press.

Rosen, J. C. (1992). Body image disorder: Definition, development, and contribution to eating disorders. In J. H. Crowther, D. L. Tennenbaum, S. E. Hobfoll, & M. A. P. Stephens (Eds.), *The etiology of bulimia: The individual and family context* (pp. 157–177). Washington, DC: Hemisphere.

Rosen, J. C. (1995). The nature of body dysmorphic disorder and treatment with cognitive behavior therapy. *Cognitive and Behavioral Practice, 2*, 143–166.

Rosen, J. C., Cado, S., Silberg, N. T., Srebnik, D., Wendt, S. (1990). Cognitive-behavior therapy with and without size perception training for women with body image disturbance. *Behavior Therapy, 21*, 481–498.

Rosen, J. C., & Cash, T. F. (1995). Learning to have a better body image. *Weight Control Digest, 5*, 409–416.

Rosen, J. C. Orosan, P., & Reiter, J. (1995). Cognitive–behavioral body-image therapy for negative body images in obese women. *Behavior Therapy, 26*, 25–42.

Rosen, J. C., & Reiter, J. (1992). *Body dysmorphic disorder examination.* Unpublished manuscript, University of Vermont, Burlington, VT.

Rosen, J. C., Reiter, J., & Orosan, P. (1995). Cognitive–behavioral body-image therapy for Body Dysmorphic Disorder. *Journal of Consulting and Clinical Psychology, 63*, 263–269.

Rosen, J. C., Saltzberg, E., & Srebnik, D. (1989). Cognitive–behavior therapy for negative body image. *Behavior Therapy, 20*, 393–404.

Rosen, J. C., Srebnik, D., Saltzberg, E., & Wendt, S. (1991). Development of a body image avoidance questionnaire. *Psychological Assessment, 3*, 32–37.

Rubin, R. T. (1982). Koro (Shook Yang): A culture-bound psychogenic syndrome. In C. T. H. Friedmann & R. A. Fauget (Eds.), *Extraordinary disorders of human behavior* (pp. 155–172). New York: Plenum Press.

Rucker, C. E., & Cash, T. F. (1992). Body images, body-size perceptions, and eating behaviors among African-American and white college women. *International Journal of Eating Disorders, 12*, 291–300.

Sank, L. I., & Shaffer, C. S. (1984). *A therapist's manual for cognitive behavior therapy in groups.* New York: Plenum Press.

Schlundt, D. G., & Johnson, W. G. (1990). *Eating disorders: Assessment and treatment.* Boston: Allyn & Bacon.

Schulman, A. H., & Kaplowitz, C. (1977). Mirror-image responses during the first two years of life. *Developmental Psychobiology, 10*, 133–142.

Scogin, F., Bynum, J., Stephens, G., & Calhoon, S. (1990). Efficacy of self-administered treatment programs: Meta-analytic review. *Professional Psychology: Research and Practice, 21*, 42–47.

Seligman, J., Joseph, N., Donovan, J., & Gosnell, M. (1987, July). The littlest dieters. *Newsweek,* 48.

Shapiro, J. P., Baumeister, R. F., & Kessler, J. W. (1991). A three-component model of children's teasing: Aggression, humor, and ambiguity. *Journal of Social and Clinical Psychology, 10*, 459–472.

Shontz, F. C. (1990). Body image and physical disability. In T. F. Cash & T. Pruzinsky (Eds.), *Body images: Development, deviance, and change* (pp. 149–169). New York: Guilford Press.

Silberstein, L. R., Striegel-Moore, R. H., Timko, C., & Rodin, J. (1988). Behavioral and psychological implications of body dissatisfaction: Do men and women differ? *Sex Roles, 19*, 219–232.

Silverstein, B., Perdue, L., Peterson, B., & Kelly, E. (1986). The role of the mass media in promoting a thin standard of bodily attractiveness for women. *Sex Roles, 14*, 519–523.

Solyom, L., DiNicola, F. F., Phil, M., Sookman, D., & Luchins, D. (1985). Is there an obsessive psychosis? Aetiological and prognostic factors of an atypical form of obsessive–compulsive neurosis. *Canadian Journal of Psychiatry, 30*, 372–380.

Stake, J., & Lauer, M. S. (1987). The consequences of being overweight: A controlled study of gender differences. *Sex Roles, 17*, 31–47.

Stein, D. J., & Hollander, E. (1992). Dermatology and conditions related to obsessive–compulsive disorders. *Journal of the American Academy of Dermatology, 26*, 237–242.

Steketee, G., & White, K. (1990). *When once is not enough: Help for obsessive–compulsives.* Oakland, CA: New Harbinger.

Striegel-Moore, R. H., Silberstein, L. R., Frensch, P., & Rodin, J. (1989). A prospective study of disordered eating among college students. *International Journal of Eating Disorders, 8*, 499–509.

Stunkard, A. J., & Burt, V. (1967). Obesity and body image: II. Age at onset of disturbances in the body image. *American Journal of Psychiatry, 123*, 1443–1447.

Stunkard, A. J., & Mendelson, M. (1967). Obesity and body image: I. Characteristics of disturbances in the body image of some obese persons. *American Journal of Psychiatry, 123*, 1296–1300.

Szymanski, M. L., & Cash, T. F. (1995). Body-image disturbances and self-discrepancy therapy: Expansion of the Body-Image Ideals Questionnaire. *Journal of Social and Clinical Psychology, 14*, 134–146.

Thompson, J. K. (1990). *Body-image disturbance: Assessment and treatment.* Elmsford, NY: Pergamon Press.

Thompson, J. K. (1992). Body image: Extent of disturbance, associated features, theoretical models, assessment methodologies, intervention strategies, and a proposal for a new DSM-IV category—Body Image Disorder. In M. Hersen, R. M. Eisler, & P. M. Miller (Eds.), *Progress in behavior modification* (vol. 28, pp. 3–54). Sycamore, IL: Sycamore Press.

Thompson, J. K., Fabian, L. J., Moulton, D. O., Dunn, M. F., & Altabe, M. N. (1991). The Physical Appearance Related Teasing Scale (PARTS). *Journal of Personality Assessment, 56*, 513–521.

Thompson, J. K., Penner, L. A., & Altabe, M. N. (1990). Procedures, problems, and progress in the assessment of body images. In T. F. Cash & T. Pruzinsky (Eds.), *Body images: Development, deviance, and change* (pp. 21–48). New York: Guilford Press.

Thompson, J. K., & Psaltis, K. (1988). Multiple aspects and correlates of body figure ratings: A replication and extension of Fallon and Rozin (1985). *International Journal of Eating Disorders, 7*, 813–818.

Tiggeman, M., & Rothblum, E. D. (1988). Gender differences in social consequences of perceived overweight in the United States and Australia. *Sex Roles, 18*, 75–86.

Tucker, L. A. (1982). Relationship between perceived somatotype and body cathexis of college males. *Psychological Reports, 50*, 983–989.

Vitiello, B., & de Leon, J. (1990). Dysmorphophobia misdiagnosed as obsessive–compulsive disorder. *Psychosomatics*, *31*, 220–222.

Wadden, T. A., Stunkard, A. J., & Liebschutz, J. (1988). Three-year follow-up of the treatment of obesity by very low calorie diet, behavior therapy, and their combination. *Journal of Consulting and Clinical Psychology*, *56*, 925–928.

Walsh, B. W., & Rosen, P. M. (1988). *Self-mutilation: Theory, research and treatment*. New York: Guilford Press.

Williamson, D. A. (1990). *Assessment of eating disorders: Obesity, anorexia, and bulimia nervosa*. Elmsford, NY: Pergamon Press.

Williamson, D. A., Davis, C. J., Bennett, S. M., Goreczny, A. J., & Gleaves, D. H. (1989). Development of a simple procedure for assessing body image disturbances. *Behavioral Assessment*, *11*, 433–446.

Wilson, G. T., & Fairburn, C. G. (1993). Cognitive treatments for eating disorders. *Journal of Consulting and Clinical Psychology*, *61*, 261–269.

Wilson, G. T., & Pike, K. M. (1993). Eating disorders. In D. H. Barlow (Ed.), *Clinical handbook of psychological disorders* (2nd ed., pp. 278–317). New York: Guilford Press.

Wilson, G. T., Rossiter, E., Kleinfield, E. I., & Lindholm, L. (1986). Cognitive–behavioral treatment of bulimia nervosa: A controlled evaluation. *Behavior Research and Therapy*, *24*, 277–288.

Wilson, G. T., & Smith, D. (1989). Assessment of bulimia nervosa: An evaluation of the Eating Disorders Examination. *International Journal of Eating Disorders*, *8*, 173–179.

Wolchik, S. A., Weiss, L., & Katzman, M. K. (1986). An empirically validated, short term psycho-educational group treatment program for bulimia. *International Journal of Eating Disorders*, *5*, 21–34.

Wolf, E. M., & Crowther, J. H. (1992). An evaluation of behavioral and cognitive–behavioral group intervention for the treatment of bulimia nervosa in women. *International Journal of Eating Disorders*, *11*, 3–16.

Wooley, S. C., & Kearney-Cooke, A. (1986). Intensive treatment of bulimia and body-image disturbance. In K. D. Brownell & J. P. Foreyt (Eds.), *Handbook of eating disorders: Physiology, psychology, and treatment of obesity, anorexia, and bulimia* (pp. 476–502). New York: Basic Books.

16

Cognitive–Behavioral Treatment of Postconcussion Syndrome

A Therapist's Manual

Robert J. Ferguson and Wiley Mittenberg

INTRODUCTION

Postconcussion Syndrome (PCS) is a disorder that occurs following about 75% to 80% of all mild head injuries (Alves, Colohan, O'Leary, Rimel, & Jane, 1986; Rimel, Girodani, Barth, Boll, & Jane, 1981). Whereas severe head injury generally produces neuropsychological deficits in memory and intellectual function, mild concussion can result in more subtle disruptions in daily functioning in the months following head trauma. This consistent cluster of postconcussive symptoms includes difficulty with attention and concentration, disturbances in memory, headache, vertigo, anxiety, depression, fatigue, irritability, blurred vision, and sensitivity to light (Mittenberg, DiGiulio, Perrin, & Bass, 1992; World Health Organization, 1978). Given that nearly 325,000 head injuries that annually occur in the United States are classified as mild (Levin, Eisenberg, & Benton, 1989), design of effective treatment for PCS appears warranted.

Research has suggested that although PCS may have an initial neurological basis, the symptoms persist primarily due to psychological factors (Cook, 1969, 1972; Levin, Benton, & Grossman, 1982; Levin et al., 1987; Miller, 1961; Mittenberg et al., 1992; Rutherford, Merrett, & McDonald, 1979). Gouvier, Cubic, Jones, Brantley, and Cutlip (1992) found that ratings of daily stress correlated with the severity (intensity, frequency, and duration) of postconcussive symptoms among head-injured patients and normal controls. Interestingly,

Robert J. Ferguson • Department of Psychiatry, Dartmouth Medical School, Dartmouth–Hitchcock Medical Center, Lebanon, New Hampshire 03756. **Wiley Mittenberg** • Center for Psychological Studies, Nova Southeastern University, Fort Lauderdale, Florida 33314.

Sourcebook of Psychological Treatment Manuals for Adult Disorders, edited by Vincent B. Van Hasselt and Michel Hersen. Plenum Press, New York, 1996.

incidence of postconcussive symptoms in head-injured groups did not differ significantly from incidence in normal controls. This implies that psychosocial stress and cognitive appraisal play a role in the manifestation and expression of PCS symptoms. Other research has indicated that the incidence of PCS appears inversely or unrelated to neuropsychological status (Levin et al., 1987; McLean, Temkin, Dikmen, & Wyler, 1983; McLean, Dikmen, Temkin, Wyler, & Gale, 1984; Mittenberg et al., 1992).

Cognitive-Behavioral Conceptualization of PCS

Although etiology of PCS appears to have a marked psychological component, few theoretical models explaining the role of psychological factors have been proposed. Mittenberg et al. (1992) presented findings that support a psychological model, with expectations of symptoms and cognitive symptom appraisal as key elements. When normal control subjects were asked to indicate types of symptoms they might experience if they had a head injury, their responses correlated highly with symptoms reported by mildly head-injured subjects ($r = .82$). Frequency of symptoms that afflicted individuals with mild head injury were essentially equivalent to the frequency expected by those without history of head injury. Expectations therefore shared as much variance with PCS as concussion itself. Mittenberg and colleagues found that mildly head-injured subjects underestimated number of premorbid daily problems with "postconcussive" symptoms. Number of everyday inconveniences of forgetfulness, concentration, anxiety, and so forth, estimated before injury on the part of mild head-trauma patients was about 50% lower than number of everyday symptoms reported by normal, uninjured controls. Apparently, mildly head injured subjects thought the incidence of these symptoms (which they believed to result from concussion) to have changed considerably. They therefore overestimated their premorbid functioning by underestimating the number of symptoms they experienced before injury.

Mittenberg et al. (1992) proposed a symptom-appraisal model that explained these findings. A consistent and accurate set of symptoms is expected to follow mild head injury by most normal adults. A concussion activates expectations and selective attention to expected symptoms. The concussion is stressful in and of itself, and increased psychosocial stress causes autonomic arousal that can interfere with cognitive processes, such as attention, concentration, and recall (Mandler, 1982). Benign, everyday occurrences of forgetting names, phone numbers, headaches, concentration difficulties, and other stress-related symptoms are unintentionally attributed to head injury. This greater awareness of and attention to symptoms in some individuals augments symptom perception. Misattribution of stress-related and normally occurring symptoms reinforces and confirms prior beliefs about mild head injury (e.g., expectations of memory disturbance, attentional difficulty, anxiety) and gives rise to increased emotional distress. Such arousal results in more cognitive interference and negative affect. The resultant cyclical reinforcement pattern causes the protracted maintenance of PCS symptoms well beyond the time of expected, normal mild head injury recovery.

Based on this model, a cognitive–behavioral treatment for PCS has been designed and implemented at our clinic. The treatment approach has two primary goals: (1) to help patients understand how PCS symptoms are intensified and maintained by anxiety or negative affect produced through misinterpretation of symptoms; and (2) to provide PCS patients with a repertoire of cognitive–behavioral stress-reduction and coping skills that reduce or eliminate stress responding, increase ability to modulate emotion, and reduce symptom incidence. Cognitive–behavior therapy (CBT) is used to improve coping with PCS symptoms through several specific steps:

1. Graded resumption of daily work and home activities.
2. Recognition and modification of self-defeating thoughts about symptoms.
3. Applied relaxation (anxiety-management training) for reduction of physiological arousal brought on by symptom distress.

The result is reduced negative emotional reactions to symptoms, and a break in the reinforcement of negative thoughts and the symptom-exacerbation cycle.

COMPONENTS OF TREATMENT

The three main components of the cognitive–behavioral treatment of PCS involves the combination of three specific procedures with demonstrated treatment efficacy:

1. Behavioral pacing of daily activities through activity scheduling.
2. Cognitive restructuring to identify, modify and/or replace self-defeating cognitions about symptoms experienced.
3. Anxiety-management training (AMT) as presented by Suinn (1990), for management of stress-related arousal brought on by symptom distress.

Activity scheduling has been used in cognitive–behavioral therapies of depression to both improve mood and motivation (Beck, Rush, Shaw, & Emery, 1979; Freeman, Pretzer, Fleming, & Simon, 1990; Lewinsohn, 1974). In its simplest form, activity scheduling involves getting the patient to engage in activity that is rewarding and reinforcing, because one behavioral conceptualization of depression is a lack of reinforcement received from the environment (Lewinsohn, 1974). The therapist systematically schedules one or two activities between treatment sessions that are reinforcing for the patient. At a gradual pace, the therapist assists the patient in scheduling more activity with each session, which increases the probability that he or she receives rewards for acting on the environment. The result is an elevation in mood and a resumption of normal activity level.

Use of activity scheduling as a treatment component of PCS appears warranted because depression is a common symptom experienced by mildly head-injured patients (Mittenberg et al., 1992; Mittenberg & Burton, 1993). In addition, gradual resumption of vocational and daily-living activities, combined with adequate rest, can increase pleasure and a sense of achievement, which improve PCS symptoms (Mittenberg & Burton, 1993). Therefore, the purpose of activity scheduling in the present treatment is twofold: first, activity scheduling can improve mood and enhance the patient's ability to more readily cope with stress that exacerbates PCS symptoms; second, resuming normal activity, if done at a sensible, moderate pace, is hypothesized to directly improve PCS symptoms and improve stress coping by not allowing the patient to become either too lethargic or too active and fatigued in recovery.

The second component of the present treatment, cognitive restructuring, plays an important role. Cognitive restructuring involves eliminating the patient's inaccurate, self-defeating automatic thoughts about symptoms and substituting them with more adaptive ones (Beck et al., 1979; W. H. Cormier & L. S. Cormier, 1985; Freeman et al., 1990). By training PCS patients to identify tendencies of negative selectivity and misattribution of stress symptoms to head injury, negative emotions evoked in response to symptom onset are likely to decrease in number and intensity. Furthermore, when more adaptive cognitions about stress symptoms are substituted for self-defeating, negative cognitions, improved coping is hypothesized to be the result.

Cognitive restructuring has also been used to reduce anxiety in social and performance situations (Elder, Edelstein, & Fremouw, 1981; Gormally, VarvilWeld, Raphael, & Sipps, 1981; Sweeney & Horan, 1982) and in the treatment of depression (Beck et al., 1979; Eifert & Craill, 1989). Because anxiety and depression are two common symptoms of PCS, cognitive restructuring appears to be a sensible treatment strategy in combating the psychological sequelea of PCS. Cognitive restructuring was associated with significantly better treatment outcome in a survey of techniques currently used to treat PCS (Mittenberg & Burton, 1993).

The third and final component of this CBT package, anxiety-management training (AMT), also has direct, theoretically sensible applications to PCS. Although AMT was originally intended as a treatment of generalized anxiety disorder, Suinn (1990) cites evidence of AMT's effectiveness with a broad range of problems that involve excessive arousal as a primary cause. AMT is effective as a treatment of anger/explosiveness (Deffenbacher, Demm, & Brandon, 1986; Hart, 1984), tension headache (Suinn & Vattano, 1979), and as a technique to enhance cognitive performance (Thompson, Griebstein, & Kuhlenschmidt, 1980). Because the present conceptualization of PCS involves emotional arousal as a key variable contributing to protracted maintenance of PCS symptoms, AMT is an effective arousal-control technique that directly addresses symptoms such as irritability, anxiety, headache, and concentration difficulty.

TREATMENT PLAN

Pretreatment

During the pretreatment examination prior to the first CBT session, a thorough assessment of the patient's present complaints and neuropsychological status should be conducted. A symptom checklist that can be used to assess the frequency, intensity, and duration of PCS appears in Sidebar 16.1. This Concussion Symptom checklist was administered to 35 head-trauma patients (mean age = 43.6, SD = 19.7; mean Glascow Coma Scale = 11.7, SD = 4.1) to establish the reliability of the measure. Coefficient alpha for frequency of the 12 symptoms experienced in the previous week was .79. Alpha for symptom duration in days per week was .81, and symptom severity on a 1 to 10 scale yielded an alpha of .83. Internal consistency reliabilities in a sample of 65 normal controls (mean age = 24.7, SD = 6.3) were .76 for symptom frequency, .82 for symptom duration, and .85 for symptom intensity. Test–retest reliabilities corrected for attenuation in a sample of 25 normal controls (mean age = 24.8, SD = 5.0) were .75 for frequency, .70 for duration, and .79 for intensity over a 1-week test–retest interval. In addition to providing an initial assessment of the presence and severity of PCS, the instrument is sensitive to symptom reduction over the course of therapy and is administered at the beginning of each treatment session.

The pretreatment examination should also include a complete neuropsychological examination, including an assessment of intelligence and memory function. Patients who have sustained a mild head injury will typically have normal cognitive abilities, although their subjective experience of PCS symptoms will lead them to believe otherwise (Levin et al., 1987). Disconfirmation of the patient's belief that he or she has suffered "brain damage" is a core component of the treatment. The therapist should explain the neuropsychological test results and indicate what the results mean with respect to the absence of cerebral dysfunction, memory impairment, and intellectual compromise. Educating the patient about the effects of mild head injury in this way, and reassurance that the symptoms are a part of the normal recovery process, appear to be effective elements of treatment for PCS (Mittenberg & Burton, 1993).

The patient is given a copy of *Recovery from Mild Head Injury: A Treatment Manual for Patients* (Mittenberg, Zielinski, & Fichera, 1993), and asked to read it before the first treatment session. This manual is based on the cognitive–behavioral model of the etiology and maintenance of PCS and includes information about the nature, incidence, and recovery course of PCS symptoms. It includes sections intended to support the cognitive reattribution of symptoms, cognitive–behavioral intervention for anxiety and depression, successive approximation of premorbid activities, and relaxation training. The patient manual explains the causes of PCS symptoms and provides simple, understandable rationales for various coping strategies. The point of the reading assignment is to introduce patients to a reinterpretation of their symptoms as normal following mild head injury. This will assist patients by introducing objective evidence of what PCS symptoms are and how worry, anxiety, and other stress responses can adversely affect symptoms. The therapist should be familiar with the content of the patient manual before implementing this treatment package.

Treatment is time-limited and will involve 12 weekly sessions, with home practice between each session. This point is made in order that the patient know how long treatment will be and that it is goal directed. It is also intended to motivate the patient to take advantage of time spent in "training" with the therapist, and thereby enhance treatment adherence. Finally, patients are informed that relaxation training is involved in treatment, and that wearing casual, comfortable clothing to therapy is helpful. If patients wear contact lenses, it is recommended that they wear glasses in therapy, as closing their eyes for 15–30 minutes with contact lenses may cause eye irritation.

The Therapist's Position

The therapist must keep in mind that the present treatment is a skills training package. Over time, the patient will master the skills with practice, and he or she will learn to incorporate these skills in daily life in order to cope effectively with symptoms. Some cases may require more than 12 sessions, and follow-up or "booster" sessions can be scheduled at the clinician's discretion. However, the emphasis in treatment is on the patient's ability to apply the skills outside of therapy, not on what is accomplished during sessions *per se*. When the skills learned in treatment are applied regularly, the symptoms are likely to be eliminated.

Therapeutic Relationship

Therapist–patient relationship factors (not outlined in this treatment manual) are vital to positive treatment outcome and should be given careful consideration by the therapist in using this treatment package. The therapist must be empathic to the patient's concerns and feelings, and establish a collaborative rather than confrontational relationship with the patient. Cognitive–behavioral approaches are only as effective as the relationship is positive. This is particularly true if the patient is to learn to think critically of his or her

Robert J. Ferguson
and Wiley Mittenberg

Sidebar 16.1

Nova Southeastern University Head Injury Treatment Program Concussion Symptom Checklist

1. Have you had *headaches* during the last week?   No = 0 Yes = 1
   How many days were you bothered by these headaches during the last week? _____
   How bad are the headaches usually, on a scale from 1 to 10? _____

2. Have you had *anxiety* during the past week?   No = 0 Yes = 1
   How many days were you bothered by this anxiety during the last week? _____
   How bad is the anxiety usually, on a scale from 1 to 10? _____

3. Have you had *depression* during the last week?   No = 0 Yes = 1
   How many days were you bothered by this depression during the last week? _____
   How bad is the depression usually, on a scale from 1 to 10? _____

4. Have you had *difficulty concentrating* during the last week?   No = 0 Yes = 1
   How many days were you bothered by concentration problems during the last week? _____
   How bad is your concentration, on a scale from 1 to 10? _____

5. Have you had *dizziness* during the last week?   No = 0 Yes = 1
   How many days were you bothered by dizziness during the last week? _____
   How bad is the dizziness, on a scale from 1 to 10? _____

negative worldviews and challenge the perceived validity of his or her appraisal and thoughts of postconcussive symptoms. The therapist should also be cognizant of a therapist–patient partnership. This partnership in cognitive therapy is referred to by Beck et al. (1979) as *collaborative empiricism*. Collaborative empiricism places emphasis on assisting the patient in discovering alternative ways of thinking about life events, rather than confronting him or her about faulty, distorted thinking, or invalid hypotheses about neuropsychological status following concussion.

Treatment Procedures in Each Session

Detailed instruction for the 12-session CBT treatment plan is presented here. The therapist can use Table 16.1 as a quick reference to summarize the steps involved in each of the 12 treatment sessions.

6. Have you had *trouble remembering things* during the last week? No = 0 Yes = 1

    How many days did you have trouble remembering things during the last week? _____

    How bad are the memory problems, on a scale from 1 to 10? _____

7. Have you had *blurry or double vision* during the last week? No = 0 Yes = 1

    How many days were you bothered by vision problems during the last week? _____

    How bad is the blurry or double vision usually, on a scale from 1 to 10? _____

8. Have you had *trouble thinking* during the past week? No = 0 Yes = 1

    How many days did you have trouble thinking during the last week? _____

    How bad is the trouble thinking usually, on a scale from 1 to 10? _____

9. Have you been *irritable* during the past week? No = 0 Yes = 1

    How many days were you irritable during the last week? _____

    How bad is the irritability usually, on a scale from 1 to 10? _____

10. Have you been *tired a lot* during the past week? No = 0 Yes = 1

    How many days were to tired a lot during the last week? _____

    How tired have you been usually, on a scale from 1 to 10? _____

11. Have you been *sensitive to bright light* during the last week? No = 0 Yes = 1

    How many days were you light sensitive during the last week? _____

    How bad is the sensitivity usually, on a scale from 1 to 10? _____

12. Have you been *sensitive to loud noise* during the last week? No = 0 Yes = 1

    How many days were you sensitive to loud noise during the last week? _____

    How bad is the noise sensitivity usually, on a scale from 1 to 10? _____

Session 1

Session 1 treatment goals include the following:

1. Administration of Concussion Symptom Checklist
2. Presentation of the treatment rationale: the 3 components of the PCS treatment package
3. Demonstration of automatic thoughts–emotion relationship with real-life data from Concussion Symptom Checklist
4. Activity scheduling
5. AMT introduction with taped relaxation induction for home practice
6. Summary and review

In Session 1, a great deal of material is covered since the session is a general introduction to cognitive–behavioral treatment of mild head-injury symptoms. The overall

Table 16.1. Summary of Treatment Protocol

Session 1

1. Administration of Concussion Symptom Checklist.
2. Presentation the treatment rationale: the three components of the PCS treatment package.
3. Demonstration of automatic thought–emotion relationship with real-life data from Concussion Symptom Checklist.
4. Activity scheduling.
5. AMT introduction with taped relaxation induction for home practice.
6. Summary and review.

Session 2

1. Administration of Concussion Symptom Checklist.
2. Cognitive restructuring
3. Review of activity schedule since Session 1.
4. AMT: Relaxation review; relaxation induction.
5. Summary and review.

Session 3

1. Administration of Concussion Symptom Checklist.
2. Cognitive restructuring
3. Review of activity schedule since Session 2.
4. AMT: Relaxation review; stress-scene development; stress induction; home practice.
5. Summary and review.

Session 4

1. Administration of Concussion Symptom Checklist.
2. Cognitive restructuring
3. Review of activity schedule since Session 3.
4. AMT: Relaxation review; stress induction; home practice.
5. Summary and review.

Session 5

1. Administration of Concussion Symptom Checklist.
2. Cognitive restructuring
3. Review of activity scheduling since Session 4.
4. AMT: Relaxation review; stress induction; home practice.
5. Summary and review.

Session 6

1. Administration of Concussion Symptom Checklist.
2. Cognitive restructuring
3. Review of activity scheduling since Session 5.
4. AMT: Relaxation review; stress induction; home practice.
5. Summary and review.

Session 7–12

Follow Session 6 format. The therapist may target new PCS symptoms for cognitive restructuring, or may develop a new stress scene in AMT if indicated.

session should take about 90 minutes in order that all six treatment goals are accomplished. The therapist must keep terms simple and use language that is understandable to the patient. Clear, concise explanations of how components of CBT work and what the patient can expect from treatment are important for treatment adherence and maximal benefit. Examples of rationales and session dialogue are provided in order to assist the therapist in conducting the introductory session.

1. Symptom Checklist Administration.   Before any other activity in Session 1, the therapist orally administers the Concussion Symptom Checklist to assess frequency and intensity of the patient's concussion symptoms of the previous week. Administering the checklist is undertaken in each of the 12 treatment sessions and has two purposes: (1) to provide a session-to-session assessment of the patient's PCS symptoms and response to treatment, and (2) to provide information about relevant, actual patient experiences with symptoms to use as data for cognitive restructuring. The therapist uses patient responses on the checklist to identify specific target symptoms for cognitive restructuring.

2. Rationale for the Three Treatment Components.   The following is a model explanation that therapists can use to introduce the CBT treatment package, the course of therapy, what can be accomplished, and what is expected of the patient:

T: The treatment approach we will be using is called cognitive–behavioral therapy. It consists of 12 weekly sessions in which the primary aim is to teach you ways to reduce stress in your life that makes your concussion symptoms worse. You will gradually learn to gain more control over your concussion symptoms as treatment progresses over our 12 meetings.

Treatment consists of three parts. First, you will begin to schedule activities so you can pace yourself at home and work to maximize improvement in your symptoms and reduce stress. This is termed *activity scheduling*. The second part of treatment involves changing thinking patterns that contribute to negative feelings, such as anxiety, irritability, and depression, and influence your daily behavior and motivation. Thinking is done entirely automatically, and often because we are so busy, we are not aware of how it influences our perceptions of ourselves, things around us, and our emotional states every waking moment we live. Identifying, becoming more aware of, and changing negative thinking patterns is called *cognitive restructuring*. In a lot of different emotional problems, cognitive restructuring is the first step to well-being. We will work on helping you begin to eliminate automatic negative thinking. This is an important part of treatment and I'll explain more about why cognitive restructuring is so important in a little while. Finally, you will also learn to cope with bodily signs and symptoms of anxiety or negative emotions caused by stress. The method we will use here is an applied relaxation technique called anxiety-management training. This technique has been used with many problems in which stress affects physical illness, and is highly effective. Hypertension, headaches, diabetes, and anxiety disorders have all been successfully treated with AMT. So, the three areas of treatment we will be covering in treatment are activity scheduling, cognitive restructuring, and anxiety-management training. Do you have any questions before I go on?

The therapist answers all questions and summarizes the three components if necessary. A demonstration of cognitive restructuring is now provided.

3. Demonstration of Thought–Emotion Relationship.   In Session 1, formal cognitive restructuring is not carried out because emphasis is placed on activity scheduling (outlined later). Rather, a demonstration of how thoughts and misattributions about concussion symptoms lead to negative arousal-inducing emotions is provided. The following is a sample therapist demonstration modeled after Beck et al. (1979):

> Now, before we make up your activity schedule and do some relaxation, let me explain the cognitive-therapy component of treatment to you. Cognitive restructuring has been shown to be useful in combating stress. And as you know, stress can make your concussion symptoms worse. First, what research has found is that when people manage the stress in their lives better, symptoms of anxiety, headache, concentration difficulties, and depression tend to be reduced and, in fact, disappear. We also know from research that stress is not something that happens to you from the outside world, such as time demands at work or bad weather conditions in heavy rush-hour traffic. Stress also comes from *within*; that is, how we think about or perceive things in life has much to do with our psychological, physical, and behavioral reactions. For example, let's say someone is home alone at night and hears a thud in another room. If he or she thinks, 'It's a burglar in the room,' how do you think he or she would feel? (See Beck et al., 1979, pp. 147–148, for use of this example.)

Patient sample answer: "Terrified," or "Scared," and so forth.

> **T:** And how might he or she behave?
> **P:** "Hide," or "Call police."
> **T:** So, in response to the *thought* that a burglar was in the other room, the person might feel scared or terrified, and behave in a way to protect him- or herself. On the other hand, let's say the person heard the exact same noise, but thought "the window was left open, and the wind knocked something over." How might that person feel then?
> **P:** She wouldn't be afraid. Might be annoyed because she had to close the window, or mad because a mess had to be cleaned up.
> **T:** And would her behavior be different?
> **P:** Yes, I suppose so. She might go see what it was.
> **T:** As opposed to calling the police or protecting one's self.
>
> So you can see how just one thought can influence feelings and behaviors. In one instance, the person's thoughts caused feelings of fear and fearful behaviors. In the other, the thoughts caused feelings of annoyance, and the person's behavior was to go solve or fix the problem. This example also shows you how many different ways there are to think about one thing, and how *automatic* and *fast* these thoughts can be.
>
> As you can see, our reactions to things that are potentially stressful all depend on our thoughts or perceptions of the situation, and how we have learned to think about things. The same goes for illness or concussion. The way we think about the symptoms can make them worse, because we can increase feelings of being stressed. In fact, many normal concussion symptoms are just like stress symptoms, such as anxiety, irritability, depression, headaches, and difficulty concentrating. Worry about these symptoms increases stress responses and makes these very symptoms worse. So it's a vicious cycle. You might have read that in the *Recovering From Head Injury* manual.

Next, the therapist provides the patient with an example of the cognition–affect relationship with a relevant PCS symptom example. A sample symptom is taken directly from the symptom checklist for this purpose. The point of this exercise is to introduce the patient to a process of examining his or her own thoughts about symptoms with the therapist and to illustrate the connection between automatic, negatively selective thinking, and symptom exacerbation. It also serves to help initiate the patient to question the validity of his or her thoughts about symptoms or negative life events.

Four steps are taken:

1. The therapist selects a target symptom.
2. The therapist, with the patient's assistance, identifies the situation in which the symptom is a problem.
3. The therapist and patient identify the patient's automatic thoughts about the symptom in the problem situation.
4. The therapist illustrates the connection between the patient's thoughts and resulting feelings, and how postconcussive symptoms are exacerbated.

A sample dialogue might proceed as follows:

T: You said on the symptom checklist that you were bothered by anxiety three times this past week. Explain to me what you were doing when the *worst* bout of anxiety occurred. (*Steps 1 and 2: Identify symptom from checklist, and identify situation.*)

P: Well, I was at work. It was a busy day and I needed to finish a report before my next customer appointment at 2:00.

T: What were you *thinking* at the time? (*Step 3: Identify automatic thought[s].*)

P: That I hated being rushed, but I also hated leaving an unfinished report when I see a new customer. I was getting nervous and was unable to concentrate due to my head injury.

T: So you were thinking 2 things. First, about the report and the deadline you don't like leaving a report unfinished when you see a customer. Second, you also were thinking that the head injury made it difficult to concentrate.

P: Yes.

T: Let's look at the first thought. Tell me, what would you think if the report was unfinished as you saw a customer?

Note: Here the therapist pursues the automatic thought of missing a deadline beyond face value. That is, what are the *consequences* of missing a deadline for this particular individual? This line of inquiry is pursued in order to get at the anxiety-provoking essence of the automatic thought. By asking the patient about the consequences of self-imposed rules such as deadlines, the basic anxiety-provoking automatic thought can be articulated. In the passage to follow, the therapist both pursues consequences of missing a deadline, and checks the external reality of the deadline itself. That is, is the deadline self-imposed, or imposed by the patient's boss?

P: I would have to finish it after the customer left, and I would feel inefficient.

T: Would your supervisor be angry if you were late? (*Therapist examines the real situation or consequence with the patient.*)

P: No, we have 24 hours to complete them. In fact I was a day early with the report.

T: So really, you were *thinking* "I must have this report in by 2:00, or I am inefficient." Is that something how that thought might have gone?

P: Yes, I guess so. Yes.

T: What feeling did you get from thinking, "I must have this report in by 2:00 or I am inefficient?" (*Step 4: Identify connection between automatic thought and evoked feeling.*)

P: Like I was under the gun. I *had* to get it done, and if I didn't, I was inefficient. I guess I made myself really nervous and rushed.

T: So, even though you really did not have a deadline, you thought about one. *And* you would have called yourself inefficient if you did not make the thought-up, self-imposed deadline. Your *thought* about the deadline led to nervous feelings. *Not* a *real* deadline. Can you see here how your thinking led to anxiety? Your own thinking about a deadline led to a feeling of being nervous and rushed.

P: Yes, I see.

T: Now, you also said you thought about how your head injury made it difficult to concentrate. What specifically did you think the instant you noticed some concentration difficulties?

P: Well, "Here it is again. I'm not thinking clearly."

T: And when you thought "Here it is again, I'm not thinking clearly," what was the feeling that you had?

P: Well, nervous! Even more so.

T: (*Step 4, again: Therapist now points out the patient's misattribution of the concentration difficulties to concussion. An alternative attribution is offered. This demonstrates to the patient how feelings and actions can vary with cognitions/thoughts about PCS symptoms.*) Okay, understand that anxiety makes concentration more difficult, even for people who have not had a concussion. Here you were thinking about a deadline that you imposed on yourself, that created some feelings of anxiety. Then, after that, you noticed concentration difficulties that you attributed to your head injury. But if you were anxious and rushed to meet the deadline, this, too, could affect your ability to concentrate and think clearly. It sounds as though the concentration trouble also arose from anxiety about the deadline.

P: Well, I guess I would have slowed things down. Taken a second to relax.

T: (*Therapist now makes connection between an alternative thought, and alternative behaving and feeling.*) So if you thought "I'm not thinking clearly due to the deadline pressure," you would have behaved differently from when you thought concentration problems were due to concussion. If you thought concentration problems were due to deadline pressure, you would have slowed down.

P: Well, I guess I would have been calmer. Not so uptight.

T: So you can see that thinking about symptoms differently changes both *feelings and behavior*. (*The therapist can then clarify the rationale of cognitive restructuring if needed.*) With cognitive restructuring, you will learn more about how your thoughts influence your stress reactions that are making your concussion symptoms worse. Together, we will examine your particular thoughts and behaviors that are most likely to produce stress and will gradually have you change habits of thinking that increase stress and produce negative feelings. It takes a little time, but it's an effective treatment. Do you have any questions at this point?

The therapist at this juncture answers all questions and clarifies main points. It should also be emphasized that the central ingredient to behavioral and emotional change is an effort on the patient's part to gradually learn skills to use in everyday life. Emphasis should be placed on at least trying a particular method for changing negative automatic thoughts without rejecting the method outright. If such rejection is allowed by patients, this only confirms that their thinking about the world and their symptoms are beyond their control, and more feelings of helplessness results. If on the other hand, the patient tries a particular strategy of changing negative thinking with the therapist without success, an alternative strategy can be used until success is obtained.

4. Activity Scheduling. Following the rationale of treatment, the patient is introduced to activity scheduling. Activity scheduling is used in a variety of cognitive–behavioral treatments of depression (Beck et al., 1979; Freeman et al., 1990; Lewinsohn, 1974). Its primary intent in treatment of depression is to elevate the mood of individuals whose inactivity contributes to excessive rumination about depressing events. It also helps provide opportunities for the individual to receive positive reinforcement from the environment through activity, thereby decreasing feelings of helplessness when acting on the environment (Lewinsohn, 1974).

Activity scheduling for PCS. For purposes of treating PCS, activity scheduling is used to involve the patient in the graded resumption of normal, everyday activities. This is done at a pace that maximizes reinforcement of the patient's actions and minimizes the negative, punishing effects of stress that led to withdrawal from social, recreational, or work activity. Withdrawal from these activities leads to more opportunity to focus on and magnify symptoms that are misattributed to head injury, whereas, in fact, the symptoms are often the common manifestations of depressed mood (e.g., concentration difficulties, trouble remembering, anxiety, etc.).

Patients with mild head-injury symptoms present behaviorally in two general manners: depressed/withdrawn or overactive. Depending on the individual's presentation, activity scheduling is carried out slightly differently. First, depressed/withdrawn patients typically withdraw from daily vocational, recreational, and social activities, and are likely to spend much time focusing on and magnifying PCS symptoms. Negative ruminating about symptoms increases negative arousal and affect, and exacerbates symptoms such as concentration and consequent memory difficulties. Emphasis in activity scheduling for these individuals is placed on *increasing* daily rewarding activities that substitutes time spent in negative rumination.

The second type of PCS behavioral presentation, the overactive type, includes individuals who may be in the early stages of mild head-injury recovery ($<$ 3 months). These individuals may try to accomplish too much in daily life following concussion and, as a result, experience feelings of general stress, fatigue, and being overwhelmed. These responses contribute to the exacerbation of PCS symptoms, and indeed may lead to depression and withdrawal from activities over the long term. In order to prevent the depression/withdrawal cycle, the therapist emphasizes a general *decrease* in work or stressful activities, and priority is given to an *increase* in rest and relaxation activities. Relaxation exercises used in this treatment manual can be used as relaxing activities.

The therapist must assist the patient in scheduling activities that can either elevate mood, increase feelings of calm and relaxation, or both. As a guideline for deciding which tasks are most appropriate for elevating mood or increasing relaxation and enjoyment, Beck et al. (1979) make the distinction between *mastery* and *pleasurable* tasks. Put simply, "Mastery refers to a sense of accomplishment when performing a specific task. Pleasure refers to pleasant feelings associated with the activity" (p. 128). The therapist should provide a clear explanation to the patient about this distinction when introducing activity scheduling. For example, scrubbing the bathroom floor may not be enjoyable, but its completion can give rise to a sense of accomplishment. The therapist can then provide more examples of mastery and pleasurable activities relevant to the patient's personal tastes, and encourage sensible increases in them. The bottom-line intent of activity scheduling is to increase the PCS patient's receipt of reinforcement resulting directly from voluntary mastery or pleasure-inducing actions.

Completing the schedule. The activity schedule itself is a simple daily record of hour to hour patient activity (see Appendix I). Activities are scheduled for specific times, emphasizing pleasure and mastery (e.g., relaxation, leisure, work activities) between meetings with the therapist. A hierarchy of activities is informally constructed by the therapist and patient in order that the most reinforcing activity is given priority. Activities given top priority will vary from patient to patient, depending on the individual PCS presentation. For example, a depressed/withdrawn patient should place priority on small housework or social activities. On the other hand, the overactive, "Type A" patient may need to put priority on relaxing activity.

The general therapist introduction to activity scheduling and step-by-step procedure carried out in Session 1 follows.

T: You may remember reading in the *Recovering From Head Injury* manual about how doing too much after a head injury can actually slow recovery. That's because your brain needs time to heal, and you may become fatigued more easily, leading to reduced ability to concentrate or remember things. At the same time, if you stop all activities, this can lead to boredom, disinterest, and feelings of depression. Depression can lead to feelings of lassitude and a general lack of motivation, and also impair your attention and concentration. It is important that you pace yourself, and schedule time for relaxation, rest, and enjoyable, fun activities to keep your mood positive. Right now, I'd like to get an idea of what your daily activities are, hour by hour, and then see if we can adjust your schedule to optimize recovery. You may also remember that I told you how managing time and stress better can eliminate some of the concussion symptoms you have been experiencing, because they flair up in response to stress. Activity scheduling is a way to manage time and stress effectively. Each week, we will review your activities together and see which activities are most beneficial to you in managing stress. It is important to note that *you* will choose your activities and we will progress at a rate which will benefit your recovery. Now, lets get an idea of your current daily routine."

The therapist should then proceed through the following steps:

1. Get an estimate of the patient's current daily hour-to-hour routine. Include typical weekdays and weekends.

2. Next, ask the patient about what enjoyable activities he or she has an interest in and encourage participation. Remember to emphasize time for relaxation and rest. Relaxation exercises seen in this manual can be used to fill in some activity. If the patient has difficulty coming up with activities that are pleasurable, the Reinforcement Survey Schedule (Cautela & Kastenbaum, 1967) may be useful in assessing this.

3. In the third step, the patient and the therapist write in the chosen activities on the Activity Schedule Form in corresponding time slots. The Activity Schedule Form is seen in Appendix I. Use the patient's daily schedule of activities from Step 1 as a guideline, and remember to emphasize a balance between *mastery* activities and *pleasurable* activities in accordance with the patient's needs. Indicate whether a given activity is a mastery or pleasurable activity by marking an "M" or "P" in the corresponding time slot on the Activity Schedule Form. Flexibility in choosing activities is emphasized.

4. Assist the patient in prioritizing activities. Some patients will be reluctant to give up extra work or housework activity, because they think it is necessary. This may be due to compulsive tendencies or secondary gain with family members. If the patient is overdoing it, and it is relatively soon after head injury (2–3 weeks), point out to the patient that he or she might hinder his or her progress, and thus hinder the ability to take care of these important matters. A "Take your time and get it right the first time" argument is usually persuasive. As a general rule, if the activity is not necessary for life (such as a job, or meal preparation), then the activity should not be given a high priority. Relaxation, enjoyable activities, and time for rest should be given strong consideration.

5. To enhance compliance with carrying out activities, the therapist can at first recommend only a minimal change in activity level. For example, for the PCS patient with depressed mood, only a single, small activity may be all he or she can handle in the first stage of treatment. For such patients it should be emphasized that mood improves *after* activity, so the difficult part is initiation of activity. However, if the task is simple, the patient may engage in the activity quite readily. One intention of increasing normal activity slowly and gradually is to provide experiences of success and reward. Too much change in

activity (even too much rest for the overactive patient) may be punishing, and the patient will not comply with activity scheduling.

6. Once the activity is complete, the patient is instructed to follow the schedule closely, and place a 0–5 rating next to the "M" and "P" in each time slot placed there in Step 3 (0 = *No Mastery or Pleasure*, 5 = *Maximum Mastery or Pleasure*). The intent of the rating is to provide an illustration of *partial* mastery or pleasure and reduce absolutist, dichotomous thinking. The therapist should drive home the point that thinking about what the patient *does not* accomplish leads to emotional distress. Conversely, ratings will serve to break down "all or nothing" thinking that sets the patient up for emotional distress.

7. The patient is instructed to bring the Activity Schedule Form to the next session so that both therapist and patient can decide on increasing or decreasing various activities.

5. Anxiety Management Training.   As previously stated, AMT is a relaxation-control technique emphasizing relaxation to combat bodily and emotional arousal brought on by stress response. The technique involves using imagery of stressful situations to induce arousal, and systematic practice of regaining relaxation control in the face of arousal. AMT can be used not only in the treatment of anxiety symptoms, but also for anger and depression, as well as medical problems (see Suinn, 1990). The patient is trained to recognize early cues of stress response, which includes bodily cues, affective cues, and cognitive cues that signal onset of intense, unpleasant emotion. Applied relaxation in the face of these cues inhibits anxious or stress-related arousal. AMT is particularly well suited for treatment of PCS, because it teaches the patient to use relaxation to control stress response in early stages before it builds and exacerbates PCS symptoms.

The AMT procedure used in the present treatment is a modified version of that presented by Suinn (1990). Several subtle procedural differences exist between Suinn's (1990) AMT approach and the present one, but the basic theoretical application of the procedure is the same. One procedural difference between Suinn's AMT and the one used in this manual is that of the relaxation procedure. In the initial two sessions, Suinn teaches the patient progressive muscle relaxation. The present treatment also uses a guided relaxation procedure, emphasizing deep, diaphragmatic breathing to provide a relaxation cue. However, the relaxation procedure used in this manual is audiotaped so the patient can practice in the office and at home, providing a greater opportunity for overlearning.

Another difference in the relaxation procedure deals with the development of a "relaxation scene." The relaxation scene is used by Suinn in the early sessions of AMT to help the patient regain relaxation after exposure to imagined stress. The present treatment eliminates this step, and has the patient focus on bodily relaxation cues instead of a relaxing "scene." This is done because cognitive restructuring, or using cognitive self-statements, is used in tandem with relaxation control in the latter stages of this treatment. Relaxation scenes may interfere with using self-statements. Moreover, Suinn eliminates the relaxation scene by Session 4 for a similar reason; imagining the relaxation scene interferes with applying physiological relaxation while using stress arousal imagery. To say the least, using imagery within imagery is confusing. Therefore, the relaxation scene is eliminated in our version of AMT.

Identification of stressful situations is carried out with the therapist in cognitive restructuring. Situations identified in cognitive restructuring can be used in AMT when the patient is ready to apply AMT relaxation control in real-life situations.

Rationale.   The rationale for AMT is provided for the patient directly following activity scheduling. The following is a therapist's introduction similar to that used by Suinn (1990):

> Now I will explain what AMT is, and how it can help you manage some of the concussion symptoms about which you have complained. AMT involves training where you learn to recognize early signs of irritability, anxiety, depression or other stress related responses so that you can control them before they affect you and make your symptoms worse. The method of control that AMT teaches is relaxation. You will first learn a very easy and straightforward relaxation exercise. Then you will learn to control your stress and concussion symptoms by applying relaxation to early warning signs of stress in real life. Being able to learn this control is a skill and requires practice. To give you this practice, we'll be having you visualize scenes of situations in which you've had problems with stress and concussion symptoms, then you practice eliminating stress reactions through relaxing. That is really all there is to it. AMT is not difficult to learn. It is an effective technique and research has shown its usefulness with treatment of anxiety disorders, anger management, and with physical problems such as headache, hypertension, diabetes, ulcer, dysmenorrhea, and recovery in coronary heart disease. (p. 219)

Relaxation induction. Once the rationale is given, the relaxation induction can begin. An audiotape of the relaxation exercise should be made prior to the session for the patient to use at home. The patient should be in a comfortable, reclining position and contact lenses should be removed. The therapist can use the following instruction:

> T: In a moment you'll be given instruction in the relaxation exercise. It's a method called *guided relaxation*, because I'll be giving you instruction on both how to relax mentally and use a breathing technique to enhance your body's relaxation. I will also give you an audiotape of the relaxation exercise, and you will use this tape for practice at home. You will find that the more you use this relaxation exercise, the better you become at relaxing, and you will generally feel more calm and at ease. You will also be able to relax more quickly with practice. Right now, just lie back, loosen any tight clothing (necktie, shirt collar), and get comfortable.

The therapist begins the relaxation exercise. A relaxation induction with deep breathing is provided by Suinn (1990). In rare cases, patients can become aroused during onset of physiological relaxation, particularly during onset of subtle yet salient relaxation cues, such as reduction in heart rate. Some patients can achieve full-blown panic (Barlow, 1988). If this is the case, the therapist can best help the patient by remaining calm. Some PCS patients who present with anxiety as a major symptom complaint may have a propensity for panic attacks or related symptoms. If the patient does become panicky during relaxation, the therapist simply asks the patient if he or she feels tense or anxious, and states that it is an occasional reaction that some people get when they first try the exercise. The therapist can have the patient open his or her eyes or sit up, but should have the patient maintain some form of the relaxation exercise. If the patient is allowed to escape the exercise completely or, in fact, leave the office, it is confirming the patient's inaccurate thoughts that something drastically awful will happen during relaxation. This only reinforces anxiety. The therapist can say the following if a patient experiences arousal or a "paradoxical response" in treatment:

> T: You appear as though you might be a little uncomfortable; is this so? (*Patient answers*). Okay, well, this is a normal response for some people when they first attempt relaxation. It's just due to anxiety.... It is also a reason why you are here—so we can work on some of these

anxiety symptoms. Let's have you take a little break by opening your eyes if you want.... That's good, and just continue to sit here a bit.... It's okay that you feel a little tense, it happens to some people. Relaxation does help these symptoms you might feel now, but it takes a little time ... and practice.... Maybe even talking about the anxiety symptoms makes them worse.... That's alright, because that is the reason you are here ... to treat these symptoms.... Just take your time ... just sit and take it easy."

(The therapist can simply acknowledge the patient's symptoms, and observe his or her reactions to the symptoms to assess coping skills. Brief questions such as "Is this how your anxiety symptoms typically come on?" or "Are these symptoms a lot like those you complain about?" are revealing. If the patient complains that the symptoms are new, reassure him or her that the exercise is in a new setting and, in fact, is a new experience for the patient. So it is alright to have these symptoms, and they will pass).

T: Now, take a slow breath with me ... going in ... pause for a second, and out slowly.... Let those shoulder muscles go as you exhale ...

The intention of this therapist's response is reassurance. Panic responses disappear in a fading manner, but can dissipate quickly. However, if others show alarm or concern that something is terribly wrong, the panic can recede slowly.

Postrelaxation. After the patient has completed the relaxation exercise, the therapist queries the patient about the experience. The therapist should ask about specific cues that indicate relaxation, such as relaxed feelings in discrete muscle groups, cognitive images, or self-statements. The therapist should know what specific sensations the patient had that indicated to that he or she was experiencing pleasant, relaxed feelings. The therapist notes and records these cues in order to modify the relaxation exercise in Session 2, if needed.

Relaxation homework. The patient is instructed to take the audiotape home and practice with it daily before the next session. As a means of circumventing compliance problems, the therapist emphasizes that without practice, it will be difficult to get the full benefit from AMT, because it involves using quick relaxation onset, which is only about a minute or so in length. In order to obtain quick, effective relaxation responses, the patient's body needs to be conditioned, just as it would for an upcoming athletic event. However, the difference between relaxation and vigorous exercise is that relaxation is easier than rigorous exercise. In fact, the patient will most likely notice an improvement in symptoms very quickly with practice. Some tips for home practice include:

1. Schedule relaxation for a quiet time of day, when there is little responsibility and the patient is at ease.
2. Practice should be done in the same place each day, free of TV, telephone, radio, or other distractions.
3. Make it known to the patient that he or she may have good and bad days, and finding it difficult to relax in the beginning is normal.

6. Summary and Review. The therapist reviews the session by summarizing the main points. The patient should understand that cognitive–behavioral treatment of postconcussive symptoms involves three components: activity scheduling, cognitive restructuring, and anxiety-management training.

Activity scheduling involves scheduling activities in order that the patient either increase daily activities to elevate mood through obtaining reinforcement, or by scheduling more time for rest and pleasurable tasks to reduce overwork and stress. The patient should also understand that cognitive restructuring involves becoming more aware of inaccurate, stress-inducing thoughts about PCS symptoms, and that these thoughts can be substituted with more adaptive, coping thoughts with practice. Formal cognitive restructuring begins in Session 2. Finally, AMT is a form of self-control training that will allow the patient to effectively cut off bodily stress or anxiety that contributes to concussion symptoms. This is done through systematic practice of relaxation, which is gradually applied to situations in which symptoms or stress are a problem. Relaxation practice is needed if effective gains are to be expected over the 12 sessions of treatment. Session 2 is then scheduled after review of these main points is complete, and the patient's questions are answered.

Session 2

Session 2 treatment goals involve the following:

1. Administration of Concussion Symptom Checklist.
2. Cognitive restructuring.
3. Review of activity schedule since Session 1.
4. AMT: Relaxation review; relaxation induction.
5. Summary and review.

In Session 2, review of activity scheduling and AMT relaxation home practice is undertaken. Another relaxation induction is also carried out. However, the most important aspect of Session 2 is cognitive restructuring immediately following administration of the symptom checklist. In fact, these two activities blend together in the session, because the checklist provides basic information about symptoms (i.e., intensity, frequency) that is used in cognitive restructuring. The entire session is approximately 90 minutes in length to accommodate all five treatment goals.

1. Symptom Checklist Administration. The Concussion Symptom Checklist is orally administered in the same manner as Session 1. This is done before anything else in the session and should take no more than 10 minutes. The therapist can note any changes in symptoms from the previous session.

2. Cognitive Restructuring. After administration of the Concussion Symptom Checklist, cognitive restructuring begins. The therapist uses the patient's responses to the checklist to identify symptoms at which cognitive restructuring can be aimed. A rationale of cognitive restructuring has already been given in Session 1, so only a brief review of it is provided here. The brief review stresses one main point: Automatic, negative, and inaccurate thoughts of symptoms cause increases in symptom intensity.

Four steps are involved in cognitive restructuring in the treatment package:

1. Identification of inaccurate, self-defeating automatic thoughts about symptoms and the situations in which they occur.
2. Introduction to refuting and replacing automatic negative thoughts with coping thoughts.
3. Shifting from automatic, negative thoughts to coping thoughts.
4. Use of coping self-statements in real situations.

Identification of inaccurate automatic thoughts. The first step in cognitive restructuring involves identifying habitual, automatic thinking about concussion symptoms that is negatively biased; that is, in what situations do symptoms arise, cause problems, and lead to the patient's negative appraisal of them, causing anxiety, anger, and so forth? The therapist identifies those symptoms that are rated greatest in intensity and frequency on the symptom checklist, then asks the patient about specific experiences with them over the previous week. The therapist should get a specific day, time, and place where the symptom occurred at its worst. A clear understanding of the environment in which the symptom occurred is essential, because social, environmental, and autonomic stimuli can act as triggers or discriminant stimuli that activate negatively biased cognitions about symptoms. The therapist can then pursue a line of inquiry to get at the automatic thought about the symptom. The therapist does not take the automatic thought reported by the patient at face value but, rather, attempts to establish the thought's idiosyncratic meaning for the patient. This identifies the underlying anxiety or stress-provoking essence of the automatic thought, and helps reveal its inaccuracy in the next step of cognitive restructuring: refuting and replacing negative thoughts with coping thoughts.

A sample dialogue of might go as follows:

T: I see here on the checklist that you were bothered by headaches on five days over the past week, more than any other symptom. You also rated the intensity quite high, an 8. Tell me about your *worst* day with headache.

P: Well, my worst day had to be Friday. It was awful. I have busy Fridays anyway, and the headache on top of it all was just bad. It lasted all day.

T: So you had one headache?

P: Yes. It began in the morning and lasted until I got home.

T: I gather you were at work when it hit. Is this true?

P: Yes.

T: Tell me, the headache started in the morning; at what time did it begin and what did you do before it started?

P: Well, on Friday morning the headache began at about 11:30. I always have busy Friday mornings, since I have to attend a long staff meeting. Then, we break down into departmental meetings and I head up my department, so I run the departmental meeting. Friday is hectic and hard to deal with anyway; I don't need a headache. I have even gotten headaches on Friday without the concussion.

T: (*Therapist summarizes events to identify the specific situation in which the headache occurred.*) So you've had headaches before the concussion on Friday, but the headache last Friday began at 11:30, after a busy morning of attending and conducting meetings. *Where were you* and *what were you doing* when you *first noticed* the onset of a headache?

P: I was at my desk, just sitting and looking at my schedule for the afternoon. Planning the rest of the day.

T: As you were planning your day, looking at the schedule on your desk, and felt the headache, what did you think about right then and there?

P: I thought, "This is bad. I have so much to do, I don't need these headaches, not now!"

T: (*Therapist confirms this automatic thought, but continues a line of inquiry to get at the meaning of the automatic thought that is the basic anxiety/stress-inducing essence of the automatic thought.*) So what you thought was "This is bad. I have so much to do and I don't need the headache." Let's look at this thought just a little closer. When you said "This is bad," what did you mean?

P: Well, just what I said. It's bad. It's inconvenient.

T: Okay, so the headache was inconvenient. What about the second part of the thought: "I have so much to do, I don't need this headache!" What does that thought mean to you?

P: Well, that this headache is in the way of my work. Ever since the concussion, it seems a headache gets me on Friday.

T: (*Therapist now has the essence and underlying* meaning *of the automatic thought and now confirms and identifies this automatic thought.*) So, your thought is something like, "This headache interferes with my work. Ever since the concussion, a headache gets me on Friday."

P: Yes, well, that's it. It's as though each Friday I have to say, "Here we go again, this Friday headache is going to get me.... Ever since the concussion it's been this way."

T: So the automatic thought you get on Fridays when a headache begins, is "Here we go again, this headache is going to get me. Ever since the concussion it's been this way."

The therapist now has identified the automatic thought. Other automatic thoughts for other situations or symptoms can be identified in the same manner. With the automatic thought identified, the therapist then records the automatic thought with its accompanying situation of occurrence on the Patient Cognition Sheet seen in Appendix II. This sheet is for the therapist's records. It will help the therapist keep track of the patient's automatic thoughts about symptoms, and the situations in which they are likely to occur. A word of caution is noted. Each week, only one or two symptom situations with automatic thoughts should be identified in the manner outlined here. Too many situations and automatic thoughts will unnecessarily complicate cognitive restructuring and make the process confusing. The point of the exercise is to make the patient more aware of his or her rapid, automatic thinking that is inaccurate and anxiety producing. This skill is best learned with one or two symptoms that are the most problematic for the patient.

Refuting and replacing automatic thoughts. Once the patient and therapist have identified negative, stress-inducing automatic thoughts about symptoms, the patient is taught to use coping thoughts or self-statements to replace the self-defeating automatic thought. In order to have the patient effectively use coping self-statements, the therapist should demonstrate the inaccurate and/or self-defeating nature of the automatic thought. This can be done through a variety of cognitive techniques, many of which are outlined in Freeman et al. (1990) or texts on cognitive therapy. However, the general technique the therapist uses to refute the patient's automatic thought and assumed validity is "examining the evidence." Simply, this technique involves testing to see if objective evidence, that outside the patient's subjective conclusions, supports the negatively biased automatic thinking. To punctuate an important point, Beck et al. (1979) indicated that negative, automatic thoughts are so habitual and so ingrained in cognitive behavior patterns that the validity of automatic thoughts is simply assumed by the patient. The therapist must therefore be the devil's advocate, questioning and examining the validity of *any* patient thought about symptoms. This is a crucial role for the therapist, and he or she must collaborate with patients in pointing out the inaccuracies of their conclusions, attributions, or other thoughts about symptoms. This is fundamental to effective cognitive restructuring.

In using this example, a dialogue outlining the second step of cognitive restructuring might go as follows:

T: So the automatic thought you get on Friday morning at your desk with a headache coming on is, "Here we go again, this headache is going to get me. Ever since the concussion it's been this way."

P: Yes.

T: Let's look at that thought, now, a little more closely. You said earlier that you usually got headaches on Friday, even before your concussion. Is this so?

P: Well, yes it is.

T: So the part of the thought that says "ever since the concussion" is not *entirely true.*

P: Well, no, it isn't.

T: Right, because if you had no headaches on Fridays before the concussion, then it might be a little more accurate. The fact is, you did have headaches on Friday, even before the concussion.

P: Yes, that's right. But it seems I get the headaches *every* Friday since the concussion. (*Here, the patient attempts to validate the negative, automatic thought. This may happen frequently, as it may be the first time the patient has ever questioned his or her own thinking about symptoms. The therapist should persist with examining the evidence in an aggressive, but not argumentative manner.*)

T: Well, is that a fact? That is, did you, for example, have a headache on the Friday before last? Just think back.

P: Let me see. Last Friday … actually, no. I didn't.

T: So, no, you don't have headaches *every* Friday, since we now know that a couple of Fridays ago you had no headache.

P: That's right.

T: So the accuracy of your automatic thought "ever since the concussion" is not very good. In fact, you have had headaches, but not *every* Friday. (*The therapist now points out the stress-related feelings resulting from the negative automatic thought.*) Can you now see how the thought "This Friday headache is going to get me. Ever since the concussion it has been this way" can lead to negative feelings. And what you were telling yourself was untrue! Your concussion didn't give you headaches *every* Friday.

P: That's right. I guess I just expected the headache on Friday, because I thought it was due to the concussion.

T: (*Therapist takes another opportunity to point out another inaccuracy: the patient misattributing Friday headache to the concussion.*) That is another inaccuracy. Why would a headache due to mild head injury just wait for each Friday to roll around? Wouldn't your head hurt constantly? You also had usual Friday headaches without head injury well before your concussion. Now you are misattributing Friday headache to head injury.

P: Well, yes, it looks as though I am. I guess I'm telling myself that Friday means a concussion headache. I know that may be untrue, but I still get the headaches on a lot of Fridays.

T: (*Therapist introduces coping self-statements.*) Yes, you do. And when you do, you tell yourself negative thoughts such as "Here we go again, this headache's going to get me … ever since the concussion." These are stress-producing thoughts. One reaction to stress is muscle tension…. This results in soreness in facial/head muscles resulting in headache. To reduce this stress response, *what could you realistically tell yourself the next time you are in the same situation, sitting at your desk telling yourself the same, inaccurate, negative thought?*

P: Well, for one thing, I could say what I'm thinking just isn't true. I might get headaches on Friday, but I can handle them, rather than worry about my concussion.

T: So you might say to yourself, "My negative thinking will only make it worse. I can handle this." Is that close to what it is that can make you feel differently about your headache?

P: Well, that's close. I just think I can handle the headache since I know it's not the concussion. I shouldn't worry, I should think positively.

T: (*Therapist directs the patient to narrow the self statement.*) So to make it a simple, reassuring statement you might say,… what? Just a few words.

P: Umm … I can handle this headache … it's just stress, so think positive.

T: (*Therapist connects selfstatement with new emotional reaction. Note also that self-statements are positive. Rather than statements such as "I should not worry," or "I should decrease this negative self-talk," the therapist encourages positive statements, such as "Think positive," or "Increase positive self-talk."*) When you say to yourself, "I can handle this headache, it's just stress, so think positive," what are some of the feelings associated with this?

P: Well, I feel a little relieved. I can relax, stay cool. Because it's not my concussion.

The therapist can then record the selfstatements on the Patient Cognition Sheet for treatment records.

Shifting automatic thoughts to coping thoughts. The therapist now assists the patient in learning how to shift from negative, inaccurate, automatic thoughts about symptoms, to coping self-statements identified in the previous step. Emphasis is placed on teaching the patient to use "early warning signs" or discriminative stimuli that might trigger negative thoughts as signals to use coping self-statements. This can be done through faded rehearsal, with the therapist modeling the "shift" using the patient's example. The therapist then has the patient repeat the model internal dialogue with therapist guidance and feedback, and again with no therapist guidance. The therapist model might go as follows:

T: We have now identified situations in which you are likely to get symptoms that are problematic for you. In your case, it is headaches on Friday mornings after meetings at work. We have found that when you notice a headache, you think negative, automatic thoughts about your headache that are inaccurate. Specifically, you say to yourself, "This Friday headache is going to get me. Ever since the concussion it has been this way." In fact, this is false. You haven't had a headache every Friday, and you also found that you blame the headache on concussion. If it was caused by concussion, it would probably not wait to bother you on Friday. So, you found that if you tell yourself, "I can handle this headache. It's just stress, think positive," you get feelings of relief. At least you will be motivated to do something about your headache, rather than simply feel helpless and do nothing.

It's important now that you pay attention to things in your immediate environment, such as things that are stressful at meetings, the time alone after Friday meetings, because these events may act as *early warning signs* that may trigger negative, automatic thinking. Negative, angry, or anxious feelings also indicate early warning to negative, automatic thinking. Your negative thinking is so ingrained that these things can trigger automatic thoughts without your being aware of them. When you sense any of the early warning signs, either at a meeting, sitting alone at your desk, or when you get a negative feeling, shift to using your positive self statement(s). It is simple to do and it is automatic with practice. Let me give you an example: Right now I am going to role play. As you would do, I am going imagine myself at my desk on Friday morning meetings. I'm sitting at the desk looking over the agenda for the day. Suddenly, I sense a headache building, right in the same place it always does. I start to feel angry and nervous at the same time I think, "Here it is again. This Friday headache is going to get me. It's been this way since the concussion.... Wait a minute, this thinking is only making me angry. I can handle this headache. Think positively, it's only stress. I get headaches on Friday regardless of the concussion."

Can you see how the process goes? You use the first cues, sitting at the desk, sensing the headache coming on, some emotional response like anger, to check for negative thinking. Then, you replace it with the thoughts that are more accurate and less stress provoking. Now you try it. Just imagine yourself at the office ..."

The therapist then has the patient provide a blow-by-blow account of the experience, relating details in a "sports announcer fashion." The therapist can ask for affective (*feeling*) or environmental cues and negative thoughts that occur, and assist the patient in using the identified positive self-statements. The process is repeated once more with no therapist guidance, but with feedback about appropriate use of coping statements at the first sign of negative thinking. The patient should be asked to "convince" themselves of the self-statement as though they were in a debate.

Use of coping statements. The next step is to have the patient use coping self-statements in real life when symptoms arise. The therapist again instructs the patient to be vigilant in identifying negative thoughts he or she uses at the first sign of symptom onset. The patient should immediately use identified coping self-statements when identified, negative automatic thoughts occur. In addition, the patient should be aware of environmental cues or social situations in which symptoms become a problem and use coping statements to preempt automatic thoughts. Patients should be encouraged to use coping self-statements regardless of whether they fully believe them. If the therapist has fully refuted the face validity of the patient's negatively biased automatic thought, believability of the coping statement will not be a problem. However, automatic, dysfunctional thinking is so habitual and reinforced that it may take some time before the replacement or self-scrutiny of such thinking becomes second nature to the patient. Only habitual use of interference brought on by coping self-statements can disrupt the reinforcement cycle of the dysfunctional, inaccurate appraisal (cognition) of symptoms. The therapist should emphasize the use of coping statements at least as an "experiment" in the face of symptoms. Each week the statements can be reviewed for their success and, if necessary, modified to suit the needs of the individual.

3. Activity Scheduling: Review and Modification. The patient and therapist review activity since Session 1. This process should take about 10 minutes. The therapist should first identify activities that were engaged in and provide verbal praise and compliments for completing the task or tasks assigned (e.g., "I am pleased that you were able to complete this activity. It shows you care about your health. It's not easy to resume activities, but you did, despite your difficulties. I am confident you will do well in the 10 remaining sessions"). If the patient did not complete the task, the patient should be encouraged for at least coming for the appointment and/or trying to complete the activity. Modifications to the graded-task assignment can be made to assure completion for next session. This means either shortening the duration of the task or finding a simpler, easier task to complete.

In the next part of the review, the therapist observes the tasks that had high and low mastery or pleasure ratings and asks the patient about his or her experiences in completing the activities. If the patient has only extreme scores, 0 or 5, this might indicate that he or she views activities dichotomously, as either all good or all bad. This may be so particularly in the early stages of treatment with patients who are depressed. The therapist should then modify activities to demonstrate a gradation of mastery or pleasure. For example, if the patient partially completed a house chore, such as vacuum cleaning two of three rooms and rated it a 0 in mastery, the therapist should point out that two thirds of the task was complete, and indeed, "mastered." A rating of 0 is thus inaccurate. The next assignment could break up the chore in segments, such as vacuuming the living room or bedroom on different days. Each task would then receive a rating, each hypothetically lower than 5 because the tasks are smaller. By demonstrating that mastery and pleasure can come in "small doses," the patient is likely to feel less overwhelmed by the activity and find the motivation to complete it.

Finally, for the PCS patient who complains of fatigue and feeling overwhelmed, yet still engages in much work activity (overactive type), more rest can be scheduled. Naps, the relaxation exercise in this manual, and a consistent bedtime can help assure adequate rest. Again, it should be pointed out to this type of patient that fatigue contributes to stress responding, which reduces attention and concentration, making PCS symptoms worse. Progress in symptom recovery is contingent on rest. Praise should be generously dispensed for any relaxation or rest the patient has demonstrated. However, assigning the patient too much rest or relaxation may lead to noncompliance, and he or she may only derive feelings of failure from activity scheduling and ignore it throughout treatment. To avoid this problem, the therapist and patient should plan small amounts of relaxation in which success is assured. The therapist can even prescribe amounts considered too small by the patient to motivate him or her to complete more relaxation/rest than that assigned. This technique of *paradoxical intention* has been used to enhance compliance in a wide variety of behavior therapies (Ascher, 1981).

Activity schedule. The activity schedule for the next session is carried out in the same manner as Session 1.

4. Anxiety Management Training: Review. The therapist reviews the patient's relaxation home practice. In order to make adequate gains in relaxation skills, the patient should have at least four practice sessions with the audiotape. If this is not the case, the patient should be praised for making efforts at whatever relaxation was accomplished and encouraged to practice more. The therapist can then offer whatever help necessary in order to assist the patient to schedule time for relaxation practice. A daily phone call as a reminder, or assisting with scheduling a specific place and time for relaxation on the part of the therapist can be helpful. Receiving a call from the therapist immediately following relaxation for feedback can also be helpful. Suinn (1990) goes so far as to offer time and space in the clinic office for patient relaxation.

The therapist should also assess the patients' responses to relaxation. For instance, what specific bodily sensations indicate deep relaxation to them? Some people may say their legs feel heavy; others notice a lightness in their arms. Whatever cues the patient mentions, these cues should be noted for possible use in later sessions in which the patient uses relaxation to combat aversive arousal. Conversely, if the patient complains about the relaxation exercise, its specific unpleasant components can be modified or eliminated. A new, modified tape can be made in Session 2.

Relaxation induction. The relaxation induction is carried out in the same manner as in Session 1. If patients feel comfortable with the exercise, the therapist can conduct the identical procedure used in Session 1, or patients can use their audiotapes. If modifications need to be made, a new tape is recorded during the induction.

5. Summary and Review. Session 2 involves using cognitive restructuring that in the present treatment package entails identifying, refuting, and replacing automatic, inaccurate thoughts about symptoms. Specific situations in which symptoms occur are identified, along with accompanying negative automatic thoughts that contribute to patient distress. The therapist then demonstrates the inaccuracy of the automatic thinking and assists the patient in finding more adaptive thinking that he or she can use as self-statements to enhance symptom coping. The patient should be urged to use self-statements, even if he or she does not fully believe them.

Activity scheduling can be modified either to increase or decrease activities, depending on the needs of the patient. Some patients may provide extreme ratings of mastery or pleasure. This may indicate dichotomous "black-or-white" thinking of a depressed individual, and tasks should be broken into segments in order to indicate to the individual that activities can be *partially* pleasurable or "masterable." Breaking up tasks can also reduce patients' feelings of being overwhelmed and improve motivation. Likewise, overactive, PCS-symptom-prone patients should schedule more rest. The relaxation exercise for AMT can be used for this purpose.

Finally, relaxation for AMT is reviewed in Session 2. If no changes are requested, the patient is praised for conducting home practice and is encouraged to continue. The patient's individual bodily responses or "relaxation signals" are noted for future AMT. If the patient has difficulty with aspects of the relaxation exercise, it can be modified and a new tape for home practice can be made in Session 2.

Session 3

Session 3 treatment goals involve:

1. Administration of the Concussion Symptom Checklist.
2. Cognitive restructuring.
3. Review of activity schedule since Session 2.
4. AMT: Relaxation review; stress-scene development; stress induction; home practice.
5. Summary and review.

Session 3 involves activity scheduling and cognitive restructuring procedures identical to Session 2. These procedures are routine for all remaining sessions. AMT involves introduction of teaching the patient relaxation control in exposure to stressful imagery about PCS symptoms. Although cognitive restructuring and activity-scheduling segments should now be shorter in length, the AMT procedure in Session 3 may require this session to be 90 minutes in length.

1. Administration of Concussion Symptom Checklist. This is completed in the same manner as the previous session. The completed checklist is used as data in cognitive restructuring.

2. Cognitive Restructuring Review. A review of the patient's ability to recognize and replace negative, inaccurate, automatic thoughts about symptoms is conducted *in vivo*. The therapist does this in four discrete steps:

a. After administering the Concussion Symptom Checklist, the therapist asks the patient about symptom experiences. The therapist should ask about those situations and symptoms identified on the previous week's Patient Cognition Sheet. For example: "I see here on the checklist you reported four days of headache as opposed to seven days last week. Tell me about your headache experiences in (the situation identified in the last session) this past week. Last week you described (the situation) as giving rise to problems with headache."

b. The therapist then inquires about the patient's ability to identify negative automatic thoughts and replace them with coping self-statements identified in the previous session (recorded on the Patient Cognition Sheet). For example: "So during (the situation), did you notice your negative automatic thoughts, such as (those listed on the Patient Cognition Sheet) as you felt the headache coming on? How about before the headache?" "When you recognized the automatic thoughts, how did you find the use of the self-statement(s) (identified self-statement in last session)?"

c. The therapist questions the patient about the *emotional consequence* of replacing the negative automatic thought (appraisal of the symptom) with the coping self-statement. For example: "After saying to yourself (self-statement), what feeling did you experience?"

d. The therapist should inquire how believable the self-statement was to the patient. If the patient reports that the statements are not believable, there are two ways to respond:

1) The therapist states that automatic negative thinking is a learned habit. After just a few experiences with replacing automatic thoughts, one cannot expect the habit to be broken completely. With practice in recognizing and replacing negative thoughts, positive thinking becomes more automatic.

2) The therapist further refutes the patient's negatively biased symptom appraisal using cognitive techniques of examining the evidence or reattribution. This strategy should be used for patients who have not shown any response to the cognitive restructuring assignment, and who believe their symptoms will never be manageable again.

More cognitive restructuring. After the four-point review of target symptoms, the therapist and patient select new symptoms and situations to target in cognitive restructuring. However, the therapist and patient may want to continue cognitive restructuring with the symptoms and situations identified in Session 2, especially if the patient experiences a great deal of distress from the symptom and does not feel he or she can effectively manage it. Cognitive restructuring follows the same steps as those seen in Session 2.

3. Activity Scheduling. Activities scheduled for the previous week are reviewed in the manner outlined in Session 2.

4. Anxiety Management Training. Session 3 introduces the patient to the heart of what makes AMT effective: exposure to arousal-inducing events through guided imagery, and control over arousal through practice of cued control relaxation. In this session, the therapist helps the patient construct a scene used for inducing arousal while the patient is in a relaxed state. Aversive imagery is referred to as the "stress scene" because the scene entails negatively valanced arousal responses to PCS symptoms that may include anxiety, irritability, or depression. The patient will also practice obtaining relaxation control over stress responses to imagined PCS symptom distress. This is done with close therapist guidance.

Relaxation review. Relaxation review is conducted in the same manner as in the previous session. Few problems are anticipated at this point in home practice, and the patient should feel reasonably comfortable with inducing relaxation. The patient should also report being able to obtain a deeply relaxed state quickly and easily. If the patient has not practiced relaxation or does not feel confident of his or her relaxation skill, the AMT stress-induction process detailed later should not be undertaken until the following week.

Stress-scene development. The stress scene is used to induce patient arousal and distress about PCS symptoms in order to provide imaginal exposure to symptom problems. During exposure to the stress scene, the patient learns to become sensitive to somatic and affective cues indicating stress responding, and to apply relaxation to regain control over aversive arousal. The same stress scene is used in successive sessions in AMT, but when sufficient progress is made, the patient and therapist construct and implement a new stress scene involving a new symptom problem. In construction of the stress scene, the therapist uses several guidelines following the AMT model (Suinn, 1990).

1. The stress scene must be a real incident. It should involve a patient experience with a PCS symptom in which the patient became upset and charged with negative affect. Feelings expressed by the patient can include anxiety, sadness, or anger. If the scene is not a real incident of experience with PCS symptoms, the patient may

fantasize about extreme responses during imaginal exposure, and arousal will increase to excessive levels, resulting in a sense of uncontrollability.

2. The scene must be of moderate to high anxiety or stress level. It should rate a 6 on a 0–10 "stress scale."

3. The scene must include *specific* detail. If it does not, the patient may inadvertently add new elements to the scene that can result in uncontrolled arousal. Essentially, the patient may add more to what is actually there. This is especially true for those patients who focus on and magnify symptoms. Specific detail should include *what* the situation was, *where* it was or *who* was there, *cognitive, behavioral, and autonomic symptoms*, and *environmental or social triggers*. Aspects of stress-scene specificity are outlined in Table 16.2.

4. The stress scene should include *no escape responses*. This includes statements such as "I felt nervous so I just left," or "I just did not listen, I put it out of my mind," or "I pretended I was elsewhere." The patient *can state the urge to escape/avoid, but the scene must entail facing the stressful event* (e.g., "I felt like leaving, but I stayed with it").

5. The stress scene should not be a composite of several real experiences with PCS symptoms. This can also lead to excessive arousal induction leading to a sense of uncontrollability. *One* stressful experience with a PCS symptom or symptoms is all that should be included in the stress scene.

6. The stress scene should be a time-limited event of just a few moments, and not a lengthy, detailed chain of events. The therapist and patient should agree on a beginning, middle, and end.

The therapist provides a *rationale* of stress-scene development and use, and also helps the patient construct the stress scene:

T: So far you've been making good progress in relaxation. You are now ready for the next step of AMT. Today, we will develop a scene or image that will help you recreate some of the

---

Table 16.2. Sample Stress Scene

Situation

It's in the morning as you leave for work. You dread having to get in your car, behind the wheel and face the traffic.

Environment

You are now walking out your front door and into the driveway toward your car. You *see* your car, a blue Saturn Coupe (describe detail), and you begin to put the keys in the lock. As you open the door to get in, you can *smell* the familiar interior as you sit behind the wheel.

Symptoms (cognitive, behavioral, somatic)

You begin to feel the tension build.... Your *heart* begins to pound; you can *feel* the *sweat* on the palm of your hands as you *grip* the wheel. You feel a little distracted as *thoughts* about not being able to concentrate on your driving well begin to race.

Cues or triggers

You now pull out on the street running through the main part of your neighborhood. The traffic begins to build.... As you pull onto the entrance ramp on the interstate, you see the rush hour traffic go by, triggering even more tension as you drive on....

same feelings (anxious, angry, depressed, etc.) you get when you sense some of your symptoms and become upset. What we will have you do with this scene is use it as imagery during your relaxation to have you experience a moderate level of stress. Then, you will use relaxation again to gain control over the stress response in your body. We will repeat this a number of times. Do you have any questions?

The therapist then answers all questions to clarify procedure.

T: Right now I would like to have you think of a real situation in which you have had some moderately unpleasant, stress-like feelings in response to your concussion symptoms. I would like you to define "moderate" as about a 6 on a 0–10 "stress" scale. Think of 0 as no stress, when you are deeply relaxed, as relaxed as you get when you are doing the relaxation home practice. On the other hand, think of 10 as a panic situation. When the stress and emotion caused by your symptom is so much you just want to explode. Five is about in between, when you may feel uncomfortable, but know you can handle things without a problem. Six is a little more stressed than this.

So, can you think of a situation in which you have had some problems with symptoms, and the stress level is about a 6?

The therapist guides the patient in creating the stress scene consistent with the guidelines listed here. A sample stress scene with areas of specificity highlighted is provided in Table 16.2. The stress scene is spoken in the second person here, but can be spoken in the first to enhance stress induction. If the patient has trouble thinking of a real incident in which symptoms have caused or contributed to emotional distress, anxiety, anger, and so forth, the therapist can ask him or her to recount a past incident from the symptom checklist that was approximately level 6 in intensity.

Stress induction. Once the stress scene has been developed the AMT stress induction-relaxation procedure can begin. The step by step procedure is outlined in Table 16.3.

Postinduction. Following the stress-induction procedure, the patient is asked about his or her ability to regain relaxation control, the most important aspect of AMT. If the patient reports difficulty, the therapist can take one of two courses of action:

1. The therapist can simply have the patient relax longer before inducing stress with the first repetition of the stress scene.
2. The therapist may only need to *mention* the stress scene in order to induce 6-level arousal in the patient.

In any case, the stress scene need not be changed but can be truncated as soon as the patient signals 6-level arousal. The therapist can also emphasize descriptions of autonomic/somatic sensations of relaxation during the patient's relaxation-control phase.

If the patient reports that the stress scene does not induce enough arousal, the therapist can emphasize autonomic and cognitive cues in the stress scene presentation. A brief review of the stress scene with the patient will enable the therapist to add more intense arousal-inducing stimuli.

Finally, the patient should not use any avoidance or escape during the imagery, such as "I got relaxed because I knew the scene wasn't real.... I just kept telling myself that," or "I just tried not to listen to you and kept relaxing" (Suinn, 1990). If the patient did use escape procedures, the steps used earlier to modify the induction procedure can be taken in order that the patient does not avoid exposure to the aversive imagery about his or her symptoms. Avoidance will maintain aversiveness of symptoms much in the same way the escape/avoidance behavior maintains anxiety in phobic patients.

Table 16.3.   AMT Stress Induction Session 3

1. The therapist uses a shortened version of relaxation instructions implemented in previos sessions. The relaxation induction should only be 10 or 12 minutes, highlighting those relaxation cues identified by the patient in Sessions 1 and 2 and home practice. The patient is instructed to raise a hand at the wrist once deep relaxation has been attained.
2. Once the *relaxation signal* is given, the therapist gives the following instructions: "Okay, I see your signal. In a moment I'll have you turn on the stress scene where (describe with brief label). Once the stress has built, just give me a signal by raising your hand. Okay, turn on the stress scene ... really imagine yourself there, you are ..." (therapist describes using detail noted in Table 16.2.).
3. *Once the patient signals the onset of arousal, the therapist maintains description of the stress scene for 10–15 seconds*: Okay I see your signal. You are in (label scene). ... Hold onto that arousal (anxiety, anger, arousal, etc.)."
4. After 10–15 seconds, the therapist turns off the stress scene and prompts the patient to relax by using deep breathing. Relaxation cues that are most effective for the patient may also be used. The patient is instructed to signal the therapist when relaxation is regained (raise hand). "Okay, now just turn off the stress scene. ... Let it disappear. ... Now just relax using the deep breathing and relax. When you are reasonably relaxed and comfortable, signal me with your hand."
5. When *relaxation* is signaled, the therapist instructs the patient to continue deep breathing and describes the relaxation body cues that are effective for the patient. This is done for *3 minutes*, during which the patient is reminded to relax various body parts (e.g., "Relax your jaw muscles, the muscles of your face" etc.).
6. *Immediately at the end of the 3-minute "body review,"* the therapist turns on the stress scene again with the *same instructions as in Step 2*. The therapist asks for a "stress signal" and maintains the stress scene this time for *20–30 seconds*. The procedure is repeated so the patient has at least 3 exposures to the stress scene.

Relaxation home practice. For home practice of AMT relaxation, the patient is taught that relaxation is easily applied to everyday situations, such as standing in line at the bank; at the desk at work; watching television; or riding a car, bus, or train. The patient is encouraged to use the breathing technique used in the relaxation exercise; the patient counts slowly to 4 (or 3) on the inhale and exhale, and relaxes muscles in various parts of the body. This can be done in a time span of 30 seconds up to 5 minutes. The patient is instructed to use this "brief relaxation" technique at any time throughout the day or evening. However, the patient is instructed not to use it for stress control yet. Rather, the patient should practice brief relaxations with breathing in times of relative calm and serenity.

The therapist can instruct the patient in "brief relaxation" while seated in a chair. Rehearsal instruction is as follows:

> **T:** For the next week, you should continue with practice of the relaxation exercise on the tape. You can also practice relaxation in short, brief periods of time that don't involve getting deeply relaxed, but involve just taking a few moments to breath deeply and relax muscles not in use. This is called *brief relaxation* and can be applied anywhere, anytime, such as standing in line, or riding in a car. Brief relaxation is a way of applying relaxation control in real life, and research has shown it to be effective with problems of anxiety control and control over high blood pressure. It's easy to do. Just sit in a chair, or, if you are standing, take a breath like you do on the tape ... from your abdomen. You can count to 3 as you inhale, 3 as you exhale. Let your shoulders and facial muscles relax as you exhale. Do this every half-hour or hour, and don't wait to use it when you feel stress. Do it even when you are calm to help keep you that way. Right now, let's just practice a brief relaxation for 30 seconds.

The therapist can demonstrate and emphasize using only abdominal muscles in breathing, keeping shoulders from lifting upward on the inhale. The patient can repeat this once or twice.

5. Summary and Review. Major points are made in Session 3 of treatment. First, cognitive restructuring involves a review of the patient's use of self-statements and ability to recognize negative automatic thoughts about symptoms *in vivo*. The therapist uses specific situations and self-statements that were identified and recorded on the Patient Cognition Sheet from the previous session. This immediately follows administration of the symptom checklist. The patient and therapist can also target new symptoms and situations for cognitive restructuring, but only if the patient appears to have reduced distress about the symptom targeted in Session 2. The therapist and patient also schedule activities for the next week, contingent on patient needs. If the patient has not been compliant with the procedure, the therapist can emphasize a limit to simple tasks as a method of motivating the client to do more in a paradoxical manner. Finally, AMT in-session introduces patients to the use of exposure to stressful imagery in order that they practice regaining relaxation control. The point of the training is to teach self-control over bodily/somatic responses caused by symptom distress. The patient is instructed to use relaxation in everyday life in the form of brief relaxations, in order to promote the generalization of relaxation skills.

Session 4

Session 4 treatment goals involve the following:

1. Administration of the Concussion Symptom Checklist.
2. Cognitive restructuring.
3. Review of activity schedule since Session 3.
4. AMT: Relaxation review; stress induction; home practice.
5. Summary and review.

Because most of the activity scheduling, cognitive restructuring, and AMT components have been thoroughly covered in the first three sessions, Session 4 should only take 1 hour. As a reminder, the therapist should indicate patient progress and the number of sessions remaining in treatment early in the session.

1. Administration of Concussion Symptom Checklist. The checklist is completed in the same manner as the previous session. Checklist data are used in cognitive restructuring.

2. Cognitive Restructuring. Cognitive restructuring is carried out in the same manner as in Session 3, immediately after symptom-checklist administration. To reiterate, first review the patient's ability to recognize negative, arousal-inducing thoughts, and replace the thoughts with self-statements (identified in the previous session and recorded on the Patient Cognition Sheet). Second, new symptoms or situations can be targeted for cognitive restructuring. Finally, the therapist should generously dispense facts about concussion symptoms cited in the patient manual, *Recovering From Head Injury: A Guide for Patients*. For example, telling the patient who is upset and worried about forgetting telephone numbers that nearly 60% of normal individuals forget telephone numbers is one way to refute inaccurate beliefs and thoughts about memory symptoms. Self-statements can be derived from this point. The therapist should see the cognitive restructuring review segment of Session 3 before proceeding with Session 4.

3. Activity Scheduling. Activities scheduled for the previous week are reviewed in the manner outlined in Session 2.

4. Anxiety Management Training. AMT in Session 4 is conducted similarly to that in Session 3, but with two changes. First, the patient carries out the initial relaxation on his or her own, without the guidance of the therapist. After 3 weeks of practice, the patient should quite easily achieve deep relaxation. Second, the patient is instructed to attend to cues or "early warning signs" of stress responding when the stress induction begins.

Relaxation review. A brief review of the patient's home practice is carried out. The therapist should inquire about the patient's experiences in applying brief relaxations *in vivo*, and identify and articulate specific relaxation strategies that were used to achieve relaxation. The patient should also be asked to identify any coping statements and compare them to those discussed in therapy.

Stress induction. The AMT stress-induction procedures is similar to that in Session 3 except for the two changes mentioned previously; patient-induced relaxation and attention to bodily "early warning signs" of stress responding. The same stress scene developed in Session 3 is used in Session 4, and will also be used in Sessions 5 and 6. Step-by-step instructions for the AMT stress-induction procedure in Session 4 are outlined in Table 16.4. However, before stress induction, the following introduction to Session 4 can be used by the therapist:

> In this session, we will have you start to initiate the relaxation without my instruction, because you have made good progress here. Then we will be doing the same thing as last session, using the stress scene to help you experience the stress of concussion symptoms, and then have you eliminate your bodily and emotional arousal with relaxation as self-control. Today, you will pay close attention to "early warning signals" of stress responses while you are in the stress scene. (see Suinn, 1990, p. 244)

Step-by-step instructions for stress induction are presented in Table 16.4.

Postinduction. The postinduction interview is carried out in the same manner as in the

---

Table 16.4. AMT Stress Induction, Session 4

1. The therapist instructs the patient to self-initiate deep relaxation: "Sit back, close your eyes so that you won't get distracted. Using whatever method works best for you, get comfortable, and begin your relaxation. Whenever you are reasonably relaxed, give me the hand signal."
2. Once the patient signals relaxation, the therapist reminds the patient to relax by breathing deeply, and directs to the patient's bodily reaction cues.
3. After *1 minute* of relaxation-cue review, the therapist turns on the stress scene: "Okay, I'll have you turn on the stress scene involving (label) now, and after you have really let the stress arousal build, signal me with your hand letting me know you are (anxious, tense, angry, etc.)." Therapist then describes stress scene.
4. Once the patient has given the signal for arousal, the therapist then instructs the patient to stay in the stress scene and *pay close attention to bodily responses that indicate arousal and responding*. The stress scene remains on for 20–30 seconds. "Okay, I see your signal. Now, let the stress response really build, allow yourself to really experience the stress of your concussion symptom.... (therapist describes for the next 20–30 seconds, and instructs patient to attend to early warning signs of arousal). "While you are in the stress scene, pay attention to areas of your body where you can feel yourself getting uncomfortable, it may be your ( ), or your ( ) getting tense.... Just notice these early warning signs of your stress responding."
5. Once the 20–30 second stress exposure is over, the therapist instructs the patient to turn off the stress scene and use deep breathing to attain relaxation. The patient is asked to signal relaxation again (raise hand at wrist briefly).
6. Once relaxation is signaled again, the therapist instructs the patient to remain in the relaxed state (reviews deep breathing and relaxation cues) for *1 minute* and *repeats the process from Step 3*. The patient should be exposed to the stress scene 3 to 5 times total, or repeated as desired.

previous session. However, the therapist should note the patient's "early warning signs" of stress arousal and emphasize them in the next session.

Relaxation home practice. Relaxation home practice is the same as in the previous session. Recommend daily practice with the relaxation tape. The patient should also continue use of brief relaxations *in vivo*. The therapist asks the patient to take note of any early warning signs of stress-related arousal in the presence of noticed concussion symptoms. The intent of the exercise is to make the patient more aware of discriminative stimuli that indicate negative affective responding and distress, which exacerbates symptoms of concussion. The patient will be instructed to apply both cognitive self-statements and brief relaxation control in response to early warning signs in future sessions. The more aware the patient is of early bodily cues and negative self-statements (inaccurate thoughts) in the arousal-symptom exacerbation cycle, the more successful he or she will be in using cognitive restructuring and AMT in stress reduction. This is a two-dimensional, preemptive stress-management technique that addresses both the cognitive and physiological aspects of stress responding and will reduce emotional distress brought about by faulty symptom appraisal.

5. Summary and Review. Session 4 continues the same as Session 3 regarding cognitive restructuring and activity scheduling. However, AMT has two changes. First, the patient induces initial relaxation without the aid of the therapist. Second, the patient is asked to attend to early warning signs or somatic/bodily cues that indicate the early onset of stress or arousal responding. The patient is asked also to be sensitive to these cues in daily life in an effort to make the patient more aware of early signs of emotional distress that could exacerbate PCS symptoms.

Session 5

Session 5 treatment goals involve the following:

1. Administration of the Concussion Symptom Checklist.
2. Cognitive restructuring.
3. Review of activity schedule since Session 4.
4. AMT: Relaxation review; stress induction; home practice.
5. Summary and review.

Session 5 is similar to Session 4 but with a little more self-control given to the patient in AMT, along with the development of a high-intensity stress scene. Also, emphasis is placed on increasing the patient's daily activity through activity scheduling. As with each session, the therapist notes the progress and reminds the patient of positive gains and the number of remaining sessions.

1. Administration of Concussion Symptom Checklist. The checklist is completed in the same manner as in the previous session. Checklist data are used in cognitive restructuring.

2. Cognitive Restructuring. Cognitive restructuring is carried out in the same manner as in the previous session. Again, new symptoms or situations can be targeted for cognitive restructuring if the symptom previously targeted is no longer a complaint.

3. Activity Scheduling. Activities scheduled for the previous week are reviewed in the manner outlined in Session 2. However by Session 5, the patient should be making some gains in the resumption of normal activities. The therapist can now put a stronger emphasis on increasing the number or duration of daily activities in the seven remaining sessions.

4. Anxiety Management Training. AMT in Session 5 involves two changes. First, a high-intensity stress scene is developed at a 9 level on the 0–10 scale. Second, the patient assumes more control over the stress scene by turning it off whenever he or she desires. This also changes the patient's hand signal for peak arousal and relaxation control. Details of this are seen in Table 16.5. An introduction to this session might go as follows:

> In this session of AMT, we will first develop a new stress scene where your concussion symptoms have caused arousal to about a level 9. Then we'll alternate that scene with the 6-level scene to promote stress-related arousal. One thing we will do differently this time is that after you get aroused and feel the stress response build (remember to pay attention to your early warning signs), you will make the decision to turn off the stress scene when you are ready. Then you use deep breathing to regain a relaxed, calm state. For signaling this time, when you get aroused and (angry, anxious, tense) raise your hand and keep it up while you retain the arousal. Once you become relaxed again, lower it. (see Suinn, 1990, p. 248)

Relaxation review. Relaxation home practice is reviewed in the same manner as in Session 4. Particular attention is devoted to the patient's ability to recognize early warning signs of anxiety, emotional distress, or excessive responding to PCS symptom onset. The therapist should note any new early warning signs and incorporate them in AMT relaxation and stress inductions.

Table 16.5. AMT Stress Induction, Session 5

1. The therapist instructs the patient to self-initiate deep relaxation: "Sit back, close your eyes so that you won't get distracted. Breath deeply, get comfortable and begin your relaxation. Whenever you are reasonably relaxed, give me the hand signal."
2. Once the patient signals relaxation (raises hand and puts it back down), the therapist reviews deep breathing and several bodily cues/"signals" of relaxation for *1 minute*; that is, the patient is reminded to relax by controlling the rate and depth of respiration, and by attending to relaxation cues (e.g., "relax the muscles in your shoulders…).
3. After *1 minute* of relaxation-cue review, the therapist turns on the stress scene. "Okay, I'll have you turn on the 6-level stress scene involving (label), and after you have really let the stress arousal build, signal me with your hand letting me know you are (anxious, tense, angry, etc.). *Pay attention to the early warning signs.* Then, keep your hand up while you are in the scene, and whenever you are ready, just turn off the scene and reinitiate relaxation. *Lower your hand when you have regained relaxation.* Okay, turn on the scene now…." (Therapist then describes stress scene).
4. Once relaxation is signaled (hand is down), the therapist says: "Okay, I see your hand is down signaling relaxation. Continue your relaxation, flowing through your body…. Take a deep breath or two … relax."
5. (*Pause*) "Now in a moment I'll have you turn on the 9-level stress scene involving (label). After you have let the stress arousal build, signal me with your hand letting me know you are (anxious, tense, angry, etc.). *Pay attention to the early warning signs.* Then, you keep your hand up while you are in the scene, and whenever you are ready, just turn off the scene and reinitiate relaxation. Lower your hand when you have regained relaxation. Okay, turn on the scene now …" (therapist then describes stress scene).
6. The alternation of the 6- and 9-level stress scenes is repeated so that the patient has minimum of four exposures to the pair of scenes.

Stress-scene development. Stress scene development is carried out in the same manner as that outlined in Session 3. However, rather than a moderate level stress scene (6), the therapist and patient develop a 9-level stress scene on the 0–10 stress scale. As with the the 6-level stress scene, the 9-level stress scene includes somatic, affective, cognitive, and behavioral elements that sufficiently detail the patient's true experience of distress during PCS symptom onset. A brief description of the setting in which symptoms are problematic is helpful as well.

Stress induction. The steps in stress induction for Session 5 are outlined in Table 16.5.

Postinduction. The postinduction inquiry concerns the patient's ability to regain relaxation over the 6- and 9-level stress scenes. Methods or strategies the patient employed in regaining relaxation, and/or cues of relaxation can be identified. The patient should have at least three trials of regaining relaxation control without struggling. If the patient has difficulty regaining relaxation, the therapist can use relaxation instruction to assist the patient (e.g., "Okay, just turn off the stress scene now … let it go … take a breath in … slowly … exhale and relax"). If this measure does not work, the session should be repeated before moving onto AMT in Session 6. The patient may also identify new warning signs of arousal; each can be identified and recorded by the therapist.

Relaxation home practice. Relaxation practice is essentially the same as in Session 4, with special attention given to the patient using early warning signs of emotional/ autonomic arousal to cue brief relaxations *in vivo*. More practice with the tape is suggested.

5. Summary and Review. Session 5 cognitive restructuring is identical to that in Session 4. However, the patient's daily activity level should increase slightly, and this is reflected in the activity schedule for the next session. Adding new activities or increasing the duration of current activities (work, social activities) is also indicated. In Session 5, a new high-intensity stress scene is developed for AMT. The high-intensity stress scene accompanies the moderate scene to induce greater negative emotional arousal about PCS symptoms in the patient. The patient is also given more control over when to shut off the stress scenes during stress induction. At least three trials (out of four attempts) of regaining relaxation control after stress-arousal induction in Session 5 are needed before the patient moves on to the AMT procedure used in Session 6. Brief relaxation periods are recommended for home practice, and the patient should become more aware of early warning signs of stress in response to PCS symptom onset.

Session 6

Session 6 treatment goals involve the following:

1. Administration of the Concussion Symptom Checklist.
2. Cognitive restructuring.
3. Review of activity schedule since Session 5.
4. AMT: Relaxation review; stress induction; home practice.
5. Summary and review.

Session 6 cognitive restructuring is carried out in the same fashion as previous sessions. Activity scheduling emphasizes an increase in daily activity, and AMT involves more intensive relaxation control. As with past sessions, the therapist informs the patient of progress made thus far in managing concussion symptoms and the number of sessions remaining (6). Session 6 can be conducted in an hour, with all remaining sessions (7–12) following the same format.

1. Administration of Concussion Symptom Checklist. The checklist is completed in the same manner as in the previous session. Checklist data are used in cognitive restructuring.

2. Cognitive Restructuring. Cognitive restructuring is carried out in the same manner as in the previous session. Again, new symptoms or situations can be targeted for cognitive restructuring if the target symptom is no longer a complaint.

3. Activity Scheduling. Activities scheduled for the previous week are reviewed in the manner outlined in Session 2. The patient should be making some gains in the resumption of normal activities. The therapist can now put a stronger emphasis on increasing the number or duration of daily activities in the remaining sessions.

4. Anxiety Management Training. AMT in Session 6 involves one major change. Instead of the patient turning off the stress scene during stress-arousal induction, he or she remains in the scene while applying relaxation control. Suinn (1990) contends that this is more akin to real life, because exposure to situations that are stressful cannot be "turned off." In the same respect, not all concussion symptoms can be "turned off." However, the patient *can* be trained in methods that enhance coping with the symptom(s) rather than allowing emotional response to escalate and exacerbate symptom episodes. This is the crux of AMT (physiological relaxation control to enhance symptom coping). An introduction to Session 6 might go as follows:

> T: This session is much like the last session. However, there is one change. Instead of "turning off" the stress scene before you initiate relaxation, you will apply relaxation *while you are still in the stress scene.* This is like real life, in which sometimes you may notice symptoms of stress, or those that you complain about in treatment, and you cannot do much about the situation. But, you *can* control your response to the situation, which is why you are practicing AMT, and the brief relaxations. In today's session, the signaling is the same: hand up to indicate your are experiencing arousal in the stress scene, hand down when you have regained relaxation control (demonstrate).

Relaxation review. Relaxation home practice is reviewed as in previous sessions. Once again, attention is devoted to the patient's ability to recognize early warning signs of anxiety, emotional distress, or excessive responding to PCS symptom onset.

Stress induction. The steps in stress induction for Session 6 are outlined in Table 16.6.

Postinduction. The postinduction inquiry concerns the patient's ability to regain relaxation over the 6- and 9-level stress scenes. The patient should have at least three trials of regaining relaxation control without struggling. If the patient has difficulty regaining relaxation, the therapist can use relaxation instruction to assist him or her (e.g., "Okay, just turn off the stress scene now … let it go … take a breath in … slowly … exhale and relax").

To reiterate a point made several times throughout this manual, the patient should not use escape or avoidance strategies in coping with stress arousal brought on through PCS symptoms used in AMT imagery. This includes using strategies, such as "I just ignored the

Table 16.6.   AMT Stress Induction, Session 6

1. The therapist instructs the patient to self-initiate deep breathing: "Using whatever method works best for you, get comfortable and begin your relaxation. Whenever you are reasonably relaxed, just lift and lower a hand" (see Suinn, P. 253)
2. Once the patient signals relaxation the therapist reminds the patient to relax by control of breathing, attending to relaxation cues. Therapist allows about 30 seconds to pass.
3. After 30 seconds, the therapist turns on the stress scene: "Okay, in a moment, I'll have you turn on the 6-level stress scene involving (label). But this time, instead of turning off the scene, you'll stay in the scene and begin to relax by breathing deeply. so while you are in the scene, eliminate the arousal … by using breathing like you do in brief relaxation … and notice the loosening in your muscles. After you have relaxed again, lower your hand and switch off the stress scene."
4. Once relaxation is signaled, the therapist says: "Okay, I see your signal. Continue your relaxation, flowing through your body…. Take a deep breath or two … relax."
5. (*Pause*) "Now in a moment I'll have you turn on the 9-level stress scene involving (label). After you have let the stress arousal build, signal me with your hand letting me know you are (anxious, tense, okay as is, etc.). *Pay attention to the early warning signs*. Then, you keep your hand up while you are in the scene, and reinstate relaxation. Lower your hand when you have regained relaxation. Okay, turn on the scene now …" (therapist then describes stress scene).
6. The alternation of the 6- and 9-level stress scenes is repeated so that the patient has a minimum of four exposures to the pair of scenes.

stress scene, and pretended I was somewhere else." As stated earlier, it is acceptable for the patient to express the *urge* to escape or avoid the stress scene, so long as he or she does not use an avoidant cognitive strategy.

Relaxation home practice. Relaxation practice is the same as in the previous session, with attention given to the use of controlled deep breathing to induce brief relaxation *in vivo*. Practice with the tape is suggested.

On a final note, the therapist emphasizes overlapping the use of cognitive self-statements and AMT relaxation control at the moment of PCS symptom onset; that is, as the patient uses self-statements in response to negative automatic thoughts about symptoms *in vivo*, he or she is instructed simply to take a deep breath and conduct a brief relaxation. This is simply the application of AMT relaxation control in real life, just as it is done in-session. The patient at this point of treatment should be quite aware of automatic thoughts that spawn negative emotional arousal, and activate physiological arousal and bodily early warning signs. The patient is simply reminded here that the two types of early warning signs are cognitive, and physiological (bodily):

1. *Cognitive.* Negative automatic thoughts about symptoms (e.g., "It's Friday, and here is the headache…. Ever since the concussion it's been terrible!") or cognitive PCS symptoms, such as concentration difficulty.
2. *Physiological.* Bodily cues or early warning signals of stress response noticed during AMT in session or *in vivo*. Onset of PCS symptoms such as headaches or tension can also act as a physiological signal.

A model introduction to using self-statements and relaxation might go as follows:

T: We've now been working well at both having you change inaccurate, stress-inducing thoughts about your symptoms, and applying relaxation control in situations in which your concussion symptoms have been giving you problems. As you know, thoughts lead to increased arousal, setting off the early warning signs we have identified in AMT. Now I would like to have you combine self-statements and brief relaxations to further your control over symptoms. All this means is that when you are in a problem situation and catch yourself using inaccurate, negative thinking about your symptoms, use the self-statement in the same way we have been working on, but also take a deep, slow breath, and relax. That's all.

Most patients may have already combined self-statements with relaxation *in vivo*. For example,

P: I knew my forgetfulness with phone numbers was normal because I read it in the book you gave me. So when I started to get upset about forgetting my friend's number, I just took a breath, and said my self-statement: "Most people forget numbers. I'm okay, this is normal." Then I went on with business, settling down a little.

If on the other hand the patient has not combined self-statements with relaxation *in vivo*, the therapist can have the patient practice this in the office. In any case, the therapist presents the task in the simplest manner possible, so that the patient finds the task easy to apply to real life.

5. Summary and Review. Session 6 comprises a format that will be followed for the remaining treatment sessions. Cognitive restructuring and activity scheduling are carried out in the same manner as in previous sessions. AMT changes for the last time in treatment. The change involves giving the patient more control over implementing relaxation in session rehearsal, but similar to real life, the patient does not "turn off" the stress scene during arousal induction. Emphasis is placed on having the patient use AMT relaxation control in the face of emotional/autonomic arousal caused by negative appraisal of PCS symptoms. The patient also is instructed to combine the use of cognitive self-statements with AMT relaxation control (brief relaxations) to provide a dual stress-management technique to reduce emotional overreacting in the face of symptom onset. The patient is instructed to use the technique the next time the symptom problem arises.

Session 7–12

Sessions 7–12 are identical to Session 6. The therapist should be sensitive to several aspects of patient progress:

1. If the patient has difficulty regaining relaxation control over stress scenes in AMT, the procedure is simply repeated, with as much therapist guidance as necessary to help the patient regain relaxation after arousal. When the patient makes sufficient progress, a second set of stress scenes (6- and 9-level) using another PCS symptom or symptom-related problem is developed and implemented. Instructions in Session 5 are followed to create the new stress scenes. AMT sessions following stress scene development simply follow the Session 6 format until 12 sessions have been completed.

2. If the patient reports difficulty in employing cognitive self-statements combined with relaxation control (brief relaxations) to reduce reactions to symptoms, the therapist and patient identify less intense situations so that success with self-control is enhanced. The 0–10 scale can be used for this purpose. A 5-level real-life situation is suitable for such experimentation; however, it is unlikely that many patients will have difficulty using self-statements and relaxation control in combination.

Notes on Termination and Relapse Prevention

Robert J. Ferguson
and Wiley Mittenberg

The present treatment follows a 12-session time-limited format. From outset of treatment, the patient is made aware of this. The therapist in each session reviews symptom progress, indicates the number of sessions undertaken, and the number of sessions remaining. This enhances expectations for progress, prepares the patient for termination, and motivates the patient to take advantage of the time spent in treatment.

Experience suggests that a minority of patients may not fully "recover" in the time spent in treatment, and some may occasionally become anxious about leaving the therapist before they are "cured." There is no need for the patient to continually report to treatment if all symptoms are not 100% relieved. In fact, individuals without a history of head injury normally report a number of daily symptoms similar to PCS (Mittenberg et al., 1992). Seemingly endless repetitions of the same procedures can foster a dependency on the therapist and, in fact, help maintain symptoms. Over time, the patient will master skills with consistent practice, and he or she will learn to incorporate the skills in daily life in order to cope effectively with symptoms. This is the prime objective of treatment. On the other hand, the therapist may continue treatment beyond 12 sessions if it can reasonably be concluded that it would benefit the patient. However, in doing so, the patient and therapist must determine the number of additional sessions scheduled and specify the goals for continuing. For example, a discernible decrease of a particular symptom that is problematic for the patient can be a goal. This can be operationalized as a specific decrease of symptom frequency, intensity, or duration, as assessed by the Concussion Symptom Checklist.

In preparing for termination, the therapist can mention in Session 9 that the last session is coming soon. An assessment of the patient's feelings and confidence in him- or herself in managing stress and PCS symptoms after treatment can be undertaken. Several points must be stressed:

1. The therapist reiterates that the symptoms experienced are normal and dissipate with time. The therapist points out to the patient that his or her progress on the Concussion Symptom Checklist over the course of treatment can provide concrete evidence of this.
2. The 12 sessions of therapy are very much a learning phase, and some additional results of treatment occur *after* the learning phase of therapy. As they become more familiar with applying skills in real life, patients will derive additional results. This means that any residual symptoms will clear up over time.
3. The skills of cognitive restructuring and relaxation training should be practiced daily and will become as automatic as the negative, automatic thoughts about symptoms they once had.
4. If the patient ever has any questions about treatment or an exacerbation of symptoms, he or she is encouraged to call the office at any time to talk with the therapist.

	Monday	Tuesday	Wednesday	Thursday	Friday	Saturday	Sunday
Hour							

0 = No pleasure   5 = Highly pleasurable
0 = No mastery   5 = High mastery

APPENDIX II: PATIENT COGNITION SHEET

Situation in which symptoms are a problem:

Specific, negative automatic thoughts about symptoms:

Positive, coping self-statements:

REFERENCES

Alves, W. M., Colohan, A. R., O'Leary, T. J., Rimel, R. W., Jane, J. A. (1986). Understanding post-traumatic symptoms after minor head injury. *Journal of Head Trauma Rehabilitation*, *1*, 1–12.
Ascher, L. M. (1981). Employing paradoxical intention in the treatment of agoraphobia. *Behavior Research and Therapy*, *19*, 533–547.
Barlow, D. H. (1988). *Anxiety and its disorders: The nature and treatment of anxiety and panic*. New York: Guilford Press.

Beck, A. T., Rush, A. J., Shaw, B. F., & Emery, G. (1979). *Cognitive therapy of depression*. New York: Guilford Press.

Cautela, J., & Kastenbaum, R. (1967). A reinforcement survey schedule for use in therapy, training, and research. *Psychological Reports, 20*, 1115–1130.

Cook, J. B. (1969). Effects of minor head injuries sustained in sports and the postconcussional syndrome. In A. E. Walker, W. F. Caveness, & M. Critchley (Eds.), *The late effects of head injury* (pp. 408–413). Springfield, IL: Thomas.

Cook, J. B. (1972). The postconcussional syndrome and factors influencing recovery after minor head injury admitted to hospital. *Scandinavian Journal of Rehabilitation Medicine, 4*, 27–30.

Cormier, W. H., & Cormier, L. S. (1985). *Interviewing strategies for helpers: Fundamental skills and cognitive behavioral interventions* (2nd ed.). Monterey, CA: Brooks/Cole.

Deffenbacher, J., Demm, P., & Brandon, A. (1986). High general anger: Correlates and treatment. *Behaviour Research and Therapy, 24*, 481–489.

Eifert, G. H., & Craill, L. (1989). The relationship between affect, behavior, and cognition in behavioral and cognitive treatments of depression and phobic anxiety. *Behavior Change, 6*, 96–103.

Elder, J. P., Edelstein, B. A., & Fremouw, W. J. (1981). Client by treatment interactions in response acquisition and cognitive restructuring approaches. *Cognitive Therapy and Research, 5*, 203–210.

Freeman, A., Pretzer, J., Fleming, B., & Simon, K. M. (1990). *Clinical applications of cognitive therapy*. New York: Plenum Press.

Garfield, S. L., & Bergin, A. E. (1986). *Handbook of psychotherapy and behavior change*. New York: Wiley.

Gormally, J., VarvilWeld, D., Raphael R. & Sipps, G. (1981). Treatment of socially anxious college men using cognitive counseling and skills training. *Journal of Counseling Psychology, 28*, 147–157.

Gouvier, W. D., Cubic, B., Jones, G., Brantley, P., & Cutlip, Q. (1992). Postconcussion symptoms and daily stress in normal and head-injured college populations. *Archives of Clinical Neuropsychology, 7*, 193–211.

Hart, K. (1984). Stress management training for Type A individuals. *Journal of Behavior Therapy and Experimental Psychiatry, 15*, 133–140.

Huey, S. R., & West, S. G. (1983). Hyperventilation: Its relation to symptom experience and to anxiety. *Journal of Abnormal Psychology, 92*, 422–432.

Levin, H. S., Benton, A. L., & Grossman, R. G. (1982). *Neurobehavioral consequences of closed head injury*. New York: Oxford Press.

Levin, H. S., Eisenberg, H. M., & Benton, A. L. (1989). *Mild head injury*. New York: Oxford University Press.

Levin, H. S., Mattis, S., Ruff, R. M., Eisenber, H. M., Marshall, L. F., & Tabaddor, K. (1987). Neurobehavioral outcome following minor head injury: A three-center study. *Journal of Neurosurgery, 66*, 234–243.

Lewinsohn, P. M. (1974). A behavioral approach to depression. In R. M. Friedman & M. M. Katz (Eds.), *The psychology of depression: Contemporary theory and research*. Washington D.C.: Winston-Wiley.

Ley, R. (1985). Blood, breath, and fears: A hyperventilation theory of panic attacks and agoraphobia. *Clinical Psychology Review, 5*, 271–285.

Mandler, G. (1982). Stress and thought processes. In L. Goldberger & S. Breznitz (Eds.), *Handbook of stress: Theoretical and clinical aspects* (pp. 88–104). New York: Free Press.

McLean, A., Dikman, S., Temkin, N., Wyler, A. R., & Gale, J. L. (1984). Psychological functioning at one month after head injury. *Neurosurgery, 14*, 393–399.

McLean, A., Temkin N. R., Dikmen, S., & Wyler, A. R. (1983). The behavioral sequelae of head injury. *Journal of Clinical Neuropsychology, 5*, 361–376.

Meichenbaum, D. H. (1977). *Cognitive behavior modification: An integrative approach*. New York: Plenum Press.

Miller, H. (1961). Accident neurosis. *British Medical Journal, 1*, 919–925.

Mittenberg, W., & Burton, D. B. (1994). A survey of treatments for postconcussion syndrome. *Brain Injury, 8*, 429–437.

Mittenberg, W., DiGiulio, D. V., Perrin, S., & Bass, A. E. (1992). Symptoms following mild head injury: Expectation as aetiology. *Journal of Neurology, Neurosurgery and Psychiatry, 55*, 157–161.

Mittenberg, W., Zielinski, R., & Fichera, S. (1993). Recovery from mild head injury: A treatment manual for patients. *Psychotherapy in Private Practice, 12*, 37–52.

Rimel, R. W., Girodani, B., Barth, J. T., Boll, T. J., & Jane, J. A. (1981). Disability caused by minor head injury. *Neurosurgery, 9*, 221–228.

Rutherford, W. H., Merrett, J. D., & McDonald, J. R. (1979). Symptoms at one year following concussion from minor head injuries. *Injury, 10*, 225–230.

Salkovskis, P. M., Warwick, H. M. C., Clark, D. M., & Wessels, D. L. (1986). A demonstration of acute hyperventilation during naturally occurring panic attacks. *Behaviour Research and Therapy, 24*, 91–94.

Schwartz, M. (1987). *Biofeedback: A practitioner's guide*. New York: Guilford Press.

Suinn, R. M. (1990). *Anxiety management training: A behavior therapy*. New York: Plenum Press.

Suinn, R., & Vattano, F. (1979). *Stress management for tension headache*. Unpublished manuscript, Colorado State University, Fort Collins, CO.

Sweeney, G. A., & Horan, J. J. (1982). Separate and combined effects of cue-controlled relaxation and cognitive restructuring in the treatment of medical performance anxiety. *Journal of Counseling Psychology, 29*, 486–497.

Thompson, J., Griebstein, M., & Kuhlenschmidt, S. (1980). Effects of EMG biofeedback and relaxation training in the prevention of academic underachievement. *Journal of Counseling Psychology, 27*, 97–106.

World Health Organization (1978). *Mental disorders: Glossary and guide to their classification in accordance with the 9th revision of the international classification of diseases*. Geneva: World Health Organization.

17

Trichotillomania Treatment Manual

Melinda A. Stanley and Suzanne G. Mouton

INTRODUCTION

Trichotillomania is a relatively understudied condition characterized by repetitive hair pulling. Diagnostic criteria for this disorder continue to evolve as new information emerges from the phenomenological and treatment literatures. However, in any discussion of pathological hair pulling, it seems important to distinguish between the syndrome of trichotillomania and the symptom of hair pulling per se. Hair pulling, for example, can occur in the context of psychotic processes and developmental disabilities, although current diagnostic criteria suggest that use of the term *trichotillomania* is not appropriate when the symptoms occur in these contexts. As such, the present chapter addresses only hair pulling that occurs when psychotic or developmental disorders are not present. In addition, the information presented here addresses only the symptoms as they occur in adults. Although trichotillomania also can be a serious disorder in childhood (Reeve, Bernstein, & Christenson, 1992), treatment of these cases is beyond the scope of this chapter. Thus, we will address the descriptive psychopathology, etiology, conceptualization, assessment, and behavioral treatment of adult trichotillomania.

Melinda A. Stanley • Department of Psychiatry and Behavioral Sciences, University of Texas Mental Sciences Institute, Health Science Center at Houston, Houston, Texas 77030.   **Suzanne G. Mouton** • Department of Educational Psychology, University of Houston, Houston, Texas 77004; and Department of Psychiatry and Behavioral Sciences, University of Texas Mental Sciences Institute, Health Science Center at Houston, Houston, Texas 77030.

Sourcebook of Psychological Treatment Manuals for Adult Disorders, edited by Vincent B. Van Hasselt and Michel Hersen. Plenum Press, New York, 1996.

Melinda A. Stanley
and Suzanne G.
Mouton

DESCRIPTION OF THE DISORDER

Diagnosis and Phenomenology

Trichotillomania was first described by a French dermatologist in the late 19th century (Hallopeau, 1889). Since that time, the disorder has been conceptualized from a range of perspectives, although it currently is classified as an impulse-control disorder. The most recent diagnostic criteria, enumerated in the fourth edition of the *Diagnostic and Statistical Manual of Mental Disorders* (DSM-IV; American Psychiatric Association, 1994), include the following: (a) recurrent pulling out of one's hair resulting in noticeable hair loss; (b) an increasing sense of tension immediately before pulling out the hair or when attempting to resist the behavior; (c) pleasure, gratification, or relief when pulling out the hair; (d) the disturbance is not better accounted for by another mental disorder and is not due to a general medical condition (e.g., a dermatological condition); and (e) the disturbance causes clinically significant distress or impairment in social, occupational, or other important areas of functioning.

Early literature describing trichotillomania was limited to dermatological data and anecdoctal case reports. Although at least one large sample of hair pullers has been described in the dermatological literature (e.g., Muller, 1990), these reports generally omit consideration of psychiatric variables. Only recently has the phenomenology of the syndrome been described in a large psychiatric sample (Christenson, Mackenzie, & Mitchell, 1991a). In this survey, pulling of scalp hair was by far the most common, although eyelash and eyebrow pulling also were reported frequently. The majority of patients reported pulling from more than one site, and the severity of resultant hair loss ranged from minimal but visible thinning of the hair to nearly total hair loss at the site. Attempts to disguise hair loss included the use of makeup, particular hair styles, or wigs. In general, data from this controlled phenomenological investigation paralleled reports from more clinically based literature (Mansueto, 1991), and preliminary data from nonclinical hair pullers (those without significant hair loss as a result of pulling) have suggested phenomenological overlap with diagnosed patients (Stanley, Borden, Bell, & Wagner, 1994). As such, a relatively consistent picture has begun to emerge.

Trichotillomania has received little attention to date in the psychiatric literature, given the tendency to minimize the potential severity of the condition and its psychosocial and medical sequelae (Winchel et al., 1992b). It recently has been recognized, however, that although mild cases of the disorder certainly can be identified, related psychosocial and medical complications can be quite severe. For example, many trichotillomania patients spend up to several hours per day engaged in pulling (Stanley, Swann, Bowers, Davis, & Taylor, 1992; Swedo & Leonard, 1992), with sometimes significant additional time spent in attempts to conceal the behavior or related hair loss from others (Mansueto, 1991). The financial costs of concealing hair loss also can be great, as are the emotional consequences of trying to hide the behavior and the concomitant feelings of guilt, humiliation, and lowered self-esteem.

Additionally, trichotillomania patients report frequent avoidance of activities wherein hair loss might be particularly obvious (Mansueto, 1991; Winchel, Jones, Stanley, Molcho, & Stanley, 1992c). At times, avoidance involves everyday activities, such as swimming or other forms of exercise, visits to hairdressers, or being in brightly lit rooms. In other cases, avoidance involves more major life functions, with patients reluctant to become involved in intimate relationships or close friendships. Medical complications also can be significant, with hair pulling sometimes causing skin irritations or infections. More serious medical complications result when patients also engage in repetitive scalp picking, which can lead to painful traumatic lesions, or trichophagia (hair ingestion), a behavior that can interfere significantly with gastrointestinal functioning (Swedo & Leonard, 1992; Winchel et al., 1992c).

Estimates of Axis I comorbidity in trichotillomania have ranged from 25% to 85%, although some studies in this regard have evaluated very small samples (Stanley et al., 1992) and others have included heterogenous groups of children, adolescents, and adults (Swedo & Leonard, 1992). In the largest samples of adult trichotillomania patients evaluated to date, comorbid Axis I diagnoses were assigned for 80% to 85% of patients (Christenson et al., 1991a; Christenson, Chernoff-Clementz, & Clementz, 1992). In these samples, affective and anxiety disorders (in particular, unipolar depression and generalized anxiety disorder) were most common, although eating disorders and substance-abuse disorders also were assigned frequently. It should be noted, however, that frequencies of comorbid Axis I diagnoses in trichotillomania were not different from those in a control group of psychiatric outpatients (Christenson et al., 1992). Comorbid Axis II diagnoses were assigned to approximately 45% of trichotillomania patients, although again the frequencies of various personality disorders were similar to those obtained in a psychiatric control group. The only exception in this regard was a lower frequency of borderline personality disorder in the trichotillomania group (Christenson et al., 1992).

The majority of chronic hair pullers do not maintain continued, focused awareness of the behavior as it is occurring (Christenson et al., 1991a; Mansueto, 1991). Rather, many patients are unaware of the symptoms, at least when an episode of pulling first begins, and others report a mixed pattern of incomplete and focused awareness. This phenomenon underlies the use of awareness training as a component of the behavioral treatment described here, and also suggests the importance of investigations regarding potential cues for the behavior. In this regard, a variety of cue types have been suggested, including environmental, sensory, cognitive, and affective.

With regard to *environmental precipitants*, virtually all hair pulling occurs primarily when patients are alone, with attempts to keep the behavior hidden from others, although some individuals have reported pulling in the presence of immediate family members (Christenson et al., 1991a). The majority of hair pulling also occurs in sedentary or contemplative situations, in particular, while patients are watching television, talking on the phone, reading, lying in bed, driving, and writing or completing paperwork (Christenson et al., 1991a; Christenson, Ristvedt, & Mackenzie, 1993; Mansueto, 1991).

Sensory stimuli also appear to be important precipitators in some cases. For example, up to 50% of trichotillomania patients indicate that pulling occurs in response to itching, burning, or otherwise increased sensitivity of the scalp (Mansueto, 1991). In addition, almost every trichotillomania patient reports that touching or stroking the hair immediately precedes pulling, and some indicate that the sensory stimulation associated with touching the hair after pulling is an important motivator for the behavior. For example, some patients report that they spend time "playing with" the hair after pulling (i.e., touching it and/or rolling it in their fingers; Mansueto, 1991). Up to 48% of chronic pullers also report various oral behaviors following pulling, including rubbing the hair around their mouths, eating the hair, or biting off the root (Christenson et al., 1991a).

Although most trichotillomania patients do not report obsessive ideation surrounding hair pulling (Stanley et al., 1992), some report *precipitating cognitions*, many of which have to do with various characteristics of the hair. For example, some patients seek certain types of hairs for pulling; they may look for short, early growth hairs or otherwise coarse, wiry, or kinky hairs (Christenson et al., 1991a; Mansueto, 1991). For other individuals, the nature of the hair follicle is important, with a number reporting a preference for roots that are large or particularly round (Mansueto, 1991). Finally, some trichotillomania patients are motivated to pull so that hair growth will be symmetrical. In all of these cases, cognitive variables seem to serve as important precipitating cues for the behavior.

Affective correlates of hair pulling also are of interest. Prior diagnostic criteria (American Psychiatric Association, 1987), in fact, required that an increasing sense of tension be reported prior to the behavior, along with feelings of gratification or relief during pulling. Christenson et al (1991a), however, demonstrated that about 20% of chronic hair pullers did not report both of these affective experiences. As a result, DSM-IV criteria were revised to broaden the scope of affective correlates, with the suggestion that tension be reported either immediately before pulling or when the individual attempts to resist the behavior. In addition, feelings of pleasure were added, along with gratification and/or relief, as affective states that can be indicated during pulling. Nonetheless, these criteria still do not represent the total range of affective experiences reported surrounding hair pulling.

When tension does precipitate pulling, it can represent a general feeling of arousal, without clear environmental precipitants, or more specific feelings of tension related to physical sensations of scalp itching or burning, cognitions about ridding the scalp of certain types of hairs, or the need to create symmetry in hair growth or appearance. However, as noted earlier, not all patients experience increasing tension prior to pulling, and other precipitative negative affective states are reported, including boredom, anger, depression, frustration, indecision, and fatigue (Mansueto, 1991). Some individuals, for example, report that pulling is calming and helps them focus more easily on tasks at hand (e.g., reading, paperwork). Others indicate that pulling actually *creates* arousal and is energizing; still others describe a somewhat dissociative state produced by hair pulling. To examine this issue in a more empirical fashion than has occurred to date, the authors and their colleagues evaluated, in a retrospective fashion, the affective correlates of pulling reported by both trichotillomania patients and nonclinical hair pullers (those without noticeable hair loss). In a sample of 17 chronic hair pullers, for example, decreases in boredom, anxiety, and tension were reported as a result of pulling (Stanley & Mouton, 1994). Pulling in these subjects also led to increased feelings of both relief and guilt. In another study, 22 nonclinical pullers reported reductions in tension, boredom, anger, and sadness as a result of pulling (Stanley, Borden, Mouton, & Breckenridge, 1995). Thus, it appears that a range of affective experiences, including but not limited to those enumerated in DSM-IV, surround hair pulling.

Epidemiology

No large-scale epidemiological investigations have been conducted to estimate the prevalence of trichotillomania, although preliminary data suggested a lifetime prevalence rate of 0.6% in a college population, using DSM-III-R criteria (Christenson, Pyle, & Mitchell, 1991c). When more liberal criteria are used, however, requiring only the presence of noticeable hair loss as a result of pulling (i.e., without requirement of the tension–gratification cycle), prevalence rates range from 2.5% to 3.0%, again in college samples (Christenson et al., 1991c; Rothbaum, Shaw, Morris, & Ninan, 1993). Estimates of point-prevalence rates of pulling that does not result in noticeable hair loss range from 10% to 15% in college populations (Graber & Arndt, 1993; Rothbaum et al., 1993; Stanley et al., 1994). Larger community-based surveys certainly are needed, particularly using the recently published DSM-IV criteria, although preliminary estimates to date suggest that trichotillomania is not a rare condition. In addition, anecdotal case studies indicate that symptoms of trichotillomania occur cross-culturally (Hussain, 1992; Shome, Bhatia, & Gautam, 1993). Although the majority of patients in U.S. studies have been Caucasian, trichotillomania patients from a range of ethnic minority groups, including African-American, Hispanic, Native American, and Asian, have been evaluated (Christenson, Mackenzie, & Mitchell, 1991a; Stanley, Prather, Wagner, Davis, & Swann, 1993a).

By far, the majority of trichotillomania patients in both dermatological and psychiatric clinics are women, with figures of 75% to 93% reported (Christenson et al., 1991a; Muller, 1987; Stanley et al., 1993a). Preliminary epidemiological surveys reviewed earlier, however, suggest that hair pulling in the community at large may be more frequent in men than figures from these clinical studies suggest, although gender ratios in community samples still suggest that women with hair pulling outnumber men 2:1 (Christenson et al., 1991c; Graber & Arndt, 1993; Stanley et al., 1994). An initial comparison of phenomenology in men and women with trichotillomania indicated more similarities than differences, however, although the sample size of male pullers was rather small (Christenson, Mackenzie, & Mitchell, 1994).

Age of onset for trichotillomania is in early adolescence, with means between 11 and 13 years reported (Christenson et al., 1991a; Stanley et al., 1993; Swedo & Leonard, 1992). The course of the disorder appears to be chronic, although significant variability can be noted in symptom severity both across and within patients (Christenson, Mackenzie, Mitchell, & Callies, 1991b).

Conceptualization

As noted earlier, trichotillomania has been conceptualized from a wide range of perspectives, with some of the earliest classifying hair pulling as a symptom of psychodynamic conflict (Greenberg & Sarner, 1965; Oguchi & Miura, 1977). In current psychiatric nomenclature, trichotillomania is characterized as an impulse control disorder, and indeed, there seems to be some overlap with other syndromes in that cluster. For example, trichotillomania patients repetitively perform a maladaptive behavior over which they report no control, and for some the behavior is pleasurable (Mansueto, 1991). However, as already mentioned, not all hair pullers report the tension-reduction cycle that is characteristic of impulse control disorders; nor do the majority describe pleasurable sensations during pulling. Relatedly, preliminary data have suggested that patients with trichotillomania do not score in the impulsive direction on a range of self-report and cognitive performance measures designed to evaluate impulse control (Stanley, Wagner, & Davis, 1993b). Thus, conceptualization of trichotillomania as an impulse control disorder is not strongly supported.

Alternative conceptualizations have suggested that trichotillomania may be a variant of obsessive–compulsive disorder (Jenike, 1990; Tynes, White & Steketee, 1990), a disorder of excessive grooming (Swedo & Leonard, 1992), or a tension–reducing habit control disorder (Azrin & Nunn, 1973). Overlap with obsessive–compulsive disorder (OCD) was posited given the following: (1) apparent similarity in the nature of symptoms (i.e., both disorders are characterized by repetitive, maladaptive behaviors over which patients perceive no control); (2) a trend toward increased rates of OCD in the families of trichotillomania probands (Lenane et al., 1992); (3) initial pharmacotherapy outcome data suggesting that clomipramine, a serotonergic reuptake inhibitor that has demonstrated preferential treatment effects in OCD, also showed superior efficacy for the treatment of trichotillomania (Swedo et al., 1989). Subsequent data have suggested, however, that although trichotillomania may exhibit some phenomenological overlap with OCD, significant differences have been noted.

First, although some trichotillomania patients report obsessive-type thoughts prior to pulling, and some report a history of or coexistent obsessive–compulsive symptoms, the disorder generally is not characterized by the presence of intrusive, repetitive thoughts that are central to a diagnosis of OCD (Stanley et al., 1993a; Stanley et al., 1992). Moreover, as noted previously, many trichotillomania patients do not report focused awareness of hair pulling during the behavior, a phenomenon that diverges greatly from the purposeful, ritualistic actions characteristic of OCD. Second, trichotillomania patients do not report multiple obsessions and compulsions, as is the case in OCD; in fact, they generally score in the normal range on standardized measures of obsessive–compulsive symptoms (Stanley et al., 1992). Third, although lifetime OCD is diagnosed in an estimated 15% of trichotillomania patients (Christenson et al., 1991a), as noted earlier, unipolar affective disorders and generalized anxiety disorder actually have been reported as the most common comorbid diagnoses. Fourth, more recent pharmacotherapy data have not supported a preferential effect for all serotonergic reuptake inhibitors in the treatment of trichotillomania. In particular, a recent controlled trial of fluoxetine found no benefit of this medication relative to placebo in a group of chronic hair pullers (Christenson et al., 1991b). Finally, data from neuropsychological and neuroanatomical studies have been mixed. An initial study in this regard indicated no differences between OCD and trichotillomania patients on two measures of visuospatial skills and spatial memory (Rettew, Cheslow, Rapoport, Leonard, & Lenane, 1991), suggesting some neurobehavioral overlap. However, another investigation using positron emission tomography demonstrated patterns of glucose metabolism in trichotillomania patients that differed from those reported in previous studies of OCD, although response to treatment with clomipramine was associated with similar patterns of hypermetabolism in the two groups (Swedo et al., 1991).

Generally, then, despite some phenomenological overlap, available data do not clearly support conceptualization of trichotillomania as a variant of OCD, although some researchers have posited that a subgroup of trichotillomania patients may be more obsessional in nature than most (Christenson et al., 1993). Nevertheless, an integration of two alternative perspectives identified earlier seems to fit more adequately the general phenomenological descriptions of chronic hair pulling. First, as Swedo and Leonard (1992) have noted, chronic hair pulling can be viewed from an ethological perspective as a disorder of excessive grooming wherein "a hard-wired grooming behavior (fixed-action pattern) ... has been released inappropriately" (p. 782). A similar hypothesis has been proposed for OCD, with compulsive rituals conceptualized as displacement behaviors (Insel & Winslow, 1990). Although this perspective has apparent face and construct validity for both disorders, it fails to account alone for all the precipitating cues described earlier.

In another model of hair pulling, the behavior is viewed as a normal reaction to stress that becomes more strongly established as it is associated with a range of internal and external cues and escapes personal and social awareness (Azrin & Nunn, 1973). This model is able to account for the relationship between hair pulling and the range of associated cues described above through a variety of conditioning mechanisms, although this perspective is lacking in its explanation of the initial origin of the behavior. As Mansueto (1993) has proposed, however, this model can be integrated smoothly with the ethological perspective described by Swedo and Leonard (1992). As such, it is plausible to presume that a fixed-action pattern (e.g., hair pulling), released initially during times of stress through some hard-wired biological mechanism, may subsequently be elicited by a wider range of cues as it becomes associated with various internal and external stimuli through processes of classical and operant conditioning. In this fashion, hair pulling may be conditioned to occur in response to various environmental, sensory, cognitive, and affective cues as it is repeatedly paired with certain stimuli, or as it serves positively or negatively reinforcing functions. It is this model that supports most strongly the use of habit reversal training for the treatment of trichotillomania.

ASSESSMENT METHODS

Goals of Assessment

As with any disorder, preparation for treatment of trichotillomania begins with a thorough assessment of target symptoms and coexistent conditions. With regard to evaluation of the symptoms *per se*, an important function of pretreatment assessment, of course, is to elicit a baseline against which to assess the impact of treatment. In this regard, frequency and duration of hair pulling are of interest, as well as degrees of distress, interference, and control. In addition, however, *pretreatment assessment* may serve a primary therapeutic function as patients become more aware of the circumstances under which they pull. Although awareness training, which is the initial component of habit-reversal training (HRT), provides more extensive and detailed attention to precipitating cues than generally is accomplished with baseline evaluations, the procedures associated with pretreatment assessment can be an initial therapeutic maneuver in this regard.

For trichotillomania, as with other disorders, it is important to assess not only the target symptoms to be treated, but also any comorbid symptoms or disorders that may impact treatment outcome. As such, conceptualization of a patient with trichotillomania should be comprehensive, with HRT serving as possibly only one component in an integrated treatment plan. Although the trichotillomania treatment literature is too premature to provide any solid information regarding predictors of efficacy, clinical expertise suggests that the presence of serious comorbid conditions (e.g., major depression, borderline personality disorder) might predict poorer prognosis following the use of HRT alone. In addition, as will be noted, the presence of comorbid symptoms may suggest that a broader range of coping responses will need to be utilitized in the context of HRT. Moreover, in cases in which serious comorbid diagnoses are appropriate, a comprehensive treatment approach that incorporates HRT along with other interventions also might be necessary. Nonetheless, the focus here will be on a review of measures designed to address the severity of trichotillomania symptoms *per se*.

Clinical Interviews

The Minnesota Trichotillomania Assessment Inventory (MTAI; Christenson et al., 1991a) is a semistructured interview that elicits detailed phenomenological data regarding hair pulling. The instrument certainly can be used to diagnose trichotillomania, but its principle utility is in the collection of descriptive data regarding clinical characteristics of the behavior. The MTAI also includes screening questions for other Axis I diagnoses, although alternative instruments probably are preferential in this regard. For example, the MTAI can be administered in conjunction with DSM-IV equivalents of the Structured Interview for DSM-III-R (SCID; Spitzer, Williams, Gibbon, & First, 1992) or the Anxiety Disorders Interview Schedule–Revised (ADIS-R; DiNardo, Moras, Barlow, & Rapee, 1993) in order to develop a comprehensive diagnostic picture of the trichotillomania patient.

A number of clinical rating scales also are available to evaluate the severity of trichotillomania symptoms, although psychometric data in support of these instruments are either weak or nonexistent. First, given the proposed overlap between trichotillomania and OCD, a version of the Yale–Brown Obsessive–Compulsive Scale (Y-BOCS; Goodman et al., 1989) was created to assess the severity of hair pulling. Specifically, the original Y-BOCS was revised such that the phrases "thoughts about hair pulling" and "hair pulling" were substituted for the words "obsessions" and "compulsions." The revised instrument, the YBOCS-TM, yields a total score and two subscale scores, TM-Thoughts and TM-Behaviors. Within each of the latter, items address time spent, interference, distress, resistance, and control. Initial psychometric data regarding the utility of the YBOCS-TM were mixed (Stanley et al., 1993a). Namely, interrater agreement, internal consistency, and test–retest reliability for the total score were adequate. However, the range of scores was somewhat restricted, and both internal consistency and test–retest reliability for the TM-Behaviors subscale were inadequate. Concurrent validity data were mixed, although the YBOCS-TM was sensitive to changes in hair pulling over treatment. These conclusions are tentative, however, given that the sample from which they were derived consisted of only 11 trichotillomania patients.

The National Institute of Mental Health-Trichotillomania Severity and Impairment Scales (NIMH-TSS, NIMH-TIS) also have been used to provide clinical ratings of hair pulling (Swedo et al., 1989). The TSS includes five questions, each of which is rated on a zero to 5 scale. Items were derived from the Y-BOCS and address frequency, resistance, intensity, distress, and interference. The TIS is a rating of the degree of damage that has resulted from hair pulling, the time expended in pulling or concealing damage, and the ability to control the behavior. Clinicians make a single rating for the TIS on a zero (*No Impairment*) to 10 (*Severe Impairment*) scale. Although both the TSS and TIS have demonstrated sensitivity to change in hair-pulling symptoms over treatment (Swedo et al., 1989), no psychometric data for either instrument are available.

The Psychiatric Institute Trichotillomania Scale (PITS; Winchel et al., 1992a, 1992b) is another clinical rating instrument that provides quantitative evaluation of the number of hair-pulling sites, severity of hair loss, duration, resistance, distress, and interference with social and/or vocational functioning. Anchors are provided to facilitate a single clinician rating (zero to 7) in each of these areas. Again, overlap with previous measures of obsessive–compulsive symptoms is evident, and no psychometric data yet are available to support the use of the PITS for the evaluation of trichotillomania.

As is apparent, a number of diagnostic and clinical rating tools are available for the evaluation of trichotillomania and its comorbid conditions. However, none of the instruments designed to assess symptom severity *per se* has been well established psychometrically. Furthermore, all measures have been developed from instruments established to assess OCD. Given the conclusions noted earlier regarding the proposed overlap between these conditions, such a strategy may have produced less than optimal measures, and new instruments may need to be generated.

As is the case for clinician-rated measures, no well-established, standardized self-report instrument yet is available to evaluate hair pulling. However, the authors and their colleagues have developed and are examining two potentially useful measures in this regard. First, the Hair-Pulling Survey (HPS; Stanley et al., 1994) was designed to investigate the epidemiology and phemonology of hair pulling in nonclinical samples. Items address the frequency and duration of symptoms, the nature of sites from which hair is pulled, situations associated with the behavior, and affective correlates of pulling. Initial use of this instrument suggested a number of areas of phenomenological overlap between clinical and nonclinical groups (Stanley et al., 1994), and provided interesting preliminary data regarding affective precipitators and consequences of the behavior (Stanley et al., 1995; Stanley & Mouton, 1994). Thorough psychometric evaluation of the HPS, however, has yet to be completed. Second, the Trichotillomania Assessment Survey (TMAS) is a self-report instrument designed to measure symptom severity in trichotillomania patients. This instrument assesses a wide range of symptoms related to hair pulling, including frequency and severity of associated hair loss, as well as affective, cognitive, and situational cues. No psychometric data regarding this instrument are yet available, although related studies currently are ongoing in the authors' clinic.

Self-monitoring procedures are utilized routinely to assess the nature and severity of hair pulling. Again, no standardized approaches are available, although patients typically are asked to record each episode of hair pulling, either as it occurs or at some regular intervals throughout the day. Often patients are asked to record the frequency and duration of episodes, along with severity of urges to pull (Azrin, Nunn, & Frantz, 1980; Christenson et al., 1991b; Stanley et al., 1993a). In addition, patients may be asked to record the number of hairs pulled, either through an estimate at the end of the day or by collecting hairs pulled throughout the day to be counted at day's end (Christenson et al., 1991b; Stanley, Bowers, Swann, & Taylor, 1991). In the authors' own work, patients also are asked to make ratings of affective experiences related to hair pulling, for example, by rating at day's end the degree of pleasure experienced as a result of hair pulling during that day (Stanley et al., 1992).

As noted earlier, any type of self-monitoring that occurs in the context of pretreatment assessment is likely to have some reactive effect on the hair pulling itself. In particular, given the potential utility of monitoring for increased awareness of the behavior, this activity may be viewed as an active ingredient of a behavioral approach. As such, its use in treatment-outcome trials as a baseline measure is of some concern (Winchel et al., 1992a). However, awareness training as described in HRT (to be discussed) provides a more extensive evaluation of precipitating cues than typically is included in any self-monitoring procedure, and the impact of various HRT components in the treatment of trichotillomania is as yet uncertain.

Behavioral Observation

There is some disagreement over the utility of behavioral-observation techniques for the assessment of trichotillomania, given that hair loss is often irregular, and patients frequently attempt to camouflage hair loss by pulling from a range of sites (Christenson et al., 1991b). In addition, rate of hair growth varies across individuals and may lag behind other indices of improvement following treatment. Furthermore, inspection of hair loss may be a difficult task, depending on the sites involved and the extent of uncovering that is required (Winchel et al., 1992a). Nonetheless, observational approaches have been used by a number of behavioral researchers, particularly in the evaluation of children with trichotillomania (Dahlquist & Kalfus, 1984; Tarnowski, Rosen, McGrath, & Drabman, 1987). Incorporation of such a strategy seems important for a broad evaluation of symptom severity.

Behavioral-observation ratings can be made by the clinician, as suggested by the Trichotillomania Impairment Scale, described earlier (Swedo et al., 1989). This type of approach, however, is subject to clinician bias and lack of standardization procedures for inspection of hair loss. To provide a more objective evaluation, sophisticated dermatological techniques can be used (Muller, 1990). Or, an attempt can be made to obtain evaluations of photographs taken in a standardized fashion. In this domain, attention needs to be given to a range of procedural variables, including distance between camera and subject, aperture of the lens, exposure and film speeds, nature of the light source, and the film development process (Winchel et al., 1992a). Although this type of process should allow for severity ratings from independent evaluators, no standardized rating scales for measuring degree of hair loss have been developed.

Summary

As noted earlier, a number of clinician-rated measures have been developed to evaluate the symptoms of trichotillomania. However, none of these has been well established psychometrically, and the majority have been derived from available measures of OCD. Thus, new measures designed specifically for the evaluation of hair pulling may need to be constructed. Furthermore, no standardized self-report measures yet are available, although two are currently under investigation by the authors and their colleagues. Self-monitoring techniques may be useful, but also provide a significant confound for evaluation of treatment effects. And strategies for behavioral observation of hair loss require significant procedural standardization, as well as the development of psychometrically sound rating scales. Thus, although a broad range of measurement strategies has been proposed for the evaluation of trichotillomania, no well-established assessment battery is available.

DETAILED TREATMENT/TRAINING PROCEDURES

Overview of Treatment–Outcome Literature

The conceptualizations of trichotillomania described earlier have led to the use of two primary treatment modalities. First, characterization of the disorder as a variant of OCD has sparked a number of investigations into the use of serotonergic reuptake inhibitors. A number of uncontrolled trials have attested to the efficacy of these compounds (e.g., Stanley et al., 1991; Winchel et al., 1992a), although only two controlled investigations have been conducted, and these produced divergent conclusions. Specifically, Swedo et al. (1989) demonstrated that clomipramine was superior to desipramine for the treatment of trichotillomania, but a more recent study by Christenson et al. (1991b) failed to demonstrate the superiority of fluoxetine relative to placebo. Thus, the utility of serotonergic reuptake inhibitors for the treatment of trichotillomania is equivocal.

Second, conceptualization of trichotillomania as a habit-control disorder has led to the development of a behavioral approach known as habit reversal training (HRT; Azrin & Nunn, 1973). This approach utilizes behavioral interventions to increase awareness and teach coping skills (e.g., competing response training, relaxation) for use in interrupting sequences of behavior. Again, a series of case studies has supported the efficacy of these procedures and related intervention packages (DeLuca & Holborn, 1984; Rosenbaum & Ayllon, 1981; Rothbaum, 1992), although only one controlled trial has demonstrated the superiority of the habit-reversal program over an alternative psychosocial intervention (Azrin et al., 1980). In this study, 34 patients were treated with a single 2-hour session of either HRT or negative practice (another behavioral intervention), followed by telephone contact over the subsequent 2 to 3 days. Results demonstrated the superiority of habit-reversal procedures over negative practice, with at least 97% reduction in hair pulling after 4 weeks. In addition, gains were maintained over an extended follow-up interval, with 87% reduction in the behavior at 22 months. Methodological limitations of this study include the use of only self-monitoring data to assess outcome, failure to document treatment integrity, and lack of standardized follow-up evaluation procedures. Nevertheless, the data strongly suggest the utility of the HRT approach. Further preliminary data also have suggested that behavioral treatment incorporating habit-reversal procedures is superior to pill placebo, with intermediate levels of response to clomipramine (Rothbaum & Ninan, 1992).

Given these initial data, the apparent efficacy of HRT for the treatment of trichotillomania is quite promising. Although the treatment-outcome literature in this domain is relatively sparse, and the central ingredients of the approach have yet to be identified, HRT procedures are consistent with a behavioral conceptualization of the disorder. Furthermore, preliminary data suggest the utility of this approach. The HRT protocol (to be described) currently is being used and tested in the authors' clinic. The approach specified involves a group format developed in an attempt to maximize education and support for participants while providing an efficient and economic means for conducting HRT. In addition, although the procedures described by Azrin et al. (1980) call for the use of a single-treatment session with subsequent phone contact, the treatment protocol described herein includes a six-session approach that allows sufficient time for practice with each component of the HRT model.

HABIT REVERSAL TRAINING—TREATMENT PROCEDURES

As noted, HRT is based on principles outlined by Azrin and his colleagues (Azrin & Nunn, 1973, 1977; Azrin et al., 1980). The treatment includes the following components: (1) *self-monitoring* of the frequency and duration of hair pulling; (2) *habit control motivation* to review the inconveniences caused by the behavior; (3) *awareness training* to identify the specific movements involved in hair pulling, the behavioral responses which immediately precede pulling (e.g., face touching, hair stroking), and situational precursors of the behavioral sequence (e.g., watching television, driving, reading); (4) *competing-response training* to identify an inconspicuous response (e.g., fist clenching) that can be used to interrupt hair pulling when it occurs or to prevent the behavior in "high-risk" situations; (5) *relaxation training* through deep breathing and postural adjustments; and (6) *generalization training* to identify and imagine high-risk situations in preparation for future episodes of hair pulling.

Several variations in the procedures described by Azrin and his colleagues are suggested here:

1. As noted earlier, treatment is conducted in six weekly sessions, each of which lasts 1½ hours.
2. Treatment is conducted in a small-group format, with 3 to 6 patients initially assigned to each group.
3. Awareness training is expanded to include examinations of cognitions and affective experiences that precede or are concurrent with hair pulling episodes.
4. Imaginal and *in vivo* exposure procedures are utilized for the practice of coping responses.

Patients also are given weekly homework assignments that take approximately 30 minutes per day.

HRT was designed to help the patient become acutely aware of the hair-pulling behavior and the inconveniences that may result, learn competing responses that can be substituted for the behavior, and practice generalization training to prepare for possible future episodes of hair-pulling. HRT is intended to reduce the frequency of hair pulling in trichotillomania. However, as noted earlier, the intervention may comprise just one part of an integrated treatment package suggested by a total conceptualization of the patient. Given the current dearth of outcome data in this domain, as well as the absence of empirical data regarding predictors of treatment response, each patient should be assessed individually to determine the relevance of HRT for that patient, as well as the need for other forms of treatment to address comorbid symptomatology.

As noted, only one controlled-outcome trial has demonstrated the efficacy of HRT, and the specific procedures described in this chapter have not yet been evaluated in an empirical fashion. Nonetheless, they are based on the rationale and techniques described by Azrin and colleagues, and represent the authors' clinical experience with treatment of the disorder. The procedures currently are being submitted to preliminary empirical evaluation, although as will be described (see Case Illustration), case report data suggest their efficacy. The six treatment sessions suggested, along with specific procedures and homework assignments, are outlined as follows:

Session 1: Introduction, Inconvenience Review, and Overview of the Treatment

The main goals of Session 1 are to help patients become comfortable discussing the symptoms and various sequelae of trichotillomania in a group setting, and to provide information about the disorder and the proposed treatment. The introduction involves a simple review of the diagnostic criteria and phenomenology of trichotillomania, followed by initial group discussion of each individual's symptoms and unique experiences with hair pulling. Issues of relevance here might include the sites from which hair is pulled, the frequency and duration of hair pulling, age and circumstances of onset, intensity of urges to pull, control over symptoms, resistance of the behavior, nature of hair loss (noticeable or hidden), types of hair pulled, and what is done with the hair after it is pulled. During this discussion, the therapist's role is to point out similarities as well as differences in the behaviors.

Next, the psychosocial and/or medical complications of the behavior should be reviewed. Each group member should be asked to share with the group at least three inconveniences or ways in which hair pulling interferes with social, occupational, or family functioning. Topics for discussion here might include time spent in pulling or covering up hair loss, expense of wigs and makeup, embarrassment or loss of self-esteem, anger or guilt, lies told to conceal behavior, avoidance of certain activities or interpersonal relationships, and medical complications (scalp irritation and infections from scalp digging).

Patients then are provided with an overview of educational information regarding hair pulling. Specifically, information regarding prevalence, onset, and theories of etiology should be presented. In this regard, a brief summary of the epidemiological information presented earlier can be useful. A review of prevalence data is particularly important, given that many patients feel they are completely alone in their experience of the disorder. Because of the shame associated with hair pulling, in fact, many patients have never discussed their symptoms with anyone.

A brief overview of etiological theories also can be useful. Conceptualization of the syndrome as a habit disorder, a problem of impulse control, and a variant of obsessive–compulsive disorder can be reviewed. Both biological and learning-based models should be mentioned, although the learning theory on which HRT is based will be reviewed in more detail. To provide a more explicit rationale for treatment, it may be helpful to paraphrase the following theoretical account by Azrin and Nunn (1973):

> A nervous habit originally starts as a normal reaction. The reaction may be to an extreme event such as physical injury or psychological trauma … , or the symptom may have started as an infrequent, but normal, behavior that has increased in frequency and has been altered in its form. The behavior becomes classified as a nervous habit when it persists after the original injury or trauma has passed and when it assumes an unusual form and unusually high frequency. Under normal circumstances the nervous habit would be inhibited by personal or social awareness of its peculiarity or by its inherent inconvenience. The [symptom] may, however, have blended into normal [behavior] so gradually as to escape personal and social awareness. Once having achieved this transformation, the [symptom] is performed so often as to become a strongly established habit that further escapes personal awareness because of its authentic nature. This analysis of nervous habits suggests several methods of treatment. The client should learn to be aware of every occurrence of the habit. Each habit movement should be interrupted so it no longer is part of a chain of normal movements. A physically competing response should be established to interfere with the habit. (p. 620)

Reactions to the theory should be elicited. The possibility that an interaction between biological variables and learning history may cause the symptoms should be noted, although the treatment to be used here will be based solely on the learning theory proposed by Azrin and Nunn (1973, 1977). An overview of subsequent sessions then should follow.

First, given the importance of full awareness of the behavior and its antecedents (Azrin & Nunn, 1973), Sessions 2 and 3 will be dedicated to *awareness training*. During these sessions, patients will become aware of (1) high-risk situations (those that elicit hair-pulling behavior), (2) the sequence of behaviors involved in pulling, and (3) the thoughts and moods that occur before, during, and after the behavior. Patients may perceive that they are already aware of their symptoms, but it is important to remind them that there are fine-tuned aspects of their behavior of which they may not be cognizant. Patients will be encouraged to begin to view hair pulling not as a single behavior, but as a series of discrete behaviors yet to be defined. Once awareness is complete, it will be important for patients to learn what is called a *competing response*—a behavior that can be used to interrupt the hair-pulling cycle or to prevent the behavior in high-risk situations. This technique will be demonstrated and practiced in Session 4. Relaxation strategies also can be useful for interrupting or preventing the behavior by diminishing stress and anxiety in high-risk situations. Session 5 is dedicated to teaching and practicing these strategies. During the final session, Session 6, patients will have the chance to review and ask questions about all treatment procedures. In addition, strategies for generalizing coping skills to new situations and extending the benefits of treatment over subsequent months will be addressed.

Homework

Patients are then asked to begin some kind of self-monitoring (see sample forms in Table 17.1), generally with instructions to rate the frequency and duration of both urges to pull and actual hair-pulling episodes at some regular interval throughout the day. In the authors' clinic, patients are asked to record these variables five times per day (8:00 A.M., 12:00 P.M., 4:00 P.M., 8:00 P.M., and bedtime). At each of these times, patients record their experiences since the prior rating. Once per day, preferably at bedtime, patients also are asked to rate the total number of hairs pulled throughout that day. In addition, patients begin to note all situations in which hair pulling occurs. A homework form, such as the one in Table 17.2, is suggested for this activity. On this form, patients are asked to record the date,

Table 17.1.   Example Self-Monitoring Form

Self-Monitoring Instructions

A. Five times daily list:
   1. Number of thoughts about hair-pulling.
   2. Time spent thinking about hair-pulling.
   3. Number of episodes of hair-pulling.
   4. Time spent hair-pulling
B. At day's end, list daily average for:
   1. Degree of pleasure from hair-pulling.
   2. Degree of anxiety prior to hair-pulling.
   3. Degree of anxiety after hair-pulling.

   0   1   2   3   4   5   6   7   8
   None Mild Moderate Marked Extreme

C. At day's end, record total number of hairs pulled.

Monitoring Form

(1) Date _____

	Thoughts about hair pulling		Hair-pulling	
	No.	Time	No.	Time
8:00 A.M.				
12:00 P.M.				
4:00 P.M.				
8:00 P.M.				
Bedtime				

Degree of pleasure (0–8) _____
Degree of anxiety prior (0–8) _____
Degree of anxiety after (0–8) _____
Number of hairs pulled _____

Table 17.2. Homework Form, Session 1

For each episode of hair-pulling during the week, please record the following:

			Situational Correlates		
Date	Day	Time	Where?	With whom?	Preceding event?

day of week, and time of day for each hair-pulling episode, and to indicate where they were, whom they were with, and what happened immediately before the pulling began.

Session 2: Awareness Training

Session 2 and all subsequent sessions begin with a review of both self-monitoring forms and the homework assignment. Questions about either of these activities are answered, and difficulties encountered with any of the assignments are addressed.

The focus of Session 2 is twofold: (1) to review the situational correlates of each patient's hair pulling, and (2) to identify preceding behaviors and the sequence of movements involved in hair pulling. The review of situational correlates generally includes some discussion of both precipitating activities (i.e., watching television, talking on the telephone, reading, driving) and temporal patterns (i.e., pulling occurs only during the work week or only in the evenings). In the context of this discussion, it may be useful to inquire about different interpersonal interactions that may be associated with hair pulling (i.e., conflict, talking to friends or strangers, acceptance of responsibility for a difficult task), again drawing conclusions regarding similarities between experiences of group members. It is also important to inquire about any other high-risk situations that may not have occurred in the past week. This part of the Session 2 discussion should lead to the conclusion that patterns of pulling are not random, and as such, the behavior is not always inevitable. Patients should begin to see that they have some degree of control over the symptoms.

To identify preceding behaviors and the sequence of movements, patients should first be asked to identify any other *secondary habits*, such as face touching, hair stroking or playing, or nail biting, that precede pulling. Providing a list of common face-touching movements, such as those suggested by Azrin and Nunn (1977), is useful in facilitating this discussion (e.g., rubbing one's chin; scratching one's face, nose, or scalp; pushing stray hairs back in place). Patients also are asked to analyze the sequence of discrete movements that lead up to and comprise the behavior. The therapist explains that one way to examine this sequence of movements is to watch oneself in the mirror as the hair pulling is performed. Another strategy is to perform the movement sequence more slowly and deliberately than usual to examine its complexity. In this regard, one might even say the movements out loud as they are being performed. Patients are then asked to perform these "assessment strategies" during the upcoming week.

To initiate the awareness of movements during Session 2, however, patients are asked to imagine themselves in a high-risk situation, and to note the preceding behaviors, secondary habits, and sequence of movements. If helpful, they may want to imagine the hair-pulling sequence occurring in slow-motion, attending carefully to the sequence of movements. When patients have reconstructed a situation clearly, a discussion of their observations is initiated. Topics for this discussion include the following: Which hand do they use to pull? What part of the hand is used? Is there an initial search for the "right hair"? Is the hair initially stroked or rolled between the fingers? How many hairs are touched at one time? Are hairs pulled or twisted until they fall out? Does hair pulling occur for the purpose of getting a root? and What happens after pulling?

Session 2 ends with a summary of the information obtained, with attention to common themes and patterns across patients. At this point, patients commonly feel an increased sense of control over their hair pulling as a result of identifying preceding behaviors and sequences of movement. Any increased sense of control should be discussed.

Homework

Patients again are asked to record the frequency and duration of hair pulling on self-monitoring forms (see Table 17.1). A new homework form is provided for continued identification of situations in which hair pulling occurs, although the assignment should be expanded to include recording of both preceding behaviors and the sequence of movements involved (see Table 17.3).

Session 3: Awareness Training

Following the usual discussion of homework and self-monitoring, any new information about precipitating situations, preceding behaviors, and sequences of movements should be identified. Patients also should be asked to note any resultant increases or decreases in symptoms.

Session 3 focuses on increasing awareness of moods and thoughts that occur along with hair pulling. The first step in this process is to make clear delineations between moods

---

Table 17.3. Homework Form, Session 2

For each episode of hair-pulling during the week, please record the following:

Date	Time	Situational correlates	Preceding behaviors	Sequence of movements

(emotions or feelings) and thoughts (interpretations or evaluations of situations). As noted earlier, surveys of both clinical and nonclinical hair pullers identify a wide range of feelings reported before hair pulling. Anxiety and tension are commonly reported, but so are boredom, anger, frustration, lethargy, and fatigue. Patients then are asked to identify feelings or moods that occur before, during, and after hair pulling. Providing a list of "feeling words" can be helpful for facilitating this discussion.

Next, a discussion of thoughts associated with hair pulling should be initiated. It is important here to emphasize that emotional reactions to situations may be profoundly influenced by one's interpretations of the situations. Identification of thoughts occurring before, during, and after hair pulling may be facilitated by providing the following possibilities:

Before:	• Inability to make a decision.
	• Perceived negative evaluation from others.
	• Negative evaluation of one's own performance.
	• Need to pull a specific type of hair.
During:	• "Now that I've started, I might as well continue."
	• "I have no control over myself."
	• "I hope no one interrupts (sees) me."
	• "I know I should stop, but I don't want to."
After:	• "I should not have done that."
	• "It will be hard to cover up the damage."
	• "I must be crazy."
	• "Next time I have the urge, I will stop myself."

Following discussion of associated thoughts and feelings, patients' reactions to these exercises are elicited. In addition, the perceived utility of this activity for increasing a sense of control over hair pulling is queried.

Homework

Group members again are asked to fill out self-monitoring forms during the coming week, and another new homework exercise is assigned (see Table 17.4). For the latter,

Table 17.4. Homework Form, Session 3

For each episode of hair-pulling during the week, please record the following:

Date/ Time	Situation	Preceding behaviors	Movement sequence	Mood			Thoughts		
				Before	During	After	Before	During	After

patients again should be asked to note precipitating situations, preceding behaviors, and movement sequences. However, they also will be asked to note the corresponding moods and thoughts that occur before, during, and after hair pulling.

Session 4: Competing-Response Training

Following the discussion of self-monitoring (difficulties, increases or decreases in hair pulling), patients are asked to discuss briefly any new information gleaned from the past week's homework assignment regarding situations, preceding behaviors, and sequences of movement. The primary focus of the homework discussion, however, is on associated thoughts and feelings. Patterns, themes, and similarities in thoughts and affect are highlighted by the therapist, and inquiries again are made about any perceived increase or decrease in sense of control over the behavior.

In Session 4, the focus of treatment shifts from awareness training to teaching strategies to interrupt or prevent the behavior. The first of these strategies is called *competing-response training*, which provides a coping response to be used to prevent the behavioral sequences (identified through the homework assignment) at any point in the cycle. The competing response most often used is fist clenching, an activity that can be done with or without an object in the hand. Variations of this response can be substituted to allow continuous performance of ongoing activities (i.e., clenching the phone receiver if patient is talking on the phone). The competing response should be compatible with ongoing activities and should not draw attention. Patients are asked to practice the clenching activity during the session, using the armrests of the chairs in the therapy room. Group members are instructed to clench their hands to a comfortable degree, and not harder. If knuckles whiten, pressure is too great. The pressure should make them aware of what their fingers are doing, but should not cause fatigue.

Patients are instructed that clenching can be initiated in high-risk situations or at any time that one becomes aware of the hair-pulling cycle. Each practice of the competing response should occur for 3 minutes. If something interrupts the clenching activity (i.e., requirements to shift gears while driving), the necessary activity should be completed with a return to clenching as soon as possible for the remainder of the 3 minutes. If the urge to pull remains upon release of the competing response, the competing response should be repeated until the urge subsides.

Imaginal exposure then can be used during the session to allow each patient to practice the competing response. Patients are asked to close their eyes and begin to imagine themselves in a high-risk situation. They are encouraged to observe the sights, sounds, and smells, and to imagine who is there, what is going on, and where their hands are. Patients are asked to look at their hands in their imaginations and notice the preceding behaviors (face touching, hair stroking) and the urge to pull. They then are asked to practice the competing response (i.e., to clench for a few seconds then release). The entire sequence is repeated at least one more time, with clenching used to interrupt the preceding behaviors. Two subsequent imaginal exposures are completed in which hair pulling is interrupted after it has already begun. Patients then are asked to open their eyes and provide feedback to the group about this experience.

Homework

Another week of self-monitoring is assigned, as well as continued recording of thoughts and moods associated with hair pulling. In addition, patients are asked to practice the competing response at least once per day during the upcoming week. To do so, they are asked to put themselves in a high-risk situation, possibly one that has been previously avoided, and practice the clenching exercise. At the start of each *in vivo* exposure experience, they are instructed to record the severity of the urge to pull on a zero to 8 scale. The competing response can be practiced at any point in the cycle, and the urge to pull following this exercise should also be recorded (see Table 17.5).

Session 5: Relaxation Training

Session 5 is opened with a brief review of self-monitoring and any new information gleaned from the past week's awareness assignment regarding moods and thoughts. Practice with the competing-response assignment is reviewed in some depth, with inquiries about both difficulties with the procedure and the utility of the technique for increasing control over symptoms. Each group member is then asked to describe at least one *in vivo* practice from the past week.

The focus of Session 5 is to provide the group members with one more coping strategy to be used in high-risk situations to prevent or stop hair pulling. Although anxiety and tension are not the only moods that precipitate hair pulling, they are among the most common. As a result, learning to relax can be a useful coping mechanism. Relaxation also can be used to combat feelings of frustration, boredom, and anger.

Two relaxation strategies are taught in this session: breathing retraining and posturing.

Table 17.5. Homework Form, Session 4

PART I

For each episode of hair-pulling during the week, please record the following:

Date/Time	Mood			Thoughts		
	Before	During	After	Before	During	After

PART II

At least once per day, practice the competing reponse procedure in a high-risk situation (preferably one that has been avoided previously).

Day	Situation	Urge to pull before (0–8)	Competing response	When used	Urge to pull after (0–8)
1.					
2.					
3.					
4.					
5.					
6.					
7.					

To introduce the former, a paraphrase of the following description from Azrin and Nunn (1977) is often helpful:

> Breathe in deeply, slowly, and evenly, and then breathe out slowly. As soon as you finish inhaling, begin exhaling, trying not to pause at the top of your breathing cycle. Do not breathe too deeply; this will cause you to pause momentarily after inhaling and create tension in your chest and stomach. The duration of the time you spend inhaling should be about the same as that spent exhaling. Count to yourself as a rough measure of whether the two durations are equal. For example, if you have counted to five slowly while exhaling, then slow down your inhaling enough so that you can count slowly to five while inhaling. (p. 69)

Patients then close their eyes and practice breathing while the therapist counts from 1 to 5 aloud. This process is repeated three times. Patients are asked to raise their index finger if they have not become more relaxed during this process. If anyone indicates failure to achieve a more relaxed feeling, the process is repeated three more times. Once everyone has become relaxed, the imaginal procedure from Session 4 is repeated, with the exception that deep breathing is used to prevent or interrupt the hair-pulling cycle. Patients are asked to practice imaginally two preventions of the behavior and two interruptions of the cycle after it has begun. Patients are then instructed to provide feedback to the group.

The second relaxation strategy involves adopting a relaxed posture by letting one's shoulders slouch forward slightly rather than remain erect. Patients are asked not to sit rigidly upright, but to lean back against the chair and slouch slightly. All group members practice this procedure and provide feedback regarding whether an increased sense of relaxation is experienced. Next, all patients are asked to practice this procedure while standing. Patients can allow their shoulders to become more rounded while relaxing their chests and stomachs. This posture can be compared with "standing at attention." After patients have practiced the use of relaxed posturing while standing, they are allowed to sit down and are led through the imaginal procedures again, interrupting the cycle twice before it begins and twice after it has started. Feedback from the group members regarding the utility of this procedure should be requested and all questions answered.

Homework

Again, self-monitoring forms should be provided for the coming week. Homework at this point should focus primarily on interruption of the hair-pulling cycle whenever it occurs, using awareness training, competing responses, and relaxation strategies (see Table 17.6). In addition, patients are asked to practice relaxation procedures more specifically, at least once per day, by placing themselves in high-risk situations. At these times, patients are instructed to record the urge to pull at the start of each *in vivo* exposure experience, and to practice the relaxation at any point in the cycle. The urge to pull following this practice should also be recorded.

Session 6: Generalization

Following a brief review of self-monitoring and any recent increases or decreases in hair pulling, patients are asked to discuss their use of all coping strategies to control the behavior during the past week. Each patient also is asked to describe at least one *in vivo* practice with relaxation procedures in high-risk situations.

The remainder of the last group focuses on general gains made in treatment, as well as

Table 17.6.   **Homework Form, Session 5**

PART I

For each episode of hair-pulling during the week, please record the following:

Date/Time	Coping Response Used	Comment

PART II

At least once per day, practice relaxation in a high-risk situation (preferably one that has been avoided previously). Record each practice below.

Day	Situation	Urge to pull before (0–8)	Competing response	When used	Urge to pull after (0–8)
1					
2					
3					
4					
5					
6					
7					

patients' plans for continued improvement. Patients are encouraged to review which aspects of the treatment were most useful for them, and which were not as helpful. Any feelings regarding termination of the group are discussed. At this point, it is important for the therapist to discuss the need for continued practice, particularly when the group is no longer available for "check in." Each member is encouraged to develop an individual plan for maintenance of gains. Such a plan might involve methods for continued awareness and use of coping skills, as well as strategies for integrating these into everyday life. Any further steps or alternative interventions that are still needed are identified. Some possibilities in this regard are reviewed here.

MAINTENANCE AND GENERALIZATION STRATEGIES

As reviewed earlier, the only controlled investigation of HRT to date demonstrated maintenance of gains over a 22-month follow-up, with 87% reduction in hair pulling at that interval (Azrin et al., 1980). However, follow-up evaluations in this study were not standardized and conducted by telephone, with data at 22 months available for only 12 of 19 subjects. Thus, although the long-term effects of HRT may be as robust as these data suggest, more well-controlled studies are needed to establish patterns of extended maintenance.

According to clinical experience and the theoretical perspective on which HRT is based, however, long-term maintenance of gains should include continued awareness of situational, affective, cognitive, sensory, and motoric cues that precede the behavior. The utility of continued self-monitoring in this regard is unclear, although one would hope that the need to record precipitating cues should dissipate once full awareness has been established. Investigations of HRT efficacy with other syndromes (e.g., nail biting) have suggested that awareness training comprises the primary active ingredient of HRT (Ladouceur, 1979). However, to the extent that competing responses assist patients in preventing or interrupting the hair-pulling cycle, continued use of these may be required for long-term maintenance of gains. Given that relatively little time in the context of HRT is devoted to training in some competing responses (e.g., relaxation), long-term maintenance may require extended treatment or practice in this regard. For example, relaxation training for other disorders is often taught over a number of weeks (e.g., Beck, Stanley, Baldwin, Deagle, & Averill, 1994). For trichotillomania patients with significant anxiety complaints, extended relaxation training also may be required. Furthermore, the competing responses delineated above may be insufficient for some patients. Specifically, for patients who experience significant maladaptive cognitions prior to pulling, an extended course of cognitive therapy may be warranted. Similarly, for patients whose hair pulling is a response to interpersonal conflict, some form of interpersonal therapy or social skills training may be necessary to interrupt the hair-pulling cycle. Finally, for those patients whose hair pulling seems to be in response to obsessional thoughts (e.g., about symmetry in hair growth or appearance), a trial of exposure and response prevention may be useful for long-term durability of gains. Thus, although HRT appears to be a promising intervention for trichotillomania, additional attention may need to be given to extending awareness training and the use of competing responses to maximize long-term outcome. The utility of support groups or self-help books for these purposes probably should be considered.

Relatedly, HRT may comprise just one component of an integrated treatment package for patients with trichotillomania. Although no empirical data have addressed the impact of comorbid conditions on outcome, clinical experience would suggest that alternative interventions targeting comorbid symptomatology may be important for long-term maintenance of gains in hair pulling. For example, patients with significant comorbid depression may benefit from extensive cognitive therapy or a trial of antidepressant medication; those with significant interpersonal difficulties might profit from the addition of social skills training or interpersonal psychotherapy.

PROBLEMS IN IMPLEMENTATION

The major obstacle that therapists encounter with HRT is noncompliance with homework assignments. Actual practice with awareness and competing-response procedures is considered central to the efficacy of HRT. However, the assignments can be time-intensive and require constant surveillance of one's behavior—which can be upsetting to some patients. In this regard, it may be helpful to discuss with patients the central role that homework plays in awareness training. Additionally, patients should be reinforced with praise when they turn in completed assignments. Sometimes, however, patients are reluctant to complete homework because it interferes with their daily routines. One example from the following case illustration is Patient 1, who had trouble completing his self-monitoring because he was "on the go" and never had time to stop and write down his hair-pulling sequences. Instead, he began to use a minicassette recorder that he carried with him throughout the day. Each time he pulled, he recorded the time, number of hairs pulled, thoughts, feelings, and situational correlates. He then transferred this information to written forms in the evenings. This strategy significantly increased Patient 1's compliance with homework assignments. Another creative approach to self-monitoring was demonstrated by a patient in a different group whose occupation involved the development of computer software. This patient reported that written homework assignments significantly disrupted his concentration, resulting in a serious inability to complete work-related tasks. As such, he felt he had to choose between completing self-monitoring procedures and working. Because he wanted to participate in the awareness training, however, he created a software program that helped him monitor his behavior while he was working. As a result, instead of having to stop his work to write down his behavior, the patient simply touched several keys which recorded the information, keeping a running log for the week. These strategies for completing monitoring assignments suggest that both patients and therapists may need to be creative in order to enhance compliance by tailoring the method of self-monitoring to each patient's lifestyle and patterns of hair-pulling behavior.

Another difficulty with the HRT procedures described here involves patients' unwillingness to participate in a group. Patients often are reluctant to come to a group and share their symptoms, particularly if they have never before talked about these behaviors. In this regard, patients should be reassured that this type of discomfort is natural, but most likely will pass as treatment progresses. Generally, after participating in a group, patients report that they think this approach was more successful than an individual format might have been. Although the relative effectiveness of group versus individual approaches has yet to be empirically determined, the authors concur that group intervention may be preferable, given the opportunity it affords patients to communicate with others who have similar symptoms.

Inconsistent attendance can be another problem in the implementation of HRT as described here. It is rare, for example, that a 6-week period will pass when every group member attends every group. Lack of attendance can be problematic, given that a significant amount of information is relayed during each session, and because each session builds on the techniques described in the prior meeting. When a patient misses a group, it is recommended that he or she be briefly "caught up" before the next group and that self-monitoring continue during the intervening week (extra forms can be handed out at Session 1 for this purpose).

Another challenge in the implementation of HRT is when patients are reluctant to accept the learning model on which the treatment is based. Sometimes, for example, patients will report that the behavior was not learned and that a biologically based physical sensation is the only cause of pulling. It is important to recognize the physical sensations that lead these individuals to pull and to acknowledge the potential role of biological variables. At the same time, however, it is important for the therapist to encourage these patients to look for patterns in the occurrence of what appear to be biologically based sensations. For example, one patient who pulled her eyelashes exclusively in response to a stinging sensation in her eyelids initially concluded that her symptoms did not fit the learning model and that HRT therefore would not be appropriate for her. When asked to attend to situations in which this stinging sensation occurred, she noticed that the feeling usually began when she was stressed (i.e., her children were crying, she had a fight with her boss, she felt anxious). As this patient examined the patterns of physical sensations, she began to understand that the learning model might be at least partially appropriate (i.e., that the hair pulling relieved a physical sensation that was a reaction to a stressful event). Thus, for patients with a strong conviction that biological variables are central, the learning model can be discussed as a potential concomitant perspective.

CASE ILLUSTRATIONS

Description of the Patients

The patients were two males and one female diagnosed with trichotillomania. All three were Caucasian and between the ages of 40 and 43. Patient 1 was a 40-year-old male who began hair pulling in college. The behavior began as simple touching, and grew into stroking and eventually pulling the hair. Patient 1 pulled his hair from the frontal portion of his scalp with relative infrequency. However, he reported that stroking of the scalp hair was pervasive throughout his day. Prior to treatment, Patient 1 described the behavior as merely a habit and did not associate the symptoms as exclusively in response to stress or tension. Hair loss was noticeable, although it was readily perceived by others as a receding hairline. Although his symptoms were rather mild, Patient 1 was included in the group because of the high level of distress that he reported as a result of the pulling. Administration of the ADIS-R and a modified version of the MTAI revealed a diagnosis of trichotillomania with a severity of 4, indicating mild symptoms that resulted in some interference with activities. Patient 1 also was given a diagnosis of simple phobia (heights), with a severity of 3.

Patient 2 was a 42-year-old male who had been hair pulling for 14 years prior to the onset of treatment. The primary hair-pulling sites for this individual were his hands and arms. At pretreatment, he exhibited almost no hair on his hands and large bald spots on his forearms. Patient 2 initially described his symptoms as occurring during "down time" while he was problem-solving or when concentrating. This individual pulled hair only while at work, and he reported complete cessation of hair pulling whenever he was on vacation. Administration of the ADIS-R and the MTAI revealed a diagnosis of trichotillomania with a severity of 4, indicating mild symptoms that resulted in some interference with activities. No comorbid diagnoses were present.

Patient 3 was a 43-year-old female who had been pulling scalp hair since she was 27, at which time she was pregnant with her second child. She had worn a wig since the onset of the symptoms and was almost completely bald, with only a few short hairs left on her head. Furthermore, she described her symptoms as a part of her daily grooming routine. Specifically, she reported sitting in front of her mirror in the morning, pulling scalp hair for extended periods of time. She explained that her pulling was in response to a burning or itching sensation in the scalp. Hair pulling caused the sensation to decrease, therefore reinforcing the behavior. Patient 3 also reported hair pulling for the sake of obtaining a large root as a secondary motivator. Administration of the ADIS-R and MTAI revealed a diagnosis of trichotillomania with a severity of 6, indicating moderate to severe symptoms that resulted in marked interference with social and/or work activities. No other disorders were diagnosed.

All three patients reported distress as a result of their symptoms and had a strong desire to stop pulling their hair. Patients 1 and 2 had never sought treatment for hair pulling, and Patient 3 had participated in a pharmacological trial of fluoxetine 1 year prior to beginning the group. None of the group members were on medication or receiving treatment for any psychological problem over the duration of the group.

Prior to the onset of treatment, all three patients expressed genuine concern about participation in the group. One of the patients (Patient 2) had never revealed to anyone that he pulled out his hair. Although the other two had shared their symptoms with others, these revelations had been limited only to family members. Furthermore, all three patients expressed that they were hesitant to discuss their symptoms with a group of strangers.

Summary of Habit-Reversal Training

Session 1 began with introductions and brief self-reported histories Although somewhat apprehensive at first, patients reported feeling more relaxed as the group progressed. Although members' symptoms were quite diverse with regard to severity, common themes and patterns became apparent nonetheless. All three patients reported that hair pulling often occurred in response to stress, anxiety, or during situations when concentration or problem solving was necessary. Furthermore, they highlighted the pleasurable or soothing feelings associated with the behavior. All three agreed that certain types of hairs were more likely to be pulled, although the types of preferred hair differed for each.

In reviewing the inconveniences of hair pulling, the most commonly reported drawback was time spent with symptoms. Other inconveniences included self-deprecation for the behavior, often leading to self-consciousness about appearance; not understanding why they had the urge to pull and feeling guilty for having pulled; and interference with interpersonal relationships. Other reported inconveniences included having to make an effort to cover up the hair loss; avoidance of many outdoor activities such as swimming, biking, and exercise; and dishonesty with professionals, such as physicians and hair stylists. Patient 3 also reported past scalp digging that had led to serious medical complications.

Patients were receptive to the various etiological theories of trichotillomania, but particularly so to the learning theory on which HRT is based. Conceptualizing the behavior as a normal reaction to an extreme event, or an infrequent behavior that persisted until it became a nervous habit, seemed to serve two purposes. First, it allowed the patients to normalize a behavior that was previously perceived as "bizarre" or "abnormal," and ruled out hypotheses that required consideration of "underlying pathology." Second, this type of explanation seemed to influence patients' perceptions of their potential ability to change and control their behaviors by "relearning" other more adaptive responses.

Following the description of HRT, patients expressed considerable enthusiasm about the proposed treatment and seemed to accept the concepts presented. Providing a convincing rationale may be paramount for the use of HRT. Specifically, much of the learning that takes place in this approach occurs outside the therapy sessions, and high expectations for improvement may facilitate active engagement in the homework assignments. To examine both credibility of the treatment and expectations for improvement, a rating form developed by Borkovec and Nau (1972) was administered at the end of Session 1, after all treatment procedures had been explained. Credibility ratings on this instrument ranged from 6.25 to 9.25 on a scale of 1 to 10, with 1 indicating *No Confidence* in the procedures described and 10 indicating *Extreme Confidence*. Ratings for expectancy of improvement ranged from 70% to 90%, indicating that subjects generally felt that this treatment would result in decreased symptoms.

Session 2 began with a review of the self-monitoring procedures and initial homework assignment. It should be noted that all patients in this group had participated previously in an assessment study that required completion of 2 weeks of self-monitoring. Thus, this activity was very familiar to them, and some symptom reduction already had been noticed as a result (see Figure 17.1). With regard to other homework, Patient 1 reported that he

Melinda A. Stanley
and Suzanne G.
Mouton

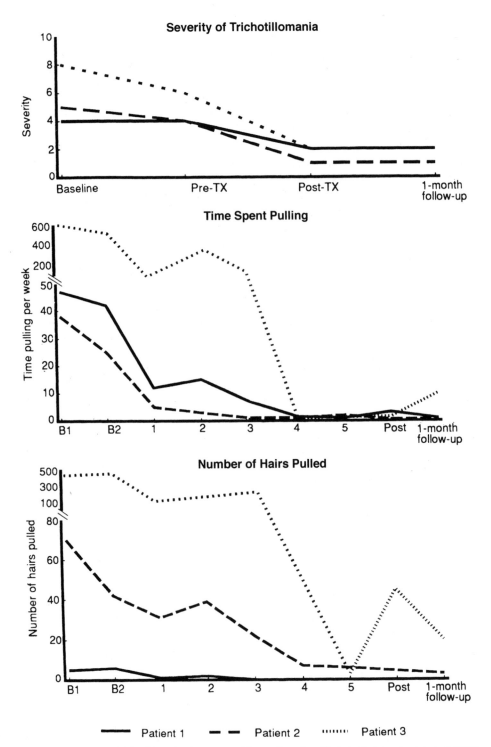

Figure 17.1 Severity of trichotillomania, time spent pulling, and number of hairs pulled at pretreatment, posttreatment, and one-month follow-up.

pulled almost exclusively in the car, while thinking about things that he needed to get done. Patient 2 found that he pulled most frequently while at the office or in the classroom, and that he pulled quite often while talking on the phone. Patient 3 reported only pulling while at home, in her bathroom. She described preceding events that included looking at her scalp, touching the stubble, and oftentimes feeling frustrated. All three group members reported pulling while they were alone or when others could not detect their behavior.

As a result of this initial awareness training, two of the group members reported that they had not realized the different situations in which they pulled. More important, they had begun to see patterns in their behavior, indicating that pulling was not always a random event. All three subjects commented that they were beginning to see the behavior as a reaction to various stimuli and that hair pulling served a distinct purpose in their lives.

The remainder of Session 2 and the resultant homework yielded much information regarding the discrete elements of each patient's pulling sequence. For example, Patient 1 described a chain of events in response to stress that began with touching his hair, proceeded to stroking and rubbing a particular spot on his scalp, and finally resulted in pulling one of the hairs with his index and little fingers. He mentioned that often the stroking behavior was "enough" and did not result in actual pulling. Patient 2 identified his primary high-risk situation as sitting at his desk at work. He described the hair pulling sequence as beginning with a visual cue, in particular, looking at his hands and arms to isolate the hair that he wanted to pull (i.e., one that was coarse, long, or out of place). This information was quite a revelation for this individual, given that he had never realized that inspection of his hands or arms always preceded pulling. Patient 3 reported pulling in situations when she was bored or anxious. As noted earlier, she described a physical sensation (itching and burning in her scalp) that always preceded the pulling behavior, and indicated that pulling helped to relieve the itching and burning feelings. All three patients reported an increased sense of control with respect to their behavior as a result of identifying patterns of hair pulling and precipitating cues.

Session 3 and the resultant homework focused on moods and thoughts associated with hair pulling. Patient 1 reported feeling anxious, agitated, worried, or depressed at every stage of hair pulling, with little change as the behavior progressed. For this individual, the only change in mood over the hair pulling sequence was an occasional feeling of guilt or disgust after having pulled. Patient 1 also reported coincident thoughts, such as "I must plan," "I need to ... ," "What would happen if ... ," "I must hurry," which also did not change over the course of the hair-pulling sequence. Patient 2 described feeling tense or uptight before pulling, soothing relief during the behavior, and disgust with himself following hair pulling. His thoughts, on the other hand, tended to stay the same throughout the sequence: He used hair pulling almost exclusively to help him concentrate at work. Patient 3 reported feeling tired prior to pulling, with a sense of relaxation during, and a feeling of contentment following the behavior. She also occasionally found that the behavior elevated her energy level, and she reported feeling more alert afterward. Associated thoughts prior to pulling were of work and things that needed to be done. During pulling, she concentrated on these same issues, and after pulling was completed, a plan generally was developed. Patient 3 also described hair pulling as helping her to concentrate and solve problems.

After additional time monitoring associated moods and thoughts, all three patients were able to "fine-tune" their reports. Each patient began reporting more specific thoughts associated with hair pulling, such as "I wish I did not pull my hair," "I can't believe I did that; I was doing so well," and "Stop pulling." Subjects also reported feeling upset with themselves more often after pulling than had been indicated previously. All three described the behavior as having come more fully into their awareness, with only isolated incidents of pulling without awareness. Relatedly, each individual described a distinct increase in perceived control over symptoms as a result of awareness training.

After Session 4 and the resultant homework, patients discussed their efforts to utilize the competing response. Patient 1 reported using objects in his surroundings (i.e., door handles, the phone, books, and the steering wheel of his car) to grip when the urge to pull manifested. He described initiating the competing response as soon as he began the sequence of movements (stroking his hair), and reported that the strategy was helpful in reducing the urge, but did not eliminate it completely. Patient 2 described using fist clenching alone or clenching the steering wheel while driving to interrupt the cycle. He noted that he used the response as soon as he found himself looking at his hands for a particular hair to be pulled. Utilizing this strategy, Patient 2 was able to eliminate the urge completely 80% of the time and to reduce the significantly the other 20% of the time. Patient 3 described using fist clenching repeatedly until the urge had subsided. She reported that she was able to eliminate the urge on every occasion utilizing the competing response.

After Session 5 and another week of practice utilizing both clenching and relaxation procedures, Patient 1 reported that he was able to reduce the urge considerably, as compared to the previous week, by using clenching and relaxation in combination. He found that relaxation only worked for him in conjunction with the fist-clenching strategy, and he employed these strategies simultaneously. Patient 2 reported using the clenching exercise as well as changing his visual cues. In particular, he forced himself to look at something other than his hand and arm hair. He commented that the clenching helped to reduce the urge, particularly while driving, but that changing his visual focus was imperative in breaking the sequence of movements. Patient 2 also used postural adjustments to eliminate the urge to pull. He described sitting at his desk and relaxing his position until the urge had passed. Patient 3 employed relaxation through deep breathing to interrupt and eliminate the urge to pull. She reported being able to feel "content" and "soothed" via relaxation instead of hair pulling.

During the final session, patients reflected on their experiences in the group and their perceptions of how helpful the strategies had been. All three subjects reported significant symptom reduction, although variability in pretreatment symptom severity across patients was high (see Figure 17.1). All patients, however, perceived increased control over their symptoms and described feeling as if they now had the "tools" to help themselves. They indicated that they had benefited from the experience, although none were sure how long the benefits would last. Suggestions were made for a "follow-up" group to monitor progress after 1 month, and all group members agreed to participate in both posttreatment and 1-month follow-up evaluations.

Posttreatment data indicated decreases in both clinician-rated severity of symptoms and time spent pulling for all three subjects, with maintenance of gains at 1-month follow-up (see Figure 17.1). Number of hairs pulled also decreased noticeably for Patients 2 and 3, although Patient 3 exhibited a slight increase in this measure at posttreatment assessment. Patient 1 completely discontinued hair pulling, although as noted earlier, number of hairs pulled for this individual at baseline was quite low. In considering outcome data for all patients, it again should be noted that each had participated in an assessment study prior to the initiation of group that required them to complete self-monitoring forms for a 2-week period. The potential impact of this simple intervention is apparent in the decreased rate of symptoms prior to the initial group session (see Figure 17.1, B1 and B2). These data are consistent with Ladouceur's (1979) conclusion that awareness training through self-monitoring may be the essential active ingredient of HRT. Although the data here suggest additional benefits over the 6-week treatment protocol, a well-controlled empirical trial will need to evaluate the relative effects of self-monitoring alone versus more extensive treatment with HRT.

SUMMARY AND FUTURE DIRECTIONS

Over the past 10 to 15 years, significant gains have been made in our understanding of trichotillomania. Recent studies with large samples of chronic hair pullers have increased dramatically our knowledge about the nature of the disorder and coexistent pathology, and preliminary treatment studies have suggested the potential utility of both pharmacological and behavioral approaches. In the behavioral arena, the most promising treatment to date is HRT, the procedures of which are detailed in this chapter. Nevertheless, relevant empirical data in this arena are sparse. Future studies will need to examine the relative utility of single- and multiple-session forms of HRT conducted in individual versus group formats. Empirical investigations also will need to identify the central active ingredients of HRT, as well as predictors of both outcome and long-term follow-up. This area is rich for future study, and the next 5 to 10 years are likely to result in further dramatic increases in our understanding of the nature and treatment of trichotillomania.

REFERENCES

American Psychiatric Association. (1987). *Diagnostic and statistical manual of mental disorders* (3rd ed., rev.). Washington, DC: Author.

American Psychiatric Association. (1994). *Diagnostic and statistical manual of mental disorders* (4th ed.). Washington, DC: Author.

Azrin, N. H., & Nunn, R. G. (1973). Habit-reversal: A method of eliminating nervous habits and tics. *Behaviour Research and Therapy, 11,* 619–628.

Azrin, N. H., & Nunn, R. G. (1977). *Habit control in a day.* New York: Simon & Schuster.

Azrin, N. H., Nunn, R. G., & Frantz, S. E. (1980). Treatment of hairpulling (trichotillomania): A comparative study of habit reversal and negative practice training. *Behavior Therapy and Experimental Psychiatry, 11,* 13–20.

Beck, J. G., Stanley, M. A., Baldwin, L. E., Deagle, E. A., & Averill, P. M. (1994). A comparison of cognitive therapy and relaxation training for panic disorder. *Journal of Consulting and Clinical Psychology, 62,* 818–826.

Borkovec, T. D., & Nau, S. D. (1972). Credibility of analogue therapy rationales. *Journal of Behavior Therapy and Experimental Psychiatry, 3,* 257–260.

Christenson, G. A., Chernoff-Clementz, E., & Clementz, B. A. (1992). Personality and clinical characteristics in patients with trichotillomania. *Journal of Clinical Psychiatry, 53,* 407–413.

Christenson, G. A., Mackenzie, T. B., & Mitchell, J. E. (1991a). Characteristics of 60 adult chronic hair pullers. *American Journal of Psychiatry, 148,* 365–370.

Christenson, G. A., Mackenzie, T. B., & Mitchell, J. E. (1994). Adult men and women with trichotillomania: A comparison of male and female characteristics. *Psychosomatics, 35,* 142–149.

Christenson, G. A., Mackenzie, T. B., Mitchell, J. E., & Callies, A. L. (1991b). A placebo-controlled, double-blind crossover study of fluoxetine in trichotillomania. *American Journal of Psychiatry, 148,* 1566–1571.

Christenson, G. A., Pyle, R. L., & Mitchell, J. E. (1991c). Estimated lifetime prevalence of trichotillomania in college students. *Journal of Clinical Psychiatry, 52,* 415–417.

Christenson, G. A., Ristvedt, S. L., & Mackenzie, T. B. (1993). Identification of trichotillomania cue profiles. *Behaviour Research and Therapy, 31,* 315–320.

Dahlquist, L. M., & Kalfus, G. R. (1984). A novel approach to assessment in the treatment of childhood trichotillomania. *Journal of Behavior Therapy and Experimental Psychiatry, 15,* 47–50.

DeLuca, R. V., & Holborn, S. W. (1984). A comparison of relaxation training and competing response training to eliminate hair pulling and nail biting. *Journal of Behavior Therapy and Experimental Psychiatry, 15*, 67–70.

DiNardo, P. A., Moras, K., Barlow, D. H., & Rapee, R. M. (1993). Reliability of the DSM-III-R anxiety disorder categories using the Anxiety Disorders Interview Schedule–Revised (ADIS-R). *Archives of General Psychiatry, 50*, 251–256.

Goodman, W. K., Price, L. H., Rasmussen, S. A., et al. (1989). The Yale–Brown Obsessive–Compulsive Scale (Y-BOCS). Part I., Development, use, and reliability. *Archives of General Psychiatry, 46*, 1006–1011.

Graber, J., & Arndt, W. B. (1993). Trichotillomania. *Comprehensive Psychiatry, 34*, 340–346.

Greenberg, H. R., & Sarner, C. A. (1965). Trichotillomania: Symptom and syndrome. *Archives of General Psychiatry, 12*, 482–489.

Hallopeau, M. (1989). Alopécie par grattage Hrichomanie ou trichotillomaniel. *Annales de Dermatologie et de Venerologie, 10*, 440–441.

Hussain, S. H. (1992). Trichotillomania: Two case reports from a similar cultural background. *Psychopathology, 25*, 289–293.

Insel, T. R., & Winslow, J. T. (1990). Neurobiology of obsessive–compulsive disorder. In M. A. Jenike, L. Baer, & W. E. Minichiello (Eds.), *Obsessive compulsive disorders: Theory and management* (2nd ed., pp. 118–131). Chicago: Year Book Medical Publishers.

Jenike, M. A. (1990). Illness related to obsessive–compulsive disorder. In M. A. Jenike, L. Baer, and W. E. Minichiello (Eds.), *Obsessive–compulsive disorders: Theory and management* (2nd ed., pp. 29–60). Chicago: Year Book Medical Publishers.

Ladouceur, R. (1979). Habit reversal treatment: Learning an incompatible response or increasing subject's awareness? *Behaviour Research and Therapy, 17*, 313–316.

Lenane, M. C., Swedo, S. E., Rapoport, J. L., Leonard, H., Sceery, W., & Guroff, J. J. (1992). Rates of obsessive–compulsive disorder in first degree relatives of patients with trichotillomania: A research note. *Journal of Child Psychology and Psychiatry, 33*, 925–933.

Mansueto, C. (1991). Trichotillomania in focus. *OCD Newsletter, 5*, 10–11.

Mansueto, C. (1993, April). *Trichotillomania and life*. Paper presented at the Massachusetts General Hospital Clinic Trichotillomania Conference, Boston, MA.

Muller, S. A. (1987). Trichotillomania. *Dermatologic Clinics, 5*, 595–601.

Muller, S. A. (1990). Trichotillomania: A histopathologic study in sixty-six patients. *Journal of the American Academy of Dermatology, 23*, 56–62.

Oguchi, T., & Miura, S. (1977). Trichotillomania: Its psychopathological aspect. *Comprehensive Psychiatry, 18*, 177–182.

Reeve, E. A., Bernstein, G. A., & Christenson, G. A. (1992). Clinical characteristics and psychiatric comorbidity in children with trichotillomania. *Journal of American Academy of Child and Adolescent Psychiatry, 31*, 132–138.

Rettew, D. C., Cheslow, D. L., Rapoport, J. L., Leonard, H. L., & Lenane, M. C. (1991). Neuropsychological test performance in trichotillomania: A further link with obsessive–compulsive disorder. *Journal of Anxiety Disorders, 5*, 225–235.

Rosenbaum, M. S., & Ayllon, T. (1981). The habit-reversal technique in treating trichotillomania. *Behavior Therapy, 12*, 473–481.

Rothbaum, B. O. (1992). The behavioral treatment of trichotillomania. *Behavioural Psychotherapy, 20*, 1–00.

Rothbaum, B. O., & Ninan, P. (1992, November). *Treatment of trichotillomania: Behavior therapy versus clomipramine*. Paper presented at the Association for the Advancement of Behavior Therapy Annual Convention, Boston, MA.

Rothbaum, B. O., Shaw, L., Morris, R., & Ninan, P. T. (1993). Prevalence of trichotillomania in a college freshman population. Letter. *Journal of Clinical Psychiatry, 54*, 72.

Shome, S., Bhatia, M. S., Gautam, R. K. (1993). Culture-bound trichotillomania. Letter. *American Journal of Psychiatry, 150*, 674.

Spitzer, R. L., Williams, J. B. W., Gibbon, M., & First, M. B. (1992). The Structured Clinical Interview for DSM-III-R (SCID). I. History, rationale, and description. *Archives of General Psychiatry, 49*, 624–629.

Stanley, M. A., Borden, J. W., Bell, G. E., & Wagner, A. L. (1994). Nonclinical hair-pulling: Phenomenology and related psychopathology. *Journal of Anxiety Disorders, 8*, 119–130.

Stanley, M. A., Borden, J. W., Mouton, S. G., & Breckenridge, J. (1995). Nonclinical hair-pulling: Affective correlates and a comparison with clinic patients. *Behaviour Research and Therapy, 33*, 179–186.

Stanley, M. A., Bowers, T. C., Swann, A. C., & Taylor, D. J. (1991). Treatment of trichotillomania with fluoxetine. Letter. *Journal of Clinical Psychiatry, 52*, 282.

Stanley, M. A., & Mouton, S. G. (1994). *Affective correlates of trichotillomania.* Manuscript in preparation.

Stanley, M. A., Prather, R. C., Wagner, A. L., Davis, M. L., & Swann, A. C. (1993a). Can the Yale–Brown Obsessive–Compulsive Scale be used to assess trichotillomania? A preliminary report. *Behaviour Research and Therapy, 31,* 171–178.

Stanley, M. A., Swann, A. C., Bowers, T. C., Davis, M. L., & Taylor, D. J. (1992). A comparison of clinical features in trichotillomania and obsessive–compulsive disorder. *Behaviour Research and Therapy, 30,* 39–44.

Stanley, M. A., Wagner, A. L., & Davis, M. L. (1993b, November). *A comparison of obsessive–compulsive disorder and trichotillomania: Self-reported and cognitive impulsivity.* Presented in F. Neziruglu, Chair, Obsessive–Compulsive and Related Disorders, Association for the Advancement of Behavior Therapy, Atlanta, GA.

Swedo, S. E., & Leonard, H. L. (1992). Trichotillomania: An obsessive–compulsive spectrum disorder? *Psychiatric Clinics of North America, 15,* 777–790.

Swedo, S. E., Leonard, H. L., Rapoport, J. L., Lenane, M. C., Goldberger, B. A., & Cheslow, B. A. (1989). A double-blind comparison of clomipramine and desipramine in the treatment of trichotillomania (hair pulling). *New England Journal of Medicine, 321,* 497–501.

Swedo, S. E., Rapoport, J. L., Leonard, H. L., Schapiro, M. B., Rapoport, S. J., & Grady, C. L. (1991). Regional cerebral glucose metabolism of women with trichotillomania. *Archives of General Psychiatry, 48,* 828–833.

Tarnowski, K. J., Rosen, L. A., McGrath, M. L., & Drabman, R. S. (1987). A modified habit reversal procedure in a recalcitrant case of trichotillomania. *Journal of Behavior Therapy and Experimental Psychiatry, 18,* 157–163.

Tynes, L. L., White, K., & Steketee, G. S. (1990). Toward a nosology of obsessive–compulsive disorder. *Comprehensive Psychiatry, 31,* 465–480.

Winchel, R. M., Jones, J. S., Molcho, A., Parsons, B., Stanley, B., & Stanley, M. (1992a). Rating the severity of trichotillomania: Methods and problems. *Psychopharmacology Bulletin, 28,* 457–462.

Winchel, R. M., Jones, J. S., Molcho, A., Parsons, B., Stanley, B., & Stanley, M. (1992b). The Psychiatric Institute Trichotillomania Scale (PITS). *Psychopharmacology Bulletin, 28,* 463–476.

Winchel, R. M., Jones, J. S., Stanley, B., Molcho, A., & Stanley, M. (1992c). Clinical characteristics of trichotillomania and its response to fluoxetine. *Journal of Clinical Psychiatry, 53,* 304–308.

18

Anger Management Training with Essential Hypertensive Patients

Kevin T. Larkin and Claudia Zayfert

INTRODUCTION

Elevations in arterial blood pressure constitute one of the major risk factors for diseases of the heart and vasculature. In fact, epidemiological data have shown that for each 10 mm Hg (millimeters in mercury) increase in blood pressure over normal values, risk for cardiovascular disease increases by 30% (Page, 1983). Normal blood pressure is typically defined as 120 mm Hg during cardiac contraction (systolic blood pressure) and 80 mm Hg during cardiac relaxation (diastolic blood pressure). According to the Joint National Committee on Detection, Evaluation, and Treatment of High Blood Pressure (1988), individuals whose resting systolic/diastolic blood pressures exceed 140/85 mm Hg are diagnosed with various forms of high blood pressure categorized in Table 18.1. This classification system replaced the previous division of hypertension into sustained high blood pressure and borderline high blood pressure, following publication of convincing evidence that even persons in the borderline hypertensive range were at increased risk for cardiovascular disease and stroke, and should be treated.

   Although the causes of elevated arterial pressures may be, in some cases, attributed to dysfunctional renal, endocrine, or cardiovascular conditions (i.e., secondary hypertension), over 90% of diagnosed hypertensive cases are of unknown origin and commonly termed *essential hypertension* (Julius & Hanson, 1983). Essential hypertension is typically asymptomatic, although in some cases diffuse complaints of headache, fatigue, dizziness, sweating, and nosebleeds have been associated with periods of excessively elevated blood pressure (Berkow, 1982). Although lack of obvious symptomatology often leads to signifi-

Kevin T. Larkin • Department of Psychology, West Virginia University, Morgantown, West Virginia 26506.
Claudia Zayfert • Dartmouth–Hitchcock Medical Center, National Center for Post-Traumatic Stress Disorder, Lebanon, New Hampshire 03756.

Sourcebook of Psychological Treatment Manuals for Adult Disorders, edited by Vincent B. Van Hasselt and Michel Hersen. Plenum Press, New York, 1996.

Table 18.1. Classification of Adult Blood Pressures by the Joint National Committee on Detection, Evaluation, and Treatment of High Blood Pressure (1988)[a]

Blood pressure range (mm Hg)	Category
Diastolic blood pressure	
< 85	Normal blood pressure
85–89	High-normal blood pressure
90–104	Mild hypertension
105–114	Moderate hypertension
≥ 115	Severe hypertension
Systolic blood pressure, when diastolic blood pressure < 90	
< 140	Normal blood pressure
140–159	Borderline isolated systolic hypertension
≥ 160	Isolated systolic hypertension

[a]From the 1988 Report of the Joint National Committee on Detection, Evaluation, and Treatment of High Blood Pressure (p. 3).

cant delays in diagnosing, assessing, and treating this disorder, great strides have been made since the 1960s in the early detection and management of elevated blood pressure problems. In fact, many epidemiological researchers now believe that improvement in diagnosing and treating high blood pressure is the single most important factor contributing to the significantly lower mortality rates from diseases of the cardiovascular system that have been observed since the 1960s (e.g., Kannel et al., 1984).

It has long been recognized that essential hypertension is a disorder resulting from multiple etiologies. Thus, although an obese patient, a patient who ingests a high-salt diet, and a patient employed in a highly stressful environment all share in common elevated arterial pressures, the etiology of the observed high blood pressures may be quite different for each of these patients. Based upon this knowledge, then, it has become clear that intervention plans aimed at regulating arterial pressure must account for the numerous etiological factors involved. This is particularly true for nonpharmacological or behavioral interventions, in which the target of treatment is to alter a specific behavior (e.g., reducing salt intake) rather than to impact directly physiological states that cause blood pressure elevations (e.g., vasoconstriction). In other words, identification of the exact etiological process involved is not as crucial for pharmacological as opposed to nonpharmacological interventions. Blood-pressure-controlling medications will lower arterial pressure regardless of the cause, whereas behavioral interventions require a better understanding of etiological processes involved in order to enhance the likelihood of treatment success.

The condition of essential hypertension has presented an interesting challenge for behavioral scientists wishing to examine the pathogenic role of various psychosocial factors with respect to both the cause and maintenance of elevated arterial pressures. Foremost among these has been examination of the hypothesized relationship between style of anger expression and blood pressure. In perhaps the earliest discussion of this relationship, Alexander (1939) proposed the "suppressed hostility" hypothesis, in which he suggested that hypertensive patients are characterized by strong dependency needs and hostile impulses. Behaviorally, this conflict may be observed in a patient's failure to express hostile impulses or angry affect, due to excessive fear that expression of anger might damage relationships with others capable of fulfilling the patient's need for nurturance. Numerous investigations have attempted to clarify the relationship between anger expression and high blood pressure and other cardiac conditions (for comprehensive reviews, see Diamond, 1982 and Chesney & Rosenman, 1985). Despite voluminous research exploring these relationships, firm conclusions about the role of anger expression in hypertension are as yet unavailable. Whereas some investigations have shown hypertensives to be more submissive in interpersonal situations in contrast to normal blood pressure controls (e.g., Gentry, Chesney, Gary, Hall, & Harburg, 1982; Keane et al., 1982), others have found high blood pressure patients to be more aggressive than normotensive controls (e.g., Baer, Collins, Bourianoff, & Ketchel, 1979; Schachter, 1957). Inconsistent findings of this nature have led some investigators to conclude that the relationship between anger expression and blood pressure is curvilinear; that is, high blood pressure is related to both "inappropriate submissiveness" and "inappropriate assertiveness" (Harburg, Blakelock, & Roeper, 1979). However, because of the uncertain psychometric properties of the instruments employed in investigations of this nature and the overreliance on self-report measures of anger expression, this argument has not been made convincingly. Incorporation of multimethod assessments with demonstrated reliability and validity will hopefully clarify the nature and direction of the anger expression–blood pressure relationship.

ASSESSMENT OF ANGER AND ANGER EXPRESSION

Recent advances in behavioral assessment have enabled researchers to examine more clearly the specific and interrelated components of anger and anger expression. In particular, domains of affect, physiology, cognition, and behavior, as they pertain to the experience and expression of anger, can now be sampled with some degree of reliability and validity. Spielberger, Johnson, Russell, Crane, Jacobs, and Worden (1985) employed the acronym AHA! (i.e., Anger–Hostility–Aggression) to describe the components of a comprehensive analysis of anger and its expression. *Anger* refers to the emotional experience typified by characteristic physiological arousal and cognitive appraisals of provocative or confrontational situations (e.g., "He bumped into me on purpose"), whereas *hostility* refers to the generalized cynical appraisals one has concerning motives of others in his or her environment (e.g., "People are generally untrustworthy"). *Aggression*, in contrast to anger and hostility, is an overtly observable verbal or physical response to the experience of anger. In general, it has been hypothesized that hostile persons tend to experience anger more frequently than nonhostile counterparts, and that persons who experience anger more frequently are more likely to exhibit aggressive social behaviors than those who rarely experience anger (Spielberger et al., 1985). For a comprehensive assessment of the experience of anger, it has been recommended that all three components of the AHA! syndrome be measured to determine their individual as well as combined contributions to increased risk for essential hypertension and subsequent cardiovascular disease.

Assessment of Anger

In general, three strategies can be employed to assess the emotional experience of anger: self-report, physiological assessment, and facial coding of emotions. Regarding the first of these, a major advance in self-report assessment of anger occurred with the publication of the Spielberger State/Trait Anger and Expression Inventory (1988). This instrument consists of separate scales to measure state anger and two factor-derived components of trait anger, trait anger–temperament (e.g., "I have a fiery temper") and trait anger–reaction (e.g., "I get angry when I'm slowed down by others' mistakes"). According to Spielberger, *trait anger–temperament* refers to "a disposition to express anger, without specifying any provoking situation or circumstance" (p. 8) whereas *trait anger–reaction* items reflect "situations that involve frustration, negative evaluations, or being treated unfairly" (p. 8). These scales have been widely employed with various clinical populations, including essential hypertensive patients, who have shown higher trait anger (specifically trait anger–reaction) scores relative to normal blood pressure controls (Crane, 1981).

Because the experience of anger, like other emotions, involves some degree of physiological arousal, measurement of anger lends itself nicely to physiological assessment strategies. Several studies have attempted to differentiate anger from other emotion states based on physiological responses (e.g., Ax, 1953; Levenson, 1992; Schachter, 1957; Schwartz, Weinberger, & Davidson, 1981). Available evidence suggests a consistent pattern of physiological arousal associated with the experience of anger. Unlike anxiety, anger is typically accompanied by a rapid secretion of norepinephrine and associated increase in diastolic blood pressure and peripheral vasodilation. In contrast, fear is more commonly associated with epinephrine secretion and increased systolic blood pressure, skin conductance, and muscle-tension activity and lowering of skin temperature. The most consistent finding, and one that may prove clinically useful as well, is that diastolic blood pressure increases more during the experience of anger than during the experience of fear. The assessment of diastolic blood pressure during provocation would provide important information to the clinician regarding the intensity of the patient's experience of anger. Such information may provide direction in treatment planning, as well as for monitoring therapeutic progress and outcome.

Although patterns of physiological reactivity may have utility for distinguishing various emotional states, a large body of literature indicates that the magnitude of cardiovascular responses should be of interest to the clinician as well. The majority of studies in this area have examined the so-called "reactivity" hypothesis. In its simplest form, this hypothesis states that individuals who consistently exhibit exaggerated cardiovascular responses to stressful or emotionally charged situations possess the greatest risk for subsequent diagnoses of essential hypertension (Wood, Sheps, Elveback, & Schirger, 1984) and other cardiac health problems (Keys, Taylor, Blackburn, Anderson, & Somonson, 1971). Certain individuals may be especially prone to excessive cardiovascular responses to stress. For example, individuals characterized as high-hostile persons show greater cardiovascular responses to anger-eliciting situations than low-hostile persons; however, high-hostile individuals cannot be distinguished from their low-hostile counterparts in their cardiovascular response to nonconfrontational, but equally challenging, stressors (e.g., Suarez & Williams, 1989). Persons exhibiting the Type A behavior pattern also show exaggerated cardiovascular responses under similar conditions in comparison with Type B individuals (e.g., Glass et al., 1980). Furthermore, investigations of persons differing with respect to family history of hypertension have established that normotensive persons with a hypertensive parent manifest greater cardiovascular reactions to anger-eliciting situations than persons with normotensive parents (e.g., Semenchuk & Larkin, 1993). A final comment regarding the comprehensive assessment of anger, however, is that the observed differences in physiological response to provocation are rarely accompanied by differential subjective reports of anger intensity (e.g., Semenchuk & Larkin, 1993). Therefore, inclusion of physiological measures permits a more comprehensive analysis of an individual's affective state during confrontation, which may have been missed if the examiner relied solely on self-report methodology.

Finally, although not commonly employed in investigations of this nature, the experience of anger has also been examined using behavioral coding of facial-muscle activity (Ekman & Friesen, 1974). In classic works describing facial displays of affect, Ekman and colleagues (Ekman, 1978; 1982; Ekman & Friesen, 1974; Ekman, Friesen, & Ellsworth, 1972) characterized the emotion of anger as one of the "basic" human emotions that could be observed both longitudinally (i.e., from early childhood to old age) and cross-culturally. According to these authors, the facial display of anger is portrayed through a furrowed, wrinkled brow, pursed lips, jaw tightness, glaring eye contact, and a slight wrinkling upward of the upper nose. Although these facial cues are important in distinguishing among specific emotions an individual may be experiencing, it is much more difficult to gain reliable indices regarding the intensity of the emotional experience based only on facial cues. Despite some of the inherent difficulties encountered in the behavioral coding of facial affect, it is an important method of assessing the experience of anger in contrived or naturalistic interpersonal encounters. Although it is unlikely that the clinician would find behavioral coding of facial affect feasible in daily practice, it is nonetheless useful to be aware of and to assess informally how affect is communicated nonverbally. Knowledge of the typical pattern of facial activity associated with anger will enable the clinician to informally assess individuals' facial expressions while discussing anger-provoking situations or during role-play interactions. In particular, it is important for the clinician to note whether facial expression is congruent with the verbal message or self-reported anger. Discordance between facial display of affect and verbal messages may signal skill deficits in assertive communication, which may be important targets for treatment.

Assessment of Hostility

Because hostility has been conceptualized as an attitude or tendency to perceive the environment from a cynical perspective, it can legitimately be accessed only through self-report methodology. Although this construct has been plagued by inherent measurement difficulties, it has known predictive validity that may of interest to the clinician. The most commonly used instruments for assessing hostility have been the Cook–Medley Hostility Questionnaire (Cook & Medley, 1954) and the Buss–Durkee Hostility Inventory (Buss & Durkee, 1957). The Cook–Medley, an MMPI-derived scale, was originally developed to assess how instructors' attitudes toward students impacted on their ability to teach. A wealth of longitudinal data subsequently linked high scores on the Cook–Medley to many forms of cardiovascular disease (e.g., Shekelle, Gale, Ostfeld, & Paul, 1983), as well as to all causes of mortality (e.g., Barefoot, Dahlstrom, & Williams, 1983). The Buss–Durkee Hostility Inventory (1957) enabled clinicians to distinguish between experiential and expressive components of hostility. *Experiential hostility* refers to the tendency to experience negative emotions, be resentful of others, and be suspicious of the motives or intentions of others, whereas *expressive hostility* refers to a generally uncooperative interpersonal style, and a tendency toward verbal aggression and antagonism. Therefore, expressive hostility may best be conceptualized as a measure of anger expression rather than hostility. In contrast to prospective studies utilizing the Cook–Medley, only a few investigations have shown relationships between Buss–Durkee-derived hostility indices and cardiovascular disease (e.g., Siegman, Dembroski, & Ringel, 1987). Despite the apparent predictive utility of these instruments, researchers continue to debate the core

Kevin T. Larkin and
Claudia Zayfert

meaning of the construct of *hostility* and its relationship to similar constructs, such as "potential for hostility" or "suspicion/mistrust" remains controversial. Thus, although measurement of hostility may be a useful indicator of cardiovascular disease risk, its utility for selecting target behaviors and planning behavioral interventions has not been adequately tested. The lack of consensus as to the specific covert or overt behaviors that comprise "hostility" may diminish the clinical utility of these measures. Furthermore, the utility of these measures as indicators of treatment outcome has not been demonstrated.

Assessment of Anger Expression

Because many forms of anger expression can be observed overtly, they can be easily measured through behavioral observation and ratings by significant others in an individual's environment, as well as by self-report. Nonetheless, self-report remains the most readily accessible method for most clinicians. The Anger Expression Scales, derived by Spielberger (1988), represent the most recent advance in standardization of self-reported style of anger expression. These scales differentiate between two common forms of anger expression: "anger-in" and "anger-out," terms originated by Funkenstein, King, and Drolette (1954). Persons characterized as anger-in were likely to withhold or suppress anger expression, whereas anger-out persons exhibited frequent displays of aggression, using both physical and verbal means (e.g., insults, threats). Although Funkenstein et al. described these styles as two ends of a continuum of anger expression, Spielberger's (1988) analysis revealed that these components were orthogonal and required separate measurement scales. Thus, individuals can score high on both anger-in and anger-out on Spielberger's scales if they employ both strategies regularly in different situations. Spielberger added a third scale, anger control, to reflect a third strategy for expressing anger, that is, the degree to which an individual monitors the experience of anger and strives to prevent the maladaptive expression of angry feelings. Thus, these scales generate information of substantial clinical utility, in that they characterize an individual's behavioral response to confrontation across a variety of stimulus contexts.

Of course, a major problem with all self-report measures of emotion lies in the obvious face validity of such instruments and the tendency for respondents to fall prey to demand characteristics of the experimental or clinical environment. Corroboration of self-report findings by friends and family members in the individuals' natural environment will provide a different perspective on their behavioral functioning. Although a person's experience of anger and the hostile attitudes represents relatively private events not amenable to reports by others, styles of anger expression lend themselves nicely to this form of measurement. Unfortunately, only a few instruments have been validated for use in this way (e.g., Lowe & Cautela, 1978). Certainly, Speilberger's Anger Expression Scales could be employed in this manner, and such an innovative use may generate clinically meaningful outcome data for treatment programs aimed at enhancing effective expression of anger. However, additional empirical work will be required to validate this instrument for this purpose.

The observation and coding of overt behavioral responses to provocation, the hallmark of behavioral assessment, represents an important, yet often neglected, component of a comprehensive analysis of anger expression. To facilitate behavioral assessment of anger expression, standardized coding schemes have been validated for use in this manner, making behavioral coding much more tolerable (e.g., Semenchuk & Larkin, 1993). Although naturalistic observation may be difficult to arrange, analogue (e.g., role-play) methods, commonly used in research (e.g., Larkin, Zayfert, Callahan, Loren, & Pope, 1991a; Morrison, Bellack, & Manuck, 1985), can yield clinically valid portrayals of an individual's level of skill. Efforts should be made to standardize presentation of stimuli as much as possible without appearing too contrived. In addition, multiple scenes are necessary to demonstrate at least minimal cross-situation generalization of behaviors. It is important to keep in mind that a thorough analogue assessment, while providing the opportunity to display skills of interest, reveals little about factors that may influence the actual performance of skills in the naturalistic environment. Self-monitoring of anger-eliciting situations can be used to guide further assessment of factors (e.g., social anxiety) that may inhibit appropriate anger expression in a patient's natural environment.

ASSESSMENT OF BLOOD PRESSURE

Casual Blood Pressure Recordings

Because of the daily (for that matter, continuous) fluctuations observed in blood pressure in response to environmental demands, it is impossible to gather a stable record of a patient's blood pressure during a single assessment session. According to the Joint National Committee on Detection, Evaluation, and Treatment of High Blood Pressure (1988), blood pressures need to be measured across multiple sessions, at least several days apart. Minimally, three blood pressure determinations should be made over a 3-week period. Equally important is the length of time persons should sit quietly at rest prior to having their blood pressure taken; five minutes is an absolute minimum and at least 30 minutes are required if the person has just run up the stairs, smoked a cigarette, or consumed caffeinated beverages. Despite the importance of these recommendations for researchers investigating nonpharmacological methods of blood pressure reduction, they are rarely followed. Thus, blood pressure reductions observed in studies of nonpharmacological interventions for essential hypertension are often criticized for inadequate measures of blood pressure at pre- and posttreatment measurement sessions (Jacob, Chesney, Williams, Ding, & Shapiro, 1991).

Measures of Cardiovascular Reactions to Anger-Provoking Situations

As stated earlier, increased attention has been focused in recent years on the previously mentioned *reactivity hypotheses*. Information observed while a person engages in a challenging or emotionally charged situation is unique and cannot be inferred from baseline levels alone. For example, two persons with identical resting blood pressures can exhibit widely disparate increases in blood pressure in response to the same environmental stimuli. It has been hypothesized that hypertensive patients with the most intense cardiovascular reactions to anger-evoking situations exhibit the greatest risk for subsequent cardiovascular disease (e.g., Williams, Barefoot, & Shekelle, 1985), and there is some evidence to suggest this might be true. Measurement of such reactions has become increasingly simple with the advent of automated blood-pressure-assessment devices, as well as ambulatory recording instrumentation. In order to assess blood pressure responses to standard laboratory role-play interactions, an automated unit can provide regular measures of cardiovascular function without disrupting the interaction. If a more individualized assessment of blood pressure reactivity to naturally occurring stressors is desired, ambulatory methods are deemed more appropriate.

In order to develop and test a comprehensive assessment of anger and anger expression among patients with high blood pressure, we enlisted 26 hypertensive volunteers to participate in a 1-hour assessment session. We assessed behavioral and cardiovascular responses to a series of neutral and confrontive role-play vignettes. Self-reported anger and anger expression were measured using the Spielberger scales (1988), and a significant-other report of social behavior was obtained using Lowe and Cautela's Social Performance Survey Schedule (1978). Preliminary analysis of these data showed significantly higher levels of self-reported angry temperament, and less eye contact and use of positive assertive verbal statements during confrontation among hypertensives when compared with normal blood pressure controls (Larkin, Zayfert, & McKittrick, 1991b). Cardiovascular reactivity measures, adjusting for baseline differences, were not different between the two groups during the confrontive scenerios. No group differences on any behavioral or cardiovascular measure were observed during the neutral role-play interactions. A multimethod assessment procedure, such as the one described here, enabled a comprehensive assessment of anger and anger expression that served to evaluate treatment efficacy for interventions aimed at modulating the experience and expression of anger among essential hypertensive patients.

OVERVIEW OF BEHAVIORAL TREATMENTS FOR ESSENTIAL HYPERTENSION

Nonpharmacological approaches for treating essential hypertension have included weight reduction (e.g., Reisin & Frohlich, 1982), dietary interventions (e.g., Wing, Caggiula, Nowalk, Koeske, Lee, & Langford, 1984), exercise programs (see Hagberg & Seals, 1986), relaxation training (e.g., Jacob, Kraemer, & Agras, 1977), biofeedback (e.g., Blanchard, Miller, Abel, Haynes, & Wicker, 1979), and the use of yoga meditation for stress reduction (Patel, 1975). Overall, observed blood pressure reductions have been more impressive for behavioral strategies aimed at losing weight through dietary interventions or exercise programs than outcome data from stress-management approaches. In fact, Jacob et al. (1991) argue quite convincingly that observed reductions in blood pressure for stress-management approaches are, for the most part, related to inadequate assessment of blood pressure at pre- and posttreatment. When pre- and posttreatment blood pressure measures were taken over multiple office visits, observed treatment effects were minimal, with reductions in blood pressure of only a few millimeters, if present at all. The 1988 Joint National Committee on Detection, Evaluation, and Treatment of High Blood Pressure corroborated this position by stating that relaxation strategies "should not be considered as definitive treatment for patients with high blood pressure" (p. 13).

Although, in general, stress-management strategies have not consistently led to significant reductions in blood pressure, behavioral-change programs that focus on coping with anger and learning to express anger effectively, have, as yet, not been subjected to rigorous empirical scrutiny. This is somewhat surprising, considering the extensive amount of investigative work examining the relationship between anger expression and blood pressure levels (see Diamond, 1982) and the fact that well established interventions for anger management have been developed (Feindler, 1987; Novaco, 1975). To illustrate the paucity of literature in this regard, Taylor and Fortmann (1983) wrote that "the most convincing studies—to change the assertive behavior in hypertensive persons and determine effects on blood pressure—have not been done" (p. 438). Almost 10 years later, Niaura and Goldstein (1992) wrote that "behavioral treatments to improve anger management in blood pressure control ... have not yet been published" (p. 151). Therefore, despite frequent calls from authorities interested in psychosocial factors in essential hypertension, no studies to date have been conducted to examine the impact of anger-management training on blood pressure levels in hypertensive patients.

The following detailed treatment protocol was devised to assess whether training in anger management would result in lower blood pressures among patients with high or moderately high blood pressures. It must be noted that the training procedures described in this treatment protocol are not new, but rather represent a combination of other well-researched clinical strategies, including relaxation training, cognitive restructuring, assertiveness training, and behavioral role-play practice. Borrowing the term *stress inoculation* from Meichenbaum (1977) and the implementation of such a program for patients with anger-expression problems devised by Novaco (1975), this training program employed an educational phase in which participants learned a conceptual model of what anger was and how to identify problems with anger and anger expression. The educational phase was followed by a skills training component, in which participants learned to regulate physiological arousal during confrontation through diaphragmatic breathing and progressive muscle relaxation and to challenge maladaptive thinking patterns that occurred throughout confrontation. These skills were practiced during the third stage of treatment, which Meichenbaum termed the *application phase*, first during imaginal practice, followed by role-play practice, and then *in vivo* encounters. The credit for the development of the specific components of this training program belong largely to Novaco (1975, 1977b) to whom we are indebted for providing us with the necessary conceptual and procedural tools for conducting this investigation of anger-management training in essential hypertension.

ANGER-MANAGEMENT TRAINING PROCEDURES

Initial (Pregroup) Meeting

Trainers met with patients for 15 minutes following completion of the preassessment (described earlier). This brief meeting served several purposes: (1) to introduce the trainer to the subject and allow an opportunity for the trainer to begin developing rapport with the patient, (2) to briefly state the purpose of the training sessions, and (3) to introduce participants to self-monitoring procedures. The trainer (T) described the treatment as follows:

> **T:** You will be meeting with me and one other participant once each week for six training sessions of approximately 1½ hours in length. The purpose of these sessions is to train you in specific ways of coping with anger and provocation. Most people are faced with stressful, anger-provoking situations from time to time in their daily lives, and research has shown that the way in which people handle their emotional response to such situations may affect their blood pressure. Therefore, we are interested in whether teaching you some new strategies for managing your reactions to provocation will affect your resting levels of blood pressure.

The trainer also obtained a statement from each patient regarding the degree to which the subject believed he or she had a problem with anger or anger expression. A rationale for self-monitoring was provided, and participants were instructed to keep track of stressful situations that occurred in their daily lives. The form depicted in Figure 18.1 was used to record all anger-provoking situations as they occurred. Participants were instructed to jot down what happened and who was involved, and to rate the intensity of anger they experienced using a 1 to 10 scale, with 10 being the most intense anger possible. Once a person reported being angry, ratings were made hourly until the level of anger toward that target diminished to 1 on the 10-point scale. If participants were provoked more than once during a given time period, ratings for each target were separated with a slash, and both targets were rated for as long as anger persisted.

Trainers emphasized the importance of self-monitoring by suggesting that record keeping would help them develop an awareness of their angry reactions to situations and would enable the trainer to monitor their use of skills learned in training. Participants were reminded that records kept throughout training would be important data for research purposes as well. Trainers informed participants that these records would be reviewed at the beginning of each training session to determine whether new anger-provoking situations had arisen during the previous week and to assess whether participants were implementing the treatment plan successfully. Trainers ended the initial meeting by emphasizing the importance of practice in acquiring new skills. This typically took the form of a statement such as "Remember that the purpose of these sessions if for you to learn skills that will help you cope with stressful situations more effectively. Learning these skills is much like

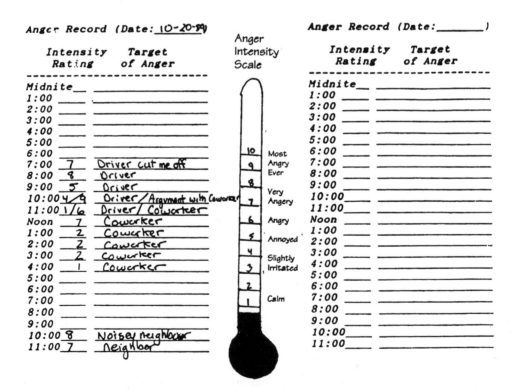

Figure 18.1. Sample anger self-monitoring record.

learning other skills, such as riding a bike or playing a musical instrument, and therefore will require regular practice."

Session 1: Assessment of Factors Affecting Anger and Didactic Presentation of Determinants of Anger

The first session began with an explanation of how training would be conducted and a discussion of confidentiality. As research participants, patients were assured further anonymity by using subject numbers in place of their name on all materials associated with the study. Participants were reminded to use their number in place of their names on all forms they completed during the training. Self-monitoring forms were collected and reviewed, and participants who had completed the homework were praised. The first 15–20 minutes of the session were used to develop rapport among participants by fostering informal conversation about each participant's personal background. As participants became familiar with one another, the trainer then introduced the rationale for the stress-inoculation program, providing participants with an overview of the training process:

> **T:** The method we are going to use to learn anger-management skills is called *stress inoculation*. Like inoculation against disease, this method works by teaching you how to handle small stressors and developing your abilities before exposing yourself to greater stressors. In this manner, success in dealing with minor irritations will enable you to learn how to deal with more challenging anger-provoking situations more successfully. Stress inoculation involves three phases: education, skills training, and practice. During the education phase, which we are conducting today, you will learn information about anger, including what it is, what it does for people, and how you can identify and control it. Then, together, we will look at how you experience and handle anger-provoking situations in your life. During the skills training phase, which begins next week, you will learn some techniques that have been shown to be helpful in dealing with anger-provoking situations. Finally, we will practice these skills in-session, first using easy situations and progressing to more difficult ones. During the practice phase, I will be asking you to try out these new skills in situations in your real life, starting with easy situations and progressing to more difficult ones.

Prior to the overview of the primary components of anger, the trainer conducted a Situation X Person X Mode of Expression analysis of each participant's anger problems as suggested by Novaco (1977b). This involved examining the range of settings in which the person functions (i.e., home, occupational setting, school, recreational location, driving), the persons involved in those settings (i.e., parents, spouse, siblings, friends, co-workers, strangers), and how anger was expressed when aroused (i.e., physical confrontation, passive–aggressive behaviors, avoidance, constructive compromise, assertive confrontation). Information from each participant's matrix was used to identify specific deficits in anger control for each patient (see Figure 18.2 for a sample matrix). Although trainers attempted to conduct a thorough analysis during this first session, assessment inevitably continued throughout the training program as participants' heightened awareness revealed additional information about their patterns of anger expression.

Didactic Presentation of Determinants of Anger

The educational component of the anger-management training began with a description of anger based on Novaco's formulation (1975, 1977b).

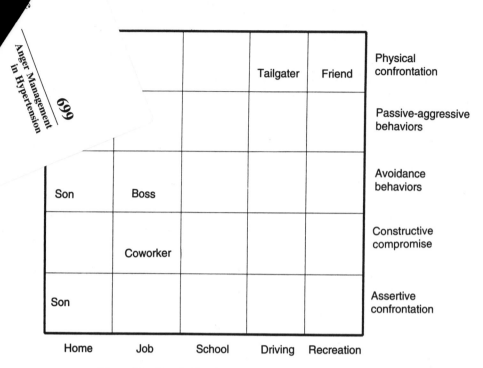

Figure 18.2. Sample Situation X Person X Mode of Expression matrix.

T: Anger is an emotion that occurs in response to certain kinds of provocative situations. Although some of these situations are nonpersonal, like hitting your thumb with a hammer, most anger-provoking situations are interpersonal in nature. Situations that evoke anger often are perceived as threatening to your physical or psychological well-being. Anger is a feeling, which is different from aggression. Aggression is one of many actions people may take in response to anger. As a feeling, anger may not be recognized by others, even when you feel it intensely. Anger expression, on the other hand, is observable, and some forms of anger expression, such as physical assault, are very obvious to others around you. In general, the more anger you feel, the greater likelihood you will engage in aggressive behavior. Aggressive behavior, in contrast, rarely occurs in persons who experience little anger. Anger, itself, is not a bad emotion. In fact, it can be very useful in motivating us to stand up for ourselves when we are being taken advantage of. It also provides us with energy to confront injustices or unfair situations in our lives. Anger becomes a problem when it is too intense or too frequent. In both cases, life can be pretty miserable, even if we know how to manage our anger appropriately. Anger management involves two things: (1) learning to control the experience of anger when it is too intense or too frequent, and (2) learning to express even mild experiences of anger through appropriate assertive means.

Next, participants selected from their self-monitoring record (or from the assessment matrix) a recent anger experience that they were willing to share with the group. The trainer instructed participants to recall the anger experience by closing their eyes and "reliving" the provocation and their response in their head. They were instructed to attend to detail (e.g., "Picture the room you are in and the individuals present") and to recall the person or situation that provoked anger and what they did, felt, and said. Participants were further prompted to recall thoughts or images that were going through their minds in response to the provocation and how angry they became. Attention was also focused on bodily sensations that participants recalled (e.g., heart pounding, sweating, muscle tension). The trainer then used an example to illustrate the response domains involved in the experience of anger (e.g., driving a car and being cut off by an inconsiderate driver). In doing this, the trainer reported cognitive responses (e.g., "They did that on purpose"), somatic responses (e.g., heart pounding), and behavioral reactions (e.g., swearing at the driver, clenching steering wheel tighter). For the purposes of this study, this standard disclosure was employed. Although in clinical settings, actual provocations that produced moderate-intensity anger and were resolved may be better to disclose, certain situations would be inappropriate for self-disclosure (e.g., an ongoing dispute between the therapist and his or her spouse).

Following the trainer's self-disclosure, each subject reported to the group the thoughts, feelings, and behaviors experienced prior to, during, and following his or her specific anger incident. Each group member then depicted the specific situation, as well as cognitive, physiological, and observable behavioral reactions to the event on a handout. Following this exercise, each component of anger was reviewed in greater detail as recommended by Novaco (1977b), referring to the participants' experiences for examples when applicable. A list of environmental events that aroused anger was created for each patient including frustrations (instances in which goal attainment is blocked), annoyances and minor irritations (e.g., interruptions, accidents such as breaking something), verbal or physical abuse, and situations involving social injustice or unfairness (e.g., discrimination). For each of these environmental events, internal cognitive and physiological responses occurring during the angry episodes were examined, including cognitive appraisals of a perceived threat or demand (e.g., "That person rammed my car with his shopping cart on purpose!"), expectations of confrontation (e.g., "That person doesn't like me and is out to get me" or "If he says 'no', I'm going to slug him"), negative self-statements (e.g., "I'm no good at this; I can't tell her off"), and physiological arousal (e.g., motor tension, autonomic arousal, sweating, choking sensations).

Next, the group examined behavioral reactions to anger-provoking events (e.g., antagonism, hostility, avoidance). Particular attention was paid to how each group member typically responded when provoked in each type of situation. Discussion spanned the range along the continuum of behavior from withdrawal and avoidance to antagonism, hostility, and aggression. Trainers also assessed whether participants felt they exhibited appropriate expression of anger or positive, assertive behavior in particular types of situations.

In addition to identifying patterns of responses to anger for each participant, the discussion included analysis of affective states subsequent to the expression of anger. Analysis of postresponse affective states included descriptions of how participants felt following their anger responses, focusing on feelings of satisfaction, guilt, and/or disappointment. The trainer also examined how others responded to the participants' expression of anger. This included a discussion of the impact of participants' responses to anger on relevant interpersonal relationships. Elucidation of the affective and interpersonal consequences of anger expression (or inexpression) set the stage for further discussion of the functions of anger according to Novaco (1977b), as follows:

T: Anger has both positive and negative functions. Although it can lead to interpersonal frustrations, disruptive or antagonistic interactions, and feelings of dissatisfaction, it can also provide us with energy to mobilize our bodies to confront injustices. Furthermore, it can serve as a signal or cue that we need to employ a coping response to remove a potential source of threat from our environment. Anger management is, therefore, not about eliminating anger, but rather about learning how to keep anger at moderate levels in order to achieve your desired goal in a given situation. This means learning to use anger to take constructive action aimed at solving a problem (i.e., take a task orientation), and to use it as a source of energy to accomplish that action. Anger management involves learning (1) to identify the internal and external cues related to your own anger, (2) to modify internal cognitive and physiological processes to keep anger at moderate levels, and (3) to maximize your ability to take constructive action. If you tend to withdraw, this course of anger-management training will encourage you to express your anger more assertively. If you tend to be aggressive, the training will introduce you to skills for expressing your anger more appropriately.

Finally, participants were instructed to continue self-monitoring and to tune in to anger-eliciting thoughts that occurred when anger was experienced during the intervening week. As homework, they were instructed to identify five situations in which they would like to improve their ability to express anger and to describe each of these situations on an index card.

Session 2: Introduction to Relaxation Training

Session 2 began with a review of patient self-monitoring and discussion of recent anger experiences in order to get a more comprehensive view of situations, persons, and modes of expression involved with anger arousal for each participant. Private speech that accompanied anger arousal was also discussed. The five index cards describing the situations that participants generated were collected for later use.

Relaxation Training

The remainder of this session was spent learning relaxation and imagery. First, trainers provided a rationale for how relaxation may help reduce physiological arousal and foster a sense of control in anger-provoking situations. A specific rationale for deep breathing and muscle relaxation was also presented (see Poppen, 1988; Bernstein & Borkovec, 1973). For example,

T: Deep breathing involves learning to use the diaphragm (muscle between lungs and stomach) rather than the shoulder and chest muscles, to draw air into the lungs. This allows more efficient breathing with less muscular work. Diaphragmatic breathing offers a unique method for effectively reducing nervous system arousal, and is particularly effective in relaxing the vascular system. This, in itself, may be useful in controlling hypertension. Diaphragmatic breathing, when used in a stressful situation, can help you to stay calm so that you can carry out strategies you will learn later in training.

Following the presentation of the rationale, each participant was instructed in the technique and guided through several minutes of deep breathing in-session, emphasizing the importance of breathing control in achieving relaxation. The instructions were as follows:

T: Place your right hand on your stomach, between the bottom of your rib cage and your navel (just above the belt line). Place your left hand on your chest, on your breast bone (sternum), just below your collar bone (clavicle). Now just breathe regularly through your nose, and notice the rise and fall of your hands as you breathe in (inhale) and breathe out (exhale). As you breathe in, imagine your stomach to be a balloon that inflates, lifting your right hand. As you breathe out, the balloon deflates, and your right hand falls. Your left hand remains still as your right hand rises and falls. Do not try to force it. Just attend to the motion of your hands and the feelings in your chest. Allow your right hand to rise and fall while your left hand remains still. Imagine that your right hand is a boat, rising and falling on the slow, rolling waves of the ocean, while your left hand sits quickly at the dock. Next slow your breathing by pausing very briefly at the top and bottom of each breath. Just a half-second or so. Do not hold your breath or pause so you are uncomfortable. Notice how there is a slight increase in tension as you breathe in, and a decrease as you breathe out. Concentrate on the tension flowing out with each breath. A slight increase in tension as you inhale, and then let go as you exhale. Each time you exhale, feel the tension leaving your body. (Adapted from Poppen, 1988, p. 67)

Using gentle shaping, positive aspects of the breathing pattern were praised, with occasional corrective feedback for negative aspects. Trainers paid close attention to the participants' use of diaphragmatic breathing and provided feedback and correction, shaping patients until they both successfully completed several minutes of breathing. Once each patient displayed proper use of the diaphragm during breathing, the rationale for muscle-relaxation training was presented (see Bernstein & Borkovec, 1973). The tension-release cycles for each of the 16 muscle groups were demonstrated for participants, as described for the initial relaxation session by Bernstein and Borkovec, followed by a complete session of progressive muscle tension–release relaxation. During the last 2 minutes of relaxation, participants were prompted to imagine a quiet and relaxing scene. Following the entire relaxation procedure, the effects of the relaxation procedures were assessed, and participants were questioned about their relaxation experience.

As homework following Session 2, participants were instructed to practice the relaxation exercises at home once each day, using a tape provided by the trainer. A record of the practice sessions was kept on the forms provided (see Figure 18.3). To assure compliance with the relaxation practice, the tapes used were marked with zero, one, or two soft tones, which patients were instructed to count and record on these forms. In addition, participants were instructed to continue identifying anger-eliciting thoughts and to continue self-monitoring during the coming week.

Session 3: Self-Statement Modification and Assertive Anger Expression

Session 3 began with a brief review of each participant's relaxation records and self-monitoring records. Difficulties with practicing relaxation were discussed. Anger experiences that had occurred since the last meeting were discussed to refine and confirm the assessment of how subjects typically handled anger. This discussion focused on self-talk that subjects engaged in during anger-provoking situations. Next, trainers provided a rationale for self-statement modification that followed the following example:

T: Managing anger means maximizing the positive functions of anger and minimizing the negative ones. Anger management involves learning to keep anger at moderate levels, and to use it as a signal to take constructive action and as a source of energy to accomplish goals. As

Kevin T. Larkin and
Claudia Zayfert

RELAXATION PRACTICE RECORD

_____ SUBJECT NO. _____

INSTRUCTIONS: Prior to practicing, rate the average level of tension that you experienced for the day. Then on a scale from 0 to 10 as indicated below, rate your level of TENSION both <u>before</u> and <u>after</u> practicing relaxation. Please bring completed form with you to your next session.

- **0 = TOTAL RELAXATION, FEELING AS RELAXED AS YOU HAVE EVER FELT**
- **2.5 = CONSIDERABLY RELAXED**
- **5 = A MID-POINT SOMEWHERE IN BETWEEN RELAXED AND TENSE**
- **7.5 = SOMEWHAT TENSE**
- **10 = EXTREMELY TENSE, AS TENSE AS YOU HAVE EVER BEEN**

DATE _____ TAPE NUMBER _____ NUMBER OF TONES HEARD _____ DAILY TENSION RATING .... _____ TENSION BEFORE RELAXATION .... _____ TENSION AFTER RELAXATION .... _____ Comments _____ _____ _____	DATE _____ TAPE NUMBER _____ NUMBER OF TONES HEARD _____ DAILY TENSION RATING .... _____ TENSION BEFORE RELAXATION .... _____ TENSION AFTER RELAXATION .... _____ Comments _____ _____ _____
DATE _____ TAPE NUMBER _____ NUMBER OF TONES HEARD _____ DAILY TENSION RATING .... _____ TENSION BEFORE RELAXATION .... _____ TENSION AFTER RELAXATION .... _____ Comments _____ _____ _____	DATE _____ TAPE NUMBER _____ NUMBER OF TONES HEARD _____ DAILY TENSION RATING .... _____ TENSION BEFORE RELAXATION .... _____ TENSION AFTER RELAXATION .... _____ Comments _____ _____ _____
DATE _____ TAPE NUMBER _____ NUMBER OF TONES HEARD _____ DAILY TENSION RATING .... _____ TENSION BEFORE RELAXATION .... _____ TENSION AFTER RELAXATION .... _____ Comments _____ _____ _____	DATE _____ TAPE NUMBER _____ NUMBER OF TONES HEARD _____ DAILY TENSION RATING .... _____ TENSION BEFORE RELAXATION .... _____ TENSION AFTER RELAXATION .... _____ Comments _____ _____ _____
DATE _____ TAPE NUMBER _____ NUMBER OF TONES HEARD _____ DAILY TENSION RATING .... _____ TENSION BEFORE RELAXATION .... _____ TENSION AFTER RELAXATION .... _____ Comments _____ _____ _____	DATE _____ TAPE NUMBER _____ NUMBER OF TONES HEARD _____ DAILY TENSION RATING .... _____ TENSION BEFORE RELAXATION .... _____ TENSION AFTER RELAXATION .... _____ Comments _____ _____ _____

PLEASE BRING COMPLETED SHEET WITH YOU TO THE NEXT SESSION

Figure 18.3. Relaxation self-monitoring record.

shown during our first session, anger is related to thoughts surrounding events that elicit it. For example, recall the driving incident I shared with you during our first session. I perceived the other driver as intentionally cutting me off, and this may have aggravated my angry feelings. Learning to challenge or question thoughts that accompanied the anger experience can help me to regulate the intensity and duration of this anger experience.

Disputing Hostile Thoughts.   Trainers used the A-B-C (Activating event–Belief–Consequence) model derived from rational–emotive therapy (Ellis, 1962) to demonstrate how different thought processes can lead to different emotional consequences. This led to a discussion of alternative ways of conceptualizing situations. The trainers introduced techniques commonly used in cognitive–behavioral therapy, such as examining the evidence for attributions, looking for alternative interpretations, identifying irrational thinking (i.e., "catastrophizing," "mind reading," "fortune-telling"), and examining the cost–benefit of getting angry. Using self-disclosure (i.e., the driving example), the trainer outlined his or her own A-B-C's and then, using the diagram in Figure 18.4, demonstrated effective disputing statements based on each of these methods. For example, such disputing self-talk included "What is the evidence that the driver was purposefully trying to cause an accident?", "What are alternative interpretations of the driver's behavior? He may be rushing his wife to the hospital," "Am I making too big a deal of this? (catastrophizing) I don't really know he was thinking he owns the road (mind reading)," and "What are the advantages and disadvantages of my continuing to get upset about the driver cutting me off. Maintaining my anger distracts me from more important things."

Following the trainer's disclosure of his or her situation, examples from participants' self-monitoring forms were used to demonstrate how to dispute hostile thoughts. Because participants had begun to identify cognitions associated with anger through their self-

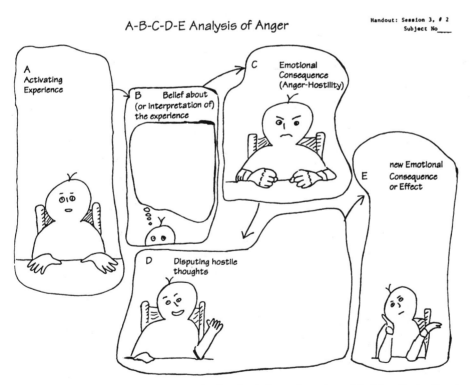

Figure 18.4. Worksheet for analyzing maladaptive thoughts during confrontation and devising effective disputing self-statements.

monitoring, translation of their internal dialogue into the A-B-C format was not very difficult. If participants had trouble generating effective disputing statements, the group helped each other in developing effective disputes.

Using Positive, Coping Self-Statements. In addition to developing skill in disputing anger-eliciting cognitions, the program introduced cognitive coping skills that would be helpful in preparing for confrontation or provocation. Borrowing from the method outlined by Novaco (1975, 1977b) and Meichanbaum (1977), trainers demonstrated positive self-talk for anticipation of confrontation, dealing with arousal during confrontation, and evaluating one's response following a provocation. The four stages of coping with provocation outlined by Novaco (1977b) were (1) preparing for provocation, (2) impact and confrontation, (3) coping with arousal and agitation, and (4) reflecting on conflict resolution (or not). The trainer referred again to the driving situation, in offering examples of effective statements for each stage of coping:

- *Preparing for provocation.* "Here it comes: I can see he's going to cut me off. I can handle it. What should I do to get out of his way?"
- *Impact and confrontation.* "Stay calm. There's nothing I can do about the way people drive."
- *Coping with arousal and agitation.* "I feel myself getting upset. It's time to take a deep breath. Try to stay relaxed and focus on what to do to avoid an accident."
- *Reflecting on conflict resolution.* "That was close; I handled it well. It could have been a lot worse. No point being aggravated, it's just going to interfere with focusing on the important things I need to do today."

Using examples from participants' self-monitoring, specific, positive self-statements were developed for each person.

Rationale for Assertive Anger Expression

Because Session 3 covered a number of important skills, it might have been advantageous for the trainer to stop here and instruct participants to practice self-statement modification during the subsequent week. However, in order to assure equivalent length of training for all participants in the present application, the rationale and overview of assertion training was also provided during this session. The rationale for assertiveness training was as follows:

T: Assertion involves standing up for personal rights and expressing thoughts, feelings, and beliefs in direct, honest, and appropriate ways that do not violate the rights of others. Assertion involves respecting your own needs and rights as well as others' needs and rights. Learning to express yourself assertively is an important skill in managing anger, because many anger provocations may be avoided by making your needs, beliefs, and feelings clear to others. Clear communication helps to avoid conflict. If others are not aware of your needs, opinions, and feelings, they cannot act in ways that demonstrate respect for them. Also, when you are provoked, assertion skills will enable you to act to solve the problem at hand, and avoid escalating conflict and increasing your anger and arousal; that is, assertion skills enable you to express your opinions and meet your needs in a diplomatic way—without offending the rights of others. (Adapted from Jakubowski & Lange, 1978)

Following this brief rationale, the trainer provided further description of the difference between passive, assertive, and aggressive responses, pointing out that aggressive behavior errs by not respecting the rights of others, and passive, nonassertive behavior does not adequately protect one's rights, because needs are not adequately communicated. Next, the trainer briefly reviewed body-language correlates of each type of behavior and then described verbal assertive responses:

> **T:** "I language" is a useful guide for helping people to express difficult negative feelings in an assertive way. In addition, the use of "I language" can be helpful in identifying whether your rights and feelings have been violated in a particular situation. Here's how to use "I language." When ... (describe other person's behavior) the effects are ... (describe how other person's behavior effects your life or feelings), I feel ... (describe feelings), and I'd prefer ... (describe what you want).

Examples such as the following were provided for a number of situations:

- *Aggressive*: "You make me so angry when you make so much noise! What's wrong with you anyway?"
- *Non-assertive*: "Um ... I'm trying to work here ... maybe you could ... uh ... keep your voice down a little?"
- *Assertive*: "When you talk loudly near my desk while I am working, I find it hard to think and concentrate on my work. I am upset about this and I would like you to go somewhere else to talk."

At the end of Session 3, participants were instructed to continue self-monitoring and relaxation practice, to practice disputing hostile thoughts using blank A-B-C worksheets, and to develop self-statements and positive, coping self-statements for each of the five situations they had described on index cards earlier in the training program. They were also asked to complete the Assertive Behavior Discrimination Test (Jakubowski & Lange, 1978) which assesses ability to distinguish assertive, nonassertive, and aggressive responses to confrontation.

Session 4: Establishment of the Anger Hierarchy and Imaginal Desensitization

As with previous sessions, the group began with a review of self-monitoring records and relaxation practice. Participants were encouraged to objectively critique the manner in which they responded to anger-provoking situations over the past week. The group reviewed each others' responses to the Discrimination Test, disputing hostile thoughts, and positive, coping self-statements during the first several minutes of the session.

Rationale for Imaginal Coping

Trainers then explained the rationale for using imaginal practice before practicing skills in real-life situations:

> **T:** Last week we covered several methods for coping constructively with anger-provoking situations. Hearing and reading about such techniques is quite different from actually using

them, however. Using them takes a good deal of preparation. Today we are going to help you prepare to use these techniques by practicing them imaginally. Imaginal practice is an extremely useful method of learning new skills. In fact, you probably do this very often without realizing you are doing it. Perhaps you have thought through what you might say to your boss when asking for a raise, or reviewed a difficult procedure or athletic skill mentally before trying it out. Today we are going to try out some of these imaginal practice techniques, focusing on what you have learned so far during this training program. Another important aspect of our approach today is that we are going to practice using easy situations first and gradually progress to more difficult ones. This is important, because a new skill requires careful attention and thought. If you are aroused from anger or anxiety, this will interfere with your ability to think things through carefully. Moreover, more difficult situations will require more sophisticated skills that you will develop with practice.

Establishment of the Hierarchy

The trainer then reviewed the anger scenarios submitted by participants in Session 2, and participants were allowed to change or substitute other scenes as they felt appropriate. Each scene was then described in detail on an index card, and participants were encouraged to write "I statements" or coping self-statements for each situation on the back of each card to serve as prompts to refer to prior to each imaginal practice scene. Anger scenarios were ordered so that a graduated series of five situations was determined for each participant. If the scenes did not reflect a gradual variation in intensity/difficulty, suggestions for modification were made as needed.

Imaginal Coping Procedure

The procedures for imaginal coping were explained as follows:

T: First we will relax for a few minutes; then I'll ask you to read over your scene. I'll ask you to close your eyes again and imagine a specific scene in detail, focusing on use of your new coping skills. It is not expected that you will imagine yourself coping successfully at first; everyone will progress at his or her own pace.

Participants then read over their descriptions of a tranquil scene and were instructed to relax using deep breathing and imagery. After having them imagine the relaxing scene for one minute, the trainer presented the first anger-hierarchy scene (e.g., a mild annoyance) using the following statement, and participants imagined it for 30 seconds:

T: Just continue relaxing like that. Now I want you to open your eyes and read over the description of your first anger-provoking scene and your coping statements. Now close your eyes again, and imagine the scene you just read in detail. See it as clearly and as vividly as you can. Imagine that you are actually in this situation, notice the feelings in your body, and pay attention to the thoughts you are thinking about the situation and people involved. Now imagine yourself coping with the situation. Imagine yourself breathing deeply, relaxing, and using your positive coping self-statements. See yourself staying composed, relaxing, settling down. Continue to imagine the scene, but see yourself handling if effectively, using the skills you have learned thus far to direct your anger constructively to achieve your goals.

To assess progress, imaginal coping with the first scene was reviewed by having participants rate how well they used their cognitive and behavioral coping skills on a 4-point scale (A = *Successful*; B = *Somewhat Successful*; C = *Somewhat Unsuccessful*; and D = *Unsuc-*

cessful). Participants were instructed to open their eyes and provide their ratings, and the group discussed the efficacy of various coping strategies that they used. Imaginal coping during the first scene was repeated until all participants gave a rating of A or B on two consecutive trials. If a participant could not imagine him- or herself coping by the third trial, the procedure was stopped and ways to enhance coping were discussed. Other group members shared how they dealt with their situations. When all participants rated coping as an A or B for two consecutive trials, the group progressed to the second scene. An identical procedure was employed for the remaining four scenes. Progression through the scenes was idiosyncratic, working at the pace of the slowest group member.

As in previous sessions, participants were instructed to continue self-monitoring and engaging in daily relaxation practice, and to take a few minutes to imaginally practice coping skills immediately following, but not during, situations that occurred during the following week. In other words, participants were not yet instructed to alter how they handled anger-provoking situations in their real lives.

Session 5: Role-Play Rehearsal

At the beginning of Session 5, homework records were checked, with a particular focus on whether patients practiced coping skills following situations that came up during the week. Subjects were questioned as to whether they were able to generate coping statements for the situations or come up with assertive alternatives, and these situations were discussed in the group.

Rationale for Role-Play Rehearsal

In presenting the rationale for role-play rehearsal, the value of practicing in the group to prepare for situations in real life was explained as follows:

T: Today we are going to try out some of your new skills by practicing them in role plays of situations we encounter. Practicing the techniques before they are needed will help you to feel comfortable using them in a real-life situation. The role plays will give you the opportunity to improve your skills, to try out different strategies for dealing with situations, and to experience the reactions of others to your new behaviors. By starting with the first situation on your hierarchy, we can work on developing skills to deal with easier situations until we feel comfortable with them, and gradually increase to the more stressful or difficult situations.

Role-Play Rehearsal Procedure

The trainer conveyed to group participants that for anger to be used in positive ways, arousal must be kept at moderate levels. The components of a problem-solving approach to conflict, as suggested by Novaco (1977b), were again reviewed, focusing on three areas during the role plays: communication of feelings, use of assertive responses, and maintenance of a task orientation.

T: Effective anger management requires knowing how to communicate feelings to others in the environment; finding a balance between a hostile, aggressive style and a passive, submissive one; sticking up for your rights without intruding on the rights of others; and keeping a task orientation.

Subjects then reviewed their self-statements and disputations in preparation for the role plays of situations from their hierarchies. Each patient started with the first situation on her or his hierarchy by participating in a reverse role play in order to experience first the other person's viewpoint in the situation. The reverse role play was followed by an actual role play, with the participant playing the role of him- or herself. Each role play was discussed in terms of use of the skills learned, with the trainer employing positive feedback when appropriate to shape better assertive statements and behaviors. Both behavioral correlates of covert skills and overt assertive behaviors were shaped (e.g., "When you took a deep breath before you spoke, I had the feeling you were keeping calm even though you were very annoyed" or "I noticed that you paused before you explained what you wanted—What were you saying to yourself then?"). The role-play practices were conducted using a successive approximations shaping process, rewarding positive gains, and providing corrective feedback in small doses.

Relaxation practice and self-monitoring were continued as homework assignments prior to the final training session. Finally, using a situation that was low on each patient's hierarchy, each participant was requested to prepare cognitive and behavioral coping strategies and to try expressing her or his anger for a relatively easy situation, or one like it, that occurred during the intervening week.

Session 6: Role-Play Rehearsal, Summary of Anger-Management Techniques, and Conclusion

In reviewing homework practice, particular attention was paid to the assignment to practice coping skills in a situation low on the patients' hierarchy. Specifically, were they able to generate coping statements for the situations? Were they able to come up with assertive alternatives? Were they able to modulate their arousal level? How confident did they feel using these skills? Did they feel more effective in handling the stressor? Remembering to praise accomplishments, the trainer employed a problem-solving approach to develop alternative solutions for any difficulties that might have arisen. The remainder of the hierarchy scenes were role-played during the final session, providing extensive feedback and shaping, as outlined in Session 5. Other problematic situations monitored during the training period that were not included in the hierarchy were also included as role-play foci. The session finished with a review of all of the skills learned during the training program:

> **T:** The anger-management program you have been through involved learning to increase awareness and be able to identify the internal and external events related to your own anger, reduce arousal by reducing physiological responses and modifying maladaptive thought processes to keep anger intensity at moderate levels, and express feelings of anger in an assertive, direct, but nonthreatening manner. Becoming proficient at all techniques taught in this training is essential to managing arousal in stressful situations and will require ongoing practice. Maintaining a repertoire of effective coping self-statements and disputations for "irrational" thoughts is essential for keeping anger from escalating, and for keeping a problem-solving, task-focused orientation to the situation. Learning to express yourself assertively is an important skill in managing anger, because clear communication of feelings helps to avoid conflict. When you are provoked, assertion skills will enable you to act to solve the problem at hand and avoid escalation of conflict.

Participants were requested to proceed at a gradual pace as they further developed and reinforced their skills through successful experiences using them in their daily lives. Subjects were cautioned to not use these techniques in situations that they were not ready for, as doing so might lead to disappointment and discouragement. However, by continuing to employ skills in appropriately challenging situations, they would be able to continue to develop them and eventually become more sophisticated in their use.

MAINTENANCE AND GENERALIZATION STRATEGIES

Obviously, interventions of this nature are of little clinical importance if the skills learned cannot be incorporated into everyday living. Although imaginal and role-play practice can resemble real-life interactions, the affect experienced *in vivo* is predictably more intense and longer lasting than that encountered in role-play practice. Therefore, use of imaginal practice and role-play rehearsal will, at best, be perceived as low-level provocation. In the present treatment protocol, patients were assigned to practice coping with provocation for one real-life situation between Sessions 5 and 6. Although there is no substitute for natural observation of actual interpersonal encounters, patients' self-report was the only information gathered regarding generalization to real-life situations. Data from a posttreatment satisfaction questionnaire were encouraging, with most patients placing a great deal of value on what they learned and reporting continued use of the skills they had developed. Maintenance of treatment gains can also be assessed through comprehensive posttreatment and follow-up assessment sessions. In the present application, posttreatment assessment methods included self-reported measures of anger, assertion, and anger expression, significant-other reports of social behaviors, heart rate and blood pressure responses that occurred during confrontation, and behavioral coding of assertive verbalizations and nonverbal facial and motoric behaviors during confrontation. At the very least, such assessment strategies affirmed that participants learned the skills; whether they continued to use them regularly is a question for future investigation.

PROBLEMS IN IMPLEMENTATION

A major problem for treatment studies of the type described herein is maintaining treatment compliance and minimizing participant attrition during training. Regarding compliance, development of an easy-to-carry booklet-type self-monitoring form appeared to facilitate compliance with that procedure. Almost all participants turned in their monitoring records on a weekly basis. The simplicity of the data being monitored and the trainer's frequent praise for compliance also helped in this regard. All other homework assignments were bound in an attractive patient handbook that the patients typically brought with them to each session. For the most part, this facilitated completion of these records as well. Compliance with relaxation training, however, represented a greater challenge due to the increased time required to practice relaxation and the lifestyle alteration that daily relaxation practice entailed. In order to best assess for compliance with relaxation instructions, specially marked relaxation tapes were created; either zero, one, or two soft tones were randomly located on the recording, and participants were instructed to monitor each tape assigned for these tones. Although compliance was extremely variable, most participants practiced relaxation on at least 18 days during the 6-week program.

Although attrition was minimal once subjects commenced training, scheduling difficulties created significant problems. Whenever one patient canceled or missed a session, the trainer had to either cancel the entire session or arrange to meet individually with the participant who canceled so he or she would have the necessary information for the next weekly session. These problems occurred in every training group at least once, forcing the consideration and eventual adoption of individual training programs for some of the participants. Although some sessions could easily be conducted individually, as well as in a group format (e.g., relaxation training), others clearly worked better in group format (e.g., role-play rehearsal). Regarding attrition, only one patient who started the training failed to complete the program. We attribute our success in maintaining our participants' interest in the training program to the fast pace of the training program and the ability to conduct training in a six-session format; an increased number of sessions, we believe, would have greatly increased our attrition rate. Also, because a significant portion of the first session was devoted to developing rapport, participants felt comfortable with one another and remarked on how useful it was to hear that others' struggles with anger expression were similar to their own.

CASE ILLUSTRATION

Reductions in casual blood pressure observed in this study were quite variable, with some persons exhibiting substantial decreases in blood pressure with training, some showing no change, and some actually showing small increases. Overall, however, significant reductions in diastolic blood pressure were observed in the treatment group in contrast to subjects in a no-treatment control condition (Larkin et al., 1991a). The variability in treatment response was expected, however, because no criterion was established to select only essential hypertensive patients who were of normal weight, consumed low salt diets, and reported having anger-expression problems. A few of our participants were obese, and blood pressures were not expected to change very much for these patients following completion of the anger-management training. To our surprise, however, none of the hypertensive subjects who had participated in the assessment phase of the project described earlier (Larkin et al., 1991b) declined treatment because they did not feel they had a problem expressing anger! These findings clearly argue for a better assessment of patient–treatment match regarding the factors involved in maintaining a patient's elevated arterial pressures. Recognizing that such variability exists, the case to be illustrated is of a woman whose blood pressure was significantly lowered through this 6-week course in anger-management training.

Donna was a 45-year-old, married, white female of normal weight, with no health problems other than a diagnosis of essential hypertension. Her recorded blood pressure of 163/88 mm Hg represents the average of nine blood pressure determinations obtained during three office visits occurring over a 3-week period. She had never received treatment for her blood pressure condition and exhibited no related cardiac risk factors (e.g., she did not smoke and had normal blood-cholesterol levels). Donna's pre- and posttreatment cardiovascular, self-report, and behavioral characteristics are depicted in Table 18.2. Regarding pretreatment information, the patient exhibited a somewhat greater-than-normal trait anger–temperament score ($T = 62$) accompanied by a less-than-average trait reactive

Table 18.2. Donna's Pre- and Posttreatment Assessment Data

	Pretreatment	Posttreatment
Cardiovascular measures		
Casual SBP (mm Hg)	163	132
Causal DBP (mm Hg)	88	85
Resting HR (bpm)	80	81
SBP reaction anger (mm Hg)	+35.5	+28.5
DBP reaction anger (mm Hg)	+5.0	+12.0
Self-report measures		
Trait anger	17	15
Trait/temperament	9	6
Trait/reaction	7	6
Anger in	11	12
Anger out	15	15
Anger control	19	22
Anger expression	23	21
Rathus Assertion	37	25
Framingham Type A	6	4
Behavioral Measures During Role-Play Provocation		
Assertive verbalization (freq./scene)	2.2	3.8
Assertive tone (1–5)	3.1	3.0
Assertive volume (1–5)	3.0	3.0
Assertive speech pace (1–5)	3.0	3.0
Assertive response latency (sec)	3.0	1.0
Assertive eye contact (sec/scene)	11.5	17.8
Nonverbal distractions (freq./scene)	8.5	8.5
Speech disturbances (freq./scene)	1.5	0.8

score ($T = 37$). Furthermore, the patient reported a greater tendency to express anger outward (anger-out: $T = 54$) than to hold it in (anger-in: $T = 40$). These self-reported findings were corroborated by the greater-than-average score on the Rathus Assertiveness Test and the Framingham measure of Type A behavior pattern. Although no normative information was available on behavioral coding data, the behaviors portrayed during role-play confrontation (e.g., poor eye contact, lengthy response latency, few assertive statements, and frequent speech disturbances (e.g., "uh", "uhm")) were also congruent with the data obtained from self-report instruments. Overall, Donna's anger problem was conceptualized as a fiery temper that was typically expressed overtly, but in an ineffective manner.

Donna was an exemplary patient who completed all homework assignments and kept excellent weekly self-monitoring records. In treatment, she identified several anger-evoking situations that she wanted to work on, including being angry at tailgating drivers, listening to sexist or racist comments made by others, and interacting with family members who were disrespectful of her. The patient practiced relaxation on 25 of the 35 days she was in treatment and readily learned to reduce her daily levels of tension. She employed both relaxation strategies and coping self-statements in dealing with all scenes on her hierarchy, first imaginally and then in role-play practice. The patient reported being able to employ the skills she had learned in training in real-life situations that evoked anger, and treatment was discontinued after the six group-training sessions.

Posttreatment data, also depicted in Table 18.2, show that Donna learned how to employ more positive assertive statements, decreased her frequency of speech disturbances, and increased her eye contact as a result of the training program. Her trait anger score decreased slightly, indicating that her temperament was somewhat less fiery at posttreatment, and that her ability to control her anger improved slightly. Her scores on the Rathus Assertiveness Test and the Framingham Type A Behavior Questionnaire also reflected these changes. Most important, both her systolic and diastolic blood pressure were reduced substantially, to the point that she no longer warranted a diagnosis of essential hypertension.

SUMMARY

For some patients, anger-management training represents a reasonable nonpharmacologic intervention that can result in substantial reductions in both systolic and diastolic blood pressure. Although some have argued that interventions of this sort should only be employed with mild or "borderline" essential hypertensive patients, our data show that even some sustained high blood pressure patients benefited greatly from this approach. The primary problem that confronts the clinician, however, is knowing who will achieve these reductions in blood pressure as a result of training, and how enduring these treatment effects might be. Given that we know very little about the characteristics of patients who get better with anger-management treatments, it is wise to be cautious about the wide clinical application of such procedures. Additional research examining the characteristics of those patients who will improve through these interventions, which components of the intervention protocol are most likely responsible for observed changes in blood pressure, and the important question of maintenance of normal levels of arterial pressure for extended periods after training need to be conducted. In summary, anger-management training works for some essential hypertensive patients through mechanisms that are presently unclear.

ACKNOWLEDGMENTS. Completion of this chapter was supported in part by a Grant-In-Aid by the American Heart Association–West Virginia Affiliate, awarded to KTL and the sabbatical leave program at West Virginia University. The authors would like to thank Ty Callahan, Kathy Pope, Brenda Loren, and Diane Garrett for serving as group trainers for this investigation. Correspondence pertaining to this chapter should be addressed to Kevin T. Larkin, Ph.D., Department of Psychology, P. O. Box 6040, West Virginia University, Morgantown, WV 26506–6040.

REFERENCES

Alexander, F. (1939). Emotional factors in essential hypertension: Presentation of a tentative hypothesis. *Psychosomatic Medicine, 1*, 173–179.

Ax, A. F. (1953). The psychophysiological differentiation between fear and anger in humans. *Psychosomatic Medicine, 15*, 433–442.

Baer, P. E., Collins, F. H., Bourianoff, G. G., & Ketchel, M. F. (1979). Assessing personality factors in essential hypertension with a brief self-report instrument. *Psychosomatic Medicine, 4*, 321–330.

Barefoot, J. C., Dahlstrom, W. G., & Williams, R. B., Jr. (1983). Hostility, CHD incidence, and total mortality: A 25 year follow-up study of 255 physicians. *Psychosomatic Medicine, 45*, 59–63.

Berkow, R. (Ed.). (1982). *The Merck manual*, (14th ed.). Rahway, NJ: Merck, Sharp, & Dome Research Laboratories.

Bernstein, D. A., & Borkovec, T. D. (1973). *Progressive relaxation training*. Champaign, IL: Research Press.

Blanchard, E. B., Miller, S. T., Abel, G. G., Haynes, M. R., & Wicker, R. (1979). Evaluation of biofeedback in the treatment of borderline essential hypertension. *Journal of Applied Behavioral Analysis, 12*, 99–109.

Buss, A. H., & Durkee, A. (1957). An inventory for assessing different kinds of hostility. *Journal of Counseling Psychology, 21*, 343–349.

Chesney, M. A., & Rosenman, R. H. (1985). *Anger and hostility in cardiovascular and behavioral disorders.* New York: Hemisphere.

Cook, W. W., & Medley, D. M. (1954). Proposed hostility and pharisaic-virtue scales for the MMPI. *Journal of Applied Psychology, 38*, 414–418.

Crane, R. S. (1981). The role of anger, hostility, and aggression in essential hypertension. *Dissertation Abstracts International, 42*, 2982B.

Delamater, A. M., Taylor, C. B., Schneider, J., Allen, R., Chesney, M., & Agras, W. S. (1989). Interpersonal behavior and cardiovascular reactivity in pharmacologically treated hypertensives. *Journal of Psychosomatic Research, 33*, 335–345.

Diamond, E. L. (1982). The role of anger and hostility in essential hypertension and coronary heart disease. *Psychological Bulletin, 92*, 410–433.

Ekman, P. (1978). Facial expression. In A. W. Siegman & S. Feldstein (Eds.), *Nonverbal behavior and communication* (pp. 97–114). Hillsdale, NJ: Erlbaum.

Ekman, P. (1982). Methods for measuring facial action. In K. Scherer & P. Ekman (Eds.), *Handbook of methods in nonverbal research* (pp. 45–90). New York: Cambridge University Press.

Ekman, P., & Friesen, W. V. (1974). Detecting deception from the body and face. *Journal of Personality and Social Psychology, 29*, 288–298.

Ekman, P., Friesen, W. V., & Ellsworth, P. (1972). *Emotion in the human face: Research and an integration of findings.* New York: Pergamon Press.

Ellis, A. (1962). *Reason and emotion in psychotherapy.* New York: Stuart.

Feindler, E. L. (1987). Clinical issues and recommendations in adolescent anger-control training. *Journal of Child and Adolescent Psychotherapy, 4*, 267–274.

Funkenstein, D. H., King, S. H., & Drolette, M. E. (1954). The direction of anger during a laboratory stress-inducing situation. *Psychosomatic Medicine, 16*, 404–413.

Gentry, W. D., Chesney, A. P., Gary, H. E., Hall, R. P., & Harburg, E. (1982). Habitual-anger-coping styles: I. Effect on mean blood pressure and risk for essential hypertension. *Psychosomatic Medicine, 44*, 195–201.

Glass, D. C., Krakoff, L. R., Contrada, R., Hilton, W. F., Kehoe, K., Mannucci, E. G., Collins, C., Snow, B., & Elting, E. (1980). Effect of harassment and competition upon cardiovascular and plasma catecholamine responses in Type A and Type B individuals. *Psychophysiology, 17*, 453–463.

Hagberg, J. M., & Seals, D. R. (1986). Exercise training and hypertension. *Acta Medica Scandinavica, 711*, 131–136.

Harburg, E., Blakelock, E. H., & Roeper, P. J. (1979). Resentful and reflective coping with arbitrary authority and blood pressure: Detroit. *Psychosomatic Medicine, 41*, 189–202.

Jacob, R. G., Chesney, M. A., Williams, D. M., Ding, Y., & Shapiro, A. P. (1991). Relaxation therapy for hypertension: Design effects and treatment effects. *Annals of Behavioral Medicine, 13*, 5–17.

Jacob, R. G., Kraemer, H. C., & Agras, W. S. (1977). Relaxation therapy in the treatment of hypertension: A review. *Archives of General Psychiatry, 34*, 1417–1427.

Jakubowski, P., & Lange, A. J. (1978). *The assertive option: Your rights and responsibilities.* Champaign, IL: Research Press.

Joint National Committee on Detection, Evaluation, and Treatment of High Blood Pressure. (1988). The 1988 report of the Joint National Committee on detection, evaluation, and treatment of high blood pressure. *Archives of Internal Medicine, 148*, 1023–1038.

Julius, S., & Hanson, L. (1983). Classification of hypertension. In J. Genest, O. Kuchel, P. Hamet, & M. Cantin (Eds.), *Hypertension: Pathophysiology and treatment* (2nd ed., pp. 679–682). New York: McGraw-Hill.

Kannel, W. B., Doyle, J. T., Ostfeld, A. M., Jenkins, C. D., Kuller, L., Podell, R. N., & Stamler, J. (1984). Optimal resources for primary prevention of atherosclerotic diseases. *Circulation, 70*, 155A–205A.

Keane, T. M., Martin, J. E., Berler, E. S., Wooten, L. S., Fleece, E. L., & Williams, J. G. (1982). Are hypertensives less assertive? A controlled evaluation. *Journal of Consulting and Clinical Psychology, 50*, 499–508.

Keys, A., Taylor, H. L., Blackburn, J., Anderson, J. T., & Somonson, E. (1971). Mortality and coronary heart disease among men studied for 23 years. *Archives of Internal Medicine, 128*, 201–214.

Larkin, K. T., Zayfert, C., Callahan, T., Loren, B., & Pope, M. K. (1991a). Anger management training in borderline essential hypertension. *Proceedings of the 12th Annual Scientific Sessions of the Society of Behavioral Medicine* (p. 79). Rockville, MD: Society of Behavioral Medicine.

Larkin, K. T., Zayfert, C., & McKittrick, T. (1991b). Assertion and cardiovascular response to confrontation in borderline essential hypertension. *Proceedings of the 12th Annual Scientific Sessions of the Society of Behavioral Medicine* (p. 94). Rockville, MD: Society of Behavioral Medicine.

Levenson, R. W. (1992). Autonomic nervous system differences among emotions. *Psychological Science, 3,* 23–27.

Lowe, M. R., & Cautela, J. R. (1978). A self-report measure of social skill. *Behavior Therapy, 9,* 535–544.

Meichenbaum, D. (1977). *Cognitive behavior modification: An integrative approach.* New York: Plenum Press.

Morrison, R. L., Bellack, A. S., & Manuck, S. B. (1985). Role of social competence in borderline essential hypertension. *Journal of Consulting and Clinical Psychology, 53,* 248–255.

Niaura, R., & Goldstein, M. G. (1992). Psychological factors affecting physical condition: Part II: Coronary artery disease and sudden death and hypertension. *Psychosomatics, 33,* 146–155.

Novaco, R. W. (1975). *Anger control: The development and evaluation of an experimental treatment.* Lexington, MA: Heath.

Novaco, R. W. (1976). Treatment of chronic anger through cognitive and relaxation control. *Journal of Consulting and Clinical Psychology, 44,* 681.

Novaco, R. W. (1977a). Stress inoculation: A cognitive therapy for anger and its application to a case of depression. *Journal of Consulting and Clinical Psychology, 45,* 600–608.

Novaco, R. W. (1977b). Therapist manual for stress inoculation therapy: Therapeutic interventions for anger problems. Unpublished manuscript, University of California at Irvine, Irvine, CA.

Novaco, R. W. (1985). Anger and its therapeutic regulation. In M. A. Chesney & R. H. Rosenman (Eds.), *Anger and hostility in cardiovascular and behavioral disorders* (pp. 203–226). New York: Hemisphere.

Page, L. B. (1983). Epidemiology of hypertension. In J. Genest, O. Kuchel, P. Hamet, & M. Cantin (Eds.), *Hypertension: Physiopathology and treatment* (2nd ed., pp. 683–699). New York: McGraw-Hill.

Patel, C. H. (1975). 12-month follow-up of yoga and biofeedback in the management of hypertension. *Lancet, 1,* 62–64.

Poppen, R. (1988). *Behavioral relaxation training and assessment.* New York: Pergamon Press.

Rathus, S. A. (1973). A 30-item schedule for assessing assertive behavior. *Behavior Therapy, 4,* 398–406.

Reisin, E., & Frohlich, E. D. (1982). Effects of weight reduction on arterial pressure. *Journal of Chronic Diseases, 35,* 887–891.

Schachter, J. (1957). Pain, fear, and anger in hypertensives and normotensives: A psychophysiologic study. *Psychosomatic Medicine, 19,* 17–29.

Schwartz, G. E., Weinberger, D. A., & Davidson, R. A. (1981). Cardiovascular differentiation of happiness, sorrow, anger, and fear following imagery and exercise. *Psychosomatic Medicine, 43,* 343–367.

Semenchuk, E. M., & Larkin, K. T. (1993). Behavioral and cardiovascular responses to interpersonal challenges among male offspring of essential hypertensives. *Health Psychology, 12,* 416–419.

Shekelle, R. B., Gale, M., Ostfeld, A. M., & Paul, O. (1983). Hostility, risk of coronary heart disease, and mortality. *Psychosomatic Medicine, 45,* 109–114.

Siegman, A. W., Dembrowski, T. M., & Ringel, N. (1987). Components of hostility and the severity of coronary artery disease. *Psychosomatic Medicine, 48,* 127–135.

Spielberger, C. D. (1988). *State-trait anger expression inventory: Professional manual.* Odessa, FL: Psychological Assessment Resources.

Spielberger, C. D., Johnson, E. H., Russell, S. F., Crane, R. J., Jacobs, G. A., & Worden, T. J. (1985). The experience and expression of anger: Construction and validation of an anger expression scale. In M. A. Chesney & R. H. Rosenman (Eds.), *Anger and hostility in cardiovascular and behavioral disorders* (pp. 5–30). New York: Hemisphere.

Suarez, E. C., & Williams, R. B., Jr. (1989). Situational determinants of cardiovascular and emotional reactivity in high and low hostile men. *Psychosomatic Medicine, 51,* 404–418.

Taylor, C. B., & Fortmann, S. P. (1983). Essential hypertension: Psychosomatic illness review: No. 9 in a series. *Psychosomatics, 24,* 433–448.

Williams, R. B. Jr., Barefoot, J. C., & Shekelle, R. B. (1985). The health consequenses of hostility. In M. A. Chesney & R. H. Rosenman (Eds.), *Anger and hostility in cardiovascular and behavioral disorders* (pp. 173–185). New York: Hemisphere.

Wing, R. R., Caggiula, A. W., Nowalk, M. P., Koeske, R., Lee, S., & Langford, H. (1984). Dietary approaches to the reduction of blood pressure: The independence of weight and sodium/potassium interventions. *Preventive Medicine, 13,* 233–244.

Wood, D. L., Sheps, S. G., Elveback, L. R., & Schirger, A. (1984). Cold pressor test as a predictor of hypertension. *Hypertension, 6,* 301–306.

Index

ISBN 0-306-45144-1

90000